A PRACTICAL APPROACH TO CARDIAC ANESTHESIA

THIRD EDITION

D1125705

A PRACTICAL APPROACH TO CARDIAC ANESTHESIA

THIRD EDITION

Editors

Frederick A. Hensley, Jr., M.D.

Department of Anesthesiology
College of Physicians and Surgeons of Columbia University
New York, New York
Anesthesiologist-in-Chief
Chief of Perioperative Services
Bassett Healthcare
Cooperstown, New York

Donald E. Martin, M.D.

Professor
Department of Anesthesiology
Pennsylvania State University School of Medicine
Associate Chair for Academic and Professional Development
Department of Anesthesiology
The Milton S. Hershey Medical Center
Hershey, Pennsylvania

Glenn P. Gravlee, M.D.

Professor
Department of Anesthesiology
Ohio State University College of Medicine and Public Health
Columbus, Ohio

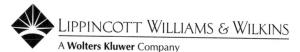

LIPPINCOTT WILLIAMS & WILKINS
A **Wolters Kluwer** Company

Philadelphia • Baltimore • New York • London
Buenos Aires • Hong Kong • Sydney • Tokyo

Acquisitions Editor: R. Craig Percy
Developmental Editor: Kerry Barrett
Production Editor: Jonathan Geffner
Manufacturing Manager: Benjamin Rivera
Cover Designer: Christine Jenny
Compositor: Circle Graphics
Printer: Maple Press

Printed in the USA

Library of Congress Cataloging-in-Publication Data

A practical approach to cardiac anesthesia / edited by Frederick A. Hensley, Jr.,
Donald E. Martin, Glenn P. Gravlee.—3rd ed.
   p. ; cm
   Includes bibliographical references and index.
   ISBN 0-7817-3444-4
   1. Anesthesia in cardiology. 2. Heart—Surgery. 3. Chest—Surgery.
   I. Hensley, Frederick A. II. Martin, Donald E. (Donald Eugene)
   III. Gravlee, Glen P.
   [DNLM: 1. Anesthesia. 2. Cardiac Surgical Procedures. 3. Heart—drug
effects. WG 460 P895 2003
   RD87.3.H43 P723 2003
   617.9'67412—dc21

                                                           2002073049

10 9 8 7 6 5 4 3 2

In memory of our mothers—Jeanette W. Hensley, Elizabeth G. Martin, and Ceci Roberts Gravlee—to whom we owe so much. They will be remembered as role models, educators, and—most importantly— wonderful human beings

CONTENTS

I. ANESTHETIC MANAGEMENT FOR CARDIAC SURGERY

II. ANESTHETIC MANAGEMENT OF SPECIFIC CARDIAC DISORDERS

III.   CIRCULATORY SUPPORT AND ORGAN PRESERVATION

IV.   THORACIC ANESTHESIA AND PAIN MANAGEMENT

CONTRIBUTING AUTHORS

Solomon Aronson, M.D.
Professor, Chief of Cardiothoracic Anesthesia, University of Chicago and University of Chicago Medical Center, Chicago, Illinois

John L. Atlee, M.D.
Professor, Department of Anesthesiology, Medical College of Wisconsin; Staff Anesthesiologist, Department of Anesthesiology, Froedtert Memorial Lutheran Hospital East, Milwaukee, Wisconsin

Hamdy Awad, M.D.
Assistant Professor, Department of Anesthesiology, The Ohio State University, Columbus, Ohio

Jeffrey R. Balser, M.D., Ph.D.
Professor, Departments of Anesthesiology and Pharmacology, Vanderbilt University; Chairman, Department of Anesthesiology, Vanderbilt University Medical Center, Nashville, Tennessee

John Butterworth, M.D.
Professor, Department of Anesthesiology, Head, Section of Cardiothoracic Anesthesiology, Wake Forest University School of Medicine; Chief, Department of Cardiothoracic Anesthesia, North Carolina Baptist Hospital, Winston-Salem, North Carolina

David B. Campbell, M.D.
William S. Pierce Professor, Department of Surgery, Division of Cardiothoracic Surgery, Pennsylvania State University; Chief, Department of Surgery, Division of Cardiothoracic Surgery, M.S. Hershey Medical Center, Hershey, Pennsylvania

Charles E. Chambers, M.D.
Professor of Medicine and Radiology, Department of Cardiology, Pennsylvania State University; Director, Cardiac Catheterization Laboratories, Department of Cardiology, Milton S. Hershey Medical Center, Hershey, Pennsylvania

Charles D. Collard, M.D.
Associate Professor, Department of Anesthesiology, Baylor College of Medicine; Department of Cardiovascular Anesthesiology, Texas Heart Institute, Houston, Texas

John R. Cooper, Jr., M.D.
Clinical Associate Professor, Department of Anesthesia, University of Texas Health Science Center at Houston; Associate Chief, Division of Cardiovascular Anesthesiology, Texas Heart Institute, Houston, Texas

Laurie K. Davies, M.D.
Associate Professor, Department of Anesthesiology, University of Florida College of Medicine; Director, Pediatric Cardiac Anesthesia, Department of Anesthesiology, Shands Hospital, Gainesville, Florida

John W. C. Entwistle III, M.D., Ph.D.
Assistant Professor, Department of Cardiothoracic Surgery, MCP–Hahnemann University; Attending Surgeon, Department of Cardiothoracic Surgery, Hahnemann University Hospital, Philadelphia, Pennsylvania

Neville M. Gibbs, M.B.B.S., M.D.
Head, Department of Anesthesia, Sir Charles Gairdner Hospital, Nedlands, Australia

Steven H. Ginsberg, M.D.
Associate Professor, Department of Anesthesia, Division of Cardiac Anesthesia, Section Chief, Cardiac Transplant, Medical Director of PACU, University of Medicine and Dentistry of New Jersey–Robert Wood Johnson Medical School; Anesthesiologist, Department of Anesthesia, Robert Wood Johnson University Hospital, New Brunswick, New Jersey

Glenn P. Gravlee, M.D.
Professor, Department of Anesthesiology, The Ohio State University College of Medicine and Public Health, Columbus, Ohio

Ronald L. Harter, M.D.
Assistant Professor, Department of Anesthesiology, The Ohio State University College of Medicine and Public Health; Anesthesiologist, Department of Anesthesiology, Mt. Carmel Medical Center, Columbus, Ohio

Charles J. Hearn, D.O.
Staff Anesthesiologist, Aultman Hospital, Canton, Ohio

Frederick A. Hensley, Jr., M.D.
Department of Anesthesiology, College of Physicians and Surgeons at Columbia University, New York, New York; Anesthesiologist-in-Chief, Chief of Perioperative Services, Department of Anesthesiology, Bassett Healthcare, Cooperstown, New York

Eugene A. Hessel, II, M.D., M.S.
Professor, Departments of Anesthesiology and Surgery (Cardiothoracic), University of Kentucky College of Medicine; Director, Cardiothoracic Anesthesia, Department of Anesthesiology, Chandler Medical Center, Lexington, Kentucky

Kane M. High, M.D.
Associate Professor, Department of Anesthesiology, Hershey Medical Center / Penn State University, Hershey, Pennsylvania

Peter G. Hild, M.D.
Clinical Associate Professor, Department of Anesthesiology, University of Kansas; Director of Cardiothoracic Anesthesia, Department of Anesthesiology, Kansas University Medical Center, Kansas City, Kansas

Jay C. Horrow, M.D., M.S.
Clinical Professor, Department of Anesthesiology, MCP–Hahnemann University, Philadelphia, Pennsylvania

Michael B. Howie, M.D.
Professor and Chair, Department of Anesthesiology, The Ohio State University College of Medicine and Public Health, Columbus, Ohio

Ivan Iglesias, M.D.
Assistant Professor, Departments of Anesthesia and Perioperative Medicine, University of Western Ontario; Consultant, Departments of Anesthesia and Perioperative Medicine, London Health Science Center, London, Ontario, Canada

Michael Jopling, M.D.
Adjunct Assistant Professor, Department of Anesthesiology, The Ohio State University College of Medicine and Public Health, Columbus, Ohio; Staff Anesthesiologist, St. Ann's Hospital, Westerville, Ohio

Daniel G. Knauf, M.D.
Associate Professor, Department of Thoracic and Cardiovascular Surgery, University of Florida; Associate Professor, Department of Surgery, Shands Hospital, Gainesville, Florida

Mark Kurusz, B.A., C.C.P.
Assistant Professor, Department of Surgery, Chief Perfusionist, Heart Center, The University of Texas Medical Branch, Galveston, Texas

David R. Larach, M.D., Ph.D.
Chief, Division of Cardiac Anesthesiology, The Heart Institute at St. Joseph Medical Center, Towson, Maryland

Jerrold H. Levy, M.D.
Professor, Department of Anesthesiology, Emory University School of Medicine; Deputy Chairman for Research, Department of Anesthesiology, Division of Cardiothoracic Anesthesiology and Critical Care, Emory Healthcare, Atlanta, Georgia

Michael G. Licina, M.D.
Associate Professor, Department of Anesthesiology, The Cleveland Clinic Foundation Health Sciences Center of the Ohio State University; Staff Anesthesiologist, Department of Cardiothoracic Anesthesia, The Cleveland Clinic Foundation, Cleveland, Ohio

Stephen R. Longo, M.D.
Associate Professor, Department of Anesthesia, Pennsylvania State University College of Medicine; The Milton S. Hershey Medical Center, Hershey, Pennsylvania

Jerry C. Luck, M.D.
Professor, Department of Medicine, Pennsylvania State University; Director, Clinical Cardiac Electrophysiology, Division of Cardiology, Milton S. Hershey Medical Center, Hershey, Pennsylvania

Donald E. Martin, M.D.
Professor, Department of Anesthesiology, Pennsylvania State University School of Medicine, Associate Chair for Academic and Professional Development, Department of Anesthesiology, The Milton S. Hershey Medical Center, Hershey, Pennsylvania

Thomas M. McLoughlin, Jr., M.D.
Clinical Associate Professor, Department of Anesthesia, Pennsylvania State University College of Medicine, Hershey, Pennsylvania; Chairperson, Department of Anesthesiology, Lehigh Valley Hospital, Allentown, Pennsylvania

Robert E. Michler, M.D.
Karl P. Klassen Professor of Surgery, Department of Surgery, The Ohio State University College of Medicine and Public Health; Chief, Cardiothoracic Surgery and Thoracic Transplantation, Department of Surgery, The Ohio State University Medical Center, Columbus, Ohio

Roger A. Moore, M.D.
Clinical Associate Professor, Department of Anesthesia, University of Medicine and Dentistry of New Jersey, Newark, New Jersey; Chair, Department of Anesthesia, Deborah Heart and Lung Center, Browns Mills, New Jersey

John M. Murkin, M.D.
Professor, Department of Anesthesiology, University of Western Ontario; Director, Cardiac Anesthesia, Department of Anesthesiology, London Health Sciences Center, London, Ontario, Canada

James G. Ramsay, M.D.
Professor, Department of Anesthesiology, Emory University School of Medicine; Chief, Anesthesiology Service, Department of Anesthesiology, Emory University Hospital, Atlanta, Georgia

Mark E. Romanoff, M.D.
Staff Anesthesiologist, Department of Anesthesiology, Carolinas Medical Center, Charlotte, North Carolina

Anne L. Rother, M.B.B.S.
Instructor in Anesthesia, Department of Anesthesiology, Harvard Medical School; Staff Anesthesiologist, Department of Anesthesiology, Brigham and Women's Hospital, Boston, Massachusetts

Sibylle A. Ruesch, M.D.
Cardiac Fellow, Department of Anesthesiology, Emory University Hospital, Atlanta, Georgia

Robert Savage, M.D.
Department of Anesthesiology, Cleveland Clinic Foundation, Cleveland, Ohio

Jack S. Shanewise, M.D.
Associate Professor, Department of Anesthesiology, Emory University School of Medicine; Director, Department of Cardiothoracic Anesthesiology, Emory Healthcare, Atlanta, Georgia

Linda Shore-Lesserson, M.D.
Associate Professor, Department of Anesthesiology, The Mount Sinai School of Medicine; Cardiothoracic Anesthesiologist, Department of Anesthesiology, The Mount Sinai Medical Center, New York, New York

Thomas M. Skeehan, M.D.
Clinical Associate Professor, Department of Anesthesia, Pennsylvania State University College of Medicine, Hershey, Pennsylvania; Associate Anesthesiologist, Department of Anesthesiology, Holy Spirit Hospital, Camp Hill, Pennsylvania

Peter Slinger, M.D.
Professor, Department of Anesthesia, University of Toronto; Anesthesiologist, Department of Anesthesia, Toronto General Hospital, Toronto, Ontario, Canada

Alann Solina, M.D.
Administrative Director, Associate Professor, Department of Anesthesiology, Chief, Division of Cardiac Anesthesia, University of Medicine and Dentistry of New Jersey–Robert Wood Johnson Medical School; Chief, Cardiac Anesthesia, Department of Anesthesiology, Robert Wood Johnson University Hospital, New Brunswick, New Jersey

Mark Stafford-Smith, M.D., C.M.
Associate Professor, Department of Anesthesiology, Duke University; Chief and Fellowship Director, Division of Cardiothoracic Anesthesia and Critical Care Medicine, Department of Anesthesiology, Duke University Medical Center, Durham, North Carolina

Alfred H. Stammers, M.S.A., C.C.P.
Adjunct Associate Professor, Department of Perfusion Sciences, University of Nebraska Medical Center, Omaha, Nebraska; Clinical Perfusionist, Department of Surgery, Geisinger Medical Center, Danville, Pennsylvania

Erin A. Sullivan, M.D.
Associate Professor, Department of Anesthesiology, Director of Thoracic Anesthesiology, University of Pittsburgh, Pittsburgh, Pennsylvania

Daniel M. Thys, M.D.
Professor, Department of Anesthesiology, College of Physicians and Surgeons, Columbia University; Chairman, Department of Anesthesiology, St. Luke's–Roosevelt Hospital Center, New York, New York

John M. Toomasian, M.S., C.C.P.
Clinical Perfusionist, Operating Room Services, Stanford University Medical Center, Stanford, California

Lee K. Wallace, M.D.
Staff, Department of Cardiothoracic Anesthesia, The Cleveland Clinic Foundation, Cleveland, Ohio

Andrew S. Wechsler, M.D.
Stanley K. Brackman Professor and Chairman, Department of Cardiothoracic Surgery, MCP–Hahnemann University; Chairman, Department of Cardiothoracic Surgery, Hahnemann University Hospital, Philadelphia, Pennsylvania

Russell P. Woda, D.O.
Associate Professor, Department of Anesthesiology, The Ohio State University College of Medicine and Public Health; Staff Anesthesiologist, Department of Anesthesiology, Mount Carmel Medical Center, Columbus, Ohio

Randall K. Wolf, M.D.
Associate Professor, Department of Surgery, The Ohio State University; Director, Minimally Invasive Cardiac Surgery and Robotics, Department of Surgery, The Ohio State University Medical Center, Columbus, Ohio

PREFACE

Since the publication of the last edition of *A Practical Approach to Cardiac Anesthesia*, in 1995, dramatic changes in the field of cardiac anesthesia and surgery have occurred. The expansion of the practice of fast-track recovery after cardiac surgery, the extensive involvement of the anesthesiologist in cardiovascular monitoring and diagnosis using transesophageal echocardiography, and anesthetic management for off-pump myocardial revascularization procedures are just a few examples of the added new dimension to our subspecialty. To accommodate the changes in the field, chapters devoted specifically to transesophageal echocardiography and alternative approaches to cardiac surgery have been included.

With the exponential growth in the literature related to cardiac anesthesiology, there is growing value in maintaining this book as a concise, "pocket-sized" daily reference for the practicing anesthesiologist, resident, certified registered nurse anesthetist, and perfusionist. Therefore, every effort has been made to include only the most relevant information, organized in a format useful to both the new resident and the seasoned clinician as they enter the cardiac operating room. A discussion of adult and pediatric extracorporeal membrane oxygenation was deleted due to their reduced role in patient treatment and the need to maintain the portability of this text. As in the previous edition, the book is divided into four main sections. Part I deals with general perioperative management of the adult patient undergoing cardiac surgery. Part II presents a detailed explanation of specific cardiac disorders. Part III deals with mechanical circulatory support and organ preservation. Part IV addresses aspects of thoracic surgery and pain management.

Many chapters are completely rewritten, while others are updated appropriately. We hope you will find this edition as valuable as the two previous editions.

F.A.H.
D.E.M.
G.P.G.

I. ANESTHETIC MANAGEMENT FOR CARDIAC SURGERY

1. THE CARDIAC PATIENT

Donald E. Martin, Charles E. Chambers, Jerry C. Luck, and
Frederick A. Hensley, Jr.

Cardiovascular disease is often considered our society's number one health problem. More than 17 million Americans have some form of cardiac disease. The majority of patients, 11 million, suffer from coronary artery disease, five million from valvular heart disease, and one million from congenital heart disease [1]. Coronary heart disease continues to be the most common cause of death among adult Americans. Furthermore, cardiovascular disease consumes more of our nation's health care resources than any other single disorder. In 1995, expenditures for circulatory disorders totaled $127.8 billion, or 17.8% of all personal health expenditures. Approximately one third of all patients undergoing any type of surgery have, or are at risk for, coronary artery disease. Of the 72 million surgical procedures performed in the United States, approximately 0.7 million are primary cardiac procedures.

By the time the anesthesiologist is consulted for patients undergoing cardiac surgery, a definitive cardiac diagnosis usually has been established, supported by invasive and non-invasive diagnostic studies, and the decision to undergo surgery has been made. The prime goals of preoperative evaluation and therapy are to quantify and reduce the patient's risk during surgery and the postoperative period.

The factors that are important in determining perioperative morbidity and anesthetic management must be assessed carefully for each patient.

I. Patient presentation
A. Age and sex
1. **Advanced age,** especially beyond 70 years, is associated with higher cardio-vascular morbidity. In patients undergoing cardiac revascularization, the Collaborative Study in Coronary Artery Surgery (CASS) found operative mortality in patients older than 70 years to be approximately 7.9% [2]. Between 1978 and 2001, several authors found age older than 70 years to be an independent predictor of cardiac death, although not necessarily of postoperative myocardial infarction, on multivariate analysis of large series of general surgical patients [3–7].
2. **Sex.** When patients of all ages are considered, operative mortality is more than twice as high among women than among men during coronary artery surgery.
B. Functional status.
For patients undergoing cardiac surgical procedures, as for most perioperative patients, perhaps the single most useful risk index is the patient's functional status, or exercise tolerance. Exercise tolerance is commonly measured in metabolic equivalents (METs). One MET is the energy consumed by the body at rest. The energy requirements, in METs, of some common daily activities are listed in Table 1.1. The capacity to climb a flight of stairs, which corresponds to a moderate exercise capacity of 4 MET, is an easily measured and sensitive index of cardiovascular risk that takes into account a wide range of specific cardiac and noncardiac factors.
C. Surgical problems and procedures.
The complexity of the surgical procedure itself may be the most important predictor of perioperative morbidity for many patients. Eighty-two percent of all cardiac surgical procedures are coronary artery bypass procedures. Valvular and other intracardiac procedures are associated with the risk of systemic and coronary air emboli. Procedures requiring ventriculotomy imply damage to ventricular muscle. Procedures on multiple heart valves, or on

Table 1.1 Energy requirements for common activities

1 MET	*Eat, dress*
↓	Walk indoors
↓	Walk a block or two on level ground
↓	Do light housework
4 MET	*Climb a flight of stairs*
↓	Run a short distance
↓	Do heavy housework, e.g., scrubbing
↓	Golf, bowling, dancing
10 MET	*Swimming, skiing, singles tennis, running*

both the aortic valve and coronary arteries, are associated with a statistical morbidity much higher than that for procedures involving only a single valve or coronary artery bypass grafting (CABG) alone. Finally, any procedure requiring more than 40 minutes on cardiopulmonary bypass is associated with greater morbidity, which increases with longer bypass duration.

II. Clinical assessment of cardiac disease. Cardiac surgery is performed commonly for one of three basic disease processes—myocardial ischemia, heart failure due to either valvular or myocardial disease, or dysrhythmias. Each of these symptom complexes has characteristics important to the anesthetic management of cardiac patients.

   A. Myocardial ischemia

   Key clinical findings
   Stable angina pectoris
   Unstable "crescendo" angina (acute coronary syndrome)
   Ischemia without angina (silent ischemia)
   Myocardial infarction

   1. **Stable angina pectoris.** Angina pectoris classically is described as an aching, heavy, or squeezing sensation in the chest behind the sternum; chest tightness; or chest pressure. Most often it affects an area about the size of a clenched fist and may radiate to the neck, jaw, either arm, back, or abdomen. It occurs most notably with exertion, after eating, or with emotion. It signifies ischemia of the cardiac muscle that occurs whenever the energy demands of the myocardium exceed the supply. Usually ischemia can be presumed to result from obstruction to coronary artery blood flow. Fixed atherosclerotic coronary disease is the most common cause. In the absence of specific coronary lesions, however, the myocardium may be rendered ischemic by coronary artery spasm, vasculitis, or trauma.

   The location, type, and severity of angina often do not indicate the extent of myocardium at risk and the anatomic coronary artery lesions. For this information, the clinician must depend on other characteristics of the anginal syndrome, such as its relationship to exercise, the progression of symptoms, and particularly the results of myocardial perfusion studies and cardiac catheterization.

   With exercise, the patient's heart rate and blood pressure rise to levels that precipitate angina. This *angina threshold* is an important guide to perioperative hemodynamic management.

   The level of exercise producing angina, described by the New York Heart Association and Canadian Cardiovascular Society classifications, will help to predict the risk of ischemic damage and operative mortality (Table 1.2). During coronary revascularization procedures, operative mortality for patients with class IV symptoms is almost double that for patients with class I angina [2].

   Angina occurring at rest implies subtotal obstruction by atherosclerotic plaque, coronary artery spasm, or spasm around a partially obstructing lesion. In patients with valvular heart disease, particularly aortic stenosis, angina at rest frequently implies coexisting coronary artery disease.

   2. **Unstable angina,** sometimes called *crescendo angina, preinfarction angina,* or *acute coronary syndrome,* describes the new onset of anginal symptoms or the rapid progression of existing symptoms. These symptoms often indicate rapid growth, rupture, or embolus of an existing plaque. Patients in this category have a higher incidence of myocardial infarction and sudden death, increased incidence of left main occlusion, and an operative mortality 3.5 times the average of that for all myocardial revascularization procedures [2].

   3. **Myocardial ischemia without angina** may be manifest by fatigue, rapid onset of pulmonary edema, cardiac arrhythmias, syncope, or an "anginal equivalent," most often characterized as indigestion or jaw pain. Anginal pain is clearly the "tip of the iceberg," occurring well after alterations in coronary flow have created ventricular dysfunction, perfusion abnormalities, and ST-segment changes. Some patients show ischemic changes on the electrocardiogram (ECG), either resting or with exercise, but no other symptoms. More than half of all patients with chronic stable angina have daily episodes of silent ischemia, and

Table 1.2 Functional classification of anginal syndrome

Functional class	New York Heart Association classification	Canadian Cardiovascular Society classification
I	Cardiac disease without limitation of physical activity	No angina with ordinary physical activity (walking or climbing stairs). Angina with strenuous or prolonged exertion
II	Slight limitation of physical activity. Fatigue or angina with ordinary physical activity	Slight limitation of ordinary activity. Limitation of walking or climbing stairs rapidly, walking uphill, after meals, and in cold wind
III	Marked limitation of physical activity. Comfortable at rest	Marked limitation of physical activity. Walking 1–2 blocks on level
IV	Angina at rest, increased with activity	Unable to carry on any physical activity without discomfort. Angina may be present at rest

these episodes are most common during the morning hours. Such silent ischemia is particularly common in the elderly and in diabetic patients and is responsible for at least 15% to 35% of all myocardial infarctions. Perhaps because of coexisting disease or because patients with silent ischemia undergo treatment only when their disease is far advanced, silent ischemia has been associated with an unfavorable prognosis. Mangano and co-workers [8] found that perioperative myocardial ischemia is common. In this series, perioperative myocardial ischemia occurred before noncoronary surgery in 20%, during surgery in 25%, and postoperatively in 40% of patients with demonstrated coronary artery disease or risk factors for coronary artery disease. **Perioperative ischemia was silent in more than 75% of the patients studied.** Ischemia on preoperative ambulatory ECG monitoring represents, along with exercise tolerance, an important predictor of postoperative cardiac events [9]. **More than half of perioperative infarctions associated with all types of surgery are believed to be "silent."**

4. **Prior myocardial infarction. Interval between prior infarction and surgery.** In patients undergoing noncardiac surgery, the risk of another infarction in the perioperative period has classically been thought to be related to the time interval between the last prior infarction and the date of surgery. In the 1970s, if the prior infarction occurred within 3 months of surgery, the risk of reinfarction at surgery was found to range from 27% to 37%, compared to approximately 4% to 6% if the infarction occurred more than 6 months preoperatively [10]. In the early 1990s, this risk was shown to be reduced with the use of aggressive invasive monitoring and intensive care unit support. More importantly, patients who suffered a preoperative myocardial infarction any time more than 1 month preoperatively no longer appear to benefit from the delay of noncardiac surgery until more than 6 months postinfarction [5]. For patients without a history of a prior infarction, the risk of perioperative infarction is only approximately 0.1% to 0.7%. Perioperative infarction occurs most often in the first 2 to 3 postoperative days and has a very high (50% to 70%) mortality, much higher than that for myocardial infarctions not occurring in the setting of surgery, perhaps because perioperative infarctions are commonly "silent" and therefore untreated.

In patients undergoing **coronary revascularization procedures,** the risk of death after perioperative infarction is lower, perhaps because the surgical procedure itself alters the course of the disease. Among patients undergoing isolated CABG surgery within 30 days of an acute myocardial infarction who were reviewed in 1989, the in-hospital death rate was 5.7%. Mortality was highest (11.0%) for those undergoing cardiac surgery in the first 3 days after infarction, decreased to 5.9% from 4 to 7 days after infarction, and was only 2.4% between 8 and 30 days after infarction. These data led to the recommendation that **elective CABG surgery be delayed until at least 1 week after myocardial infarction** [11].

Perioperative myocardial infarction in patients with *prior coronary bypass.* In patients who have undergone coronary artery bypass surgery and have returned to the operating room for noncardiac procedures, the risk of perioperative infarction (0% to 1.2%) and perioperative cardiac death (0.5% to 0.9%) is low and is similar to that in patients with no prior infarction. In contrast, **higher mortality is associated with noncardiac surgery performed at the same time** as CABG surgery [12].

Location and extent of infarction. An anterior infarction is more likely to be associated with left ventricular failure, whereas an inferior infarction is likely to be associated with bradycardia and heart block. A history of complications, such as heart failure or dysrhythmias, in the early postinfarction period may help further in predicting perioperative problems. The location of a prior infarction may influence the risk of reinfarction associated with anesthesia and surgery.

B. Congestive heart failure

Key clinical findings
Fatigue
Dyspnea on exertion
Orthopnea
Nocturnal dyspnea
History of congestive heart failure
Presence of valvular heart disease
Jugular venous distention
Rales

1. **Clinical assessment of ventricular function.** An estimate of the patient's preoperative exercise tolerance may provide a reasonably sensitive index of his or her ventricular function. An exercise capacity of approximately 4 MET, equivalent to climbing a flight of stairs, indicates preserved ventricular function. It sometimes is difficult, however, to assess ventricular function based solely on history, particularly in a patient whose exercise capacity is limited by noncardiac factors. Valvular and congenital heart diseases usually are characterized by gradual progression of congestive heart failure. In contrast, patients with coronary artery disease may not manifest symptoms of heart failure until the occurrence of an ischemic "event." Ventricular dysfunction can occur almost immediately in association with an ischemic event and may be permanent after myocardial infarction.

2. **Perioperative morbidity.** Evidence of congestive heart failure or ventricular dysfunction preoperatively is associated with increased operative mortality. Recent series showed a two-fold to three-fold greater risk of postoperative morbidity or mortality in CABG patients with preoperative congestive heart failure and a 30-fold greater risk in patients with preoperative cardiogenic shock [13,14].

C. Dysrhythmias

Key clinical findings
Palpitations—chronic or acute
Dizziness
Syncope or near-syncope

1. **Incidence.** Cardiac dysrhythmias are common in patients presenting for cardiac surgery. In the perioperative period, abnormal rhythms occur in more than 75% of patients. However, those dysrhythmias are life threatening in less than 1%.

2. **Supraventricular tachycardia.** Supraventricular tachycardias (SVTs) appear most often in the preoperative history as palpitations or near-syncope. Atrial fibrillation and flutter, the most common SVTs, increase in frequency with age and in association with organic heart disease. Atrial fibrillation and flutter are nonspecific signs of generalized cardiac disease. Paroxysmal SVT is seen frequently in young individuals without apparent heart disease. These dysrhythmias usually cause no direct hemodynamic deterioration. However, in patients with ventricular dysfunction, mitral valve or aortic valve disease, a hypertrophied left or right ventricle, or pulmonary disease, loss of atrial contribution to ventricular filling caused by an SVT may reduce cardiac output severely. In patients with an intraaortic balloon pump, the presence of SVT may make it difficult for the device to inflate at the appropriate time.

In the series reported by Magovern et al. [13] and Higgins et al. [14], preoperative dysrhythmias were associated with a small but significant increase in morbidity after CABG surgery.

3. **Ventricular tachycardia.** Ventricular dysrhythmias may lead directly to ventricular fibrillation, especially if they occur in the setting of acute or recent infarction. Ventricular dysrhythmias that have been present for many years, especially in elderly patients, and dysrhythmias that improve with exercise are more likely to be benign. The frequency of ventricular dysrhythmias is increased by metabolic derangement (hypokalemia), digitalis intoxication, and progressive heart failure.

4. **Bradycardia.** Anesthetics frequently affect sinus node automaticity but rarely cause complete heart block. Asymptomatic patients with ECG-documented atrioventricular conduction disease (PR prolongation or single or bifascicular bundle branch block) rarely require temporary pacing perioperatively. However, symptomatic patients, or patients with Mobitz II or complete heart block, require preoperative evaluation for permanent pacing.

For patients with left bundle branch block in whom a Swan–Ganz catheter is being placed, a transcutaneous pacemaker may need to be available because of the risk of induction of right bundle branch block, and thus complete heart block, during passage of the pulmonary artery catheter. Patients with a left bundle branch block and right coronary artery disease may be at particular risk during passage of a Swan–Ganz catheter.

D. **Cyanosis.** Cyanosis is a bluish discoloration of the skin caused by the presence of deoxygenated hemoglobin in the blood. It is important to note that it is not the ratio of oxygenated to deoxygenated hemoglobin that determines cyanosis but rather the absolute amount of deoxygenated hemoglobin. More than 5 g of deoxygenated hemoglobin per 100 mL of blood is required to produce visible cyanosis. Thus, cyanosis is a common finding in some forms of congenital heart disease and in secondary polycythemic states. However, in anemic states, tissue hypoxemia may exist in the absence of cyanosis. Both blood flow and skin thickness in various regions of the body affect the degree of cyanosis that is present clinically. Thus, cyanosis is most apparent in the fingers and nail beds (poorly perfused tissue), lips, and mucous membranes (thin skin).

Cyanosis may be secondary to a number of cardiorespiratory dysfunctional states, such as low-output states (cardiogenic shock), pneumonia, and adult respiratory distress syndrome. However, congenital, acquired, or physiologic intracardiac right-to-left shunts (e.g., atrial or ventricular defects, thebesian veins) most commonly cause detectable cyanosis.

E. **Multifactorial risk indices.** Multifactorial indices, which combine and assign relative importance to many clinical parameters, are more useful than any single factor in determining a patient's cardiovascular risk, or risk of overall morbidity. Since the 1970s, many of these indices have been proposed [3–6] for patients undergoing noncardiac surgery as well as cardiac surgery, particularly CABG [13–15]. Although these risk indices differ in details, they are remarkably similar, in their broad conclusions, for both cardiac and noncardiac procedures.

The clinical risk factors for noncardiac surgery and the relative importance assigned to them by five of the major multifactorial indices are listed in Table 1.3.

Table 1.3 Multifactorial indices of perioperative cardiovascular risk for noncardiac surgical procedures: summary of significant risk factors in recent multivariate analyses

Risk factor	Goldman et al. 1978 [3]	Detsky et al.1986 (modified index) [4]	American College of Cardiology/ American Heart Association 2002 [5]	American College of Physicians 1997 [6]	Boersma et al. 2001 [7]
Age >70 yr	X	X	X	X	X
Angina		X	X	X	X
Acute coronary syndrome		XX	XX	XX	
Myocardial infarction	XX	X	X	X	X
Pulmonary edema		X	XX	X	
Heart failure	XX		X		X
Exercise tolerance			XX		
Valvular aortic stenosis	X	XX	X	XX	
Supra-ventricular dysrhythmias	X	X	X	X	
Ventricular dysrhythmias	X	X	X	X	
Hypertension			X		
Pulmonary disease	X	X		X	
Renal disease	X	X	X	X	
Liver disease	X	X		X	
Stroke			X		XX
Diabetes mellitus				X	
Surgical site	X		XX		
Emergency surgery	X	X		X	
β-Blocker therapy					X

X, risk factor; XX, major risk factor

Most of these indices contain some factors that assess the severity of ischemic heart disease, congestive heart failure, valvular heart disease, general medical status, and type of surgery. A recent index, developed by Boersma and colleagues [7] in 2001, includes for the first time the preoperative use of β-blocker therapy as an independent factor reducing risk. Gilbert and colleagues [16] compared the ability of four indices to predict cardiovascular morbidity in 2,035 patients and found no significant difference.

In 1997, the American College of Cardiology and the American Heart Association joined forces to craft a simple three-tiered scheme, using only data from the patient history and physical examination, and perhaps resting ECG, to guide preoperative noninvasive testing and therapy for cardiac patients undergoing noncardiac surgery. This scheme emphasizes the importance of the patient's exercise tolerance and surgical procedure to perioperative risk. An updated version of this scheme, published in 2002, is shown schematically in Figure 1.1 [5].

The preoperative clinical factors that affect hospital survival after CABG surgery were studied, retrospectively and prospectively, by Magovern et al. [13], Higgins et al. [14], and Jones et al. [15]. The most important risk factors in these studies are compared in Table 1.4. In most of the series, important factors were patient age; coexisting valvular heart disease; left ventricular function; prior cardiac surgery; the urgency of the procedure; and systemic pulmonary, renal, and vascular disease, as well as diabetes.

III. Noninvasive cardiac diagnostic studies
A. Electrocardiogram

Key clinical findings
Atrioventricular block
Atrial flutter/fibrillation
Wolff–Parkinson–White syndrome
Ischemia (ST-segment elevation or depression, T-wave inversion)
Infarction (diagnostic Q waves)
Hypertrophy

ECG abnormalities are common, occurring in 2% to 45% of patients undergoing noncardiac surgery. Even "significant" or "key" findings, such as those discussed earlier, are found in 10% to 15% of patients. Gloyna et al. [17] found similar rates of ECG abnormalities in patients undergoing CABG surgery and those undergoing noncardiac surgery, thus calling into question the predictive value of the ECG, particularly for patients with known coronary disease. On the other hand, several authors showed a close relationship between the presence of ischemic changes detected by ECG monitoring before and during surgery and postoperative cardiac morbidity after noncardiac surgery [8,12].

Furthermore, in patients with known ischemic heart disease, plaque rupture and the acute coronary syndrome can occur suddenly. Therefore, preoperative ECG should be performed within 24 to 48 hours before the procedure to rule out any silent preoperative ischemic changes or infarction. Obviously, if the patient has a prolonged episode of chest pain before the surgical procedure, regardless of the time interval, this patient should undergo ECG immediately.

FIG. 1.1 Eight-step approach to preoperative assessment of cardiac disease based on clinical risk factors, patient exercise tolerance, and the nature of the surgical procedure. "High surgical risk" procedures include aortic and other vascular procedures, and prolonged procedures with anticipated large fluid shifts and/or blood loss. "Intermediate surgical risk" procedures include carotid endarterectomy, as well as major head and neck, intrathoracic, intraperitoneal, orthopedic, and prostate surgery. "Low surgical risk" procedures include superficial, extremity, and endoscopic procedures. (From American College of Cardiology/American Heart Association Task Force. ACC/AHA guideline update for perioperative cardiovascular evaluation for noncardiac surgery. *Circulation* 2002;105:1257–1267, with permission.)

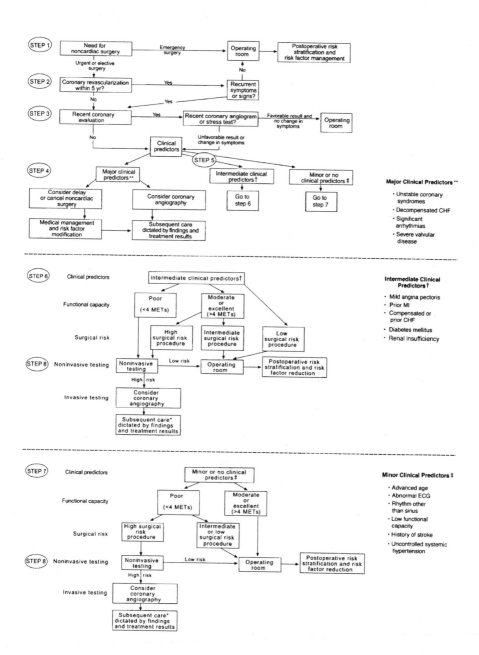

Table 1.4 Multifactorial indices of cardiovascular risk for cardiac surgical procedures: summary of significant risk factors in recent multivariate analyses

Risk factor	Jones et al. 1996 [15][a]	Magovern et al. 1996 [13][b]	Higgins et al. 1997 [14][b,c]
Age	XX	3	3
Cardiac factor			
Previous cardiac operation	XX	1	2
Urgency of surgery	XX	5	6
Catheter-induced coronary closure		4	
Severity of angina	X		
Number of previous myocardial infarctions	X		
Cardiogenic shock		7	3
Congestive heart failure	X	1	
Ventricular arrhythmias	X		
Systemic factor			
Cerebrovascular disease	X	1	1
Peripheral vascular disease	X	2	3
Chronic obstructive pulmonary disease	X	1	2
Insulin-dependent diabetes mellitus		2	1
Renal insufficiency		2	4
Anemia		1	2
Albumin <4.0		1	5
Gender		1	
Low body mass index		1	1

[a] Jones et al.: X, risk factor; XX, major (core) risk factor.
[b] Magovern et al., Higgins et al.: clinical risk score (1 = lowest risk to 7 = highest risk).
[c] Higgins et al.: only preoperative factors included.

B. Chest roentgenogram

Key clinical findings
Heart size
Pulmonary vascular markings

Routine preoperative chest films have not been found to be cost-effective for most noncardiac or nonthoracic procedures. However, specific information derived from these studies in cardiac and thoracic patients justifies their routine preoperative use. In patients with coronary artery disease, cardiomegaly with a cardiothoracic ratio greater than 0.5 reliably predicts a low ejection fraction (EF). In contrast, in patients with valvular disease, an abnormal cardiac silhouette may occur even in the face of preserved ventricular function, but normal heart size is a highly specific index of good ventricular function.

Important surgical landmarks visible on a chest roentgenogram can be used by the surgeon during the operation. Inspection of a lateral chest roentgenogram before a cardiac reoperation will show the relationship of the right ventricular free wall to the sternum and may change the technique for surgical opening of the chest.

C. Exercise tolerance testing

Key clinical findings
Ischemic threshold
ST depression
Hypotension
Angina
Dysrhythmias

The exercise tolerance test (ETT) is the most useful and least expensive diagnostic test for the initial evaluation of chest pain of unknown etiology. It also is performed to determine functional capacity and for prognostic stratification in patients with evidence of ischemic disease before therapeutic interventions such as coronary bypass surgery. In addition, ETT is used to risk-stratify patients after myocardial infarction and to monitor the effect of antianginal medications. **ETT rarely is useful as a screening test in asymptomatic patients.**

1. Many protocols exist for ETT. The primary goal of the test is to increase the workload of the heart to provoke maximal increase of myocardial blood flow, which may be as high as four times resting levels. Limitation in this blood flow increase occurs with 50% to 70% reduction in vascular cross-sectional area.

   a. The level of exercise is dependent on expected patient performance. The Naughton protocol utilizes a low initial workload and small increments and is used for patients who had a recent infarction, for debilitated patients, and for those with reduced functional capacity due to moderate angina pectoris.

   b. The Bruce protocol has a higher initial workload and greater increments and is excellent for patients with mild symptoms but no physical disability. Symptom-limited testing is preferable to submaximal exercise testing.

   c. The amount of work can be expressed in METs, which are multiples of resting oxygen consumption in milliliters per kilogram per minute.

   d. A MET level of 4 corresponds to the ability to perform daily activities, such as housework. Patients who, on preoperative ETT, can exercise at a level of at least 4 MET appear less likely to die of, or suffer from, perioperative infarction than patients who cannot achieve this exercise level.

   e. ETT has the most predictive value when flat or down-sloping ST depression of at least 1.5 mm occurs at early stages of exercise and persists into the recovery period. The occurrence of angina or dysrhythmias increases the prognostic significance of the test. These changes would predict a three-fold to seven-fold increase in the risk of ischemic disease. Unfortunately, an absence of changes does not guarantee the absence of disease, as approximately one third of patients with demonstrable coronary artery disease have a negative or nondiagnostic ETT.

   ETT is considered strongly positive and strongly suggestive of left main or three-vessel coronary artery disease when (a) the systolic blood pressure falls by 10 mm Hg or more; (b) more than five leads show positive ST-segment changes; and (c) ischemic changes occur within 3 minutes and (d) take longer than 9 minutes to resolve.

   If the exercise test elicits ischemia (angina pectoris, dysrhythmias, or ST-segment depression) at a certain heart rate, an **anginal threshold** has been established. One then has a rough idea that ischemic changes or dysrhythmias can be expected at a similar heart rate in the operating room. When ischemia or dysrhythmias occur at rest after exercise, the prognosis is more ominous.

2. **Limitations of ETT**

   a. Inability to exercise because of systemic disease, particularly peripheral vascular disease

   b. Abnormal resting ECG precluding ST-segment analysis (left bundle branch block, left ventricular hypertrophy, digoxin therapy)

   c. β-Blocker therapy that prevents the patient from achieving 85% of his or her maximum permissible heart rate

D. **Echocardiography**

Key clinical findings
Segmental wall motion
Ejection fraction
Valvular function
Congenital anatomic defects

Transthoracic echocardiography is a completely noninvasive test that provides specific preoperative assessment of several types of cardiac abnormalities. First, two-dimensional (2D) and Doppler echocardiography together provide quantitative assessment of the severity of valvular stenosis or insufficiency, and of pulmonary hypertension. Second, assessment of regional wall motion provides more sensitive and specific assessment of the existence and extent of myocardial infarction than surface ECG. Third, 2D echocardiography provides quantitative assessment of global ventricular function or EF. Fourth, echocardiography can detect even small pericardial effusions. Fifth, echocardiography can detect anatomic cardiac abnormalities, from atrial septal defects (ASDs) and ventricular septal defects (VSDs) to aneurysms and mural thrombi.

Injected contrast agents increase the sensitivity and accuracy of echocardiography, allow visualization of coronary arteries, and allow use of the technique in obese patients or those with poor acoustic windows.

E. Stress echocardiography. Stress echocardiography can use exercise stress or pharmacologic stress, with dobutamine, to increase myocardial work. Abnormally contracting myocardial segments seen on stress echocardiography are classified as either *ischemic,* if their reduced contraction pattern is in response to stress, or *infarcted,* if their contractility remains consistently depressed before, during, and after stress.

Dobutamine stress echocardiography (DSE) has indications similar to pharmacologic perfusion imaging with comparable sensitivity but possibly increased specificity. In a meta-analysis comparing the ability of dipyridamole thallium perfusion imaging, radionuclide ventriculography, ambulatory ECG, and DSE to predict adverse outcomes in preoperative patients, Mantha et al. [18] found DSE to be most predictive.

For patients with poor acoustic windows due to body habitus or severe lung disease, myocardial contrast agents now are available to improve imaging. Still, for some patients, a difficult echocardiographic window or poor global ventricular function may preclude its use. Furthermore, this test cannot be used in those patients in whom a recent myocardial infarction, an aneurysm, or other vascular malformation would make tachycardia or hypertension risky.

F. Radionuclide imaging. Radionuclide stress imaging is used to assess the perfusion and viability of areas of myocardium. This technique cannot provide an anatomic diagnosis of a cardiac lesion. It is a more sensitive and specific test than ETT and can provide assessment of global left ventricular function as well. Myocardial perfusion imaging is a nuclear technique using intravenous radioisotopes, either thallium-201 or the cardiac-specific technetium-99 perfusion agents sestamibi (Cardiolite) or tetrofosmin (Myoview), as an indicator of the presence or absence of coronary artery disease.

Exercise stress or pharmacologic stress is necessary to increase coronary blood flow for the test. Pharmacologic vasodilators are preferable but contraindicated in patients with severe bronchospastic lung disease, in which case dobutamine may be used. The available pharmacologic vasodilators adenosine and dipyridamole (Persantine) are used to produce maximal coronary vasodilation of approximately four to five times resting values.

Vessels with fixed coronary stenoses will not dilate; thus, less perfusion agent can reach the myocardium. Myocardium perfused by these vessels will show up as a "defect" on stress scans when compared to surrounding myocardium supplied by nonobstructed coronaries. When compared to the images acquired at rest, any defects still present—*fixed* or *persistent defects*—are suggestive of nonviable or infarcted myocardium. Defects present on stress and not at rest, termed *reversible defects,* suggest viable myocardium at risk for ischemia when stressed.

The technique used to acquire these images is single photon emission computed tomography (SPECT). Compared to ETT, the sensitivity for the detection of coronary artery disease increases to approximately 85% to 90%. A slightly higher false-positive rate, however, limits specificity in unselected patients to about 75% to 80% [19]. The sensitivity and specificity of nuclear perfusion imaging are similar for pharmacologic and stress-based techniques.

The predictive value of the test can be improved by using it in high-risk subgroups. Selective use of pharmacologic perfusion imaging in patients who have at least one of two clinical risk factors for ischemic disease (age more than 70 years and congestive heart failure) can maximize the usefulness of this procedure in predicting cardiac outcome in patients undergoing noncardiac surgery of all types [9].

Contraindications are as follows:

Unstable angina or myocardial infarction within 48 hours
Severe primary bronchospasm
Methylxanthine ingestion within 24 hours
Allergy to dipyridamole or aminophylline

Pharmacologic vasodilators should be used in patients who cannot exercise or who have a medical condition such as a cerebral aneurysm, which would contraindicate exercise.

G. Specialized imaging techniques

1. **Positron emission tomographic scan.** Positron emission tomographic scanning techniques use different radioisotopes than SPECT imaging. These isotopes have a higher energy decay and a shorter half-life, and they can assess both regional myocardial blood flow and myocardial metabolism on a real-time basis. The higher cost of this technique, which also includes a cyclotron to produce the isotopes, often precludes its widespread use.

2. **Magnetic resonance imaging.** Magnetic resonance imaging (MRI) is used to provide both high-resolution and three-dimensional imaging of cardiac structures, including coronary angiography. Changes in molecular composition of the myocardium can change its magnetic moment and MRI signal, allowing MRI to detect lipid accumulation, edema, fibrosis, rate of phosphate turnover, and intracellular pH in ischemic areas. Finally, MRI imaging can be gated to the cardiac cycle, allowing rapid and accurate assessment of myocardial function. The clinical application of MRI is limited by its cost and the length of the tests.

IV. Cardiac catheterization

Key clinical findings
Coronary anatomy
Ventricular function
Valvular anatomy and function
Pulmonary vascular resistance

A. **Overview.** Cardiac catheterization still is considered the gold standard for diagnosis of cardiac pathology before most open heart operations and for definition of lesions of the coronary vessels. More than 95% of patients undergoing open heart operations have catheterization before the procedure. The remaining 5% are assessed only by noninvasive techniques, such as echocardiography and Doppler flow studies. They have pathologic findings, such as ASD or VSD, which are adequately defined by noninvasive means.

The following general description of catheterization data and their interpretation is an introduction to the general concepts of catheterization reporting and the types of information available from cardiac catheterization. Most formal catheterization reports contain the following:

- Brief summary of indications for the catheterization procedure
- Description of the catheterization procedure itself
- Hemodynamic data, including chamber pressures and cardiac output
- Descriptive information on coronary anatomy, ventricular function, and valvular regurgitation
- Calculation of derived parameters, including valve areas, EF, and pulmonary and systemic vascular resistances

If only coronary anatomy is to be delineated, often only a systemic–arterial or left-sided catheterization will be performed. However, if any degree of left ventricular dysfunction, valvular abnormality, pulmonary disease, or impaired right ventricular function exists clinically, a right-sided (Swan–Ganz) catheterization also will be performed. A range of normal hemodynamic values obtained from right-sided and left-sided catheterizations is listed in Table 1.5.

Interpretation of catheterization data emphasizes the following areas:

B. **Assessment of coronary anatomy**

1. **Procedure.** Radiopaque dye is injected through a catheter placed at the coronary ostia to delineate the anatomy of both the right and left coronary arter-

Table 1.5 Normal hemodynamic values obtained at cardiac catheterization

Parameter	Measurement	Value
Peripheral arterial or aortic pressure	Systolic/diastolic	≤140/90 mm Hg
	Mean	≤105 mm Hg
Right atrial pressure	Mean	≤6 mm Hg
Right ventricular pressure	Systolic/end-diastolic	≤30/6 mm Hg
Pulmonary artery pressure	Systolic/diastolic	≤30/15 mm Hg
	Mean	≤22 mm Hg
Pulmonary artery wedge pressure	Mean	≤12 mm Hg
Left ventricular pressure	Systolic/end-diastolic	≤140/12 mm Hg
Cardiac index		2.5–4.2 L·min^{-1}·m^{-2}
End-diastolic volume index		<100 mL/m^{-2}
Arteriovenous O$_2$ content difference		≤5.0 mL/dL
Pulmonary vascular resistance		20–130 dyne·s·cm^{-5}
		or
		0.25–1.6 Woods units
Systemic vascular resistance		700–1600 dyne·s·cm^{-5}
		or
		9–20 Woods units

ies. Multiple views are important to define branch lesions best, decrease artifacts at points of tortuosity or vessel overlap, and determine more clearly the degree of stenosis, particularly in eccentric lesions. Two common projections of the coronary arteries are the right anterior oblique (RAO) and the left anterior oblique (LAO) views (Fig. 1.2).

2. **Interpretation.** The degree of vessel stenosis generally is assessed by the percentage reduction in vessel diameter, which in turn correlates with the reduction in cross-sectional area of the vessel at the point of narrowing. Lesions that reduce vessel diameter by greater than 50%, reducing the cross-sectional area by greater than 75%, are considered significant. Lesions also are characterized as either focal or segmental. There is a great deal of interobserver variability in interpretation of the degree of stenosis in the range from 40% to 70%.

C. **Assessment of left ventricular function.** Both global and regional measures of ventricular function can be obtained from catheterization data.

   1. **Global ventricular measurements**

      a. **Left ventricular end-diastolic pressure (LVEDP).** An elevated value above 15 mm Hg **usually** indicates some degree of ventricular dysfunction. LVEDP is an index that may reflect either systolic or diastolic dysfunction and is acutely affected by preload and afterload. Without examining other indices of function, an isolated measurement of elevated LVEDP simply indicates that something is abnormal. An elevated LVEDP measurement associated with a normal left ventricular contractile pattern and cardiac output may indicate a decrease in left ventricular compliance.

      b. **Forward cardiac output–cardiac index.** Forward cardiac output is the total amount of blood pumped past the aortic valve into the systemic circulation. It generally is determined by the thermodilution method.

      c. **Left ventricular ejection fraction**

         (1) **Calculation.** EF is defined as the volume of blood ejected (stroke volume) per beat divided by the volume in the left ventricle before ejection [end-diastolic volume (EDV)]. The stroke volume (SV) is equal to EDV minus the end-systolic volume (ESV). The equation for EF determination is therefore:

$$EF = \frac{[EDV - ESV]}{EDV} = \frac{SV}{EDV}$$

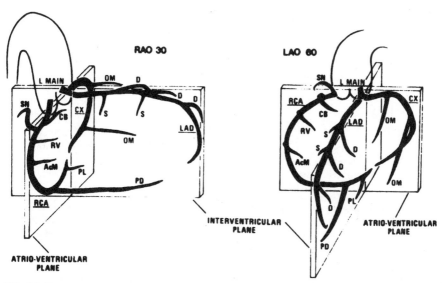

FIG. 1.2 Representation of coronary anatomy relative to the interventricular and atrioventricular valve planes. Coronary branches are left main (*L Main*), left anterior descending (*LAD*), diagonal (*D*), septal (*S*), circumflex (*CX*), obtuse marginal (*OM*), right coronary (*RCA*), conus branch (*CB*), sinus node (*SN*), acute marginal (*AcM*), posterior descending (*PD*), and posterolateral left ventricular (*PL*). (From Baim DS, Grossman W. Coronary angiography. In: Grossman W, ed. *Cardiac catheterization and angiography,* 3rd ed. Philadelphia: Lea & Febiger, 1986:185, with permission.)

ESV and EDV determinations are extrapolated from data gained from left ventriculography. In this procedure, radiopaque dye is used to define the left ventricle, and motion pictures (cines) are taken for several cardiac cycles. The cines are analyzed, either by computer or by hand, by tracing the 2D **areas** highlighted by the radiopaque dye. The areas are calculated during both systole and diastole. These areas then are converted to **volumes** based on a formula for an ellipse that most closely represents the ventricular chamber dimension. Volume measurements are most accurate when two views are used (i.e., RAO and LAO) for the calculations. An EF calculation using the volume measurements calculated from just one projection (RAO) frequently is misleading. Furthermore, EF, like any other indirect measurement of contractility, is reflective of only one point in time and can be influenced by heart rate, preload, and afterload.

(2) **Angiographic versus forward cardiac output.** The ejected volume of blood (EF) can either pass forward through the aorta or, in the presence of valvular lesions, proceed in a retrograde direction through the mitral valve or the aortic valve. Hence, the **angiographic** or **total cardiac output** calculated as stroke volume times heart rate takes into account both **forward** and **backward** flow. With valvular regurgitation, the **angiographic** cardiac output will be greater than the forward cardiac output.

(3) **Mitral regurgitation.** EF greater than 50% is normal in the presence of normal valvular function. However, in the presence of significant mitral regurgitation, EF of 50% to 55% suggests moderate left ventricular dysfunction, because part of the volume is ejected backward into a low-resistance pathway (i.e., into the left atrium).

    d. Diastolic volume index. EDV indexed to the patient's body surface area is another global measure of ventricular performance. It can, however, be elevated in patients with regurgitant or volume overload lesions with preserved left ventricular function (similar to the LVEDP). A normal index is considered less than 100 mL/m².

    e. Arteriovenous O₂ content difference. The Fick equation relates cardiac output to oxygen extraction by the body as follows:

$$\text{Cardiac output} = \frac{O_2\,\text{consumption}}{O_2\,\text{content difference}}$$

    Thus, cardiac output is inversely related to arteriovenous O₂ content difference, assuming that oxygen consumption is constant. A normal value of arteriovenous O₂ difference is less than 5 mL/dL. A low-cardiac output state would be represented by an increased extraction of oxygen, resulting in a widened arteriovenous O₂ content difference.

  2. Regional assessment of ventricular function. Uniform rapid inward contraction of the entire left ventricle (observed during left ventriculography) represents a normal contractile pattern. This observation provides qualitative assessment of overall ventricular function but is not as specific as the calculated EF.

    Qualitative regional differences in contraction may be evident. For examination, the heart is divided into segments. The anterior, posterior, apical, basal, inferior (diaphragmatic), and septal regions of the left ventricle are examined (Figs. 1.3 and 1.4). Motion of each one of these particular regions is defined as normal, hypokinetic (decreased inward motion), akinetic (no motion), or dyskinetic (outward paradoxical motion) in relation to the other normally contracting segments.

    One wall (e.g., the anterior wall) may appear hypokinetic and the rest of the ventricle may contract normally. Despite this one area of abnormal motion, however, global ventricular function may still be preserved. Obviously, if half of the left ventricle is mildly hypokinetic, global measurements of ventricular function also should be depressed.

    Regional wall-motion abnormalities usually are secondary to previous infarction or acute ischemia. However, very infrequently myocarditis as well as

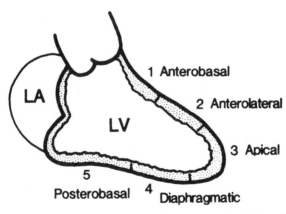

FIG. 1.3 Terminology for left ventricular segments *1* to *5* analyzed from the right anterior oblique ventriculogram. *LA*, left atrium; *LV*, left ventricle. (From CASS Principal Investigators and Associates. National Heart, Lung, and Blood Institute Coronary Artery Surgery Study [part II]. *Circulation* 1981;63[Suppl]:1–14, with permission.)

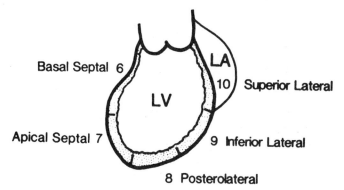

FIG. 1.4 Terminology for left ventricular segments *6* to *10* analyzed from the left anterior oblique ventriculogram. *LA,* left atrium; *LV,* left ventricle. (From CASS Principal Investigators and Associates. National Heart, Lung, and Blood Institute Coronary Artery Surgery Study [part II]. *Circulation* 1981;63[Suppl]:1–14, with permission.)

    rare infiltrative processes by myocardial tumors lead to regional wall-motion abnormalities.

D. Assessment of valvular function. This section will be limited to a brief discussion of the methods used to study lesions of the aortic and mitral valves. The specific hemodynamic patterns of acute and chronic valvular disease will be discussed in Chapter 12.

  1. Regurgitant lesions

    a. Qualitative assessment. A relative scale of 1+ to 4+ (with 4+ being the most severe) is used to quantitate the severity of valvular incompetence during the injection of dye. Visual inspection is used to determine the intensity and rapidity of washout of dye from the left ventricle after aortic root injection (aortic regurgitation) or from the left atrium after ventricular injection (mitral regurgitation).

    b. Calculation of regurgitant fraction. The percentage of regurgitant blood flow can be calculated by the following equation:

$$\text{Regurgitant fraction} = \frac{\text{SV angiographic} - \text{SV forward}}{\text{SV angiographic}}$$

where forward stroke volume is the volume calculated from the thermodilution method divided by simultaneous heart rate. The angiographic stroke volume is determined during left ventriculography. If there is a large difference in heart rate when the two different output measurements are obtained, this calculation would be erroneous. If aortic and mitral regurgitation occur in combination, the amount contributed by each valve to the total amount of regurgitation can be detected only by viewing the cineangiograms qualitatively.

    c. Pathologic V waves. In patients with mitral regurgitation, the pulmonary capillary wedge trace may manifest giant V waves. Normal or physiologic V waves are seen in the left atrium at the end of systole and are secondary to filling from the pulmonary veins against a closed mitral valve. With valvular incompetence, the regurgitant wave into the left atrium is superimposed on a physiologic V wave, producing a giant V wave (Fig. 1.5). One would expect this giant V wave to occur earlier in the cardiac cycle. However, transmission of the wave to the pulmonary artery catheter depends on a number of factors, including compliance of the left atrium and the pulmonary venous circuit. With chronic regurgitation, the left atrium dilates

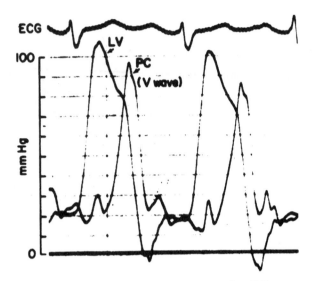

FIG. 1.5 Left ventricular (*LV*) and pulmonary capillary wedge (*PC*) pressure tracings obtained from a patient with ruptured chordae tendineae and acute mitral insufficiency. The giant V wave results from regurgitation of blood into a relatively small and noncompliant left atrium. The electrocardiogram (*ECG*) illustrates the timing of the PC V wave, whose peak follows ventricular repolarization, as manifest by the T wave of the ECG. (From Grossman W. Profiles in valvular heart disease. In: Grossman W, Baim DS, eds. *Cardiac catheterization, angiography, and intervention,* 4th ed. Philadelphia: Lea & Febiger, 1991:564, with permission.)

due to volume overload, and it becomes highly compliant and absorbs the back-pressure wave. Thus, a giant V wave need not be present even with severe regurgitation if there is a huge compliant left atrium.

2. **Stenotic lesions.** The severity of valvular stenosis can be determined only by knowing the size of the pressure drop across the stenotic valve **and** the amount of flow across the stenosis during either systolic ejection or diastolic filling. One cannot uniformly assess the severity of stenosis solely by examining the pressure gradient (either peak to peak or mean) across the valve.

Gorlin and Gorlin [20] developed an equation for determining valve area based on these two factors. A simplified version of this equation is as follows:

$$\text{Valve area} = \frac{\text{cardiac output (L/min)}}{\sqrt{\text{mean pressure gradient}}}$$

If the mean pressure gradient and cardiac output are given on the catheterization report, a quick estimate of either aortic or mitral valve area can be made.

When examining combined regurgitant and stenotic lesions of the same valve, the total or angiographic cardiac output must be used in the calculation; otherwise, the severity of stenosis will be overestimated. Values for normal and abnormal valve areas are discussed in Chapter 12.

E. **Assessment of pulmonary hemodynamics.** Pulmonary artery hypertension can be a result of increased anterograde pulmonary flow or elevated pulmonary venous pressures. Increased anterograde pulmonary flow is characteristic of ASDs or VSDs. An increase in pulmonary venous pressure occurs with left ventricular failure, mitral valve disease, and, less commonly, aortic valve disease. Either situation (i.e., an increased anterograde flow or elevated pulmonary venous pressure) may induce pulmonary vascular changes and result in elevated pulmonary vascular resistance. Normal values for pulmonary artery pressure and resistance are listed in Table 1.5.

Remember that catheterization data represent only *one* point in time, and medical management may have changed the hemodynamic pattern and catheterization results at the time of cardiac operation.

V. Systemic disease
A. Atherosclerotic vascular disease

Key clinical findings
Carotid bruits
Transient ischemic attack
Cerebrovascular accident
Claudication
Hypertension
Azotemia

Aortic, carotid, and peripheral vascular disease frequently are associated with coronary artery disease. Furthermore, the presence of major vascular disease certainly affects the morbidity and anesthetic management of patients scheduled to undergo cardiopulmonary bypass procedures.

1. **Carotid disease.** Symptoms of transient ischemic attack or visual disturbance should be sought in all preoperative cardiac patients. The presence of these symptoms or of an asymptomatic carotid bruit should warrant at least noninvasive Doppler carotid flow studies before cardiac surgery. Patients with symptoms and greater than 80% stenosis may benefit from endarterectomy before cardiac, as before noncardiac, surgery. There is no clear answer for those patients who either are asymptomatic or have lesions of lesser severity. Neurologic outcome has been studied in relatively few patients with high-grade carotid stenosis during and after cardiopulmonary bypass. However, cardiopulmonary bypass, or cardiac surgery, appears to confer little additional risk of stroke in patients with carotid stenosis. Even in the absence of symptoms, it is wise to assume that every patient older than 70 years with coronary artery disease also has some cerebrovascular disease, and intraoperative blood pressure management should be planned accordingly.

2. **Renovascular disease.** Severe recent-onset or recently progressive hypertension, abdominal bruits, or renal insufficiency should prompt thorough investigation of the renal vasculature, including renin measurement. Preoperative use of angiotensin-converting enzyme inhibitors in patients with renal artery stenosis can induce renal insufficiency. Further, renal vascular disease, if present, requires that the physician exercise increased care in patients with hypotension on cardiopulmonary bypass and in those with radiopaque dye loads in the immediate preoperative period. Mannitol and other diuretics may be needed to preserve renal function intraoperatively.

3. **Peripheral vascular disease.** Symptoms of claudication should be sought and peripheral pulses should be examined in both arms and legs in patients with generalized vascular disease. Preoperative assessment of pulse strength is necessary to form a baseline for postoperative evaluation, to determine the most appropriate sites for arterial cannulation, and to locate the best peripheral insertion site for an intraaortic balloon pump or arterial cardiopulmonary bypass cannula should the need arise.

B. Hypertension

Key clinical findings
Range of resting and admission blood pressures
Duration of hypertension
Antihypertensive therapy
Azotemia
Hypokalemia
Palpitations
Headache

Table 1.6 Patients at high risk of secondary hypertension

Blood pressure >180 systolic or >110 diastolic
Blood pressure not controlled by two or more agents
Increase in previously well-controlled blood pressure
Sudden onset, labile, or paroxysmal hypertension
Hypertension with onset before age 25 yr or after age 50 yr

The contribution of hypertension to perioperative morbidity and the implications for anesthetic management depend on (a) the etiology of hypertension; (b) blood pressure level, both with stress and at rest; (c) preexisting complications of hypertension; and (d) physiologic changes due to drug therapy.

1. **Etiology.** From 85% to 95% of patients have so-called primary or essential hypertension, probably related to an alteration of membrane handling of sodium, potassium, or calcium. It is important to exclude preoperatively the 5% to 15% of patients with treatable causes of secondary hypertension, especially patients who are at greater than average risk of secondary hypertension, as listed in Table 1.6. Common causes of secondary hypertension usually are renal or endocrine and account for an additional 5% to 10% of hypertensive patients. Other rare disorders are found in less than 1% of patients (Table 1.7). When indicated, a search for secondary hypertension should include urinalysis; determination of creatinine, glucose, and electrolyte levels; ECG, and chest films. Pheochromocytoma, although very rare, is particularly important because of its potential morbidity in association with anesthesia. It should be ruled out preoperatively in patients with headache, labile or paroxysmal hypertension, abnormal pallor, or perspiration.

2. **Severity.** Evaluation of all cardiac patients, and hypertensive patients in particular, should include determination of the *range* of blood pressures within which the patient usually functions. Intraoperative cardiac morbidity in the form of dysrhythmias and ischemic ECG changes has been observed more frequently in hypertensive patients with awake diastolic blood pressures greater

Table 1.7 Causes of hypertension

Medical cause (Incidence)	Drug-induced hypertension
Essential hypertension (85%–95%)	Caffeine
Secondary hypertension	Cocaine
Common causes	Chlorpromazine
Renal (2%–6%)	Cyclosporine
Renal parenchymal disease	Ethanol
Renovascular disease	Monoamine oxidase inhibitors
Endocrine (1%–2%)	Nicotine
Pheochromocytoma	Nonsteroidal antiinflammatory drugs
Cushing disease	Oral contraceptives
Hyperaldosteronism	Steroids
Sleep apnea (1%)	Sympathomimetics
Rare causes	Nasal decongestants
Adrenogenital syndrome	Weight loss regimens
Acromegaly	
Aortic coarctation	
Hypercalcemia	
Familial dysautonomia, porphyria, neuropathies	
Renin-producing tumors	

than 110 mm Hg. Increased perioperative risk in patients with diastolic blood pressures between 90 and 110 mm Hg is more controversial.

3. **"Pseudonormotension."** It is rare for essential hypertension to resolve without treatment. The hypertensive patient who becomes normotensive for no apparent reason presents a special dilemma. A myocardial ischemic event or progression of stenotic valvular disease may cause this apparent resolution of hypertension in which the patient becomes normotensive only because his or her heart can no longer generate sufficient cardiac output to produce hypertension. The patient's response to any surgical or anesthetic stress may be immediate cardiac failure.

4. **Sequelae of hypertension.** The hypertensive state can lead to sequelae that are most evident in the heart, central nervous system, and kidney. In particular, patients with established hypertension may exhibit (a) left ventricular hypertrophy leading to decreased ventricular compliance; (b) neurologic symptoms, such as headache, dizziness, tinnitus, and blurred vision that may progress to cerebral infarction; and (c) renal vascular lesions leading to proteinuria, hematuria, and decreased glomerular filtration progressing to renal failure.

5. **Sequelae of antihypertensive therapy.** Most antihypertensive agents have beneficial effects in the perioperative period, reducing vascular reactivity and myocardial workload. They should be continued until the morning of the operation. β-Blockers and clonidine, in particular, must be continued throughout the perioperative period to avoid a "rebound" phenomenon. Antihypertensive therapy, however, often leads to hypovolemia and hypokalemia, which must be recognized and treated preoperatively. Preoperative use of angiotensin II receptor antagonists also has been shown in some series to be associated with hypotension upon induction of anesthesia. Most current antihypertensives have other hemodynamic effects that may be important to intraoperative management (Table 1.8).

C. **Pulmonary disease**

Key clinical findings
History of cigarette smoking
Sputum production
Dyspnea
Wheezing
Recent respiratory infection

Cardiac surgery requires thoracotomy, which leads to increased risk of postoperative ventilatory complications. Furthermore, cardiopulmonary bypass itself, and therapy with drugs such as amiodarone, can lead to postoperative pulmonary damage. Risk factors for postoperative pulmonary insufficiency and the need for prolonged mechanical ventilation should be sought on preoperative evaluation. Risk factors include the following:

1. **History of smoking.** A history of smoking is common in adults with heart disease and raises several questions. Does smoking in the absence of other risk factors increase surgical risk? Is recent smoking a more important risk factor than chronic smoking? If so, how long of a smoke-free interval is necessary to reduce risk?

A history of smoking in the absence of any signs or symptoms of respiratory disease does little to increase anesthetic risk. However, a history of prolonged smoking is associated almost invariably with signs and symptoms of bronchitis or obstructive pulmonary disease, and it increases the significance of these symptoms. Discontinuing smoking 1 to 3 days preoperatively confers little beneficial effect, except that it allows carbon monoxide levels in the blood to decrease. Warner and colleagues [21] found that the risk of postoperative pulmonary complications requiring therapy in the hospital after CABG, in fact, **increased** from approximately 33% in current smokers to 57% in patients who had stopped smoking for less than 8 weeks. However, the risk decreased to 14% in patients who stopped smoking more than 8 weeks before surgery and decreased to the nonsmoker's rate of 11% in patients who had stopped smoking for more than 6 months.

(*text continues on page 26*)

Table 1.8 Common antihypertensives

Classification	Agents	Side effects
Diuretics		
Saluretic	Indapamide Metolazone (Mykrox, Zaroxolyn)	Mild hypokalemia Orthostasis Decreased response to norepinephrine Hypercholesterolemia Hyperglycemia
Loop	Bumetanide Ethacrynic acid (Edecrin) Furosemide (Lasix) Chlorthalidone	Hypovolemia Hypokalemia Ototoxicity
Potassium-sparing	Amiloride (Midamor, Moduretic) Spironolactone Triamterene (Dyrenium, Maxzide)	Hyperkalemia Azotemia Sensitivity to muscle relaxants
Thiazides	Bendroflumethiazide Chlorothiazide (Diuril) Hydrochlorothiazide (HydroDIURIL) Hydroflumethiazide (Diucardin) Methyclothiazide (Aquatensen)	Hypovolemia Hypokalemia Azotemia
Catecholamine-depleting	Reserpine	Orthostatic hypotension Sensitivity to direct-acting pressors Sensitivity to anesthetics (some authors recommend stopping 48–72 h preoperatively)
Central-acting α_2-agonists	Clonidine (Catapres) Guanabenz Guanfacine (Tenex) Methyldopa (Aldomet)	Hepatic dysfunction Withdrawal hypertension Potentiate sedatives Hemolytic anemia
Central-acting α_1-inhibitors	Prazosin (Minipress)	Resistance to indirect-acting pressors Orthostatic hypotension
Direct vasodilators	Hydralazine Minoxidil (Loniten)	Hypotension Reflex tachycardia Orthostasis
α_1-Adrenergic blockers	Doxazosin (Cardura) Terazosin (Hytrin)	
Angiotensin-converting enzyme inhibitors	Benazepril (Lotensin) Captopril Enalapril (Vasotec) Fosinopril (Monopril) Lisinopril (Prinivil, Zestril) Moexipril (Univasc) Perindopril (Aceon) Quinapril (Accupril) Ramipril (Altace) Trandolapril (Mavik)	Hypotension Pancytopenia Hyperkalemia Angioedema Exacerbate renal insufficiency Cough

continued

Table 1.8 *Continued*

Classification	Agents	Side effects
Angiotensin II receptor antagonists	Candesartan (Atacand) Eprosartan (Teveten) Irbesartan (Avapro) Losartan (Cozaar) Telmisartan (Micardis) Valsartan (Diovan)	Hypotension Impaired renal function Impaired hepatic function
β-Adrenergic blockers		
Nonselective	Nadolol (Corgard) Propranolol (Inderal) Timolol (Blocadren) Penbutolol (Levatol)	Bradycardia Orthostasis Hypoglycemia Bronchospasm Congestive heart failure
β₁-selective	Acebutolol (Sectral) Atenolol (Tenormin) Betaxolol (Kerlone) Bisoprolol (Zebeta) Metoprolol (Lopressor, Toprol XL)	Bradycardia Orthostasis Congestive heart failure
Intrinsic sympathomimetic activity	Pindolol	Bradycardia Orthostasis Hypoglycemia Bronchospasm Congestive heart failure
α- and β-Blockers	Labetalol (Normodyne, Trandate) Carvedilol (Coreg)	Orthostasis Hepatic failure
Ganglionic blocker	Mecamylamine (Inversine)	Orthostasis Choreiform movement Sensitivity to pressor amines

Calcium channel blockers	Dihydropyridines
	  Amlodipine (Norvasc)
	  Felodipine (Plendil)
	  Isradipine (DynaCirc)
	  Nicardipine (Cardene)
	  Nifedipine (Adalet, Procardia)
	  Nisoldipine (Sular)
	  Nimodipine (Nimotop)
		Coronary vasodilation
		Peripheral vasodilation

	Benzothiazepine Diltiazem (Cardizem, Tiazac)	Coronary vasodilation Suppress sinus node automaticity Suppress atrioventricular nodal conduction

	Phenylalkylamine
	  Verapamil (Calan, Covera, Isoptin, Verelan)
	  Bepridil (Vascor)
		Coronary vasodilation
		Suppress sinus node automaticity
		Suppress atrioventricular nodal conduction
		Decrease contractility
		Vasodilation
		Bradycardia
		Ventricular dysrhythmias
		Torsades de pointes

2. Patients with chronic lung disease manifest by dyspnea on exertion or at rest, sputum production, or audible wheezes on physical examination have two to six times the rate of pulmonary complications found in normal patients after thoracic surgery.

3. **Recent respiratory infection.** Controversy exists about the need to postpone surgery in a patient with an upper respiratory infection who is undergoing a peripheral surgical procedure. In a cardiac or major thoracic procedure, however, the difficulty encountered in clearing an increased volume of tenacious bronchial secretions can easily lead to postoperative atelectasis or pneumonia. Especially in infants and young children, purulent secretions can lead to mucous plugging of the bronchi and, in our experience, recurrent occlusion of a small endotracheal tube requiring emergency reintubation in the early postoperative period. For these reasons, we recommend postponement of elective cardiac surgery in patients, especially children, with evidence of an upper or lower respiratory infection manifest by cough, hoarseness, or purulent nasal discharge within 2 weeks of surgery. In patients undergoing emergent surgery, special efforts to clear secretions by suctioning or bronchoscopy will be needed in the early postoperative period.

4. **Age.** Resting Po_2 decreases almost linearly with age. However, the risk of pulmonary complications increases significantly only after age 70 to 80 years in patients with no other pulmonary risk factors.

5. **Weight.** Obesity, or weight in excess of 10% above ideal body weight, is sufficient to increase the chances of atelectasis. With further increases in body weight, severe chronic atelectasis can occur. In the extreme case of the morbidly obese patient with pickwickian syndrome, such atelectasis can lead to pulmonary hypertension and right ventricular failure.

6. **Cardiac disease.** Valvular heart disease, particularly mitral valve disease, and chronic congestive heart failure are associated with postoperative respiratory failure and the need for prolonged ventilation. Pulmonary hypertension from these or other causes is one mechanism by which cardiac disease contributes directly to perioperative pulmonary insufficiency.

7. **Pulmonary function testing.** In patients judged to be at increased perioperative risk based on clinical criteria, and especially in patients with aortic or mitral valve disease, spirometry is indicated to evaluate perioperative lung function. Shapiro divided patients into groups with low, moderate, or high risk of acute respiratory failure in the first postoperative 24 hours based on preoperative spirometry (Table 1.9).

D. **Hepatic dysfunction**

Key clinical findings
History of hepatitis
Ascites

Table 1.9 Risk indices based on spirometry

Low risk
 FVC (% predicted) + FEV$_1$ (% FVC) > 150
Moderate risk
 150 > (FVC [% predicted] + FEV$_1$ [% FVC]) > 100
High risk
 FVC (% predicted) + FEV$_1$ (% FVC) < 100
    or
 FVC < 20 mL/kg
    or
 Postbronchodilator FEV$_1$/FVC < 50%

FVC, forced vital capacity; FEV$_1$, forced expiratory volume in 1 sec.
From Shapiro BA. *Clinical application of respiratory care,* 3rd ed. Chicago: Year Book, 1985: 524, with permission.

Serum bilirubin greater than 3
Serum albumin less than 3
Elevated prothrombin time (PT)

1. **Acute hepatitis.** Acute viral, alcoholic, or toxic hepatitis is associated with high perioperative morbidity for approximately 1 month after onset of the disease or until aspartate aminotransferase level returns to normal. Therefore, no elective surgery should be performed during this period. If patients with acute hepatitis must undergo emergency surgery, higher morbidity and mortality must be expected.

2. **Chronic hepatic disease.** The severity of liver function impairment and its impact on operative outcome can be gauged from criteria such as those developed by Child (Table 1.10). The laboratory abnormalities listed in the table can be simplified into the "rule of threes," which states that there is a high risk of liver failure if:

Serum albumin < 3 < serum bilirubin.

3. **Clotting abnormalities.** Patients with severe liver dysfunction often have an elevated PT due to deficits of clotting factors II, VII, IX, and X, which are manufactured in the liver. In these patients, vitamin K therapy should be used first. If the liver still cannot produce sufficient clotting factors, transfusions of fresh frozen plasma are indicated before and during surgery, keeping in mind the danger of fluid overload in patients with congestive heart failure or poor left ventricular function. Also, use of intravenous vitamin K in an attempt to correct coagulopathy quickly can cause severe hypotension and a life-threatening anaphylactic response. In any patient with liver function that is limited enough to prolong PT, a slowed drug metabolism should be expected. Vasoactive drugs (lidocaine and aminophylline in particular) must be infused at a reduced rate.

4. **Abnormal electrolyte measurements.** Hyponatremia, hypokalemia, and metabolic acidosis occur with liver dysfunction and often are secondary to hyperaldosteronism or diuretic use.

E. **Renal disease**

Key clinical findings
Daily urine output
Serum creatinine
Albuminemia
Serum electrolytes
Hematocrit

1. **Microalbuminuria and cardiovascular risks.** Recent evidence shows that the risks of major cardiovascular morbidity is increased 1.5 to 2 times in patients with microalbuminuria, considering both patients with and patients without diabetes mellitus [22]. Thus, even early stages of renal disease represent systemic disturbances that are associated with cardiovascular disease.

Table 1.10 Child's criteria for classification of hepatic function

	Low risk	Moderate risk	High risk
Functional impairment	Minimal	Moderate	Severe
Serum bilirubin (mg/dL)	<2	2–3	>3
Serum albumin (g/dL)	>3.5	3.0–3.5	<3
Ascites	None	Easily controlled	Poorly controlled
Neurologic disorder	None	Minimal	Moderate to severe
Nutrition	Good	Adequate	Poor, wasted

From Child CG III. *The liver and portal hypertension.* Philadelphia: WB Saunders, 1964: 50, with permission.

2. **Renal failure and cardiopulmonary bypass.** Renal disease impairs the ability to maintain body fluid, electrolyte, and acid–base balance in the face of operative stress and to excrete waste products and drug metabolites. For patients undergoing cardiopulmonary bypass, particular concern exists because of (a) the large fluid load typically administered with a crystalloid cardiopulmonary bypass prime and (b) the potassium usually administered as part of the cardioplegic solution. Oliguric patients usually are in more danger from both fluid and potassium administration than are polyuric patients.

3. **Metabolic acidosis.** Most patients with established renal failure have some degree of metabolic acidosis. When preoperative acidosis becomes severe (plasma bicarbonate less than 18 mEq/L), the extra acid load that may be generated during surgery may lead to acidemia and a subsequent decrease in myocardial function.

4. **Anemia.** Patients with chronic renal failure are anemic. Hemoglobin ranging between 7 and 8 g/dL is associated with increased cardiac output and myocardial oxygen demand. Therefore, use of a crystalloid cardiopulmonary bypass prime could reduce hemoglobin to levels that would seriously reduce O_2-carrying capacity in these patients.

5. **Pericarditis.** Patients with chronic renal failure have a high incidence of pericarditis, which may lead to adhesions and make the surgical procedure more difficult, longer, and more bloody.

F. **Diabetes mellitus**

Key clinical findings
Duration
Insulin requirement
Fasting blood glucose
Autonomic instability
Renal insufficiency

1. **Silent ischemia.** Diabetic patients, particularly those with proteinuria or other evidence of diabetic nephropathy and autonomic neuropathy, are at increased risk of ischemic heart disease, even at a young age. Diabetics are more likely to suffer myocardial infarction and, if infarction does occur, it is more likely to be fatal than in nondiabetics. Because of autonomic neuropathy, an infarction, if it occurs, is more likely to be **silent.**

2. **Glucose management.** Perioperative hyperglycemia, with blood glucose greater than 200 mg/dL, has been associated with an increased infection rate and slower wound healing in patients after cardiac surgical procedures [23]. Cardiopulmonary bypass is a strong stimulus to hyperglycemia. Therefore, aggressive management of blood glucose, often with an insulin infusion, is required intraoperatively and in the first 2 postoperative days. At Penn State University, we found that an insulin infusion, established as listed in Table 1.11 and titrated based on the patient's hourly blood glucose, has provided better blood glucose control than alternative subcutaneous or "sliding scale" insulin regimens. Most patients in whom this infusion was used had blood glucose levels less than 200 mg/dL, except during and immediately after cardiopulmonary bypass. No episodes of hypoglycemia requiring more than discontinuation of the infusion occurred.

3. **Autonomic neuropathy.** Autonomic instability, manifest by either orthostatic hypotension or lack of heart rate variation with deep breathing, is the single manifestation of diabetes mellitus most closely associated with cardiovascular risk. Patients with autonomic neuropathy are at increased risk for sudden death and for aspiration of gastric contents because of delayed gastric emptying.

4. **NPH insulin.** Because NPH (neutral protamine hagedorn) contains the protamine moiety, patients taking NPH insulin are at increased risk of allergic reaction to protamine received after cardiopulmonary bypass.

Table 1.11 Perioperative insulin infusion[a] protocol, Penn State University

Most recent blood glucose (mg/dL)[b]	Regimen 1[c]	Regimen 2[d]	Regimen 3[e]
<70	Administer 50 mL of D50, stop infusion, and recheck in 15 min. If again <70, discontinue protocol. If >70, restart infusion.		
70–100	0 U/h	0.8 U/h	1 U/h
101–120	0.5 U/h	1 U/h	1.5 U/h
121–150	1 U/h	1.5 U/h	3 U/h
151–200	1.5 U/h	2.5 U/h	4 U/h
201–250	2 U/h	4 U/h	6 U/h
251–300	3 U/h	5 U/h	8 U/h
301–350	4 U/h	6 U/h	10 U/h
351–400	5 U/h	8 U/h	12 U/h
>400			Bolus of 10 U of regular insulin; Infusion at 12 U/h

[a] The insulin infusion should be prepared by adding 25 units of regular insulin to 250 mL of normal saline solution (NSS), producing a final concentration of 0.1 U/mL. Fifty milliliters should be run through the intravenous tubing before starting the infusion. For patients requiring high insulin doses and with low maintenance fluid requirements, a concentrated infusion may be substituted containing 100 units of regular insulin in 100 mL of NSS, producing a final concentration of 1 U/mL.
If the patient's blood sugar remains >200 for 2 hours (two determinations in a row) and has increased in the past hour, he or she should be advanced to the next higher regimen. Similarly, if blood sugar remains 70–100 for 2 hours, they should be placed on the next lower regimen.
If blood glucose remains >200 for 2 hours on regimen 3, titrate infusion as needed to maintain glucose <200.
[b] Blood glucose should be measured at least hourly, beginning 1 h preoperatively.
[c] Initial regimen for patients using <30 U/d of insulin or patients using only oral agents whose glycohemoglobin is <7, or if no glycohemoglobin is available, whose resting preoperative blood glucose is <150.
[d] Initial regimen for patients using ≥30 U/d of insulin or more or patients using only oral agents whose glycohemoglobin is ≥7, or if no glycohemoglobin is available, whose resting preoperative blood glucose is ≥150.
[e] For use only in patients who do not respond to the other two regimens; with blood glucose >200; two times consecutively on regimen 2.

G. Coagulation disorders

Key clinical findings
Patient or family history of abnormal bleeding
Drugs inhibiting coagulation
Liver dysfunction
Abnormal coagulation studies
   PT
   Partial thromboplastin time (PTT)
   Platelet count
   Fibrinogen level

1. **History of bleeding.** A personal or family history of abnormal bleeding is perhaps the best indicator of an underlying hemostatic defect. A history of small bruises, petechiae, epistaxis, and gastrointestinal bleeding is common in patients with platelet disorders. Large bruises and hematomas, hemarthrosis, and hematuria are common in patients with defects of the intrinsic or extrinsic coagulation pathway.

2. **Anticoagulants.** Most perioperative bleeding disorders in our current patient population are drug induced. Preparations containing aspirin and nonsteroidal antiinflammatory agents are commonly taken by patients who require cardiac surgery. It is not sufficient to inquire about aspirin. Each patient also should

be asked about Bufferin, Ecotrin, or any other pain or arthritis medication (Table 1.12). A more complete discussion of the factors surrounding perioperative coagulation defects is given in Chapter 18. In patients taking warfarin (Coumadin), particularly patients with prosthetic valves in place, the drug should be stopped 4 to 5 days before surgery and low-molecular-weight heparin substituted until 24 hours before the operation. Coagulation status should be checked using PT and PTT immediately before surgery.

3. **Screening studies.** In patients planning to undergo cardiopulmonary bypass, three screening tests are indicated: (a) platelet count, (b) PT, and (c) PTT. These tests will detect virtually all significant coagulopathies and will ensure that any bleeding after cardiopulmonary bypass is not due to a preexisting condition. Only if the result of one of these tests is abnormal is it necessary to pursue further laboratory studies. In the absence of any personal or family history of abnormal bleeding, PTT may be the only "screening" test necessary to detect a significant, but occult, coagulopathy.

4. **Platelet (glycoprotein IIb/IIIa) inhibitors.** An increasing number of patients are undergoing cardiac surgery after having received glycoprotein IIb/IIIa inhibitors in the setting of an acute coronary syndrome or percutaneous coronary intervention. These agents inhibit platelet aggregation by preventing the binding of fibrinogen, von Willebrand factor, to platelet glycoprotein IIb/IIIa receptors. Three of these inhibitors currently are available:

Abciximab (ReoPro). As an antibody to the platelet receptor, this long-acting agent can produce low levels of platelet inhibition for up to 10 days and can be reversed only with platelet transfusion. However, bleeding time returns to less than 12 minutes (75% of normal) in most patients after 24 hours. Some patients undergoing CABG after administration of abciximab require platelet transfusion, and the risk of excessive bleeding is about 3% to 5%.

Eptifibatide (Integrilin). One of two synthetic small molecular IIb/IIIa glycoprotein receptor drugs whose effects cannot be reversed with platelet transfusion, this agent causes platelet inhibition that decreases to 30% to 50% within 4 hours of administration, with bleeding time returning to 1.5 times normal within 6 hours. Because eptifibatide is excreted by the kidneys, dose adjustment is needed in patients with serum creatinine greater than 2 to 2.5.

Tirofiban (Aggrastat). The other synthetic small molecular agent, tirofiban, has a plasma half-life of about 2 hours. Platelet function returns to 90% of nor-

Table 1.12 Drugs that induce hemostatic defects

Platelet inhibitors
   Aspirin
   Indomethacin
   Nonsteroidal antiinflammatory drugs
   Phenylbutazone
   Tricyclic antidepressants
Warfarin potentiators
   Alcohol
   Amiodarone
   Cimetidine
   Clofibrate
   Mefenamic acid
   Methyldopa
   Nalidixic acid
   Phenformin
   Phenylbutazone
   Sulfonamide
   Tolbutamide

mal within 4 to 8 hours of administration. Duration of action is not prolonged by moderate liver disease, but it is prolonged in patients with renal disease.

These agents are associated with a small but significant risk of persistent thrombocytopenia, with attendant risk of excess bleeding. They have been used frequently along with anticoagulants, including warfarin and heparin, as well as other platelet inhibitors. However, use in conjunction with thrombolytics is not recommended.

The need to delay surgery after use of these agents has not been established, but delay of 24 to 48 hours, if feasible, would be optimum.

VI. **Management of preoperative cardiac medications**
   A. **Calcium channel blockers.** Calcium channel blockers are used to treat ischemic heart disease, supraventricular dysrhythmias, and systemic hypertension. They improve the myocardial oxygen supply–demand ratio by both increasing the supply and reducing the demand. Calcium channel blockers reduce coronary vascular resistance and are especially useful in relieving coronary vasospasm. Simultaneously, they reduce inotropy, dilate the systemic vasculature, and possibly provide direct protection to the ischemic myocardium from calcium-related injury. Therefore, administration of calcium channel blockers—diltiazem, nifedipine, and verapamil—should be continued preoperatively, and the last dose should be given the morning of surgery.

   B. **β-Adrenergic blockers.** β-Adrenergic blockers are used primarily for the treatment of hypertension and stable exercise-induced angina without coronary vasospasm in patients with good ventricular function. These drugs also can be used to treat SVT, including that due to preexcitation syndromes; hypertension; and the manifestations of systemic disease, which range from hyperthyroidism to migraine headaches. β-Blocker therapy is beneficial in the perioperative period, and abrupt withdrawal of β-blockers can lead to a rebound phenomenon, which is manifest by nervousness, tachycardia, palpitations, hypertension, and even myocardial infarction, ventricular arrhythmias, and sudden death. Mangano et al. [24], Raby et al. [25], as well as many other authors, found that preoperative treatment with β-blocking agents reduces perioperative tachycardia and lowers the incidence of ischemic events. Therefore, administration of β-blockers should continue until the morning of surgery and even intraoperatively. Postoperatively, reinstitution of β-blocker therapy is essential to avoid the rebound phenomenon.

   C. **Digitalis.** Digitalis is used preoperatively both as an inotropic agent in patients with chronic symptoms of congestive heart failure and to control the ventricular rate in patients with atrial flutter or fibrillation.
      1. The risks of digitalis toxicity are increased by fluid shifts, hypokalemia, and hyperventilation in the perioperative period. Furthermore, the benefit of digitalis in treating heart failure often is marginal, and more effective intravenous inotropes with a wider margin of safety are available. Therefore, digitalis used preoperatively as an inotrope should not be given on the day of surgery; other inotropes can be substituted if needed.
      2. Digitalis used to treat a rapid ventricular response to atrial fibrillation or flutter, on the other hand, is very effective and is easy to titrate using the heart rate as a guide. Preoperatively, the adequacy of digitalization can be assessed by observing the changes in heart rate that result from exercise, such as walking in the hall. Stability of the heart rate indicates adequate digitalization. Administration of digitalis should be continued in these patients until the morning of the operation and should be supplemented intraoperatively with small intravenous doses if needed to keep the ventricular rate under 100. Serum potassium must be monitored carefully in patients maintained on digitalis therapy.

   D. **Antidysrhythmics.** Preoperative dysrhythmias may require any of a large number of oral antidysrhythmic agents, including amiodarone, or calcium channel blockers. Therapy for ventricular dysrhythmias should be continued perioperatively. Disopyramide, in particular, has been associated with difficulty in terminating cardiopulmonary bypass in our patients. Therefore, we recommend that another agent be substituted, if at all possible, even on the day before the operation. Similarly, encainide and flecainide should be used only for life-threatening dysrhythmias, as there is increased mortality in postmyocardial infarction patients treated with these drugs.

Amiodarone has been reported to cause intractable hypotension and bradycardia, unresponsive to catecholamines, in noncardiac surgery patients, as well as an inability to wean from cardiopulmonary bypass during cardiac surgery. However, patients often require continued therapy for intractable dysrhythmias. We have successfully anesthetized an increasing number of patients treated with amiodarone up until the day of surgery without untoward effects.

VII. Premedication. Premedication in any surgical patient is given for one of four reasons: relief of anxiety, amnesia, analgesia, and protection from secretions and noxious reflexes.

For adults, analgesia, sedation, and amnesia for painful preoperative procedures are of greatest importance. Oral benzodiazepines, such as diazepam 10 to 15 mg orally or lorazepam 0.5 to 1.0 mg orally, given upon the patient's arrival at the hospital, followed by intravenous lorazepam, midazolam, or fentanyl once an intravenous infusion is established, have been found most effective. Oral midazolam 0.5 to 0.75 mg/kg is effective for pediatric patients.

Complete preoperative evaluation and proper premedication, including especially the use of β-blockade in appropriate patients with good ventricular function, smooth the patient's transition into the operating room and may reduce the incidence of perioperative ischemia in susceptible patients.

References

1. **Mangano DT. Preoperative assessment of cardiac risk. In: Kaplan JA, Reich DL, Konstadt SN, eds. *Cardiac anesthesia,* 4th ed. Philadelphia: WB Saunders, 1999:3.**
2. Kennedy JW, Kaiser GC, Fischer LD, et al. Clinical and angiographic predictors of operative mortality from the Collaborative Study in Coronary Artery Surgery (CASS). *Circulation* 1981;63:793–802.
3. Goldman L, Caldera DL, Southwick FS, et al. Cardiac risk factors and complications in noncardiac surgery. *Medicine* 1978;57:357–370.
4. Detsky AS, Abrams HB, McLaughlin JR, et al. Predicting cardiac complications in patients undergoing non-cardiac surgery. *J Gen Intern Med* 1986;1:211–219.
5. **American College of Cardiology/American Heart Association Task Force. Guideline update for perioperative cardiovascular evaluation for noncardiac surgery. *Circulation* 2002;105:1257–1267.**
6. **American College of Physicians. Guidelines for assessing and managing the perioperative risk from coronary artery disease associated with major noncardiac surgery. *Ann Intern Med* 1997;127:309–312, 313–328.**
7. Boersma E, Poldermans D, Bax JJ, et al. Predictors of cardiac events after major vascular surgery, role of clinical characteristics, dobutamine echocardiography, and β-blocker therapy. *JAMA* 2001;285:1865–1873.
8. Mangano DT, Browner WS, Hollenberg M, et al. Association of perioperative myocardial ischemia with cardiac morbidity and mortality in men undergoing noncardiac surgery. *N Engl J Med* 1990;323:1781–1788.
9. **Mangano DT, Goldman L. Preoperative assessment of patients with known or suspected coronary disease. *N Engl J Med* 1995;333:1750–1756.**
10. Steen PA, Tinker JH, Tarhan S. Myocardial reinfarction after anesthesia and surgery. *JAMA* 1978;239:2566–2570.
11. Kennedy JW, Ivey TD, Misbach G, et al. Coronary artery bypass graft surgery early after acute myocardial infarction. *Circulation* 1989;79[Suppl I]:I-73–I-78.
12. Mangano DT. Perioperative cardiac morbidity. *Anesthesiology* 1990;72:153–184.
13. Magovern JA, Sakert T, Magovern GJ, et al. A model that predicts morbidity and mortality after coronary artery bypass graft surgery *J Am Coll Cardiol* 1996;28:1147–1153.
14. Higgins TL, Estafanous FG, Loop FD, et al. ICU admission score for predicting morbidity and mortality risk after coronary artery bypass grafting. *Ann Thorac Surg* 1997;64: 1050–1058.
15. Jones RH, Hannan EL, Hammermeister KE, et al. Identification of preoperative variables needed for risk adjustment of short-term mortality after coronary artery bypass graft surgery. *JACC* 1996;28:1478–1487.

16. Gilbert K, Larocque BJ, Patrick LT. Prospective evaluation of cardiac risk indices for patients undergoing noncardiac surgery. *Ann Intern Med* 2000;133:356–359.
17. Gloyna DF, Morton GH, Hoffer JL, et al. The incidence of an abnormal ECG in the surgical patient: is a positive history predictive? *Anesthesiology* 1998;89:A1349.
18. Mantha S, Roizen MF, Barnard J, et al. Relative effectiveness of four preoperative tests for predicting adverse cardiac outcomes after vascular surgery: a meta-analysis. *Anesth Analg* 1994;79:422–433.
19. Lee TH, Boucher CA. Noninvasive tests in patients with stable coronary artery disease. *N Engl J Med* 2001;344:1840–1845.
20. Gorlin R, Gorlin SG. Hydraulic formula for calculation of the area of the stenotic mitral valve, other cardiac valves, and central circulatory shunts. *Am Heart J* 1951;41:1–29.
21. Warner MA, Offord KP, Warner ME, et al. Role of preoperative cessation of smoking and other factors in postoperative pulmonary complications: a blinded prospective study of coronary artery bypass patients. *Mayo Clin Proc* 1989;64:609–616.
22. Gerstein HC, Mann JFE, Yi Q, et al. Albuminuria and risk of cardiovascular events, death, and heart failure in diabetic and nondiabetic individuals. *JAMA* 2001;286:421–426.
23. Furnary AP, Zerr KJ, Grunkemeier GL, et al. Continuous intravenous insulin infusion reduces the incidence of deep sternal wound infection in diabetic patients after cardiac surgical procedures. *Ann Thorac Surg* 1999;67:352–362.
24. Mangano DT, Layug EL, Wallace A, et al. Effect of atenolol on mortality and cardiovascular morbidity after noncardiac surgery. *N Engl J Med* 1996;335:1713–1720.
25. Raby KE, Brull SJ, Timimi F, et al. The effect of heart rate control on myocardial ischemia among high-risk patients after vascular surgery. *Anesth Analg* 1999;88:477–482.

2. CARDIOVASCULAR DRUGS

Jeffrey R. Balser and John Butterworth

Numerous potent drugs are used to manage hemodynamic derangements before, during, and after cardiovascular and thoracic operations. This chapter reviews the indications, mechanisms, dosing, drug interactions, and common adverse events for these agents.[1] Drug errors repeatedly have been shown to be one of the more common causes of accidental injury to patients, particularly in hospitalized, critically ill patients. Therefore, we suggest that the package insert or *Physicians' Desk Reference* [1] (which contains the package insert information) be consulted before any unfamiliar drug is prescribed or administered [2]. Fortunately, it has never been easier to obtain drug information. Convenient sources of drug information include numerous books and web sites, some of which are provided at the end of this chapter [2–5]. With the increasing capacity and convenience of personal digital assistants, many physicians now maintain an updateable library of drug information in their hand or pocket at all times.

I. **Drug dosage calculations**
  A. **Conversions to milligrams or micrograms per milliliter**
     1. Drugs are administered in milligrams, micrograms, or units. Unfortunately, not all drugs are labeled in a uniform manner. Conversion of units often is necessary.
     2. A drug labeled $z\%$ contains z g/dL; $10 \times z$ equals the number of grams per liter, numerically equivalent to the number of milligrams per milliliter.
        a. Example: Mannitol 25% solution contains 25 g/dL, which equals 250 g/L or 250 mg/mL.
        b. Example: Lidocaine 2% contains 2 g/dL, or 20 g/L, or 20 mg/mL.
     3. Concentrations given as ratios are converted to milligrams or micrograms per milliliter as follows:

        1:1,000 = 1 g/**thousand** mL = 1 **milli**gram/mL

        1:1,000,000 = 1 g/**million** mL = 1 **micro**gram/mL

        a. Example: Epinephrine is packaged for resuscitation in 1:10,000 dilution. Thus, it is one tenth as concentrated as 1:1,000; therefore, 1:10,000 is 0.1 mg/mL (or 100 µg/mL).
        b. Example: A brachial plexus block is to be performed with 0.5% bupivacaine to which epinephrine 1:200,000 must be added. Because the desired concentration is five times greater than 1:1,000,000, 5 µg of epinephrine should be added for each milliliter of bupivacaine.
  B. **Calculating infusion rates using standard drip concentrations (adults)**
     1. Step 1. Dose rate (µg/min): Calculate the desired per minute dose. Example: A 70-kg patient who is to receive dopamine at 5 µg/kg/min needs a 350-µg/min dose rate.
     2. Step 2. Concentration (µg/mL): Calculate how many micrograms of drug are in each milliliter of solution. To calculate concentration (µg/mL), simply multiply the number of milligrams in 250 mL by 4. Example: When nitroglycerin is diluted 100 mg/250 mL, there are $100 \times 4 = 400$ µg/mL. Example: Dopamine, 200 mg, added to 250 mL fluid = 200/250 mg/mL = 800 mg/L = 800 µg/mL concentration.
     3. Step 3. Volume infusion rate (mL/min): Divide the dose rate by the concentration (µg/min ÷ µg/mL = mL/min). The infusion pump should be set for this volume infusion rate. Example: 350 µg/min ÷ 800 µg/mL = 0.44 mL/min. Conversion of volume rate from milliliters per minute to milliliters per hour simply involves multiplying by 60 min/hour (0.44 mL/min × 60 = 26 mL/hour).
     4. Table 2.1 can be consulted as an alternative means for determining vasoactive drug infusion rates for patients of different weights.
     5. Finally, and perhaps most importantly, the wide availability of micropressor-controlled, programmable infusion pumps has virtually eliminated the need for complex calculations at the bedside.

---

[1] We have freely adapted and incorporated sections of the extraordinarily detailed and complete chapter authored by Drs. Larach and Solina from the preceding edition of this textbook.

Table 2.1 Vasoactive drug infusion rates

Drug	Add (to 50 mL)	Dilution (μg/mL)	Starting dose (μg·kg⁻¹·min⁻¹)	Patient weight (kg)														
				5	10	15	20	25	30	40	50	60	70	80	90	100	120	140
Epinephrine or norepinephrine	3 mg	60	0.1	0.5	1.0	1.5	2.0	2.5	3.0	4.0	5.0	6	7	8	9	10	12	14
Dopamine	400 mg	8,000	5	0.2	0.4	0.6	0.8	1	1.2	1.6	1.8	2.2	2.6	3	3.4	3.8	4.6	5.2
Dobutamine	250 mg	5,000	5	0.3	0.6	0.9	1.2	1.5	1.8	2.4	3.0	3.6	4.2	4.8	5.4	6.0	7.2	8.4
Inamrinone[a]	250 mg	5,000	5	0.3	0.6	0.9	1.2	1.5	1.8	2.4	3.0	3.6	4.2	4.8	5.4	6.0	7.2	8.4
Milrinone[a]	50 mg	1,000	0.5	0.2	0.3	0.5	0.6	0.8	0.9	1.2	1.5	1.8	2.1	2.4	2.7	3.0	3.6	4.2
Nitroprusside	50 mg	1,000	0.5	0.2	0.3	0.5	0.6	0.8	0.9	1.2	1.5	1.8	2.1	2.4	2.7	3.0	3.6	4.2
Nitroglycerin	100 mg	2,000	0.5	0.1	0.2	0.3	0.3	0.4	0.5	0.6	0.8	0.9	1.1	1.2	1.4	1.5	1.8	2.1

Values under patient weight heading show the drug infusion rate in milliliters per hour.
[a] Both inamrinone and milrinone are not diluted, except in very small infants.

C. Preparation of drug infusions for pediatric patients
   1. Most pediatric anesthesia departments, critical care units, and pharmacies have specific preferences as to how drugs should be mixed prior to infusion. We strongly recommend that practitioners adhere to the predominant practice in their unit, whether or not they perceive it to be optimal. Unless there is a clear medical advantage to use of another dilution technique, patient safety is maximized when variation is minimized. We mention two of the more common ways in which drugs are diluted for pediatric patients in succeeding sections.
   2. **Technique A: Standard, single drug concentration for all patients.**
      a. **Advantages** are that it is simple (no arithmetic calculations are required) and the fluid volume administered scales upward appropriately with weight.
      b. **Disadvantages** are that the standard dilution for each drug must be remembered, and volume infusion rates may be too excessive in critically ill infants.
   3. **Technique B: Custom drug dilution based on patient weight.** This method permits infusion of a single fluid volume rate to patients of any weight. Our opinion is that this technique seems to maximize the possibility for drug dilution mistakes.
      a. Step 1. Decide on a starting dose per kilogram for the drug. Some standard values are as follows:

Dopamine } Dobutamine	5 µg/kg/min
Nitroprusside	0.5 µg/kg/min
Epinephrine Norepinephrine } Isoproterenol	0.04 µg/kg/min

      b. Step 2. Multiply **starting dose** (in µg/kg/min) by **weight** (in kg) to give starting dose rate in µg/min.
      c. Step 3. Decide on **volume rate** of fluid that should carry this starting dose of drug into the patient:

For most children weighing >5 kg	0.1 mL/min (6 mL/hour)
For babies	0.05 mL/min (3 mL/hour)

      These volumes may be decreased substantially if a continuous carrier infusion is utilized.

      d. Step 4. Divide starting dose rate (step 2) by volume rate (step 3) to give desired **concentration** of drug. Units cancel: (µg/min)/(mL/min) = µg/mL. Example: In a 6.3-kg baby:
         (1) Select standard starting dosages of dopamine and isoproterenol.
         (2) Calculate starting dose rate:
            (a) Dopamine: 5 µg/kg/min × 6 kg = 30 µg/min.
            (b) Isoproterenol: 0.1 µg/kg/min × 6 kg = 0.6 µg/min.
         (3) Choose volume rate: 0.05 mL/min.
         (4) Calculate concentration:
            (a) Dopamine: 30 µg/min ÷ 0.05 mL/min = 600 µg/mL.
            (b) Isoproterenol: 0.6 µg/min ÷ 0.05 mL/min = 12 µg/mL.
         (5) Dilute drugs:
            (a) Dopamine: 600 mg/L (or 150 mg/250 mL).
            (b) Isoproterenol: 12 mg/L (or 3.0 mg/250 mL).
D. Pediatric bolus doses. We find it convenient to prepare syringes of certain drugs (e.g., epinephrine and atropine) so that a standard emergency dose equals a 1-mL volume.
II. Drug–receptor interactions
   A. Receptor activation. Can responses to a given drug dose be predicted? The short answer is: *partially*. The more accurate answer is: *not with complete certainty*.

Many factors determine the magnitude of response produced by a given drug at a given dose.
   1. **Pharmacokinetics** relates the dose to the concentrations that are achieved in plasma or at the effect site. In brief, these concentrations are affected by the drug's volume of distribution and clearance, and, for drugs administered orally, by the fractional absorption [6,7].
   2. **Pharmacodynamics** relate drug concentrations in plasma or at the effect site to the drug effect.
      a. **Concentration of drug at the effect site (receptor)** is influenced by the concentration of drug in plasma and by tissue perfusion; lipid solubility and protein binding; diffusion characteristics, including state of ionization (electrical charge); and local metabolism.
      b. **Number of receptors** per gram of end-organ tissue may vary.
         (1) Up-regulation (increased density of receptors) is seen with a chronic **decrease** in receptor stimulation. Example: Chronic administration of β-adrenergic receptor antagonists increases the number of β-adrenergic receptors.
         (2) **Down-regulation** (decreased density of receptors) is caused by a chronic **increase** in receptor stimulation. Example: Chronic treatment of asthma with β-adrenergic receptor agonists reduces the number of β-adrenergic receptors.
      c. **Drug receptor affinity and efficacy may vary.**
         (1) Receptor binding and activation by an agonist produces a biochemical change in the cell. Example: α-Adrenergic receptor agonists increase protein kinase C concentrations within smooth muscle cells. β-Adrenergic receptor agonists increase intracellular concentrations of cAMP.
         (2) The biochemical change may produce a cellular response. Example: Increased intracellular protein kinase C produces an increase in intracellular [Ca^{2+}], and this results in smooth muscle contraction. Conversely, increased intracellular concentrations of cAMP relax vascular smooth muscle but increase the inotropic state of cardiac muscle.
         (3) **Receptor desensitization** may occur when prolonged agonist exposure to receptor leads to loss of cellular responses with agonist-receptor binding. An example of this is the reduced response to β$_1$-adrenergic receptor agonists that occurs in patients with chronic heart failure, as a result of the increased intracellular concentrations of β-adrenergic receptor kinase, an enzyme that leads to uncoupling of the receptor from its effector enzyme adenylyl cyclase.
         (4) Other factors, including acidosis, hypoxia, and drug interactions, can reduce cellular response to receptor activation.
III. **Vasopressors**
   A. **α-Adrenergic receptor pharmacology (Fig. 2.1)**
      1. **α$_1$-Postsynaptic receptors** mediate peripheral vasoconstriction (arterial plus venous), especially with neurally released norepinephrine (NE). Cardiac α$_1$-receptors increase inotropy while **decreasing** heart rate (HR). (Positive inotropy can only be seen with selective administration in coronary arteries where peripheral effects cannot supervene.)
      2. **α$_2$-receptors** on presynaptic nerve terminals decrease NE release through negative feedback. Activation of **brain α$_2$-receptors** (e.g., with clonidine) produces an antihypertensive action by decreasing sympathetic nervous system activity and causes sedation. **Postsynaptic α$_2$-receptors** mediate constriction of vascular smooth muscle.
      3. **Drug interactions**
         a. **Reserpine interactions.** Reserpine depletes intraneuronal NE and with chronic use induces a "denervation hypersensitivity" state. Indirect-acting sympathomimetic drugs show diminished effect because of depleted stores, whereas direct-acting or mixed-action drugs may produce exaggerated responses because of receptor up-regulation. The best approach is to start

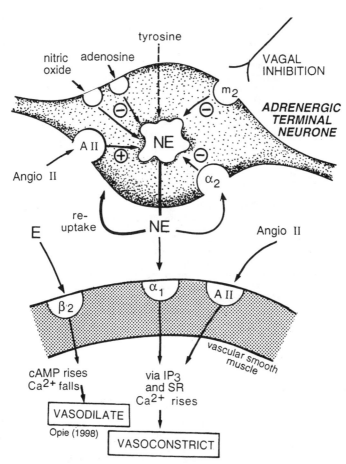

FIG. 2.1 Schematic representation of the adrenergic receptors present on the sympathetic nerve terminal and vascular smooth muscle cell. Norepinephrine (NE) is released by electrical depolarization of the nerve terminal; however, the quantity of NE release is *increased* by neuronal (presynaptic) β_2-receptor or muscarinic-cholinergic stimulation and is *decreased* by activation of presynaptic α_2-receptors. On the *postsynaptic* membrane, stimulation of α_1- or α_2- adrenergic receptors causes vasoconstriction, whereas β_2-receptor activation causes vasodilation. Prazosin is a selective α_1-antagonist drug. Note that NE does not stimulate β_2-receptors, but epinephrine (E) does. (From Opie LH. Control of the circulation. In: *The heart: physiology, from the cell to circulation.* Third Edition. Philadelphia: Lippincott Williams & Wilkins, 1998:17–41, with permission.)

with small dosages of direct-acting drugs while carefully monitoring blood pressure (BP). Fortunately, reserpine is rarely prescribed.

   b. Tricyclic and tetracyclic antidepressant or cocaine interactions. These drugs increase the catecholamine concentration at receptors by blocking the reuptake of catecholamines by prejunctional neurons. Interactions between these drugs and sympathomimetic agents can be very severe and likely represent a greater danger than the widely feared monoamine oxidase (MAO) inhibitor reactions. In general, if sympathomimetic drugs are required, small dosages of direct-acting agents with careful monitoring of BP and electrocardiogram (ECG) are most effective.

4. **Specific agents**
   a. **Selective agonists**
      (1) **Methoxamine (Vasoxyl)**
         (a) **Methoxamine is a synthetic noncatecholamine.**
         (b) **Actions.** The drug is a direct α_1-agonist, devoid of β or α_2 effects, that produces vasoconstriction.
         (c) **Offset.** A longer duration of action than phenylephrine [1.0 to 1.5 hours intramuscularly (IM)] and is not metabolized by either MAO or catechol-O-methyl transferase (COMT).
         (d) **Indications for use**
            (i) Hypotension due to low systemic vascular resistance (SVR) states: regional anesthesia or sepsis.
            (ii) Emergency therapy of hypovolemic hypotension until circulating blood volume is restored.
         (e) **Clinical use**
            (i) Methoxamine dose (adult): 1- to 5-mg intravenous (IV) bolus; 10 to 20 mg IM.
            (ii) The long duration of action of methoxamine makes it difficult to titrate the dosage to rapidly changing hemodynamic conditions. We prefer phenylephrine or NE.
      (2) **Phenylephrine (Neo-Synephrine)** [8]
         (a) **Phenylephrine is a synthetic noncatecholamine.**
         (b) **Actions.** The drug is a selective α_1-agonist devoid of β effects. It causes vasoconstriction, primarily arteriolar and minimally venous.

Phenylephrine

HR	Decreased (reflex, caused by BP elevation)
Contractility	No effect
Cardiac output (CO)	No change or decreased
BP	Increased
SVR	Increased
Preload	Minimal direct

         (c) **Offset** occurs by rapid metabolism by MAO; there is no COMT metabolism.
         (d) **Advantages.** A direct agonist with short duration (less than 5 minutes), it increases perfusion pressure for the brain, kidney, and heart in the presence of low SVR states. When used during hypotension, phenylephrine will increase coronary perfusion pressure without increasing myocardial contractility. If *hyper*tension is avoided, myocardial oxygen consumption (MVO_2) does not rise substantially. If contractility is depressed due to ischemia, drug may produce an increased CO. It is useful for correcting hypotension in patients with coronary artery disease, hypertrophic subaortic stenosis, or valvular aortic stenosis.
         (e) **Disadvantages.** It may decrease stroke volume (SV) secondary to increased afterload; it may increase pulmonary vascular resistance (PVR); it may decrease renal and mesenteric perfusion. Urine output and limb perfusion must be monitored. Reflex bradycardia can occur, but usually it is not severe and it will respond to atropine. In rare patients, phenylephrine may induce coronary artery spasm or spasm of an internal mammary, radial, or gastroepiploic artery bypass graft.
         (f) **Indications for use.**
            (i) Hypotension due to peripheral vasodilation, low SVR states (e.g., septic shock, vasodilator excess).

(ii) For patients with supraventricular tachycardia (SVT), re-flex vagal stimulation in response to increased BP may terminate the arrhythmia; phenylephrine treats both the hypotension and the arrhythmia.

(iii) It can oppose right-to-left shunting during acute cyanotic spells in tetralogy of Fallot.

(iv) Temporary therapy of hypovolemia until blood volume is restored, although a drug with positive inotropic action (e.g., ephedrine) usually is a better choice in patients without coronary disease, and in general, vasoconstrictors should be avoided in hypovolemia.

(g) Administration. IV infusion (central line preferable) or IV bolus.

(h) Clinical use

(i) **Phenylephrine dose**

(a) IV infusion: 0.5 to 10 µg/kg/min.

(b) IV bolus: 1 to 10 µg/kg, increased as needed (some patients with peripheral vascular collapse may require larger bolus injections to raise SVR).

(c) For tetralogy of Fallot spells in children: 5 to 50 µg/kg IV as a bolus dose.

(ii) **Mixing**

(a) IV infusion: Usually mix 15 mg in 250 mL of IV fluid (60 µg/mL).

(b) IV bolus: Dilute to 60 to 100 µg/mL.

(iii) Nitroglycerin may be added to reduce preload while maintaining or increasing arterial BP with phenylephrine. This combination may maximize myocardial oxygen supply while minimizing increases in MVo_2.

(iv) Phenylephrine is the vasopressor of choice for short-term use in most patients with coronary artery disease or aortic stenosis without severe congestive heart failure (CHF).

b. Mixed agonists

(1) Dopamine (Intropin) [8]

See Section **IV:** Positive inotropic drugs.

(2) Ephedrine

(a) Ephedrine is a plant-derived alkaloid with sympatho-mimetic effects.

(b) Actions

(i) Mild direct α, β_1, and β_2-agonist

(ii) Indirect NE release from neurons

Ephedrine

HR	Slightly increased
Contractility	Increased
CO	Increased
BP	Increased
SVR	Slightly increased
Preload	Increased (mobilization of blood from viscera and lower body)

(c) Offset. Five to 10 minutes IV; no metabolism by MAO or COMT; renal elimination

(d) Advantages

(i) Mild, easily administered and titrated pressor and inotrope

(ii) Short duration of action with IV administration (3 to 10 minutes); lasts up to 1 hour with IM administration

(iii) Limited tendency to produce tachycardia

(iv) Does not reduce blood flow to placenta; safe in pregnancy *(v)* Nearly ideal to correct sympathectomy-induced relative hypovolemia and decreased SVR after spinal or epidural anesthesia

    (e) Disadvantages

        (i) Efficacy is blunted effect when NE stores are depleted.

        (ii) There is a high risk of malignant hypertension with MAO inhibitors.

        (iii) Tachyphylaxis with repeated doses.

    (f) Indications

        (i) Hypotension due to low SVR or low CO, especially if HR is low, and particularly with spinal or epidural anesthesia.

        (ii) Temporary therapy of hypovolemia until circulating blood volume is restored, although, as previously noted, in general vasoconstrictors should not substitute for definitive treatment of hypovolemia.

        (iii) Transient myocardial depression (anesthetic overdose).

    (g) Administration. IV, IM, subcutaneous (SC), by mouth (PO)

    (h) Clinical use

        (i) Ephedrine dose: 5- to 10-mg bolus IV, repeated or increased as needed; 25 to 50 mg IM.

        (ii) Ephedrine is conveniently mixed in a syringe (5 to 10 mg/mL) and can be given as an IV bolus into a freely running IV line.

        (iii) Ephedrine is a useful, quick-acting, titratable IV pressor that can be administered via peripheral vein during anesthesia.

(3) Epinephrine (Adrenaline)

See Section **IV:** Positive inotropic drugs.

(4) NE (noradrenaline, Levophed) [8]

    (a) NE is the primary physiologic postganglionic sympathetic neurotransmitter; it also is released by adrenal medulla and central nervous system (CNS) neurons.

    (b) Actions

        (i) Direct α_1 and α_2 actions and β_1-agonist action

        (ii) Limited β_2 effect *in vivo,* despite NE being a more powerful β_2-agonist than dobutamine *in vitro.*

Norepinephrine

HR	Variable; unchanged or may decrease if BP rises (reflex); increases if BP remains low
Contractility	Increased
CO	Increased or decreased (depends on SVR)
BP	Increased
SVR	Markedly increased
PVR	Increased

    (c) Offset is by neural uptake and metabolism by MAO and COMT.

    (d) Advantages

        (i) Direct adrenergic agonist. Equipotent to epinephrine at β_1-receptors.

        (ii) Redistributes blood flow to brain and heart because all other vascular beds are constricted.

        (iii) Elicits intense α_1 and α_2 vasoconstriction; may be effective when phenylephrine (α_1 only) is not.

    (e) Disadvantages

        (i) Reduced organ perfusion: risk of ischemia of kidney, skin, liver, bowel, and extremities.

        (ii) Myocardial ischemia possible; increased afterload, HR, contractility. Coronary spasm may be precipitated.

       (iii) Pulmonary vasoconstriction.

       (iv) Arrhythmias.

       (v) Great risk of skin necrosis with SC extravasation.

(f) Indications for use

       (i) Peripheral vascular collapse when it is necessary to increase SVR [e.g., septic shock or "vasoplegia" after cardiopulmonary bypass (CPB)].

       (ii) Conditions in which a rise in SVR is desired together with cardiac stimulation.

       (iii) Need for increased SVR in which phenylephrine has proved ineffective.

(g) Administration. IV only, by central line only

(h) Clinical use

       (i) Usual NE starting infusion doses: 15 to 30 ng/kg/min IV (adult); usual range, 50 to 300 ng/kg/min.

       (ii) Minimize duration of use; monitor closely for oliguria and metabolic acidosis.

       (iii) NE can be used with vasodilator (nitroprusside or phentolamine) to counteract α stimulation while leaving β_1 stimulation intact; however, if intense vasoconstriction is not required, we recommend that a different drug be used.

       (iv) For treating severe right ventricular (RV) failure, the simultaneous infusion of NE into the *left atrium* (through a left atrial catheter placed intraoperatively) plus inhaled nitric oxide (NO) is useful. The left atrial NE reaches the systemic vascular bed first and is largely metabolized peripherally before it reaches the lung (Table 2.2).

(5) Interactions with monoamine oxidase inhibitors

(a) MAO is an enzyme that inactivates (deaminates) NE, dopamine, and serotonin. The MAO inhibitors treat severe depression by increasing catecholamine concentrations in the brain by inhibiting catecholamine breakdown. Administration of indirect-acting adrenergic agonists or meperidine to patients taking MAO inhibitors can produce a life-threatening hypertensive crisis. Ideally, 2 to 3 weeks should elapse between discontinuing the hydrazine drug phenelzine and elective surgery. Nonhydrazine MAO inhibitors (isocarboxazid, tranylcypromine) require 3 to 10 days for offset of effect. Selegiline at doses 10 mg or less per day has little MAO-A effect and should present fewer adverse drug interactions than other MAO inhibitors.

(b) The greatest risk of inducing a hyperadrenergic state occurs with indirect-acting sympathomimetic drugs (such as ephedrine), because they release the MAO-inhibiting increased intraneuronal stores of NE. Because dopamine releases NE, it should be initiated with caution in the MAO-inhibited patient.

(c) In MAO-inhibited patients, preferred drugs are those with purely direct activity: epinephrine, NE, isoproterenol, phenylephrine, and dobutamine. All pressor drugs should be used cautiously, in small dosages, with BP monitoring and observation of ECG for arrhythmias.

B. Vasopressin pharmacology and agonists [9,10]

  1. Actions

    a. Vasopressin is an endogenous antidiuretic hormone that in high concentrations produces a direct peripheral vasoconstriction through activation of smooth muscle V1 receptors. Vasopressin has no actions on β-adrenergic receptors, so it may have benefit over epinephrine during resuscitation after cardiac arrest. Vasopressin has been administered intraarterially in a selective fashion to control bleeding esophageal varices.

Table 2.2 Acute treatment of pulmonary hypertension and right ventricular failure

Pulmonary hypertension

Hyperventilation	Maintain P_aCO_2 at 25–28 mm Hg
Oxygen	Prevents hypoxic vasoconstriction
Nitric oxide	Inspired, 0.05–80 ppm
Nitroprusside	0.1–4 µg/kg/min
Nitroglycerin	0.1–7 µg/kg/min
Alprostadil	0.05–0.4 µg/kg/min
Epoprostenol	9 ng/kg/min[a]
Tolazoline	Bolus 0.5–2 mg/kg, then 0.5–10 mg/kg/h
Phentolamine	1–20 µg/kg/min
Isoproterenol	0.02–20 µg/kg/min
Diltiazem	Effective orally; no data on intravenous use

Right ventricular failure
(*use therapies listed for pulmonary hypertension to reduce pulmonary artery pressure; in addition, the following may be used:*)

Dobutamine	2–20 µg/kg/min
Dopamine	≤5 µg/kg/min
Epinephrine[b]	0.05–0.2 µg/kg/min
Inamrinone	5–20 µg/kg/min (maintenance)
Milrinone	0.5–0.75 µg/kg/min (maintenance)
Norepinephrine[b]	0.05–0.2 µg/kg/min (maintain coronary perfusion pressure)
Right ventricular assist device	Rest right heart
Pulmonary artery balloon counterpulsation	Unload right heart
Intraaortic balloon counterpulsation	Unload left heart, improve coronary perfusion to left and right heart

[a] Used mainly for chronic management of primary pulmonary hypertension.
[b] May be administered via left atrial line to reduce actions on pulmonary vasculature.

   b. Vasopressin produces relatively more vasoconstriction of skin, skeletal muscle, intestine, and adipose tissue than of coronary or renal beds. Vasopressin causes cerebrovascular dilation.
 2. Advantages
   a. Vasopressin is a very potent agent that acts independently of adrenergic receptors.
   b. Some studies suggest that vasopressin may be effective at maintaining adequate SVR in severe acidosis, sepsis, or after CPB, even when agents such as NE or phenylephrine have proven ineffective.
   c. Vasopressin may restore coronary perfusion pressure after cardiac arrest without also producing tachycardia and arrhythmias, as is common when epinephrine is used successfully for this purpose.
 3. Disadvantages
   a. Vasopressin produces a variety of unpleasant signs and symptoms in awake patients, including pallor of skin, nausea, abdominal cramping, bronchoconstriction, and uterine contractions.
   b. Decreases in splanchnic blood flow may be of concern in patients receiving vasopressin for more than a few hours, particularly when it is coadministered with agents such as α-adrenergic agonists and positive inotropic drugs. Increases in serum concentrations of bilirubin and of "liver" enzymes are common.
   c. Vasopressin may be associated with a decrease in platelet concentration.
   d. Lactic acidosis is common in patients receiving vasopressin infusion (admittedly, these patients are generally critically ill and already receiving other vasoactive agents).

   4. Clinical use
   a. Vasopressin is considered to be an acceptable alternative to epinephrine in treating countershock-refractory ventricular fibrillation (VF) in adults according to the Guidelines for Emergency Cardiac Care of the American Heart Association [10]. The evidence was judged to be insufficient (as of 2001) to support an active recommendation to use vasopressin rather than epinephrine at the present time. Vasopressin may be helpful in patients who remain in cardiac arrest after receiving appropriate doses of epinephrine, but the data supporting this indication remain inadequate. Typical resuscitation doses used were 40 units as an IV bolus.
   b. Vasopressin has been used in a variety of conditions associated with vasodilatory shock, including sepsis and the "vasoplegic" syndrome after CPB. Typical adult doses range from 4 to 6 units/hour. We have found this drug to be effective, but sometimes associated with a troublesome metabolic acidosis that we speculate may be the result of inadequate visceral perfusion.

IV. Positive inotropic drugs
A. Treatment of low CO [8]
   1. Goals. Increase organ perfusion and oxygen delivery to tissues
   a. Increase CO by increasing SV or HR (when appropriate) or both.
   b. Maximize myocardial oxygen supply [increase diastolic arterial pressure, diastolic perfusion time, and blood O_2 content; decrease left ventricular end-diastolic pressure (LVEDP)].
   c. Provide an adequate mean arterial pressure (MAP) for perfusion of other organs.
   d. Minimize myocardial oxygen demand by avoiding tachycardia and LV dilation.
   e. Treatment of metabolic disturbances, arrhythmias, or cardiac ischemia will nearly always be indicated.
   f. Drug treatment of critically ill patients with intrinsic myocardial failure may include:
      (1) β_1-Adrenergic stimulation
      (2) Phosphodiesterase inhibition
      (3) Dopaminergic stimulants
      (4) Calcium sensitizers (increase calcium sensitivity of contractile proteins)
      (5) Calcium salts
      (6) Digitalis
      (7) Liothyronine
   2. Monitoring. Positive inotropic drug dosing is most effectively regulated using data from arterial line, pulmonary artery (PA) catheter with thermodilution CO capability, and/or echocardiography. In addition, mixed venous oxygen saturation monitoring can be extremely valuable. The inotropic drug dosage is titrated to CO and BP, together with assessment of organ perfusion, e.g., urine output and concentration.

B. cAMP-Dependent agents
   1. β-Adrenergic and dopaminergic receptor agonists
   a. Similarities among sympathomimetic drugs
      (1) β_1-Agonist effects are primarily stimulatory.

β_1-Agonists

HR	Increased
Contractility	Increased
Conduction velocity	Increased
Atrioventricular (AV) block	Decreased
Automaticity	Increased
Risk of arrhythmias	Increased

(2) **β_2-Agonists** cause vasodilation and bronchodilation, as well as increasing HR and contractility (albeit with less potency than β_1-agonists).

(3) **Postsynaptic dopaminergic receptors** mediate renal and mesenteric vasodilation, increase renal salt excretion, and reduce gastrointestinal motility. Presynaptic dopaminergic receptors inhibit NE release.

(4) **Diastolic ventricular dysfunction.** Cardiac β-receptor activation enhances diastolic ventricular relaxation by facilitating the active, energy-consuming process that pumps free intracellular Ca^{2+} into storage sites. Abnormal relaxation occurring in ischemia and other myocardial disorders leads to increased diastolic stiffness. By augmenting diastolic relaxation, β-adrenergic receptor agonists reduce LVEDP and heart size [LV end-diastolic volume (LVEDV)], improve diastolic filling, reduce left atrial pressure (LAP), and improve the myocardial oxygen supply/demand ratio.

(5) **Systolic ventricular dysfunction.** More complete ventricular ejection during systole will reduce the LV end-systolic volume. This reduces heart size, LV systolic wall tension (by LaPlace law), and MVo_2.

(6) **Myocardial ischemia.** The net effects of β-receptor stimulation on myocardial O_2 supply and demand are multifactorial and may be difficult to predict. MVo_2 tends to increase as HR and contractility rise, but MVo_2 is reduced by lowering LVEDV. β-Agonists improve O_2 supply when LVEDP is decreased, but can worsen the supply/demand ratio particularly if HR rises or diastolic BP is lowered.

(7) **Hypovolemia** should be treated aggressively; however, volume overload may lead to myocardial ischemia by restricting subendocardial perfusion. Treatment may include positive inotropes, nitroglycerin, and diuretics.

(8) **There is a risk of tissue damage or sloughing when vasoconstrictor drugs are extravasated outside of a vein.** In general, catecholamine vasoconstrictors should not be infused for long periods of time through a peripheral IV line because of the risk of extravasation or infiltration. These drugs may be given through peripheral IV lines provided that:

    (a) No central venous catheter is available.

    (b) The drug is injected only into a free-flowing IV line.

    (c) The IV site is observed closely during and after the injection.

b. **Dobutamine (Dobutrex)** [8]

(1) **Dobutamine is a synthetic catecholamine distributed as a racemic mixture.**

(2) **Actions**

    (a) Direct β_1-agonist, with limited β_2 and α_1 effects. Dobutamine has no α_2 or dopaminergic activity.

    (b) On the heart, dobutamine increases inotropy via both β_1 and perhaps α_1 activities, but HR is increased only by the β_1 effect.

    (c) On blood vessels, dobutamine is predominantly a vasodilator drug. Mechanisms for vasodilation include:

        (i) β_2-Mediated vasodilation that is only partially counteracted by (−) dobutamine's α_1 constrictor effects

        (ii) The (+) dobutamine enantiomer and its metabolite, (+)-3-O-methyldobutamine, are α_1 *antagonists*. Thus, as dobutamine is metabolized, any α_1-agonist actions of the drug could diminish over time.

Dobutamine

HR	Increased
Contractility	Increased
CO	Increased
BP	Usually increases, may remain unchanged
LVEDP	Decreased
LAP	Decreased
SVR	Decreased by dilating all vascular beds; slight increase may be seen at low dosages (α) or in β-blocked patients
PVR	Decreased

(3) **Offset.** Offset of action is achieved by redistributing metabolism by COMT, and by conjugation with glucuronide in liver; an active metabolite is generated. Plasma half-life is 2 minutes.

(4) **Advantages**

   (a) At low doses there is generally less tachycardia than with equivalent doses of isoproterenol or dopamine.

   (b) Afterload reduction (SVR and PVR) may improve LV and RV systolic function, which can benefit the heart with single or dual ventricular failure.

   (c) Renal blood flow may increase (due to a β₂ effect), but not as much as with comparable (but low) doses of dopamine.

(5) **Disadvantages**

   (a) Tachycardia and arrhythmias are dose related and can be severe.

   (b) Hypotension may occur if the reduction in SVR is not fully offset by an increase in CO; dobutamine is an inotrope but is not a pressor.

   (c) Coronary steal similar to that occurring with isoproterenol is possible, leading to ischemia.

   (d) The drug is a nonselective vasodilator: Blood flow may be shunted from kidney and splanchnic bed to skeletal muscle.

   (e) Tachyphylaxis has been reported when infused for more 72 hours.

   (f) Mild hypokalemia may occur.

   (g) As a partial agonist, dobutamine can inhibit actions of full agonists (e.g., epinephrine) under certain circumstances.

(6) **Indications.** Low CO states (cardiogenic shock), especially with increased SVR or PVR.

(7) **Administration.** IV only (central line is preferable, but dobutamine has little vasoconstrictor activity, minimizing risk of extravasation).

(8) **Clinical use**

   (a) Dobutamine dose: IV infusion, 2 to 20 µg/kg/min. Some patients may respond to initial doses as low as 0.5 µg/kg/min and, at such low doses, HR usually does not rise.

   (b) Dobutamine increases CO with a lesser increment in MVo_2 and higher coronary blood flow compared with dopamine as a single drug. However, addition of nitroglycerin to dopamine may be equally effective.

   (c) Dobutamine acts similar to a fixed-ratio combination of an inotropic drug and a vasodilator drug. These two components cannot be titrated separately.

   (d) In patients undergoing coronary surgery, dobutamine produces more tachycardia than epinephrine when administered to produce the same increase in SV [11].

   (e) When dobutamine is given to β-blocked patients, SVR may increase. Invasive hemodynamic monitoring is required to ascertain the drug's effect on CO and SVR.

c. Dopamine (Intropin) [8]

(1) **Dopamine is a catecholamine precursor to NE and epineph-rine in nerve terminals and the adrenal medulla.**

(2) **Actions**

(a) Direct action: α_1, β_1, β_2, and dopaminergic (DA_1) agonist

(b) Indirect action: Induces release of stored neuronal NE.

(c) The dose versus response relationship often is given as follows; however, the relationship between dose and concentration and between dose and response is highly variable from patient to patient.

Dopamine

Dose (µg/kg/min)	Receptor activated	Effect
1–3	Dopaminergic (DA_1)	Increased renal and mesenteric blood flow
3–10	$\beta_1 + \beta_2$ (plus DA_1)	Increased HR, contractility, and CO; decreased SVR; PVR may rise from early α vasoconstriction
>10	α (plus β plus DA_1)	Increased SVR, PVR; decreased renal blood flow; increased HR, arrhythmias. Increased afterload may decrease CO

(3) **Offset** is achieved by uptake by nerve terminals plus metabolism by MAO and COMT. Small quantities of dopamine can be metabolized to NE in nerve terminals.

(4) **Advantages**

(a) Increased renal perfusion and urine output at low-to-moderate dosages (partially due to a specific DA_1-agonist effect).

(b) Blood flow shifts from skeletal muscle to kidney and splanchnic beds.

(c) BP response is easy to titrate because of its mixed inotropic and vasoconstrictor properties.

(5) **Disadvantages**

(a) There is a significant indirect-acting component; response can diminish when neuronal NE is depleted (e.g., in patients with chronic CHF or during reserpine treatment).

(b) Sinus, atrial, or ventricular tachycardia and arrhythmias may occur.

(c) Less maximal inotropic effect than epinephrine.

(d) Skin necrosis may result from extravasation.

(e) Renal vasodilating effects are overridden by α-mediated vaso-constriction at dosages >10 µg/kg/min with risk of renal, splanch-nic, and skin necrosis. Monitor urine output.

(f) Pulmonary vasoconstriction is possible.

(g) MVO_2 increases, and myocardial ischemia may occur if coronary flow does not increase commensurately.

(h) Increased BP at increased doses may be detrimental to a failing heart, indicating need for adding a vasodilator.

(6) **Indications**

(a) Hypotension due to low CO or low SVR (although other agents are superior for the latter indication).

(b) Temporary therapy of hypovolemia until circulating blood vol-ume is restored (but dopamine should not substitute or delay primary treatment of hypovolemia).

(c) Renal failure or insufficiency (widely used for this purpose, but limited evidence basis).

(7) Administration. IV only (preferably by central line)

(8) Clinical use

    (a) Dopamine dose: 1 to 20 µg/kg/min IV.

    (b) Often mix 200 mg in 250 mL of IV solution (800 µg/mL).

    (c) Good first choice for temporary treatment of hypotension until intravascular volume can be expanded or until a specific diagnosis can be made.

    (d) Correct hypovolemia if possible before use (as with all pressors).

    (e) Switch to a direct-acting agonist such as epinephrine or switch to or add milrinone if inotropic response is not adequate at dopamine doses of 5 to 10 µg/kg/min.

    (f) Consider adding a vasodilator (e.g., nitroprusside) when BP is adequate and afterload reduction would be beneficial.

d. Dopexamine [8]

(1) Actions

    (a) Dopexamine is a synthetic analogue of dobutamine with vasodilator action. Its cardiac inotropic and chronotropic activity is caused by direct β_2-agonist effects and by NE actions (due to baroreceptor reflex activation and neuronal uptake-1 inhibition) that *indirectly* activate β_1-receptors. In CHF, there is selective β_1 down-regulation, with relative preservation of β_2-receptor number and coupling. The latter assume greater than normal physiologic importance, making dopexamine of theoretically greater utility than agents with primary β_1-receptor activity.

    (b) Receptor activity

        α_1 and α_2: minimal

        β_1: little *direct* effect; β_2: direct agonist

        DA_1: potent agonist (increases renal blood flow)

    (c) Inhibits neuronal catecholamine uptake-1, increasing NE actions

    (d) Hemodynamic actions

Dopexamine

HR	Increased
CO	Increased
SVR	Decreased
MAP	Little change or decrease
Preload	No change or slight decrease
PA pressure	No change or slight decrease

(2) Offset. Half-life: 6 to 11 minutes. Clearance is by uptake into tissues (catecholamine uptake mechanisms) and by hepatic metabolism.

(3) Advantages

    (a) Lack of vasoconstrictor activity avoids α-mediated complications.

    (b) Decreased renovascular resistance might *theoretically* help preserve renal function after ischemic insults.

(4) Disadvantages

    (a) Less effective than other agents.

    (b) Dose-dependent tachycardia may limit therapy.

    (c) Tachyphylaxis.

    (d) Not approved by the U.S. Food and Drug Administration for release in the United States.

(5) Indications. Treatment of low CO states

(6) Administration. IV

(7) Clinical use

    (a) Dopexamine dose: 0.5 to 4.0 µg/kg/min IV (maximum 6 µg/kg/min).

(b) Therapeutic effects similar to the combination of variables doses of dobutamine with dopamine 1 to 2 µg/kg/min (renal dose) or fenoldopam 0.05 µg/kg/min.

e. **Epinephrine (Adrenaline)** [8]

(1) **Epinephrine is a catecholamine produced by the adrenal medulla.**

(2) **Actions**

(a) Direct agonist at α_1, α_2, β_1, and β_2-receptors

(b) Dose response (adult, approximate)

Epinephrine

Dose (ng/kg/min)	Receptors activated	SVR
10–30	β	May decrease
30–150	β and α	No change or increase
>150	α and β	Increased

(c) Increased contractility and HR with all dosages, but SVR may decrease, remain unchanged, or increase dramatically depending on the dosage. CO usually rises but, at high dosages, α-receptor–mediated vasoconstriction may cause a lowered SV due to high afterload.

(3) **Offset** occurs by uptake by neurons and tissue and by metabolism by MAO and COMT (rapid).

(4) **Advantages**

(a) This drug is direct acting; its effects are not dependent on release of endogenous NE.

(b) Potent α and β stimulation result in greater maximal effects and equivalent increases in SV; less tachycardia after heart surgery than dopamine or dobutamine.

(c) It is a powerful inotrope with variable (and adjustable) α effect. Lusitropic effect (β_1) enhances the rate of ventricular relaxation.

(d) If BP rises, tachycardia may be diminished due to reflex vagal stimulation.

(e) It is an effective bronchodilator and mast cell stabilizer, useful for primary therapy of severe bronchospasm, anaphylaxis, or anaphylactic reactions.

(f) If diastolic BP rises and heart size decreases, myocardial ischemia may be reduced. However, as with any inotropic drug, epinephrine may induce or worsen myocardial ischemia.

(5) **Disadvantages**

(a) Tachycardia and arrhythmias.

(b) Organ ischemia, especially kidney, secondary to vasoconstriction, may result. Urine output must be closely monitored.

(c) Pulmonary vasoconstriction may occur, which can produce pulmonary hypertension and possibly RV failure; addition of a vasodilator may reverse this.

(d) There is a risk of myocardial ischemia. Positive inotropy and tachycardia increase myocardial oxygen demand and reduce oxygen supply.

(e) Extravasation from a peripheral IV cannula can cause necrosis; thus, a central line is preferable.

(f) As with most adrenergic agonists, elevation of plasma glucose and lactate occurs. This may be accentuated in diabetics.

(g) Initial increases in plasma K^+ occur due to hepatic release, followed by decreased K^+ due to skeletal muscle uptake.

(6) Indications
   (a) Cardiac arrest (especially asystole or VF); electromechanical dissociation. Epinephrine's efficacy is believed to result from increased coronary perfusion pressure during cardiopulmonary resuscitation. Recently, the use of high-dose (0.2 mg/kg) epinephrine has been debated, but there is no demonstrable outcome benefit to conventional resuscitation doses.
   (b) Anaphylaxis and other systemic allergic reactions; epinephrine is the agent of choice.
   (c) Cardiogenic shock, especially if a vasodilator is added.
   (d) Bronchospasm.
   (e) Reduced CO after CPB.
   (f) Hypotension with spinal or epidural anesthesia can be treated with low-dose (1 to 4 µg/min) epinephrine infusions as conveniently and effectively as with ephedrine boluses [12].
(7) Administration. IV (by central line); via endotracheal tube (rapidly absorbed by tracheal mucosa); SC
(8) Clinical use
   (a) Epinephrine dose
      (i) SC: 10 µg/kg (maximum of 400 µg or 0.4 mL 1:1,000) for treatment of mild-to-moderate allergic reactions or bronchospasm.
      (ii) IV: Low-to-moderate dose (for shock, hypotension): 0.03 to 0.2 µg/kg bolus (IV), then infusion at 0.01 to 0.30 µg/kg/min.
         Resuscitation dose (for cardiac arrest): 0.5- to 1.0-mg IV bolus; pediatric, 5 to 15 µg/kg (may be given intratracheally in 1- to 10-mL volume). Larger doses are used when response to initial dose is inadequate.
         Resuscitation doses of epinephrine may produce extreme hypertension with stroke or myocardial infarctions. A starting dose of epinephrine exceeding 150 ng/kg (10 µg in an adult) IV bolus should be given only to a patient in extremis!
   (b) Watch for signs of excessive vasoconstriction. Monitor SVR, urine output, and extremity perfusion.
   (c) Addition of a vasodilator (e.g., nitroprusside or phentolamine) to epinephrine can counteract the α vasoconstriction, leaving positive cardiac inotropic effects undiminished. Alternatively, addition of milrinone or inamrinone may permit lower doses of epinephrine to be used. We find combinations of epinephrine and milrinone particularly useful in cardiac surgical patients.
f. Norepinephrine (noradrenaline, Levophed)
   See Section **III:** Vasopressors.
g. Isoproterenol (Isuprel)
   (1) Isoproterenol is a synthetic catecholamine.
   (2) Actions
      (a) Direct β_1- plus β_2-agonist
      (b) No α effects

Isoproterenol

HR	Increased
Contractility	Increased
CO	Increased
BP	Variable
SVR	Markedly decreased; all vascular beds dilated; dose related
PVR	Decreased

   (3) Offset. Rapid (half-life, 2 minutes); uptake by liver, conjugat d, 60% excreted unchanged; metabolized by MAO, COMT.

(4) Advantages
   (a) Isoproterenol is a potent direct β-receptor agonist.
   (b) It increases CO by three mechanisms:
      (i) Increased HR
      (ii) Increased contractility → increased SV.
      (iii) Reduced afterload (SVR) → increased SV.
   (c) It is a bronchodilator (IV or inhaled).
(5) Disadvantages
   (a) It is not a pressor! BP often falls (β_2 effect) while CO rises.
   (b) Hypotension may produce organ hypoperfusion, hypotension, and ischemia.
   (c) Tachycardia limits diastolic filling time.
   (d) Proarrhythmic.
   (e) Dilates all vascular beds and is capable of shunting blood away from critical organs toward muscle and skin.
   (f) Coronary vasodilation can reduce blood flow to ischemic myocardium while increasing flow to nonischemic areas producing coronary "steal."
   (g) May unmask preexcitation in patients with an accessory AV conduction pathway [e.g., Wolff–Parkinson–White (WPW) syndrome].
(6) Indications
   (a) Bradycardia unresponsive to atropine, when electrical pacing is not available.
   (b) Low CO, especially for situations in which increased inotropy is needed and tachycardia is not detrimental, such as:
      (i) Pediatric patients with fixed SV.
      (ii) After resection of ventricular aneurysm (small fixed SV).
      (iii) Denervated heart (after cardiac transplantation).
   (c) Pulmonary hypertension or right heart failure.
   (d) AV block: Use as temporary therapy to decrease block or increase rate of idioventricular foci. Use with caution in second-degree Mobitz type II heart block because block may increase in degree.
   (e) Status asthmaticus: Intravenous use mandates continuous ECG and BP monitoring.
   (f) β-Blocker overdose.
   (g) Isoproterenol should not be utilized for therapy of cardiac asystole. Cardiopulmonary resuscitation (CPR) with epinephrine or pacing is the therapy of choice because isoproterenol-induced vasodilation results in reduced carotid and coronary blood flow during CPR.
(7) Administration. IV (safe through peripheral line, will not necrose skin); PO
(8) Clinical use and isoproterenol dose. IV infusion is 20 to 500 ng/kg/min.
2. Phosphodiesterase inhibitors
   a. Inamrinone (Inocor) [8]
      (1) Inamrinone is a bipyridine derivative that inhibits the cGMP-inhibited cAMP-specific phosphodiesterase (PDE III), increasing cAMP concentrations in cardiac muscle (positive inotropy) and in vascular smooth muscle (vasodilation).

Inamrinone

HR	Generally little change (tachycardia at high doses)
MAP	Variable (frequently the decrease in SVR is offset by the increase in CO)
CO	Increased
LAP	Decreased

Inamrinone (*continued*)

SVR	Decreased
PVR	Decreased
MVo$_2$	Generally little change or decrease (increase in CO is offset by the decrease in wall tension)

    (2) Offset
        (a) The elimination half-life is 2.5 to 4 hours but is 6 hours with CHF.
        (b) Offset occurs by hepatic conjugation, with 30% to 35% excreted, unchanged, in the urine.
    (3) Advantages
        (a) As a vasodilating inotrope, inamrinone increases CO by augmenting contractility *and* decreasing cardiac afterload.
        (b) As a single agent, inamrinone has favorable effects on MVo$_2$ (little increase in HR; decreases afterload, LVEDP, and wall tension).
        (c) It does not depend on activation of β-receptors and therefore retains effectiveness despite β-receptor down-regulation or uncoupling (e.g., chronic CHF) and in the presence of β-blockade.
        (d) Low risk of tachycardia or arrhythmias.
        (e) Inamrinone acts synergistically with β-adrenergic receptor agonists and dopaminergic receptor agonists.
        (f) Pulmonary vasodilator.
        (g) Positive lusitropic properties (ventricular relaxation) at even very low dosages.
    (4) Disadvantages
        (a) Thrombocytopenia after chronic (more than 24 hours) administration.
        (b) Will nearly always cause hypotension from vasodilation if given by rapid bolus administration. Hypotension is easily treated with intravenous fluid and α-agonists.
        (c) Increased dosages may result in tachycardia (and therefore increased MVo$_2$)
    (5) Indications
        (a) Low CO syndrome, especially in the setting of increased LVEDP, pulmonary hypertension, and RV failure.
        (b) To supplement/potentiate β-adrenergic receptor agonists.
        (c) As a bridge to cardiac transplantation.
    (6) Administration. IV infusion only. Do not mix in dextrose-containing solutions.
    (7) Clinical use
        (a) Inamrinone loading dose is 0.75 to 1.5 mg/kg. When given during or after CPB, usual dosage is 1.5 mg/kg.
        (b) IV infusion dose range is 5 to 20 μg/kg/min (usual dosage is 10 μg/kg/min).
        (c) In patients who are anticipated to need intensive positive inotropic drug support, it is convenient to administer a bolus dose while they are still on CPB, when vasodilation is easier, to counteract with increased pump flow.
  b. Milrinone (Primacor) [8]
    (1) Actions
        (a) Milrinone, like inamrinone, has powerful cardiac inotropic and vasodilator properties. Milrinone increases intracellular concentrations of cAMP by inhibiting its breakdown. Milrinone inhibits the cyclic GMP-inhibited, cAMP-specific phosphodiesterase (type III) in cardiac and vascular smooth muscle cells. In cardiac myocytes, increased cAMP causes positive inotropy, lusitropy (enhanced diastolic myocardial relaxation), chronotropy, and dromotropy

(AV conduction), as well as increased automaticity. In vascular smooth muscle cells, increased cAMP causes vasodilation.

(b) Hemodynamic actions

Milrinone

HR	Usually no change; may have slight increase at increased doses
CO	Increased
BP	Variable
SVR and PVR	Decreased
Preload	Decreased
MVo$_2$	Often unchanged

(2) **Onset and offset.** When administered as an IV bolus, milrinone rapidly achieves its maximal effect. The elimination half-life of milrinone is considerably shorter than that of inamrinone.

(3) **Advantages**

(a) Used as a single agent, milrinone has favorable effects on the myocardial oxygen supply/demand balance, due to reduction of preload and afterload, and lack of marked tachycardia.

(b) Milrinone does not act via β-adrenoceptors, and it retains efficacy when β-adrenergic receptor coupling is compromised, as in chronic CHF.

(c) It induces no tachyphylaxis.

(d) Milrinone has a reduced proarrhythmic effect compared to β-adrenergic receptor agonists.

(e) When compared to dobutamine at equipotent doses, milrinone is associated with a greater decrease in PVR, greater augmentation of RV ejection fraction, less tachycardia, fewer arrhythmias, and lower MVo$_2$.

(f) This drug may act synergistically with drugs that stimulate cAMP production, such as β-adrenergic receptor agonists.

(g) With chronic use, milrinone, unlike inamrinone, does not cause thrombocytopenia.

(4) **Disadvantages**

(a) Vasodilation and hypotension are predictable with rapid IV bolus doses.

(b) As with other positive inotropic drugs, including epinephrine and dobutamine, independent manipulation of cardiac inotropy and SVR cannot be achieved using only milrinone.

(c) Arrhythmias may occur.

(5) **Clinical use**

(a) Milrinone loading dose: 25 to 75 μg/kg (usual dose is 50) given over 1 to 10 minutes. Often it is desirable to administer the loading dose before separating the patient from CPB so that hypotension can be managed more easily [13].

(b) Maintenance infusion: 0.375 to 0.75 μg/kg/min. Dosage must be reduced in cases of renal failure.

(c) Oral preparation available for chronic use.

3. **Glucagon.**

a. **Glucagon is a peptide hormone produced by the pancreas.**

b. **Actions.** Glucagon increases intracellular cAMP, acting via a specific receptor.

Glucagon

Contractility	Increased
AV conduction	Increased
HR	Increased
CO	Increased, with a variable effect on SVR

    c. Offset of action of glucagon occurs by redistribution and proteolysis by the liver, kidney, and plasma. Duration of action is 20 to 30 minutes.

    d. Advantages. Glucagon has a positive inotropic effect even in the presence of β-blockade.

    e. Disadvantages
- **(1)** Consistently produces nausea and vomiting
- **(2)** Tachycardia
- **(3)** Hyperglycemia and hypokalemia
- **(4)** Catecholamine release from pheochromocytomas
- **(5)** Anaphylaxis (possible)

    f. Indications for the use of glucagon include:
- **(1)** Hypoglycemia (especially if no IV access) from insulin overdosage
- **(2)** Spasm of sphincter of Oddi
- **(3)** β-Blocker toxicity
- **(4)** Refractory CHF

    g. Administration. IV, IM, SC

    h. Clinical use
- **(1)** Glucagon dose: 1 to 5 mg IV slowly; 0.5 to 2.0 mg IM or SC
- **(2)** Infusion: 25 to 75 µg/min
- **(3)** Rarely used (other than for hypoglycemia) due to gastrointestinal side effects and severe tachycardia

C. cAMP-Independent agents

    1. Calcium [8]

        a. Calcium is physiologically active only as the free calcium ion (Ca_i).
- **(1)** Normally, approximately 50% of the total plasma calcium is bound to proteins and anions and the rest remains as free calcium ions.
- **(2)** Factors affecting ionized calcium concentration
  - **(a)** Alkalosis (metabolic or respiratory) decreases Ca_i.
  - **(b)** Acidosis increases Ca_i.
  - **(c)** Citrate binds (chelates) Ca_i until citrate is metabolized.
  - **(d)** Albumin binds Ca_i.
- **(3)** Normal plasma concentration: $[Ca_i] = 1.0$ to 1.3 mmol/L

        b. Actions of calcium salts

Calcium

HR	No change or decrease (vagal effect)
Contractility	Increase (especially during hypocalcemia)
BP	Increase
SVR	Increase (may decrease if hypocalcemia present)
Preload	Little change
CO	Variable

        c. Offset. Calcium is incorporated into muscle and bone and binds to protein, free fatty acids, heparin, and citrate.

        d. Advantages
- **(1)** Calcium increases cardiac inotropy *in vitro* without increasing HR; however, there is minimal evidence that it produces a measurable sustained increase in CO in patients.
- **(2)** It has rapid action with a duration of approximately 10 to 15 minutes (7-mg/kg dose).
- **(3)** It reverses hypotension caused by the following conditions:
  - **(a)** Halogenated anesthetic overdosage
  - **(b)** Calcium-channel blockers (CCBs)
  - **(c)** Hypocalcemia
  - **(d)** CPB, especially with dilutional or citrate-induced hypocalcemia, or when cardioplegia-induced hyperkalemia remains present

(administer calcium salts only after heart has been well reperfused to avoid augmenting reperfusion injury)

      (e) β-Blockers (watch for bradycardia!)

    (4) It reverses cardiac toxicity from hyperkalemia (e.g., arrhythmias, heart block, and negative inotropy).

e. Disadvantages

    (1) Calcium can provoke digitalis toxicity in patients who are therapeutically digitalized. This toxicity can present as ventricular arrhythmias, AV block, or asystole.

    (2) Calcium potentiates the effects of hypokalemia on the heart (arrhythmias).

    (3) Severe bradycardia or heart block occurs rarely.

    (4) When extracellular calcium concentration is increased while the surrounding myocardium is being reperfused or is undergoing ongoing ischemia, increased cellular damage or cell death occurs.

    (5) Post-CPB coronary spasm may occur rarely.

    (6) Associated with pancreatitis when given in large doses to patient recovering from CPB.

    (7) Calcium may inhibit sympathomimetic amines, such as epinephrine and dobutamine [14].

f. Indications for use

    (1) Hypocalcemia

    (2) Hyperkalemia (to reverse AV block or myocardial depression)

    (3) Intraoperative hypotension due to decreased myocardial contractility from hypocalcemia, calcium channel blockers, or protamine

    (4) Anesthetic overdose

    (5) Counteract effects of hypermagnesemia.

g. Administration

    (1) Calcium chloride: IV, preferably by central line (causes peripheral vein inflammation and sclerosis)

    (2) Calcium gluconate: IV, preferably by central line

h. Clinical use

    (1) Calcium dose

        (a) 10% calcium chloride 10 mL (contains 272 mg of elemental calcium or 13.6 mEq): adult, 200 to 1,000 mg slow IV; pediatric, 10 to 20 mg/kg slow IV

        (b) 10% calcium gluconate 10 mL (contains 93 mg of elemental calcium or 4.6 mEq): adult, 600 to 3,000 mg slow IV; pediatric, 30 to 100 mg/kg slow IV

    (2) During massive blood transfusion (more than one blood volume replaced), a patient receives a large load of citrate, which binds calcium. In normal situations, hepatic metabolism quickly eliminates citrate from plasma, and hypocalcemia does not occur. However, hypothermia and shock may decrease citrate clearance with resultant severe hypocalcemia.

    (3) Ionized calcium levels should be measured frequently to guide calcium salt therapy.

    (4) Calcium formerly was used to treat asystole, despite no evidence that calcium has any beneficial effect on asystole. It is not recommended for treating asystole or electromechanical dissociation unless hypocalcemia, hyperkalemia, or hypermagnesemia is present.

    (5) Calcium should be used with care in situations of ongoing myocardial ischemia or during reperfusion of ischemic tissue. "Routine" administration of large doses of calcium to all adult patients at the end of CPB is unnecessary and may be deleterious if the heart has been reperfused only minutes earlier.

    (6) Hypocalcemia is frequent in children emerging from CPB.

2. Digoxin (Lanoxin)
  a. Digoxin is one of many glycosides derived from the foxglove plant.
  b. Actions
      (1) Mechanism of action: Digoxin inhibits the integral membrane protein Na,K-ATPase, causing Na^+ accumulation in cells, leading to increased intracellular Ca_i, which leads to increased Ca^{2+} release from the sarcoplasmic reticulum into the cytoplasm with each heartbeat, ultimately causing increased myocardial contractility.
      (2) Hemodynamic effects
          (a) Digoxin

Contractility	Increased
AV conduction	Decreased
Ventricular automaticity	Increased rate of phase 4 depolarization
Refractory period	Decreased (in atria and ventricles); increased in AV node

          (b) Hemodynamics in CHF

Digoxin	
HR	Decreased
SV	Increased
SVR	Decreased
MVO_2	Decreased

  c. Offset. Digoxin elimination half-life is 1.7 days (renal elimination). In anephric patients, half-life is more than 4 days.
  d. Advantages
      (1) Supraventricular antiarrhythmic action
      (2) Reduced ventricular rate in atrial fibrillation or flutter
      (3) An orally active positive inotrope that is not associated with increased mortality in CHF
  e. Disadvantages
      (1) Digoxin has an extremely low therapeutic index; 20% of patients show toxicity at some time.
      (2) Increased MVO_2 and SVR occur in patients without CHF (angina may be precipitated).
      (3) The drug has a long half-life, and it is difficult to titrate dosage.
      (4) There is large interindividual variation in therapeutic and toxic serum levels and dosages. The dose response is nonlinear; near-toxic levels may be needed to achieve a change in AV conduction.
      (5) Toxic manifestations may be life threatening and difficult to diagnose. Digoxin can produce virtually any arrhythmia. For example, digitalis is useful in treating SVT, but digitalis toxicity can trigger SVT.
      (6) Digoxin may be contraindicated in patients with accessory pathway SVT (see digoxin use for SVT in Section **VIII.E**).
  f. Indications for use
      (1) Supraventricular tachyarrhythmias (see Section **VIII.E**)
      (2) Chronic ventricular contractile dysfunction
  g. Administration. IV, PO, IM
  h. Clinical use (general guidelines only)
      (1) Digoxin dose (assuming normal renal function; decrease maintenance dosages with renal insufficiency)
          (a) Adult: loading dose IV and IM, 0.25- to 0.50-mg increments (total 1.00 to 1.25 mg or 10 to 15 µg/kg); maintenance dose, 0.125 to 0.250 mg/day based on clinical effect and drug levels
          (b) Pediatric digoxin (IV administration)

Age	Total digitalizing dose (DD) (μg/kg)	Daily maintenance dose (divided doses, normal renal function)
Neonates	15–30	20%–35% of DD
2 mo–2 yr	30–50	25%–35% of DD
2–10 yr	15–35	25%–35% of DD
>10 yr	8–12	25%–35% of DD

(2) Digoxin has a gradual onset of action over 15 to 30 minutes or more; peak effect occurs 1 to 5 hours after IV administration.

(3) Use with caution in presence of β-blockers, calcium channel blockers, or calcium.

(4) Always consider the possibility of toxic side effects.

   (a) Signs of toxicity include arrhythmias, especially with features of both increased automaticity and conduction block (e.g., junctional tachycardia with 2:1 AV block). Premature atrial or ventricular depolarizations, AV block, accelerated junctional tachycardia, ventricular tachycardia (VT) or VF (may be unresponsive to countershock), or gastrointestinal or neurologic toxicity may be apparent.

(5) Factors potentiating toxicity

   (a) Hypokalemia, hypomagnesemia, hypercalcemia, alkalosis, acidosis, renal insufficiency, quinidine therapy, and hypothyroidism may potentiate toxicity.

   (b) Beware of calcium salt administration to digitalized patients! Malignant ventricular arrhythmias (including VF) may occur, even if the patient has received no digoxin for more than 24 hours. Follow ionized calcium levels to permit use of smallest possible doses of calcium. Monitor carefully. Fortunately, bolus dosing of calcium salts is rarely indicated.

(6) Therapy for digitalis toxicity

   (a) Increase serum [K+] to upper limits of normal (unless AV block is present).

   (b) Treat ventricular arrhythmias with phenytoin or lidocaine or amiodarone.

   (c) Treat atrial arrhythmias with phenytoin or amiodarone.

   (d) β-Blockers are effective for digoxin-induced arrhythmias, but ventricular pacing may be required if AV block develops.

   (e) Beware of cardioversion. VF refractory to countershock may be induced. Use low-energy synchronized cardioversion and slowly increase energy as needed.

(7) Serum digoxin levels

   (a) Therapeutic: approximately 0.5 to 2.5 ng/mL. Values of less than 0.5 ng/mL rule out toxicity. Values exceeding 3.0 ng/mL are definitely toxic.

   (b) Increased serum concentrations may not produce clinical toxicity in children or hyperkalemic patients, or when digitalis is used as an atrial antiarrhythmic agent.

   (c) Reduced serum concentrations may produce clinical toxicity in patients with hypokalemia, hypomagnesemia, hypercalcemia, myocardial ischemia, or hypothyroidism, or those recovering from CPB.

(8) Because of its long duration of action, long latency of onset, and increased risk of toxicity, digoxin is not used to treat acute heart failure.

3. **Triiodothyronine (T₃, liothyronine IV)** [8]. T_3 is the active form of thyroid hormone. It has multiple cellular actions on the nucleus and on mitochondria, affecting gene transcription and oxidative phosphorylation. There is evidence that CPB induces a state of low plasma thyrotropin (T_3), termed the "euthyroid

sick" syndrome. Laboratory studies demonstrate T_3 stimulates cardiac inotropy and lusitropy even in the face of overwhelming β-adrenergic receptor blockade and without increasing intracellular concentrations of cAMP. Some reports suggest that exogenous replacement may facilitate the separation from CPB of patients who could not be weaned using conventional therapies. Other clinical trials have failed to identify efficacy of T_3. Doses that have been suggested include a bolus of 0.4 µg/kg IV followed by 0.4 µg/kg infused over 6 hours. T_3 is advocated over thyroxine because of the very slow onset time of the latter hormone and the reduced ability of critically ill patients to convert T_4 to T_3.

   4. **Levosimendan** [15]
      a. **Actions**
         (1) Binds in Ca-dependent manner to cardiac troponin C, shifting the Ca^{2+} tension curve to the left. Levosimendan may stabilize Ca^{2+}-induced confirmational changes in troponin C.
         (2) Its effects are maximized during early systole when intracellular Ca^{2+} concentration is greatest and least during diastolic relaxation when Ca^{2+} concentration is low.
         (3) Levosimendan inhibits phosphodiesterase III activity.
         (4) Hemodynamic actions

Levosimendan

HR	increased
CO	increased
SVR	decreased
MAP	unchanged
Pulmonary capillary wedge pressure (PCWP)	unchanged
MVo_2	unchanged

      b. **Advantages**
         (1) Does not increase intracellular Ca^{2+}
         (2) Associated with improved outcome in some study of CHF
      c. **Disadvantages**
         (1) Unknown potency relative to other agents
         (2) Limited clinical data currently available
      d. **Indications**
         (1) Treatment of low CO
      e. **Administration**
         (1) Intravenous
      f. **Clinical use**
         (1) 8 to 24 µg/kg/min
         (2) Similar hemodynamic profile to PDE inhibitors
         (3) Despite its biochemical actions on PDE, levosimendan is not associated with increased cAMP, so it may have reduced tendency for arrhythmias relative to sympathomimetics.
 V. **β-Adrenergic receptor blocking drugs** [3,8]
   A. **Actions.** These drugs bind and antagonize β-adrenergic receptors typically producing the following cardiovascular effects:

Heart rate	Decreased
Contractility	Decreased
Blood pressure	Decreased
SVR	Increased [unless drug has intrinsic sympathomimetic activity (ISA)]
AV conduction	Decreased
Atrial refractory period	Increased
Automaticity	Decreased

B. Advantages
1. Reduce MVo$_2$, and decrease HR and contractility.
2. Increase the duration of diastole, during which most blood flow and oxygen are delivered to the LV.
3. Show synergism with nitroglycerin for treating myocardial ischemia; blunt the reflex tachycardia and increase contractility secondary to nitroglycerin, nitroprusside, or other vasodilator drugs.
4. Have an antiarrhythmic action, especially against atrial arrhythmias. β-Blockers also reduce catecholamine-induced ventricular arrhythmias.
5. Decrease LV ejection velocity (useful in patients with asymptomatic septal hypertrophy or aortic dissection).
6. Have antihypertensive action.
7. Reduce dynamic ventricular outflow tract obstruction (e.g., tetralogy of Fallot, hypertrophic cardiomyopathy).
8. Use of these agents is associated with reduced mortality after myocardial infarction, chronic heart failure, chronic hypertension, and with vascular surgery.

C. Disadvantages
1. Severe bradyarrhythmias are possible.
2. Heart block (first-, second-, or third-degree) may occur, especially before cardiac conduction abnormalities are present, or when IV β-blockers and certain IV calcium channel blockers are coadministered.
3. Bronchospasm is possible in patients with reactive airways.
4. CHF can occur in patients with reduced ejection fraction. Elevated LVEDP may induce myocardial ischemia due to elevated systolic wall tension.
5. Signs and symptoms of hypoglycemia (except sweating) are masked in diabetics.
6. SVR is increased due to inhibition of β$_2$ vasodilation; use with care in patients with severe peripheral vascular disease or in patients with pheochromocytoma without α-blockade treatment.
7. Risk of coronary artery spasm is present in rare susceptible patients.

D. Distinguishing features of β-blockers (Table 2.3)
1. Selectivity (β$_1$). Selective β-blockers possess a higher potency at β$_1$-receptors than at β$_2$-receptors. They are less likely to cause bronchospasm or to increase SVR than a nonselective drug. However, β$_2$ selectivity is dose dependent (drugs lose selectivity at higher dosages). Caution must be exercised when an asthmatic patient receives any β-blocker.
2. Intrinsic sympathomimetic activity (ISA). These drugs possess "partial agonist" activity. Thus, drugs with ISA will block β-receptors (preventing catecholamines from combining with a receptor) but also will cause mild stimulation of the same receptors. A patient receiving a drug with ISA would be expected to have a higher resting HR and CO (which shows no change with exercise) but a lower SVR compared to a drug without ISA.
3. Duration of action. In general, β-blockers with longer durations of action are eliminated by the kidneys, whereas propranolol and the drugs of 4 to 6 hours' duration undergo hepatic elimination. Esmolol, the ultrashort-acting β-blocker (plasma half-life, 9 minutes), is eliminated within the blood by a red blood cell esterase. After abrupt discontinuation of esmolol infusion (which we do not recommend), most drug effects are eliminated within 5 minutes. The duration of esmolol is not affected when plasma pseudocholinesterase is inhibited by echothiophate or physostigmine.

E. Clinical use
1. β-Blocker dosage
   a. See Table 2.3.
   b. Begin with a low dosage and slowly titrate dosage to effect.
   c. For metoprolol IV dosage use 0.5- to 1.0-mg increments every 2 to 5 minutes (for adults) as needed while constantly monitoring the ECG, PCWP (if PA catheter is in place), BP, and lung sounds. Intravenous dosage is much smaller than oral dosage because first-pass hepatic extraction is bypassed. The usual acute IV metoprolol dose is 0.015 to 0.07 mg/kg.

2. If β-blockers must be given to a patient with bronchospastic disease, choose a selective β_1-blocker such as metoprolol or esmolol and consider concomitant administration of an inhalation β_2-agonist (such as albuterol).

3. Treatment of toxicity. β-Agonists (e.g., isoproterenol, possibly in large doses) and cardiac pacing are the mainstays. Calcium, inamrinone, milrinone, glucagon, or liothyronine may be effective because these agents do not act via β-receptors.

4. Assessment of β-blockade. When β-blockade is adequate, a patient should not demonstrate an increase in HR with exercise.

5. Use of α-agonists in β-blocked patients. When agonist drugs with α or both α and β actions are administered to patients who are β blocked, e.g., with an epinephrine-containing IV local anesthetic test dose, a greater elevation of BP can be expected owing to α vasoconstriction unopposed by β_2 vasodilation. This may produce deleterious hemodynamic results (increased afterload with little increased CO).

6. Esmolol is given by IV injection (loading dose), often followed by continuous infusion (for details on esmolol dosing for SVT, see Section **VIII.E**). It is of greatest use when the required duration of β-blockade is short (i.e., to attenuate a short-lived stimulus). Esmolol's ultrashort duration of action plus its β_1 selectivity and lack of ISA make it a logical choice when it is necessary to administer a β-blocker to patients with asthma, heart failure, or another relative contraindication. It also is useful in critically ill patients with changing hemodynamic status.

7. Labetalol is a combined α- and β-antagonist (α/β ratio $= 1:7$), which produces vasodilation without reflex tachycardia. Labetalol is useful for preoperative or postoperative control of hypertension. During anesthesia, its relatively long duration of action makes it less useful than other agents for minute-to-minute control or HR and BP. However, treatment with labetalol will reduce the dosage of nitroprusside or other short-acting vasodilator required.

8. β-Adrenergic receptor antagonist withdrawal. Abrupt withdrawal of chronic β-blocker therapy may produce a withdrawal syndrome including tachycardia and hypertension. Myocardial ischemia or infarction may result. Thus, chronic β-blocker therapy should not be abruptly discontinued perioperatively. We have seen this syndrome after abrupt discontinuation of esmolol when it had been administered for only 48 hours!

F. Specific Agents
    1. See Table 2.3.

VI. Vasodilator drugs [8]
  A. Comparison
    1. Sites of action

Arterial (decreased SVR)	Both arterial and venous
Calcium channel blockers	Angiotensin-converting enzyme (ACE) inhibitors
Hydralazine	Nitroglycerin
Phentolamine	Nitroprusside
	Prazosin
	Alprostadil
	Trimethaphan

    2. Mechanisms of action
      a. Direct vasodilators: calcium blockers, hydralazine, minoxidil, nitroglycerin, nitroprusside, trimethaphan
      b. α-Adrenergic blockers: labetalol, phentolamine, prazosin, terazosin, tolazoline
      c. Ganglionic blockers: trimethaphan
      d. ACE inhibitors: enalaprilat, captopril, enalapril, lisinopril
      e. Central α_2-agonists (reduce sympathetic tone): clonidine, guanabenz, guanfacine
      f. Calcium channel blockers (see Section **VII**: Calcium channel blockers)

Table 2.3 β-Adrenergic blocking drugs

	Acebutolol (Sectral)	Atenolol (Tenormin)	Betaxolol (Kerlone)	Carteolol (Cartrol)	Esmolol (Brevibloc)	Labetalol (Trandate)
Bioavailability[c]	40	55	89	85	—	25
β Half-life[d] (h)	3–4	6–9	14–22	6	9 min	3–8
Elimination	H (60%–70%)	R (85%)	H (85%)	R (50%–70%)	Blood	H
Active metabolites	Yes	No	No	No	No	No
β₁ Selectivity	Yes	Yes	Yes	Yes	Yes	No
ISA	Yes	No	No	No	No	No
α-Antagonist	No	No	No	No	No	Yes
Intravenous use	No	No	No	No	Yes	Yes
Initial PO dose[e] (mg)	400 qd	50 qd	10 qd[f]	2.5 qd[f]	—	100 bid
Maximum PO dose[e] (mg)	600 bid[f]	100 qd[f]	40 qd	10 qd	—	1,200 bid
Maximum usual IV[g] dose (mg)	—	—			0.25–0.5 mg/kg load, then 50–200 µg/kg/min	20 mg load, then 40–80 q10min to max 300

(continued)

Table 2.3 Continued

	Metoprolol (Lopressor)	Nadolol (Corgard)	Penbutolol (Levatol)	Pindolol (Visken)	Propranolol (Inderal)	Sotalol[a] (Betapace)	Timolol[b] (Blocadren)
Bioavailability[c]	50	20	100	>90	33	95	75
β half-life[d] (h)	3–4	14–24	5	3–4	3.5–6.0	7–15	3–4
Elimination	H	R (75%)	H	H (60%) R (40%)	H	R	H (80%) R (20%)
Active metabolites	No	No	No	No	Yes	No	No
β₁ selectivity	Yes	No	No	No	No	No	No
ISA	No	No	Minimal	Yes	No	No	No
α-Antagonist	No	No	No	No	No	No	No
Intravenous use	Yes	No	No	No	Yes	No	No
Initial PO dose[e] (mg)	50 qd	40 qd	20 qd	5 bid	10–20 bid–qid	80 bid[f]	10 bid
Maximum PO dose[e] (mg)	200 bid[f]	320 qd[f]	40 qd	30 tid[f]	80 qid	640 qd	30 bid[f]
Maximum usual IV[g] dose (mg)	15 in 5-mg increments	—	—	—	4–8 in 0.5- to 1.0-mg increments		—

[a] Sotalol also has class III antidysrhythmic activity.
[b] Timolol eye drops can produce systemic β blockade.
[c] In percentage after oral dose.
[d] Half-life may not be predictive of clinical duration of action.
[e] Usual dosages for adults.
[f] Decrease dosage in renal failure.
[g] IV doses must be given in small, divided doses with careful monitoring. Adult dosages are given.
Modified from Larach DR, Kofke WA. Cardiovascular drugs. In: Kofke WA, Levy JH, eds. Postoperative critical care procedures of the Massachusetts General Hospital. Boston: Little, Brown and Company, 1986:469.
H, hepatic elimination; ISA, intrinsic sympathomimetic activity; IV, intravenous; PO, by mouth; R, renal elimination.

3. Indications for use

a. Hypertension, increased SVR states. Use arterial or mixed drugs.

b. Controlled hypotension. Short-acting drugs are most useful (e.g., nitroprusside, nitroglycerin, nicardipine, trimethaphan, and volatile inhalational anesthetics).

c. Valvular regurgitation. Reducing SVR will tend to improve oxygen delivery to tissues.

d. CHF. Vasodilation reduces MVO_2 by lowering preload and afterload (systolic wall stress, due to reduced LV size and pressure). Vasodilation also improves ejection and compliance.

Type of CHF	Preferred vasodilator class
Elevated filling pressures	Venous
Elevated SVR	Arterial
Both	Mixed (or combination)

e. Thermoregulation. Vasodilators are used during the cooling and rewarming phases of CPB to facilitate uniform tissue perfusion and accelerate core and shell temperature equilibration. This is especially important during pediatric CPB procedures involving total circulatory arrest where increased CBF promotes brain cooling.

f. Pulmonary hypertension. Vasodilators can improve pulmonary hypertension that is not anatomically fixed. Presently, inhaled NO is the only truly selective pulmonary dilator.

g. Myocardial ischemia. Vasodilator therapy can improve myocardial O_2 balance by reducing MVO_2 (decreased preload and afterload), and nitrates and calcium channel blockers can dilate conducting coronary arteries to affect favorably the distribution of myocardial blood flow.

h. Intracardiac shunts. Vasodilators are used in the setting of nonrestrictive cardiac shunts, especially ventricular septal defects and aortopulmonary connections, to manipulate the ratio of pulmonary artery to aortic pressures. This allows control of the direction and magnitude of shunt flow.

4. Cautions

a. Hyperdynamic reflexes. All vasodilator drugs decrease SVR and BP and may activate baroreceptor reflexes. This cardiac sympathetic stimulation produces tachycardia and increased contractility. Myocardial ischemia due to increased myocardial O_2 demands can be additive to ischemia produced by lowering BP, which reduces coronary blood supply. Addition of a β-blocker can attenuate these reflexes.

b. Ventricular ejection rate. Reflex sympathetic stimulation will increase the rate of ventricular ejection of blood (dP/dt) and raise the systolic aortic wall stress. This may be detrimental with aortic dissection. Thus, addition of β-blockade or use of a ganglionic blocker is beneficial in patients with aortic dissection, aortic aneurysm, or recent aortic surgery.

c. Stimulation of the renin-angiotensin system is implicated in the "rebound" increased SVR and PVR when some vasodilators are discontinued abruptly. Renin release can be attenuated by concomitant β-blockade, and the actions of renin are attenuated by ACE inhibitors.

d. Intracranial pressure (ICP). Most vasodilators will adversely affect ICP, except for trimethaphan and fenoldopam.

B. Specific agents

1. Direct vasodilators

a. Hydralazine (Apresoline)

(1) Actions

(a) This drug is a direct vasodilator. It may inhibit peripheral conversion of dopamine to NE.

(b) It primarily produces an arteriolar dilatation, with little venous (preload) effect.

Hydralazine

HR	Increased (reflex)
Contractility	Increased (reflex)
CO	May increase
BP	Decreased
SVR and PVR	Decreased
Preload	Little change

(2) **Offset** occurs by acetylation in the liver. Patients who are slow acetylators (up to 50% of the population) may have higher plasma hydralazine levels and may show a longer effect, especially with oral use.

(3) **Advantages**

    (a) Selective vasodilation. Hydralazine produces more dilation of coronary, cerebral, renal, and splanchnic beds than of vessels in the muscle and skin.

    (b) Maintenance of uterine blood flow (if hypotension is avoided).

(4) **Disadvantages**

    (a) Slow onset (5 to 15 minutes) after IV dosing; peak effect should occur by 20 minutes. Thus, doses should be separated by at least 10 to 15 minutes.

    (b) Reflex tachycardia or coronary steal can precipitate myocardial ischemia.

    (c) A lupuslike reaction, usually seen only with chronic PO use, may occur with chronic high doses (more than 400 mg/day) and in slow acetylators.

(5) **Clinical use**

    (a) Hydralazine dose

        (i) IV: 2.5- to 5.0-mg bolus every 15 minutes (maximum 20 to 40 mg)

        (ii) IM: 20 to 40 mg every 4 to 6 hour

        (iii) PO: 10 to 50 mg every 6 hours

        (iv) Pediatric dose: 0.02 to 0.05 mg/kg IV every 4 to 6 hours, slowly

    (b) Latency of onset limits its usefulness in acute hypertensive crises.

    (c) Doses of nitroprusside or trimethaphan can be reduced by the addition of hydralazine. This decreases the risk of cyanide toxicity from nitroprusside or prolonged ganglionic blockade from trimethaphan.

    (d) Because duration of action is a few hours, intraoperative administration to hypertensive patients will help control postoperative hypertension.

    (e) Addition of a β-blocker attenuates reflex tachycardia.

    (f) Patients with coronary artery disease should be monitored for myocardial ischemia.

    (g) Enalaprilat is replacing hydralazine for use in many patients.

b. Nitroglycerin (glyceryl trinitrate) [8]

  (1) **Actions**

    (a) Nitroglycerin is a direct vasodilator, producing greater venous than arterial dilation. A nitric acid-containing metabolite activates vascular cyclic guanosine monophosphate (cGMP) production.

Nitroglycerin

HR	Increased (reflex)
Contractility	Increased (reflex)
CO	Variable; often decreased, due to decreased preload (unless ischemia is reduced)
BP	Decreased (high dosages)
Preload	Marked decrease
SVR	Decreased (high dosages)
PVR	Decreased

    (b) Peripheral venous effects. Venodilation and peripheral pooling reduce venous return to the heart, decreasing heart size and preload. This effect usually reduces MVO_2 and increases diastolic coronary blood flow.

    (c) Coronary arterial effects.

        (i) Spasm is relieved.

        (ii) Flow redistribution provides more flow to ischemic myocardium and increases endocardial-to-epicardial flow ratio.

        (iii) There is increased flow to ischemic regions through collateral vessels.

    (d) Myocardial effects

        (i) Improved pump function due to reduced ischemia

        (ii) Antiarrhythmic action (VF threshold in ischemic myocardium is raised because the drug makes the effective refractory period more uniform throughout the heart)

    (e) Arteriolar effects (higher dosages only)

        (i) Arteriolar dilatation decreases SVR. With reduced systolic myocardial wall stress, MVO_2 decreases, and ejection fraction and SV may improve.

        (ii) Arteriolar dilating effects often require very large doses, exceeding 10 µg/kg/min in many patients, whereas much lower doses give effective venous and coronary arterial dilating effects. When reliable peripheral arteriolar dilation is needed, nitroprusside usually is a better choice (it can be used together with nitroglycerin).

  (2) Offset occurs by metabolism in smooth muscle and liver. Half-life in humans is 1 to 3 minutes.

  (3) Advantages

    (a) Selective preload reduction (lowers LV and RV end-diastolic and atrial pressures).

    (b) Virtually no metabolic toxicity

    (c) Effective for myocardial ischemia

        (i) Decreases infarct size after coronary occlusion

        (ii) Effective prophylactically before an ischemia-producing stress

        (iii) Maintains arteriolar autoregulation, so coronary steal is unlikely

    (d) Useful in acute CHF to decrease preload and reduce pulmonary vascular congestion

    (e) Increases vascular capacity; allows infusion of residual pump blood after CPB is terminated

    (f) Not readily degraded by light

    (g) Dilates the pulmonary vascular bed and can be useful in treating acute pulmonary hypertension and right heart failure

    (h) Attenuates biliary colic and esophageal spasm

(4) Disadvantages

(a) It decreases BP as preload and SVR decrease at higher dosages. This may result in decreased coronary perfusion pressure. Monitor BP and ECG, especially when using IV nitroglycerin.

(b) Reflex tachycardia and reflex increase in myocardial contractility are dose related. Consider administering IV fluids or β-blockers.

(c) It inhibits hypoxic pulmonary vasoconstriction (but to a lesser extent than nitroprusside). Monitor Po_2 or supplement inspired gas with oxygen.

(d) It may increase ICP.

(e) It is adsorbed by polyvinyl chloride IV tubing. Titrate dosage to effect; increased effect may occur when tubing becomes saturated. Special infusion sets that do not adsorb drug are available but unnecessary.

(f) Tolerance. Chronic continuous therapy (for longer than 24 hours) can result in tolerance and reduced hemodynamic and antianginal effects. Tolerance during chronic therapy may be avoided by discontinuing the drug (if appropriate) for several hours daily.

(g) Dependence. Coronary spasm and myocardial infarction have been reported after removal of patients from chronic industrial exposure.

(h) Methemoglobinemia. Avoid using more than 7 to 10 µg/kg/min for prolonged periods.

   (i) Pancuronium neuromuscular blockade may be slightly prolonged.

(5) Clinical use

(a) Nitroglycerin dose

   (i) IV bolus: A bolus of 50 to 100 µg may be superior to infusion for acute ischemia. Rapidly changing levels in blood cause more vasodilation than a constant infusion (and may be more likely to produce hypotension).

   (ii) Infusion: dose range, 0.1 to 7.0 µg/kg/min.

   (iii) Sublingual: 0.15 to 0.60 mg.

   (iv) Topical: 2% ointment (Nitropaste), 0.5 to 2.0 inches every 4 to 8 hours; or controlled-release transdermal preparation (Transderm-Nitro, Nitrodisc), 5 to 10 mg (or more) every 24 hours or as needed.

(b) Unless Tridilset (or other nonpolyvinyl chloride tubing) is used, infusion requirements may decrease after the initial 30 to 60 minutes.

(c) Nitroglycerin is better stored in bottles than in bags if storage for more than 6 to 12 hours is anticipated.

(d) When administered during CPB, venous pooling may cause large decreases in pump reservoir volume.

c. Nitroprusside (Nipride) [8,16]

(1) Actions

(a) Nitroprusside is a direct-acting vasodilator. The nitrate group is converted into NO in vascular smooth muscle, which causes increased cGMP levels in cells.

(b) It has balanced arteriolar and venous dilating effects.

Nitroprusside

HR	Increased (reflex)
Contractility	Increased (reflex)
CO	Variable
BP	Markedly decreased (dose-dependent)
SVR	Markedly decreased
PVR	Decreased

(2) Advantages
- **(a)** Nitroprusside has a very short duration of action (1 to 2 minutes) permitting precise titration of dose.
- **(b)** It has pulmonary vasodilator in addition to systemic vasodilator effects.
- **(c)** This agent is highly effective for virtually all causes of hypertension except a high CO state.
- **(d)** A greater decrease in SVR (afterload) than preload is produced at low dosages.

(3) Disadvantages
- **(a)** Cyanide and thiocyanate toxicity may occur.
- **(b)** The solution is unstable in light and so must be protected from light. Photodecomposition inactivates nitroprusside over many hours but does not release cyanide ion.
- **(c)** Tachycardia and increased inotropy are reflex effects that respond to β-blockade. These effects are undesirable with aortic dissection due to increased shearing forces.
- **(d)** Hypoxic pulmonary vasoconstriction is blunted and may produce arterial hypoxemia.
- **(e)** Vascular steal. All vascular regions are dilated equally. Although total organ blood flow may increase, flow may be diverted from ischemic regions (previously maximally vasodilated) to nonischemic areas that have been appropriately vasoconstricted. Thus, myocardial ischemia may be worsened. However, severe hypertension is clearly dangerous in ischemia, and the net effect often is beneficial. ECG monitoring is important.
- **(f)** Chronic hypertension shifts autoregulation to a higher pressure range. Sudden BP lowering may induce myocardial, cerebral, or renal ischemia and is not recommended.
- **(g)** Rebound systemic or pulmonary hypertension may occur if nitroprusside is stopped abruptly (especially in patients with CHF). Nitroprusside should be tapered.
- **(h)** Mild preload reduction due to venodilation occurs; fluids often need to be infused if CO falls.
- **(i)** Risk of increased ICP exists (although it often decreases with resolution of hypertension).
- **(j)** Platelet function is inhibited (clinical consequences are uncertain).

(4) Toxicity
- **(a)** Chemical formula of nitroprusside is $Fe(CN)_5NO$. Nitroprusside reacts with hemoglobin to release highly toxic free cyanide ion (CN^-).
- **(b)** Nitroprusside + oxyhemoglobin → four free cyanide ions + cyanomethemoglobin (nontoxic).
- **(c)** Cyanide ion produces inhibition of cytochrome oxidase, preventing mitochondrial oxidative phosphorylation. This produces tissue hypoxia despite adequate Po_2.
- **(d)** Cyanide detoxification.
    - *(i)* Cyanide + thiosulfate (and rhodanase) → thiocyanate. Thiocyanate is much less toxic than cyanide ion. Availability of thiosulfate is the rate-limiting step in cyanide metabolism. Adults typically can detoxify 50 mg of nitroprusside using existing thiosulfate stores. Thiosulfate administration is of critical importance in treating cyanide toxicity. Rhodanase is an enzyme found in liver and kidney that promotes cyanide detoxification.
    - *(ii)* Cyanide + hydroxocobalamin → cyanocobalamin (vitamin B_{12}).
- **(e)** Patients at increased risk of toxicity

(i) Those resistant to vasodilating effects at low dosages (if an initial dose greater than 3 µg/kg/min is necessary for effect).

(ii) Those receiving a high-dose infusion (greater than 8 µg/kg/min). Whenever the dosage approaches this value for any period of time, frequent blood gas measurements must be performed, and consideration must be given to the following:

  (a) Decrease dosage by adding a different vasodilator (such as enalaprilat, labetalol, hydralazine, or trimethaphan) or a β-blocker.

  (b) Consider using a PA catheter to monitor mixed venous oxygenation (see Section f.2 following).

(iii) Those receiving a high total dose (greater than 1 mg/kg) over 24 hours.

(iv) Those in whom either severe renal or hepatic dysfunction is present.

(f) Signs of nitroprusside toxicity.

(i) Tachyphylaxis occurs in response to vasodilating effects of nitroprusside (larger doses are necessary to produce the same effect).

(ii) Elevated mixed venous Po_2 (due to decreased cellular O_2 utilization) occurs in the absence of a rise in CO.

(iii) There is metabolic acidosis.

(iv) No cyanosis is seen with cyanide toxicity (cells cannot utilize O_2; therefore, blood O_2 saturation remains high).

(v) Chronic toxicity is due to elevated thiocyanate levels and is a consequence of long-term therapy or thiocyanate accumulation in renal failure. Thiocyanate is excreted unchanged by the kidney (elimination half-life, 1 week). Elevated thiocyanate levels (greater than 5 mg/dL) can cause fatigue, nausea, anorexia, miosis, psychosis, hyperreflexia, and seizures.

(g) Therapy of cyanide toxicity.

(i) Cyanide toxicity should be suspected when a metabolic acidosis or unexplained rise in mixed venous Po_2 appears in any patient receiving nitroprusside.

(ii) As soon as toxicity is suspected, nitroprusside must be discontinued and substituted with another agent; lowering the dosage is not sufficient because clinically evident toxicity implies a marked reduction in cytochrome oxidase activity.

(iii) Ventilate with 100% O_2.

(iv) Treat severe metabolic acidosis with bicarbonate.

(v) Mild toxicity (base deficit less than 10, stable hemodynamics when nitroprusside stopped) can be treated by sodium thiosulfate, 150 mg/kg IV bolus (hemodynamically benign).

(vi) Severe toxicity (base deficit greater than 10, or worsening hemodynamics despite discontinuation of nitroprusside:

  (a) Create methemoglobin that can combine with cyanide to produce nontoxic cyanomethemoglobin, removing cyanide from cytochrome oxidase:

    (i) Give 3% sodium nitrite, 4 to 6 mg/kg by slow IV infusion. (Repeat one-half dose 2 to 48 hours later as needed), or

    (ii) Give amyl nitrite: Break 1 ampule into breathing bag. (Flammable!)

(b) Sodium thiosulfate, 150 to 200 mg/kg IV over 15 minutes, should also be administered to facilitate metabolic disposal of the cyanide. Note that thiocyanate clearance is renal dependent.

(c) Consider hydroxocobalamin (vitamin B_{12}) 25 mg/hour. Note: These treatments should be administered even during CPR; otherwise, O_2 cannot be utilized by body tissues.

(5) Clinical use

(a) Nitroprusside dose: 0.1 to 2.0 µg/kg/min IV infusion. Titrate dose to BP and CO. Avoid doses greater than 2 µg/kg/min. Doses as high as 10 µg/kg/min should be infused for no more than 10 minutes.

(b) Supplement inspired gas with O_2 or monitor oxygenation.

(c) Solution in a bottle or bag must be protected from light by wrapping in metal foil. Solution stored in the dark retains significant potency for 12 to 24 hours. It is not necessary to cover the administration tubing with foil.

(d) Because of the high potency of nitroprusside, it is best administered by itself into a central line using an infusion pump. If other drugs are being infused through the same line, use a carrier flow so that changes in one drug's infusion rates do not affect the quantity of other drugs entering the patient per minute (the "bolus effect").

(e) Continuous BP monitoring with an arterial catheter is recommended.

(f) Infusions should be tapered gradually—not stopped abruptly—to avoid rebound increases in systemic and PA pressures.

(g) Use this drug cautiously in patients with concomitant hypothyroidism or severe liver or kidney dysfunction.

d. Nitric oxide

(1) Actions

(a) NO is a vasoactive gas naturally produced from L-arginine primarily in endothelial cells. It was formerly known as *endothelium-derived relaxing factor*. NO diffuses from endothelial cells to vascular smooth muscle, where it increases cGMP and effects vasodilation, in part by decreasing cytosolic calcium. It is an important physiologic intercellular signaling substance, and NO or its absence is implicated in pathologic conditions such as reperfusion injury and coronary vasospasm.

(b) It is administered by inhalation for treatment of pulmonary hypertension, particularly for respiratory distress syndrome in infancy.

Nitric oxide

PVR	Decreased
SVR	No change
RVSWI[2]	Decreased

(2) Offset. NO rapidly and avidly binds to the heme moiety of hemoglobin, forming the inactive compound nitrosylhemoglobin, which in turn degrades to methemoglobin. The biologic half-life of NO in blood is approximately 6 seconds.

(3) Advantages

(a) NO appears to be the long-sought "selective" pulmonary vasodilator. It is devoid of systemic actions.

[2] Right-ventricular stroke work index.

      (b) Unlike parenterally administered pulmonary vasodilators, inhalational NO favorably affects lung V/Q relationships, because it vasodilates primarily those lung regions that are well ventilated.

      (c) There is low toxicity, provided stringent safety precautions are taken.

  (4) Disadvantages

      (a) Stringent safety precautions are required to prevent potentially severe toxicity, such as overdose or catastrophic nitrogen dioxide-induced pulmonary edema.

      (b) Methemoglobinemia may become clinically significant, and blood levels must be monitored at daily intervals.

      (c) Chronic administration may cause ciliary depletion and epithelial hyperplasia in terminal bronchioles.

      (d) NO is corrosive to metal parts during chronic use.

  (5) Clinical use

      (a) NO is administered inhalationally by blending dilute NO gas into the ventilator inlet gas. Therapeutic concentrations range from 0.05 to 80 parts per million (ppm). The lowest effective concentrations should be utilized, and responses should be monitored carefully. The onset of action for reducing PVR and RVSWI is 1 to 2 minutes in patients with pulmonary hypertension that is not anatomically fixed.

      (b) NO must be purchased prediluted in nitrogen in assayed tanks, and an analyzer must be used intermittently to assay the gas stream entering the patient for NO and nitrogen dioxide. NO usually is not injected between the ventilator and the patient (to avoid overdose), and it must never be allowed to contact air or oxygen until it is used (to prevent formation of toxic nitrogen dioxide). Use of soda lime in the inspiratory limb to absorb nitrogen dioxide has been advocated.

      (c) NO has been used to treat persistent pulmonary hypertension of the newborn and other forms of pulmonary hypertension, and the adult respiratory distress syndrome (with variable success).

2. α-Adrenergic blockers [3]

  a. Labetalol (Normodyne, Trandate)

  See section **V** on β-adrenergic receptor blockers.

  b. Phentolamine (Regitine)

    (1) Actions

      (a) Competitive antagonist at α_1, α_2, and 5-hydroxytryptamine (5-HT, serotonin) receptors.

      (b) Primarily arterial vasodilation with little venodilation.

Phentolamine

HR	Increased
Contractility	Increased
BP	Decreased
SVR	Decreased
PVR	Decreased
Preload	Little change

    (2) Offset occurs by hepatic metabolism, in part by renal excretion. Offset after IV bolus occurs after 10 to 30 minutes.

    (3) Advantages

      (a) Good for increased NE states such as pheochromocytoma.

      (b) Antagonizes undesirable α stimulation. For example, reversal of deleterious effects of NE extravasated into skin is achieved by local infiltration with phentolamine 5 to 10 mg in 10-mL saline.

(c) Sometimes combined with NE for positive inotropic support after CPB.

(4) **Disadvantages**

(a) Tachycardia arises from two mechanisms:

(i) Reflex via baroreceptors.

(ii) Direct effect of α_2-blockade. Blockade of presynaptic receptors eliminates the normal feedback system controlling NE release by presynaptic nerve terminals. As α_2 stimulation decreases NE release, blockade of these receptors allows increased presynaptic release. This results in increased β_1 sympathetic effects only, as the α-receptors mediating postsynaptic α effects are blocked by phentolamine. Myocardial ischemia or arrhythmias may result. Thus, the tachycardia and positive inotropy are β effects that will respond to β-blockers.

(b) Gastrointestinal motility is stimulated and gastric acid secretion increased.

(c) Hypoglycemia occurs.

(d) Epinephrine may cause hypotension in α-blocked patients ("epinephrine reversal") via a β_2 mechanism.

(e) Arrhythmias occur.

(f) There is histamine release.

(5) **Clinical use**

(a) Phentolamine dose

(i) IV bolus: 1 to 5 mg (adult) or 0.1 mg/kg IV (pediatric)

(ii) IV infusion: 1 to 20 µg/kg/min

(b) When administered for pheochromocytoma, β-blockade generally also is instituted.

(c) β-Blockade will attenuate tachycardia.

(d) Phentolamine promotes uniform cooling of infants during CPB (dose, 0.1 to 0.5 mg/kg).

c. **Prazosin (Minipress)**

(1) **Actions.** A selective α_1 competitive antagonist, prazosin's main cardiovascular action is vasodilation (arterial and venous) with decreased SVR and decreased preload. Reflex tachycardia is minimal.

(2) **Offset** occurs by hepatic metabolism. The half-life is 4 to 6 hours.

(3) **Advantages**

(a) Virtual absence of tachycardia makes this a more useful antihypertensive drug than nonselective α-blockers such as phentolamine.

(b) The only important cardiovascular action is vasodilation.

(4) **Disadvantages.** Postural hypotension with syncope may occur, especially after the initial dose.

(5) **Indications.** Oral treatment of chronic hypertension.

(6) **Administration.** PO

(7) **Clinical use**

(a) Prazosin dose: initially 0.5 to 1.0 mg bid (maximum 40 mg/day).

(b) Prazosin is closely related to two other α_1-blockers with which it shares a common mechanism of action:

(i) Doxazosin (Cardura). Half-life, 9 to 13 hours. Dose: 1 to 4 mg/day (maximum 16 mg/day)

(ii) Terazosin (Hytrin). Half-life, 8 to 12 hours. Dose: 1 to 5 mg/day (maximum 20 mg/day)

d. **Tolazoline (Priscoline)**

(1) **Actions**

(a) Tolazoline, an imidazoline derivative, is a competitive α-adrenergic antagonist belonging to the same family as phentolamine.

(b) In addition to blocking α_1- and α_2-receptors, tolazoline stimulates muscarinic cholinergic receptors (enhancing gastrointestinal motility and salivary secretions), causes histamine release from mast cells, and displays a sympathomimetic effect.

Tolazoline

HR	Increased, often marked
CO	Increased
BP	Decreased
SVR	Decreased
PVR	Decreased
PVR/SVR ratio	Variable

(2) Offset occurs by hepatic metabolism and renal excretion, with a half-life in neonates of 3 to 10 hours.

(3) Disadvantages

(a) There is little evidence that tolazoline is a selective pulmonary vasodilator. Generally, substantial systemic vasodilation also occurs, with hypotension. If PVR is fixed and SVR decreases, then the PVR/SVR ratio actually may increase.

(b) Sympathomimetic effect (possibly due to enhanced neuronal NE release) plus reflex sympathetic activation lead to marked tachycardia and arrhythmias. Pulmonary vasoconstriction may occur in some patients.

(c) Peptic ulceration, abdominal pain, and nausea may occur.

(d) Hypotension may occur.

(e) Thrombocytopenia may occur.

(4) Clinical use

(a) Tolazoline is used primarily as a pulmonary vasodilator in neonates with persistent pulmonary hypertension.

(b) Tolazoline dose: bolus 0.5 to 2.0 mg/kg; infusion 0.5 to 10 mg/kg/hour.

3. ACE inhibitors

a. Benazepril (Lotensin)

(1) This is an oral ACE inhibitor used primarily to treat hypertension; it is largely similar to captopril (see following Section b: Captopril). The drug must first be converted to an active metabolite in the liver.

(2) Benazepril dose: 10 to 20 mg PO bid.

b. Captopril (Capoten)

(1) Actions

(a) In common with all ACE inhibitors, captopril blocks the conversion of angiotensin I (inactive) to angiotensin II in the lung. This decrease in plasma angiotensin II levels causes vasodilation, generally without reflex increases in HR or CO.

(b) Many tissues contain ACE (including heart, blood vessels, and kidney), and inhibition of the local production of angiotensin II may be important in the mechanism of action of ACE inhibitors.

(c) Plasma and tissue concentrations of kinins (e.g., bradykinin) and prostaglandins increase with ACE inhibition and may be responsible for some side effects.

(d) Captopril, enalaprilat, and lisinopril inhibit ACE directly, but benazepril, enalapril, fosinopril, quinapril, and ramipril are inactive and must undergo hepatic metabolism into the active metabolites.

(2) Offset occurs primarily by renal elimination with a half-life of 1.5 to 2.0 hours. Dosages of all ACE inhibitors (except fosinopril) should be reduced with renal dysfunction.

(3) **Advantages** (in common with all ACE inhibitors)
   (a) Oral vasodilator with high efficacy in chronic hypertension.
   (b) No tachyphylaxis or reflex hemodynamic changes.
   (c) Improved symptoms and survival in CHF, hypertension, and after MI.
   (d) May retard progression of renal disease (e.g., in diabetes).
   (e) Improves LV remodeling after myocardial infarction
(4) **Disadvantages** (in common with all ACE inhibitors)
   (a) There is reversibly decreased renal function, due to reduced renal perfusion pressure. Patients with renal artery stenosis bilaterally (or in a single functioning kidney) are at particular risk of renal failure.
   (b) Increased plasma K^+ and hyperkalemia may occur, due to reduced aldosterone secretion.
   (c) Allergic phenomena (including angioedema and hematologic disorders) occur rarely. Captopril may induce severe dermatologic reactions.
   (d) Chronic nonproductive cough is frequent.
   (e) Reduced coronary perfusion pressure during exercise may exacerbate exercise-induced angina.
   (f) Severe fetal abnormalities and oligohydramnios may occur during second- and third-trimester exposure.
(5) **Indications**
   (a) Chronic hypertension
   (b) Chronic heart failure or following myocardial infarction
   (c) Renal insufficiency
(6) **Administration.** PO
(7) **Clinical use**
   (a) Captopril dose
      (i) Adults: 6.25 to 100 mg PO bid or tid, with the lower doses being used for treatment of heart failure
      (ii) Infants: 50 to 500 µg/kg daily in three doses
      (iii) Children older than 6 months: 0.5 to 2.0 mg/kg/day divided into three doses
   (b) A diuretic often is added to increase antihypertensive efficacy. Hyperkalemia may result from use of a K^+-sparing diuretic or K^+ supplementation.
   (c) Interactions. ACE inhibitors interact with digoxin (reduced digoxin clearance) and with lithium (Li intoxication). Greater reductions in BP may occur with general anesthetics. Captopril interacts with allopurinol (hypersensitivity reactions), cimetidine (central nervous system changes), and insulin or oral hypoglycemic drugs (hypoglycemia).

c. Enalapril (Vasotec)
(1) **Actions.** An oral ACE inhibitor used primarily to treat hypertension and CHF, enalapril is very similar to captopril (see Section b). The drug must first be converted to an active metabolite in the liver.
(2) **Clinical use.** Enalapril dose: 2.5 to 40 mg/day PO in one or two divided doses.

d. Enalaprilat (Vasotec-IV)
(1) **Actions.** Enalaprilat is an IV ACE inhibitor that is the active metabolite of enalapril. It is used primarily to treat severe or acute hypertension and is very similar to captopril (see Section b).
(2) **Offset** is by renal elimination, with a half-life of 11 hours.
(3) **Advantages**
   (a) This drug has a longer duration of action than nitrates, thereby avoiding the need for continuous infusion. It can help extend BP control into the postoperative period.
   (b) Unlike hydralazine, reflex increases in HR, CO, and MVo_2 are absent.

(4) Disadvantages

   (a) There is a longer onset time (15 minutes) than with IV nitro-prusside. Peak action may not occur until 1 to 4 hours after the initial dose.

   (b) Pregnancy. Oligohydramnios and fetal abnormalities may be induced. Use during pregnancy should be limited to life-threatening maternal conditions.

(5) Enalaprilat IV dose

   (a) Adults: 1.25 mg IV slowly every 6 hours (maximum 5 mg IV every 6 hours). In renal insufficiency (creatinine clearance less than 30 mL/min), initial dose is 0.625 mg, which may be repeated after 1 hour, then 1.25 mg every 6 hours.

   (b) Pediatrics: A dosage of 250 µg/kg IV every 6 hours has been reported to be effective in neonates with renovascular hypertension.

e. Fosinopril (Monopril)

   (1) An oral ACE inhibitor used primarily to treat hypertension, fosinopril is very similar to captopril (see Section b). The drug must first be converted to an active metabolite in the gastrointestinal tract and liver.

   (2) Unlike other ACE inhibitors, substantial biliary excretion occurs, so doses do not need to be altered with renal insufficiency.

   (3) Fosinopril dose: 10 to 80 mg PO once daily.

f. Lisinopril (Prinivil, Zestril)

   (1) Lisinopril is an oral ACE inhibitor used primarily to treat hypertension. It is very similar to captopril (see Section b). The drug must first be converted to an active metabolite in the liver.

   (2) Lisinopril dose: 20 to 80 mg PO once daily.

g. Quinapril (Accupril)

   (1) An oral ACE inhibitor used primarily to treat hypertension, quinapril is very similar to captopril (see Section b). The drug must first be converted to an active metabolite in the liver.

   (2) Quinapril dose: 10 to 80 mg PO daily in one or two divided doses.

h. Ramipril (Altace)

   (1) An oral ACE inhibitor used primarily to treat hypertension, ramipril is very similar to captopril (see Section b). The drug must first be converted to an active metabolite in the liver.

   (2) Ramipril dose: 1.25 to 10.0 mg PO once daily.

4. Central α_2-agonists

a. Clonidine (Catapres)

   (1) Actions

   (a) CNS. Clonidine reduces sympathetic outflow by activating central α_2-receptors and by reducing NE release by peripheral sympathetic nerve terminals.

   (b) Clonidine is a partial agonist (activates receptor submaximally but also antagonizes effects of other α_2-agonists).

   (c) There is some direct vasoconstrictor action at α_2-receptors on vascular smooth muscle, but this effect is outweighed by the vasodilation induced by actions in the CNS.

   (2) Offset

   (a) Long duration (β half-life, 12 hours)

   (b) Peak effect 1.5 to 2.0 hours after an oral dose

   (3) Advantages

   (a) α_2-Agonists potentiate general anesthetics and narcotics through a central mechanism. This effect can reduce substantially doses of anesthetics and narcotics required during anesthesia for myocardial revascularization surgery.

   (b) There are no reflex increases in HR or contractility.

   (c) Clonidine reduces sympathetic coronary artery tone.

(d) It attenuates hemodynamic responses to stress.

(e) Prolongs duration of regional anesthesia

(4) Disadvantages

(a) Rebound hypertension prominent after abrupt withdrawal.

(b) Clonidine may potentiate opiate drug effects on CNS.

(c) Sedation is dose dependent.

(5) Clinical use

(a) Clonidine dose

(i) Adult: 0.2 to 0.8 mg/day PO (maximum, 2.4 mg/day). When used as anesthetic premedication, the usual dose is 5 µg/kg PO.

(ii) Pediatrics: 3 to 5 µg/kg every 6 to 8 hours.

(b) Rebound hypertension frequently follows abrupt withdrawal. Clonidine should be continued until immediately before the operation, and either it should be resumed soon postoperatively (by skin patch, nasogastric tube, or PO) or another type of antihypertensive drug should be substituted. Alternatively, clonidine can be replaced by another drug 1 to 2 weeks preoperatively.

(c) Intraoperative hypotension may occur.

(d) Transdermal clonidine patches require 2 to 3 days to achieve therapeutic plasma drug levels.

(e) Guanabenz and guanfacine are related drugs with similar effects and hazards.

(f) Use of clonidine may improve hemodynamic stability during coronary bypass surgery.

(g) Clonidine attenuates sympathetic outpouring during drug addiction withdrawal.

(h) It may reduce postoperative shivering.

(i) Commonly added to local anesthetic solutions before peripheral nerve blocks to prolong the duration of action.

b. Guanabenz (Wytensin)

(1) This oral α_2-agonist is similar to clonidine (see Section a).

(2) Guanabenz dose: 4 mg PO bid (maximum 32 mg PO bid).

c. Guanfacine (Tenex)

(1) This oral α_2-agonist is similar to clonidine (see Section a).

(2) Actions. Guanfacine has a longer duration of action than clonidine due to renal elimination (half-life, 15 to 20 hours).

(3) Guanfacine dose: 1 mg PO daily (maximum 3 mg daily).

d. Other vasodilators

(1) Fenoldopam (Corlopam)

(a) Actions

(i) Fenoldopam is a short-acting DA-1 agonist that causes profound peripheral vasodilation. The mechanism appears to be through stimulation of cAMP.

(ii) The drug has no α- or β-adrenergic receptor activity at clinical doses and thus no direct actions on HR or cardiac contractility.

(iii) Fenoldopam stimulates diuresis and natriuresis.

(b) Advantages

(i) Relative to other short-acting IV vasodilators, fenoldopam has almost no systemic toxic effects.

(ii) Fenoldopam alone among vasodilators stimulates diuresis and natriuresis; thus, it should provide "renal protective" effects comparable to "renal dose" (1 to 2 µg/kg/min) dopamine.

(iii) Fenoldopam, unlike dopamine, reduces global and regional cerebral blood flow.

(c) Disadvantages

(i) As is true for other dopaminergic agonists, fenoldopam will commonly induce nausea in awake patients.

(d) Clinical use
- (i) Fenoldopam is an appropriate single agent to use whenever a combination of a vasodilator and "renal dose" dopamine is used. For example, many patients recovering from aortic valve replacement for aortic stenosis have postoperative hypertension. These patients also may benefit from the diuretic effects of fenoldopam to eliminate the multiple kilograms of excessive extracellular water they accumulate intraoperatively and in the first few postoperative hours.
- (ii) Fenoldopam carries no risk of cyanide or of methemoglobinemia and may have theoretical advantages over both nitroprusside and nitroglycerin for control of acute hypertension.
- (iii) For treatment of urgent or emergent hypertension in adults, we initiate fenoldopam at 0.05 µg/kg/min and double the dose at 5- to 10-minute intervals if it should prove ineffective. Doses of up to 1.0 µg/kg/min may be required.
- (iv) The limited data available in pediatrics suggest that weight-adjusted doses at least as great as those used in adults are necessary.
- (v) For inducing diuresis and natriuresis, we have found that doses of 0.05 µg/kg/min are effective in adults.

(2) Alprostadil (Prostaglandin E_1, PGE_1, Prostin VR)
- **(a) Actions.** This drug is a direct vasodilator acting through specific prostaglandin receptors on vascular smooth muscle cells.
- **(b) Offset** occurs by rapid metabolism to inactive substances by enzymes located in most body tissues, especially the lung.
- **(c) Advantages**
  - (i) Alprostadil selectively dilates the ductus arteriosus (DA) in neonates and infants. May maintain patency of an open DA for as long as approximately 60 days of age and may open a closed DA up to 10 to 14 days of age.
  - (ii) Metabolism by lung endothelium reduces systemic vasodilation compared with its potent pulmonary vascular dilating effect.
- **(d) Disadvantages**
  - (i) Systemic vasodilation, producing hypotension.
  - (ii) May produce apnea in infants (10% to 12%), especially if birth weight is less than 2 kg. Also, fever or seizures possible.
  - (iii) Extremely expensive (synthetic drug).
  - (iv) Inhibits platelet function (reversible).
- **(e) Administration.** Infused IV or through umbilical arterial catheter
- **(f) Indications for use**
  - (i) Cyanotic congenital heart disease with reduced pulmonary blood flow
  - (ii) Severe pulmonary hypertension with right heart failure
- **(g) Clinical use**
  - (i) Alprostadil dose: Usual IV infusion starting dose is 0.05 µg/kg/min. The dose should be titrated up or down to the lowest effective value. Doses as high as 0.4 µg/kg/min may be required.
  - (ii) Intravenous alprostadil is used in combination with left atrial NE for treatment of severe pulmonary hypertension with right heart failure.

(3) Epoprostenol (PGI_2) is used for the long-term treatment of primary pulmonary hypertension and pulmonary hypertension associated with scleroderma. The acute treatment of pulmonary hypertension and RV failure is summarized in Table 2.2.

VII. Calcium Channel Blockers [3]

A. General considerations

1. **Tissues utilizing calcium.** Calcium is required for cardiac contraction and conduction, smooth muscle contraction, neuromuscular transmission, and hormone secretion.

2. **How calcium enters cells.** Calcium ions (Ca^{2+}) interact with the intracellular machinery in two ways, by entering the cell from outside or by being released from intracellular storage sites. These two mechanisms are related because Ca^{2+} crossing the sarcolemma acts as a trigger, releasing sequestered Ca^{2+} from the sarcoplasmic reticulum into the cytoplasm. These processes can raise intracellular free Ca^{2+} concentrations 100-fold.

3. **Myocardial effects of calcium.** The force of myocardial contraction is directly related to the cytoplasmic ionized calcium concentration [(Ca^{2+})], high levels causing contraction and low levels permitting relaxation. At the end of systole, energy-dependent pumps transfer Ca^{2+} from the cytoplasm back into the sarcoplasmic reticulum, causing free cytoplasmic Ca^{2+} to decrease. If ischemia prevents sequestration of cytoplasmic Ca^{2+}, diastolic relaxation of myocardium is incomplete. This abnormal diastolic stiffness of the heart raises LVEDP and produces symptoms of CHF.

4. **Myocardial effects of CCBs.** CCBs owe much of their usefulness to their ability to reduce the entry of the "trigger" current of Ca^{2+}. This reduces the amount of Ca^{2+} released from intracellular stores with each heartbeat. Therefore, all CCBs in high enough doses reduce the force of cardiac contraction, although this effect often is counterbalanced by reflex actions in patients. Clinical dosages of some CCBs, such as nifedipine and nicardipine, do not produce myocardial depression in humans.

5. **Vascular smooth muscle and the cardiac conduction system are particularly sensitive to Ca^{2+} channel blockade.**

6. **Site selectivity.** CCBs affect certain tissues more than others. Thus, verapamil in clinical dosages depresses cardiac conduction, whereas nifedipine does not. However, all CCBs cause vasodilation.

7. **Direct versus indirect effects.** Selection of a particular CCB for clinical use is based primarily on its relative potency for direct cellular effects in the target organ and its relative potency for inducing cardiovascular reflexes.

B. Clinical effects common to all calcium blockers

1. **Peripheral vasodilation**
   a. **Arterial vasodilation reduces LV afterload,** and this vasodilation helps offset any direct negative cardiac inotropic action.
   b. **Venous effects.** Preload usually changes little because venodilation is minimal, and negative inotropy often is offset by reduced afterload. However, if CCBs reduce myocardial ischemia and diastolic stiffness, filling pressures may decrease.
   c. **Regional effects.** Most vascular beds are dilated, including the cerebral, hepatic, pulmonary, splanchnic, and musculoskeletal beds. Renal blood flow autoregulation is abolished by nifedipine, making flow pressure-dependent.
   d. **Coronary vasodilation is induced by all CCBs.** These drugs are all highly effective for coronary vasospasm.
   e. **CCBs versus nitrates.** Unlike nitrates, CCBs do not incite tachyphylaxis.
   f. **Reversal of vasodilation.** α-Agonists such as phenylephrine often restore BP during CCB-induced hypotension, but calcium salts usually are ineffective.

2. **Depression of myocardial contractility.** The degree of myocardial depression that occurs following administration of a CCB is highly variable, depending on the following factors:
   a. **Selectivity.** The relative potency of the drug for myocardial depression compared with its other actions is an important factor. Nifedipine and other

dihydropyridines are much more potent as vasodilators than as myocardial depressants; clinical dosages that cause profound vasodilation have minimal direct myocardial effects. Conversely, vasodilating dosages of verapamil may be associated with significant myocardial depression in some patients.

  b. **Health of the heart.** A failing ventricle will respond to afterload reduction with improved ejection. An ischemic ventricle will pump more effectively if ischemia is reversed. As CCBs reduce afterload and ischemia, CO may rise with CCB therapy in certain situations. Direct negative inotropic effects may not be apparent.

  c. **Sympathetic reflexes** can counteract direct myocardial depression and vasodilation due to CCBs.

  d. **Reversal of myocardial depression.** Calcium chloride, β-agonists, and inamrinone all can be used to help reverse excessive negative inotropy and heart block, but pacing may be needed.

3. **Improving myocardial ischemia**

  a. **Oxygen supply** can be improved by:

    (1) Reversing coronary artery spasm.

    (2) Vasodilating the coronary artery, increasing flow to both normal and poststenotic regions. Diltiazem and verapamil appear to preserve coronary autoregulation, but nifedipine may cause a coronary steal.

    (3) Increasing flow through coronary collateral channels.

    (4) Decreasing HR (prolonging diastolic duration during which subendocardium is perfused) with verapamil and diltiazem.

  b. **Oxygen consumption** can be reduced by:

    (1) Diminishing contractility.

    (2) Decreasing peak LV wall stress (afterload reduction).

    (3) Decreasing HR (by verapamil and diltiazem).

4. **Electrophysiologic depression**

  a. **Spectrum of impairment of AV conduction**

    (1) **Verapamil and diltiazem.** At one end of the spectrum, clinical doses of verapamil or diltiazem usually produce significant electrophysiologic effects. Thus, verapamil has a high relative potency for prolonging AV refractoriness compared with its vasodilating potency.

    (2) **Dihydropyridines.** On the other hand, nifedipine and other drugs of this class in dosages that produce profound vasodilation do not change AV conduction.

  b. **AV node effects.** The depression of AV nodal conduction by CCBs may be beneficial for its antiarrhythmic effect.

  c. **Sinoatrial (SA) node effects.** Diltiazem and verapamil decrease sinus rate, whereas nifedipine and nicardipine often increase HR slightly.

  d. **Ventricular ectopy** due to mitral valve prolapse, atrial or AV nodal disease, halothane–epinephrine interactions, and some types of digitalis toxicity may respond to CCBs.

5. **Clinical uses**

  a. **Myocardial ischemia**

  b. **Hypertension** (although outcome benefits remain controversial)

  c. **Hypertrophic cardiomyopathy** by relieving LV outflow obstruction

  d. **Cerebral vasospasm following subarachnoid hemorrhage** (nimodipine)

  e. **Possible reduction of cyclosporine nephrotoxicity with concomitant CCB therapy in transplant recipients.** Also, CCBs may potentiate the immunosuppressive action of cyclosporine.

  f. **Migraine prophylaxis**

C. **Specific Agents**

  1. **Amlodipine (Norvasc)**

    a. **Actions.** A dihydropyridine CCB with actions closely resembling those of nifedipine (see Section 7), amlodipine is primarily a vasodilator without clinically important negative cardiac inotropy. It is used most commonly for oral treatment of hypertension or angina pectoris.

    b. Amlodipine dose. 5 to 10 mg PO once daily; decrease with hepatic dysfunction.

2. Bepridil (Vascor)

    a. Actions. In addition to blocking calcium channels, bepridil inhibits membrane sodium channels, prolongs cardiac repolarization, and causes additional negative cardiac inotropy by a noncalcium channel mechanism. Its vasodilator actions are more selective for the coronary than for other vessels, but hypotension may be induced.

    b. Offset is by hepatic metabolism (with active metabolites). The elimination half-life is 33 hours.

    c. Advantages

        (1) Effective in the oral treatment of angina pectoris that is not controlled adequately by other medical therapies.

        (2) Does not cause clinically apparent myocardial depression but is not recommended for use with severe LV dysfunction.

    d. Disadvantages

        (1) Proarrhythmic action. Bepridil can increase QT intervals, which may cause ventricular arrhythmias; torsades de pointes occurs rarely. For this reason, bepridil is contraindicated in patients with a prolonged QT interval, conduction abnormalities, or elevated K^+.

        (2) T-wave abnormalities may be induced.

    e. Bepridil dose. 200 to 400 mg PO once daily

3. Diltiazem (Cardizem)

    a. Diltiazem is a benzothiazepine calcium blocker.

    b. Actions. Diltiazem has a selective coronary vasodilating action, causing a greater increase in coronary flow than in other vascular beds.

Diltiazem

HR	Slight decrease
Contractility	No change or small decrease
BP	Decreased
Preload	No change
SVR	Decreased
AV conduction	Slowed

    c. Offset occurs by hepatic metabolism (60%) and renal excretion (35%). Plasma elimination half-life is 3 to 5 hours. The active metabolite is desacetyldiltiazem.

    d. Advantages

        (1) Diltiazem often decreases HR during sinus rhythm.

        (2) It is highly effective in treating and preventing classic or vasospastic myocardial ischemia.

        (3) Used in rate control for SVT (see Section VIII, E).

        (4) Perioperative hypertension can be controlled with IV diltiazem. Of particular benefit to the myocardium is the lack of reflex tachycardia, improved diastolic compliance, and antiischemic action.

    e. Disadvantages

        (1) Sinus bradycardia and conduction system depression are possible.

    f. Indications

        (1) Myocardial ischemia, both classic angina and coronary artery spasm

        (2) Hypertension, acute or chronic

        (3) SVT, including atrial fibrillation or flutter (see Section VIII, E)

        (4) Sinus tachycardia, especially intraoperative or postoperative

    g. Diltiazem dose (adult) (see Section VIII, E)

4. Felodipine (Plendil)

    a. **Actions.** A dihydropyridine CCB with actions closely resembling those of nifedipine (see Section 7), felodipine is primarily a vasodilator without clinically important negative cardiac inotropy. It is used most commonly for oral treatment of hypertension.

    b. **Felodipine dose.** 5 to 10 mg PO once daily.

5. Isradipine (DynaCirc)

    a. **Actions.** A dihydropyridine CCB with actions closely resembling those of nifedipine (see Section 7), isradipine is primarily a vasodilator without clinically important negative cardiac inotropy. It is used most commonly for oral treatment of hypertension or angina pectoris.

    b. **Isradipine dose.** 2.5 to 10.0 mg PO bid.

6. Nicardipine (Cardene)

    a. **Actions.** A dihydropyridine calcium blocker with actions closely resembling those of nifedipine (see Section 7), nicardipine is primarily a vasodilator without clinically important negative cardiac inotropy. It is used most commonly for treatment of hypertension or myocardial ischemia.

    b. Intravenous nicardipine

        (1) The IV preparation is a highly effective vasodilator in anesthetized patients, causing only minimal HR increase and no increase in ICP. Nicardipine lacks the rebound hypertension that can occur with nitroprusside and causes less venodilation than does nitroglycerin.

        (2) **Offset.** Metabolism occurs in the liver, with plasma α and β half-lives of 3 and 14 minutes, respectively. When IV administration is stopped, 50% offset vasodilation occurs in approximately 30 minutes.

        (3) **Clinical use.** Nicardipine IV is effective for control of perioperative hypertension. It also can improve diastolic LV function during ischemia by acceleration of myocardial relaxation (lusotropy). Nicardipine may prove to be of particular benefit in the treatment of coronary spasm, especially in patients with LV dysfunction. Nicardipine can elevate plasma cyclosporine levels.

    c. **Nicardipine dose.** PO: 20 to 40 mg tid; IV: 1 to 4 µg/kg/min in adults, titrated to BP. The drug causes phlebitis when infused for more than 12 hours through a peripheral IV catheter.

7. Nifedipine (Adalat, Procardia)

    a. **Nifedipine is a dihydropyridine calcium channel blocker.**

    b. **Actions**

Nifedipine

HR	Increased (reflex)
Contractility	Increased (reflex)
BP	Decreased
Preload	No change, or slightly decreased
SVR	Markedly decreased
AV conduction	Increased (reflex)

    c. **Offset** occurs by hepatic metabolism. Plasma elimination half-life is 1.5 to 5.0 hours, and there are no active metabolites.

    d. **Advantages**

        (1) Profound vasodilation is the predominant effect.

           (a) Coronary vasodilation and relief of coronary vasospasm reduce myocardial ischemia.

           (b) Peripheral vasodilation can improve CO via LV unloading.

        (2) Virtually no myocardial depression occurs in clinical dosages. Therefore, nifedipine can be used in patients with poor ventricular function.

        (3) Generally this drug is devoid of conducting system toxicity.

        (4) It may be combined with β-blockers without increased risk of AV block or with nitrates provided that the patient is monitored for excessive vasodilation.

   e. Disadvantages
      (1) It is extremely light sensitive; thus, no IV preparation is available.
      (2) Administration must be PO or via mucosa of the nose or mouth.
      (3) Severe hypotension is possible due to peripheral vasodilation.
      (4) No significant antiarrhythmic effect occurs unless relief of myocardial ischemia decreases ischemia-induced arrhythmias.
      (5) Peripheral edema is possible (not due to heart failure).
      (6) The drug must be avoided in hypertrophic cardiomyopathy due to increased aortic outflow tract obstruction.
      (7) Short-acting versions of this drug have been associated with *worsened* outcome in treatment of essential hypotension.
   f. Clinical use
      (1) Nifedipine dose: PO, 10 to 40 mg tid; sublingual, 10 to 20 mg liquid (extracted from capsule).
      (2) Nifedipine generally is selected for its vasodilator and antianginal properties.
      (3) The sublingual (or intranasal) route is useful in treatment for hypertensive emergencies when no IV is present.
      (4) If excessive vasodilation with hypotension occurs, phenylephrine may be used (high dosages may be required).
      (5) In rare patients, angina is exacerbated with nifedipine. This may be related to hypotension or to a coronary steal phenomenon.
8. Nimodipine (Nimotop)
   a. Actions. A dihydropyridine CCB with actions closely resembling those of nifedipine, nimodipine lacks clinically important negative cardiac inotropy. It is a more effective dilator of cerebral arteries compared with other CCBs. Its primary use is in patients with subarachnoid hemorrhage for oral treatment and prophylaxis of cerebral vasospasm and neurologic deficits.
   b. Nimodipine dose. 60 mg PO (or by nasogastric tube) every 4 hours.
9. Verapamil (Calan, Isoptin) (see Section VIII, E).
VIII. Pharmacologic control of heart rate and rhythm
   A. Overview of arrhythmias [17–19]
      1. Conduction pathway. Drug interactions with the cardiac rhythm depend upon the structure and physiology of the cardiac conduction pathway. The cardiac impulse normally arises in the SA node and passes through the atria to enter the AV node. Impulses then transit the specialized conduction system, including the His bundle, the major bundle branches, and the Purkinje fiber network, before spreading into the ventricular myocardium. Agents that inhibit conduction from the sinus node to (or through) the AV node prolong the interval from the P wave (which represents atrial systole) to the QRS complex (which represents ventricular systole), manifest as the "PR" interval on the ECG (Fig. 2.2). Conversely, agents that prolong conduction through the specialized conduction system or the ventricle lengthen the QRS complex.
      2. The role of the conduction system in arrhythmias. Drugs that suppress AV nodal conduction (β-blockers, calcium channel blockers, adenosine; see following) terminate SVTs that originate in the AV node or involve the AV node in a reentrant pathway (Table 2.4). Conversely, rhythms that originate in atrial tissue above the AV node, including atrial flutter or fibrillation, as well as paroxysmal rhythms stimulated by unopposed catecholamines (common in perioperative patients), respond to AV nodal blockade with slowing of the ventricular response rate, because the passage of impulses from the atrium to the ventricle through the AV node is slowed. Junctional tachycardias, common during the surgical period, arise in the specialized conduction system and may convert to sinus rhythm in response to AV nodal blockers only if they originate very close to the AV node, but are otherwise unresponsive. Ventricular arrhythmias usually exhibit no beneficial response to AV nodal blockade, because these rhythms originate in tissues distal to the AV node.

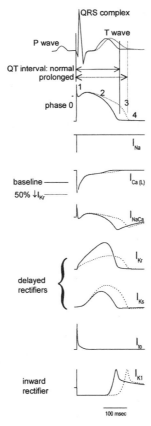

FIG. 2.2 Relationship between the electrocardiogram (***top***), the action potential in the ventricle (***second panel***), and individual ion currents. The amplitudes of the currents are not on the same scales. The *solid lines* represent the baseline; the *dotted lines* the computation when I_{Kr} is reduced by 50%. Note that this change not only prolongs the action potential duration (APD) (as expected); it also generates changes in the time course of I_{Ca-L}, I_{Ks} and the sodium–calcium exchange current, each of which thus also modulates the effect of reduced I_{Kr} on the APD. (From Roden DM, Balser JR, George AL Jr, et al. Cardiac ion channels. *Annu Rev Physiol* 2002;64:431–475, with permission. © 2002 by Annual Reviews www.annualreviews.org.)

3. **Initiating the cardiac action potential.** The effects of drugs on the surface ECG can be predicted from their effects on the ion channel currents that compose the cardiac action potential (AP in Fig. 2.2). The action potential represents the time-varying transmembrane potential of the myocardial cell during the cardiac cycle. The AP is divided into five distinct phases; the channels responsible for "phase 0" initiate the AP and underlie impulse propagation. In the atria and the ventricles, the phase 0 current is generated by sodium channels and is inhibited by the local anesthetic-type drugs (lidocaine, procainamide) that prolong the QRS complex. In AV and SA nodal cells (not shown in Fig. 2.2), phase 0 is produced by L-type calcium channels, so drugs that suppress calcium channels (β-blockers and calcium channel blockers) slow the HR by acting on the SA node and prolong the PR interval by slowing conduction through the AV node. The latter effect renders the AV node a more

Table 2.4 Response of common supraventricular tachyarrhythmias
to intravenous adenosine

Supraventricular tachycardia	Mechanism	Adenosine response
AV nodal reentry	Reentry within AV node	Termination
AV reciprocating tachycardias (orthodromic and antidromic)	Reentry involving AV node and accessory pathway (Wolff–Parkinson–White syndrome)	Termination
Intraatrial reentry	Reentry in the atrium	Transiently slows ventricular response
Atrial flutter/fibrillation	Reentry in the atrium	Transiently slows ventricular response
Other atrial tachycardias	Abnormal automaticity cAMP-mediated triggered activity	Transient suppression of the tachycardia Termination
AV junctional rhythms	Variable	Variable

AV, atrioventricular.
Adapted from Balser JR. Perioperative management of arrhythmias. Barash PG, Fleisher LA, Prough DS, eds. *Problems in anesthesia.* Lippincott–Raven, Philadelphia, 1998;10(2):201.

efficient "filter" for preventing rapid trains of atrial beats from passing into the ventricle; hence, the rationale for AV nodal blockade during SVT.

4. **The later phases of the AP** (Fig. 2.2) [17–19] reflect repolarization and are modulated by a number of outward (mainly K) and inward (mainly Ca) currents. In general, the long plateau (phase 2) is maintained by L-type calcium current and is terminated (phase 3) by potassium currents. Hence, the QT interval on the ECG reflects the length of the AP and is determined by a delicate balance between these currents. Drugs that reduce calcium current tend to abbreviate the AP plateau, shorten the QT, and reduce the inward movement of calcium calcium ions into the cardiac cell (hence, the negative inotropic effect). Conversely, agents that block outward potassium current prolong the action potential and the QT interval on the ECG (example shown in Fig. 2.2).

5. **Reentry** underlies a wide variety of supraventricular and ventricular arrhythmias, and implies the existence of a pathologic circus movement of electrical impulses around an anatomic loop (accessory pathway or infarct scar) or a "functional" loop (ischemia or drug-induced dispersion of AP duration). Fibrillation, in either the atrium or ventricle, is believed to involve multiple coexistent reentrant circuits of the functional type. Drugs may terminate reentry through at least two mechanisms. Agents that suppress currents responsible for initiation of the AP, the sodium current in the ventricle (Fig. 2.2) or the calcium current in the AV node, may slow or block conduction in a reentrant pathway and thus terminate an arrhythmia. Interventions that prolong the AP, such as potassium channel blockade (Fig. 2.2), in turn prolong the refractory period of cells in a reentrant circuit and thus "block" impulse propagation through the circuit. Agents operating through the latter mechanism are more effective in suppressing fibrillation in the atrium and ventricle.

6. **Triggered automaticity** may occur during phase 2 or 3 [early afterdepolarization (EAD)] or phase 4 [delayed afterdepolarization (DAD)]. Drugs that block potassium channels prolong the duration of the AP, lengthening the QT interval on the ECG (Fig. 2.2), and thereby stimulate EADs. In addition, low serum potassium, hypomagnesemia, and slow HR synergistically prolong the QT and precipitate EADs. EADs in turn elicit a polymorphic VT known as *"torsades de pointes."* At the same time, inherited mutations that suppress potassium channel function provoke the congenital long QT syndrome, an inherited condition where the QT interval is prolonged and risk for torsades

de pointes is increased. Moreover, "silent" mutations in potassium channels may provoke QT prolongation and torsades only during exposure to potassium-channel blocking drugs; hence, the "acquired" and congenital long QT syndromes are mechanistically related and represent distinct points on a continuum of ion channel dysfunction. Commonly used drugs that may prolong the QT and provoke torsades are listed in Table 2.5.

DADs are most common during conditions of intracellular calcium ion (Ca^{2+}) overload. Common clinical entities are digitalis toxicity, excess catecholamine states (exercise, acute myocardial infarction, perioperative stress), and heart failure. Arrhythmias provoked by DADs are responsive to maneuvers aimed at lowering intracellular Ca^{2+}, such as calcium channel blockade.

B. **Nonsustained ventricular tachycardia (NSVT)** [17,20]

   1. **Definition and etiology:** NSVT is three or more premature ventricular contractions (PVCs) occurring at a rate exceeding 100 beats/min and lasting 30 seconds or less without hemodynamic compromise. These arrhythmias occur in up to 50% of patients during or after thoracic and major vascular surgeries, often in the absence of cardiac disease.

   2. **Management.** The rhythms do not influence early or late mortality in patients with preserved LV function and do not require suppressive drug therapy in most circumstances. However, NSVT with normal LV function may be the first sign of a reversible, life-threatening condition, such as hypoxemia or cardiac ischemia; therefore, its presence should always trigger a thorough evaluation. Among patients with low CO following coronary artery bypass grafting (requiring pressor support), NSVT is an independent predictor of more serious, life-threatening arrhythmias. Similarly, patients who undergo aortic valve replacement and have NSVT are at increased risk for sustained ventricular arrhythmias. There are no studies available to guide therapy in these circumstances, so clinical management is empiric. Hemodynamically unstable patients with marginal perfusion may deteriorate with recurrent episodes of NSVT (problematic ventricular pacing or intraaortic balloon counterpulsation) and may benefit from suppression with IV lidocaine or β-blockade if hemodynamically tolerated. Repletion of postbypass hypomagnesemia (2 g $MgCl_2$ IV) reduces the incidence of NSVT after cardiac surgery.

C. **Sustained ventricular arrhythmias** [17,21]

   1. **Monomorphic VT.** The mechanism for monomorphic VT is a reentrant pathway around scar tissue from a healed myocardial infarction, producing a constant QRS morphology. Patients may have a stable (perfusing) BP with this rhythm, and procainamide or amiodarone often are preferred over lidocaine for chemical cardioversion. In cases of hemodynamic instability, DC countershocks should be utilized for cardioversion and antiarrhythmic drug therapy considered as a means to maintain sinus rhythm. Monomorphic VT is less common during surgery than the polymorphic VTs (discussed later).

   2. **Long QT polymorphic VT (torsades de pointes).** As discussed earlier, this rhythm usually is an acquired complication of therapy with drugs that prolong

Table 2.5 QT-prolonging drugs

Antiarrhythmics	Quinidine, procainamide, disopyramide, sotalol, amiodarone, ibutilide, dofetilide
Antipsychotics	Haloperidol, risperidone
Antihistamines	Terfenadine, astemizole
Antifungal	Ketoconazole, fluconazole, itraconazole
Antibiotics	Trimethoprim-sulfamethoxasole, pentamidine, erythromycin(s)
Antidepressants	Amitriptyline, imipramine, doxepin
Phenothiazines	Chlorpromazine, thioridazine
Gastrointestinal	Cisapride, droperidol

Modified from Murray KT, Roden DM. Disorders of cardiac repolarization: the long QT syndromes. In: Crawford MH, DiMarco JP, eds. Cardiology. London: Mosby, 2001:15.7.

the QT interval (Table 2.5). The management of torsades is distinctive. After administering DC countershocks to achieve conversion, additional maneuvers are aimed at shortening the QT interval in order to maintain sinus rhythm. This includes IV magnesium sulfate and maneuvers to increase HR (atropine, isoproterenol, or ventricular pacing). Antiarrhythmic drug therapy is considered when the rhythm is refractory to these measures, and agents devoid of potassium channel blockade, such as lidocaine or phenytoin, should be chosen to avoid further prolongation of the QT interval. Among the antiarrhythmic agents that prolong the QT interval, the incidence of torsades de pointes is lowest with amiodarone; hence, IV amiodarone is a rational alternative therapy for polymorphic VT of unclear etiology that is refractory to other therapies.

3. **Normal QT polymorphic VT and VF** are the most common, life-threatening ventricular arrhythmias in perioperative patients and may occur in patients with ischemic or structural heart disease. Intravenous antiarrhythmic agents are common adjuncts to DC countershocks, and the agents used for this purpose include lidocaine, bretylium, procainamide, and more recently amiodarone. There are no prospective clinical data evaluating the efficacy of antiarrhythmic agents during cardiac arrest in perioperative patients, and randomized, prospective trials in all settings are scarce. In a recent blinded, randomized, prospective trial, IV amiodarone was shown to produce a short-term survival benefit over placebo (44% vs. 34%, $p = 0.03$) when treating out-of-hospital cardiac arrest refractory to DC cardioversion [22]. Amiodarone and procainamide both carry "2b" designations (acceptable, not harmful, supported by fair evidence) in the revised, year 2000 American Heart Association ACLS guidelines for treatment of VF or pulseless VT. There are no human clinical trials to indicate whether lidocaine is effective for treating shock-resistant VT/VF, and the agent now carries an "indeterminate" recommendation in the published guidelines. Bretylium has been removed from the ACLS treatment guidelines because of a high occurrence of side effects (postganglionic adrenergic blockade, orthostatic hypotension with continuous infusion), limited supply and availability from the manufacturer, and the availability of safer agents. In all cases, defibrillation is the means to achieve conversion to sinus rhythm, and these antiarrhythmic agents should be viewed as supplements to help maintain sinus rhythm.

4. **Specific agents available in IV form** [21,23]
   a. **Procainamide (Pronestyl, Procan-SR)**
      (1) **Dosing**
         (a) **Loading dose**
            (i) IV: 10 to 50 mg/min (or 100 mg every 2 to 5 minutes) up to 17 mg/kg
            (ii) Pediatric IV: 3 to 6 mg/kg given slowly
         (b) **Maintenance dose**
            (i) Adult: IV infusion, 2 mg/kg/hour; PO, 250 to 1,000 mg every 3 hours
            (ii) Children: IV infusion, 20 to 50 µg/kg/min; PO, 30 to 50 mg/kg/day divided in four to six doses
      (2) **Pharmacokinetics**
         Therapeutic plasma level is usually 4 to 10 µg/mL. With bolus administration, the duration of action is 2 to 4 hours. Metabolism is both hepatic (50%, N-acetylprocainamide) and renal. Slow acetylators are more dependent on renal elimination. Patients with reduced renal function require lower maintenance doses and need close monitoring of serum levels and the ECG QT intervals.
      (3) **Adverse effects**
         (a) High serum levels or rapid loading may cause negative inotropic and chronotropic effects, leading to hypotension and hypoperfusion. Overdose may require pacing and/or β-agonist therapy.
         (b) High serum levels of procainamide and/or its principal active metabolite (N-acetylprocainamide) induce QT prolongation and

torsades de pointes. Discontinuation of therapy should be considered if the corrected QT interval exceeds 450 msec.

(c) CNS excitability may occur, with confusion and seizures.

(d) A lupuslike syndrome may be seen with long-term therapy.

b. Amiodarone (Cordarone)

(1) **Dosing**

(a) PO: 800 to 1,600 mg/day for 1 to 3 weeks, gradually reducing dosage to 400 to 600 mg/day for maintenance.

(b) Intravenous:

(i) Loading: For patients in a perfusing rhythm, 150 mg over 10 minutes in repeated boluses until sustained periods of sinus rhythm occur. For patients in pulseless VT/VF, more rapid bolus administration may be warranted. Patients often require two to four or more boluses for a sustained response.

(ii) Maintenance: 1 mg/min for 6 hours, then 0.5 mg/min thereafter, with the goal of providing approximately 1 g/day.

(2) **Pharmacokinetics.** The drug is metabolized hepatically, but has very high lipid solubility that results in marked tissue accumulation. The elimination half-life is 20 to 100 days. Hence, for patients treated chronically, it usually is unnecessary to "reload" amiodarone when doses are missed during surgery, and postoperatively patients usually resume their preoperative dosing.

(3) **Adverse effects**

(a) Amiodarone is an α- and β-receptor noncompetitive antagonist; therefore, it has potent vasodilating effects and can render negative inotropic effects. Hence, vasoconstrictors, IV fluid, and occasionally β-agonists are required for hemodynamic support, especially during the IV amiodarone loading phase.

(b) Amiodarone blocks potassium channels and typically prolongs the QT interval, but is only rarely associated with torsades de pointes. The risk of torsades on amiodarone therapy is poorly correlated with the QT interval, and QT prolongation on amiodarone, if not excessive, usually does not require cessation of therapy.

(c) Amiodarone use may cause sinus bradycardia or heart block due to β-receptor blockade, and patients requiring sustained IV amiodarone therapy sometimes require pacing or low doses of supplemental β-agonists.

(d) The side effects of long-term oral dosing (subacute pulmonary fibrosis, hepatitis, cirrhosis, photosensitivity, corneal microdeposits, hypothyroidism, or hyperthyroidism) are of little concern during short-term (days) of IV therapy.

(e) This drug may increase the effect of oral anticoagulants, phenytoin, digoxin, diltiazem, quinidine, and other drugs.

c. Lidocaine (lignocaine, Xylocaine)

(1) **Dosing**

(a) Loading dose: 1 mg/kg IV, a second dose may be given 10 to 30 minutes after first dose. Loading dose is sometimes doubled for patients on CPB who are experiencing VF before separation. The total dose should not exceed 3 mg/kg.

(b) Maintenance dose: 15 to 50 µg/kg/min (i.e., 1 to 4 mg/min in adults).

(2) **Pharmacokinetics.** Duration of action is 15 to 30 minutes after administration of a bolus dose. Metabolism is hepatic, and 95% of metabolites are inactive. However, for infusions lasting more than 24 hours, serum levels should be monitored. Many factors that reduce hepatic metabolism will increase serum levels, including CHF, α-agonists, liver disease, and advanced age.

(3) **Adverse effects**
  (a) CNS excitation may result from mild-to-moderate overdose, producing confusion or seizures. At higher doses, CNS depression will ensue, producing sedation and respiratory depression.
  (b) Lidocaine, like other antiarrhythmics with sodium channel-blocking properties (amiodarone, procainamide), slows ventricular excitation. Hence, patients with AV nodal block who are dependent upon an idioventricular rhythm may become asystolic during lidocaine therapy.

  d. Bretylium
  (1) **Dosing**
    (a) Loading dose: 5 to 10 mg/kg every 15 to 30 minutes, to a maximum of 30 mg/kg.
    (b) **Maintenance (adults).** IV 5 to 10 mg/kg infused over 10 to 20 minutes every 6 hours, or as a constant infusion 1 to 2 mg/min.
  (2) **Pharmacokinetics.** Duration of action is 6 to 24 hours after a single IV loading dose. Elimination is almost entirely renal excretion of unchanged drug; hence, maintenance dosages should be reduced with renal insufficiency. Plasma level monitoring is not helpful in patient management.
  (3) **Adverse effects**
    (a) Bretylium has complex effects on the autonomic nervous system, causing a transient initial catecholamine release (with a positive inotropic effect and chronotropic effect), followed by postural hypotension, which requires that patients be kept supine.
    (b) The therapeutic effects of IV bretylium may be delayed up to 10 to 20 minutes after a bolus injection.

D. Bradyarrhythmias [7]
  1. Asystole
    a. CPR with cardiac compressions should be instituted immediately. As hypoxemia is a common cause of asystole, efforts to secure the airway and provide oxygenation may be the most critical resuscitation measures.
    b. The ECG recording of VF is sometimes "fine" (low amplitude) and may be confused with asystole. If this is suspected, DC countershocks should be applied.
    c. Definitive therapy consists of ventricular pacing and/or transcutaneous pacing if immediately available (see Chapter 16).
    d. For pharmacologic therapy, useful drugs include atropine (1 mg IV, repeat every 3 to 5 minutes) and epinephrine (1 mg IV push, repeat every 3 to 5 minutes). Isoproterenol infusion may be a poor choice for asystole because of reduced coronary perfusion pressure during CPR.
  2. Heart rate below 40 beats/min
    a. Cardiac compressions may induce VF, so if possible, pharmacologic agents or pacing should be utilized to increase the HR.
    b. Certain persons (i.e., trained athletes) may tolerate HRs near 40 beats/min. Patients with reduced diastolic compliance (aortic stenosis, hypertensive cardiomyopathy, ongoing ischemia) cannot increase SV in response to bradycardia and poorly tolerate extreme bradycardia.
    c. For pharmacologic therapy, useful drugs include atropine, isoproterenol, and epinephrine. *Avoid antiarrhythmics such as lidocaine, procainamide, bretylium, or amiodarone because these agents may slow a ventricular escape rhythm, worsening the bradycardia.*
  3. Drug therapies for bradyarrhythmias [23,24]
    a. Atropine
      (1) **Dosing.** IV bolus: In adults, use 0.4 to 1.0 mg (may repeat); in children, use 0.02 mg/kg (minimum 0.1 mg, maximum 0.4 mg, may repeat).
      (2) **Pharmacokinetics.** The heart rate effects of IV atropine appear within seconds, and the effects last as long as 15 to 30 minutes. When given IM, SC, or PO, offset occurs in approximately 4 hours. There is

minimal metabolism of the drug, and 77% to 94% of it undergoes renal elimination.

    (3) Adverse effects. Atropine is a competitive antagonist at muscarinic cholinergic receptors, and its adverse effects are largely systemic manifestations of this receptor activity.

        (a) Tachycardia (undesirable with coronary disease).

        (b) Exacerbation of bradycardia by low dosages (0.2 mg or less in an adult).

        (c) Sedation (especially in pediatric and elderly patients).

        (d) Urinary retention.

        (e) Increased intraocular pressure in patients with closed-angle glaucoma. Atropine may be safely given, however, if miotic eye drops are given concurrently.

b. Glycopyrrolate (Robinul)

    (1) Dosing (adults). 0.1 mg IV, repeated at 2- to 3-minute intervals.

    (2) Differences from atropine. Less likely to cause sedation, but also less likely to produce tachycardia. This agent often is chosen to manage mild intraoperative bradycardia or as an antagonist to the heart rate slowing effects of neostigmine when reversing neuromuscular blockade. Atropine remains the drug of choice in severe or life-threatening bradycardia.

c. Isoproterenol (Isuprel)

    (1) General features. Isoproterenol is a synthetic catecholamine with direct β_1- and β_2-agonist effects and thus has both positive inotropic (through β_1-mediated enhanced contractility plus β_2-mediated vasodilation) and positive chronotropic effects.

    (2) Dosing. IV infusion is 0.02 to 0.50 µg/kg/min.

    (3) Pharmacokinetics. The agent is used as a continuous infusion and has a short half-life (2 minutes), making it titratable. It is partly metabolized in the liver (MAO, COMT) and partly excreted unchanged (60%).

    (4) Adverse effects

        (a) The major potential adverse effect of isoproterenol is myocardial ischemia in patients with coronary artery disease, because the combination of tachycardia, positive inotropy, and hypotension may create a myocardial oxygen supply/demand mismatch.

        (b) The agent may provoke supraventricular arrhythmias or may unmask preexcitation in patients with an accessory AV conduction pathway (e.g., Wolff–Parkinson–White syndrome).

E. Supraventricular arrhythmias [17]

    1. Therapy-based classification

      a. General. SVT is among the anesthesiologist's most valuable warning signs, often foreshadowing life-threatening conditions that may be correctable. Hence, the initial management of the surgical patient who suddenly develops SVT should not be on heart-directed pharmacologic therapies, but rather on correctable etiologies that may include hypoxemia (O_2 saturation), hypoventilation (end tidal CO_2), hypotension (absolute or relative hypovolemia due to bleeding, anaphylaxis), light anesthesia, electrolyte abnormalities (K^+ or Mg^{2+}), or cardiac ischemia (HR, nitroglycerin).

      b. Hemodynamically unstable patients. Patients with low BP (e.g., systolic BP less than 80 mm Hg), cardiac ischemia, or other evidence of end-organ hypoperfusion require immediate *synchronous* DC cardioversion. Although some patients may only respond transiently to cardioversion in this setting (or not at all), a brief period of sinus rhythm may provide valuable time for correcting the reversible causes of SVT (see earlier) and/or instituting pharmacologic therapies (see later). During cardiac or thoracic surgery, patients may experience SVT during dissection of the pericardium, placement of atrial sutures, or insertion of the venous cannulae required for CPB. If hemodynamically unstable SVT occurs during open thoracotomy, the surgeon should attempt open synchronous cardioversion.

Patients with critical coronary lesions or severe aortic stenosis with SVT may be refractory to cardioversion and thus enter a malignant cascade of ischemia and worsening arrhythmias that requires the institution of CPB. Hence, early preparation for CPB is recommended before inducing anesthesia in cardiac surgery patients judged to be at exceptionally high risk for SVT and consequent hemodynamic deterioration.

c. Hemodynamically stable patients.

    (1) Adenosine therapy (Table 2.4)

        (a) In certain patients, the SVT involves a reentrant pathway involving the AV node. These rhythms typically have a regular R-R interval and are common in relatively healthy patients. Adenosine administered as a 6-mg IV bolus (repeated with 12 mg if no response) may terminate the SVT.

        (b) Many of the rhythms commonly seen in the perioperative period do not involve the AV node in a reentrant pathway, and AV nodal block by adenosine in such cases will produce only transient slowing of the ventricular rate. This may lead to "rebound" speeding of the tachycardia following the adenosine effect. Hence, in cases where the rhythm is recognizable and known to be refractory to adenosine (atrial fibrillation, atrial flutter), adenosine therapy should be avoided. The hallmark of atrial fibrillation is an irregularly irregular R-R interval.

        (c) Junctional tachycardias are common during the surgical period and sometimes convert to sinus rhythm in response to adenosine, depending on the proximity of the site of origin to the AV node. Ventricular arrhythmias exhibit no response to adenosine since these rhythms originate in the ventricle.

    (2) Rate control therapy

        (a) Rationale for rate control. In most cases, ventricular rate control is the mainstay of therapy.

            (i) Lengthening diastole serves to enhance LV filling, thus enhancing SV.

            (ii) Slowing the ventricular rate reduces MVO_2 and lowers the risk of cardiac ischemia.

        (b) Rationale for drug selection. The most common selections are IV β-blockers or calcium channel blockers due to their rapid onset.

            (i) Among the IV β-blockers, esmolol has the most rapid elimination properties, rendering it titratable on a minute-to-minute basis and allowing meaningful dose adjustments during periods of surgery that provoke changes in hemodynamic status (i.e., bleeding, abdominal traction). The drug has obligatory negative inotropic effects that are problematic for patients with severe LV dysfunction.

            (ii) Both IV verapamil and IV diltiazem are calcium channel blockers that are less titratable than esmolol, but nonetheless provide rapid slowing of the ventricular rate in SVT within minutes. Moreover, IV diltiazem has less negative inotropic action than verapamil or esmolol and therefore is preferable in patients with heart failure.

            (iii) IV digoxin slows the ventricular response during SVT through its vagotonic effects at the AV node, but should be temporally supplemented with other IV agents due to its slow onset (approximately 6 hours).

        (c) Accessory pathway rhythms. AV nodal blockade can reduce the ventricular rate in WPW and improve hemodynamic status. However, 10% to 35% of patients with WPW eventually develop atrial fibrillation. In this case, the rapid rate of atrial excitation (greater than 300 impulses/min), normally transmitted to the ventricle after "filtering" by the AV node, instead is transmitted to the ventricle via the accessory bundle at a rapid rate. The danger of inducing VT/VF in this scenario is exacerbated by treatment with classic AV nodal blocking agents (digoxin, calcium channel blockers, β-blockers, adenosine) because they reduce the accessory bundle refractory period. Hence, WPW patients who experience atrial fibrillation should not receive AV nodal blockers. IV procainamide slows conduction over the accessory bundle and is an option for treating AF in patients with accessory pathways.

d. Specific rate control agents [17,23,25]

  (1) Esmolol (Brevibloc)

   (a) Dosing. During surgery and anesthesia, the standard 0.25 to 0.5 mg/kg load (package insert) may be accompanied by marked hypotension. In practice, reduced IV bolus doses of 12.5 to 25 mg are be administered repeatedly and titrated to effect, followed by an infusion of 50 to 200 μg/kg/min. Transient hypotension during the loading phase usually can be managed with IV fluid or vasoconstrictors (phenylephrine).

   (b) Pharmacokinetics. Esmolol is rapidly eliminated by a red blood cell esterase, making it titratable on a minute-to-minute basis. After discontinuation of esmolol, most drug effects are eliminated within 5 minutes. The duration of esmolol action is not affected when plasma pseudocholinesterase is inhibited by echothiophate or physostigmine.

   (c) Adverse effects

    (i) Esmolol is a potent, selective β₁-receptor antagonist. It may cause hypotension through both vasodilation and negative inotropic effects.

    (ii) Compared to nonselective β-blockers, esmolol is less likely to elicit bronchospasm, but should still be used with caution in patients with known bronchospastic disease.

  (2) Verapamil (Isoptin, Calan)

   (a) Dosing

    (i) IV loading (adults): 5 to 15 mg, consider administering in 1- to 2-mg increments during surgery and anesthesia, or in unstable patients. Dose may be repeated after 30 minutes.

    (ii) Maintenance IV: 5 to 15 mg/hour

    (iii) PO (adults): 40 to 80 mg tid to qid (maximum 480 mg/day).

    (iv) Pediatric dose: 75 to 200 μg/kg IV; may be repeated.

   (b) Pharmacokinetics. Elimination occurs by hepatic metabolism, and plasma half-life is 3 to 10 hours, so lengthy intervals (hours) between dose increments for IV infusions should be utilized to avoid cumulative effects.

   (c) Adverse effects

    (i) Verapamil blocks L-type calcium channels and may cause hypotension due to both peripheral vasodilation and negative inotropic effects, especially during the IV loading phase. The vasodilatory effects may be mitigated by administration of IV fluid or vasoconstrictors (i.e., phenylephrine). Patients with severe LV dysfunction may not tolerate IV verapamil and may be better candidates for IV diltiazem (see later).

    (ii) Verapamil (given chronically) reduces digoxin elimination and can raise digoxin levels, producing toxicity.

  (3) Diltiazem (Cardizem)

   (a) Dosing (adult)

    (i) IV loading: 20 mg IV over 2 minutes. May repeat after 15 minutes with 25 mg IV if HR exceeds 110 beats/min. Smaller doses or longer loading periods may be used in patients who have myocardial ischemia or hemodynamic instability, or who are anesthetized.

        (ii) Maintenance: Infusion at 5 to 15 mg/hour, depending on HR control.

        (iii) PO dose: 120 to 360 mg/day (sustained-release preparations are available).

    (b) Pharmacokinetics. Metabolism is both hepatic (60%) and renal excretion (35%). Plasma elimination half-life is 3 to 5 hours, so lengthy intervals (hours) between dose increases for IV infusions should be utilized to avoid cumulative effects.

    (c) Adverse effects

        (i) Diltiazem, like all calcium channel blockers, elicits vasodilation and may evoke hypotension. At the same time, partly due to its afterload reducing properties, IV diltiazem is less likely to compromise CO in patients with reduced LV function (relative to other AV nodal blockers) and is the drug of choice for rate control in this circumstance.

        (ii) Sinus bradycardia is possible, so diltiazem should be used with caution in patients with sinus node dysfunction or those also receiving digoxin or β-blockers.

  (4) High-dose IV magnesium

    (a) Dosing. Regimens including a 2- to 2.5-g initial bolus, followed by a 1.75 g/hour infusion, are described.

    (b) Issues with use. High-dose magnesium is used rarely for SVT, but nonetheless may successfully provide rate control for patients with SVT. In some cases, rates of conversion to sinus rhythm exceeding placebo or antiarrhythmic agents have been noted. *The use of these high magnesium doses requires close monitoring of serum levels and should be avoided in patients with renal insufficiency.* An increased requirement for temporary pacing due to the AV nodal blockade also has been noted.

2. Cardioversion of SVT [17]

  a. Limitations of pharmacologic or "chemical" cardioversion

    (1) The 24-hour rate of spontaneous conversion to sinus rhythm for recent-onset perioperative SVT exceeds 50%. Many patients who develop SVT under anesthesia will remit spontaneously within hours of emergence.

    (2) Most of the antiarrhythmic agents with activity against atrial arrhythmias have limited efficacy when utilized in IV form for rapid chemical conversion. Although 50% to 80% efficacy rates are cited for many IV antiarrhythmics in uncontrolled studies, these findings are largely an artifact of high placebo rates of conversion (approximately 60% over 24 hours). Although improved rates of chemical cardioversion are seen with high doses of IV amiodarone (about 2g/day), the potential for undesirable side effects in the perioperative setting requires further study.

    (3) Most agents have adverse effects, including negative inotropic effects or vasodilation (amiodarone, procainamide, bretylium). In addition, these agents may provoke polymorphic ventricular arrhythmias (torsades de pointes). Although less common with amiodarone, newer IV agents that exhibit high efficacy for converting atrial fibrillation (i.e., ibutilide) exhibit rates of torsades as high as 8%.

  b. Rationale for cardioversion. In the operating room, chemical cardioversion should be aimed mainly at patients who cannot tolerate (or do not respond to) IV rate control therapy, or who fail DC cardioversion and remain hemodynamically unstable. Intraoperative elective DC cardioversion in an otherwise stable patient with SVT also carries inherent risks (VF, asystole, stroke). Moreover, the underlying factors provoking SVT during or shortly after surgery are likely to persist beyond the time of cardioversion, inviting recurrence. Hence, when elective DC cardioversion is considered, it may be prudent to first establish a therapeutic level of an antiarrhythmic agent that maintains sinus rhythm (i.e., procainamide, amiodarone), with a view to preventing SVT recurrence following electrical cardioversion. Guidelines for administration of IV procainamide and amiodarone were provided earlier (see Section VIII, C4).

3. **SVT prophylaxis for postoperative patients** [17,26]
SVT may occur during the days following surgery and occurs within the first 4 postoperative days in up to 40% of cardiac surgeries. Many postoperative prophylaxis regimens have been evaluated and are discussed in recent reviews. Prophylactic administration of a number of drugs typically used to slow AV nodal conduction (β-blockers, calcium channel blockers) may slightly reduce the incidence of postoperative atrial fibrillation but by no means eliminate the problem. At the same time, the antiarrhythmic agents (sotalol, amiodarone) may be more effective, but concerns regarding adverse effects and/or cost have limited their use, and risk/benefit analyses from multicenter trials are needed. Nonetheless, antiarrhythmic prophylaxis should be considered in selected patients at high risk for hemodynamic or ischemic complications from postoperative SVT. **Table 2.6 summarizes treatment for cardiac arrhythmias.**

IX. **Diuretics** [23,24].
A. **Actions.** Most IV diuretics act at the loop of Henle in the kidney to block resorption of electrolytes from the tubule. This action increases excretion of water and electrolytes (Na, Cl, K, Ca, Mg) from the body.
B. **Effects shared by all loop diuretics**
  1. **Hypokalemia**
  2. **Metabolic alkalosis**
  3. **Increased serum uric acid**
  4. **Ototoxicity.** Deafness, temporary or permanent, occurs rarely with ethacrynic acid but has also been reported with furosemide or bumetanide. Coadministration with an aminoglycoside antibiotic may increase risk. One possible

Table 2.6 IV drug therapy for arrhythmias

Cardiac origin	Arrhythmia subtype	Intravenous drug therapy
Supraventricular	SVTs (regular R-R interval)	Trial of adenosine, then other AV blockers (caution in WPW patients with AF); consider procainamide or amiodarone
	Atrial fibrillation, atrial flutter	1. Rate control with AV blockers (diltiazem, verapamil, β-blockers) 2. Maintenance of SR (in combination with synchronous cardioversion): amiodarone, procainamide 3. Ibutilide for rapid cardioversion (caution: risk of polymorphic VT)
Ventricular	Nonsustained VT	1. No drug therapy if HD stable 2. Lidocaine, β-blockade (if tolerates), or amiodarone if NSVT causes HD instability
	Monomorphic VT	Amiodarone, procainamide
	Polymorphic VT (long QT)	Mg^{2+}, K^+, and isoproterenol or pacing to raise HR. Discontinue offending QT-prolonging agent.
	VF, polymorphic VT (normal QT)	Amiodarone, procainamide

AV, atrioventricular; HD, hemodynamics; HR, heart rate; SR, sinus rhythm; SVT, supraventricular tachycardias; VF, ventricular fibrillation; VT, ventricular tachycardia; WPW, Wolff–Parkinson–White syndrome.

mechanism for this is drug-induced changes in endolymph electrolyte composition.

C. Specific drugs

1. Furosemide (Lasix)

a. **Pharmacokinetics.** Renal tubular secretion of unchanged drug and of glucuronide metabolite. Half-life of 1.5 hours.

b. **Clinical use**

(1) **Dosing**

(a) Adults: The usual IV starting dose for patients not currently receiving diuretics is 2.5 to 5.0 mg, increasing as necessary to a 200-mg bolus. Patients already receiving diuretics usually require 20- to 40-mg initial doses to produce a diuresis. A continuous infusion (0.5 to 1.0 mg/kg/hour) at approximately 0.05 mg/kg/hour in adults produces a more sustained diuresis with a lower total daily dose compared with intermittent bolus dosing.

(b) Pediatric: 1 mg/kg (maximum, 6 mg/kg). The pediatric infusion rate is 0.2 to 0.4 mg/kg/hour.

(2) Because furosemide is a sulfonamide, allergic reactions may occur in sulfonamide-sensitive patients (rare).

(3) Furosemide often causes transient vasodilation of veins and arterioles, with reduced cardiac preload.

2. Bumetanide (Bumex)

a. **Pharmacokinetics.** Combined renal and hepatic elimination. Half-life is 1 to 1.5 hours.

b. **Clinical use**

(1) **Dosing.** 0.5 to 1.0 mg IV, may be repeated every 2 to 3 hours to a maximum dose of 10 mg/day.

(2) Myalgias may occur.

3. Ethacrynic acid (Edecrin)

a. **Pharmacokinetics.** Combined renal and hepatic elimination.

b. **Clinical use**

(1) **Dosing.** 50 mg IV (adult dose) or 0.5 to 1.0 mg/kg (maximum 100 mg) titrated to effect.

(2) Usually reserved for patients who fail to respond to furosemide or bumetanide.

4. Mannitol

a. **Mechanism/pharmacokinetics.** Mannitol is an osmotic diuretic that is eliminated unchanged in urine. It also is a free-radical scavenger.

b. **Clinical use**

(1) Unlike the loop diuretics (e.g., furosemide), mannitol retains its efficacy even during low glomerular filtration states (e.g., shock).

(2) Diuresis with this agent may have protective effects in some clinical scenarios (i.e., CPB, poor renal perfusion, hemoglobinuria, or nephrotoxins).

(3) As an osmotically active agent in the bloodstream, it is sometimes used to reduce cerebral edema.

c. **Dosing.** Initial dose is 12.5 g IV to a maximum of 0.5 g/kg.

d. **Adverse effects**

(1) May produce hypotension if administered as a rapid IV bolus.

(2) May induce transient CHF as intravascular volume may expand before diuresis begins.

References

1. *Physician's desk reference, 55th ed.* Montvale, NJ: Medical Economics Company, 2001.
2. Epocrates: http://**www.epocrates.com**.
3. Hardman JG, Limbird LE. *Goodman & Gilman's: the pharmacological basis of therapeutics,* 9th ed. New York: McGraw-Hill, 2001.
4. **Drug Facts and Comparisons 2001 (an annual publication).**

5. *The Medical Letter.* New Rochelle, NY: The Medical Letter, Inc. (biweekly publication).
6. **Shargel L, Yu ABC. *Applied biopharmaceutics and pharmacokinetics,* 4th ed. Stamford, CT: Appleton & Lange, 1999.**
7. Gibaldi M, Perrier D. *Pharmacokinetics,* 2nd ed, rev. New York: Marcel Dekker, 1982.
8. Butterworth JF IV, Prielipp RC, MacGregor DA, et al. Pharmacologic cardiovascular support. In: Kvetan V, Dantzker DR, eds. *The critically ill cardiac patient: multisystem dysfunction and management.* Philadelphia: Lippincott-Raven, 1996:167–192.
9. Chugh SS, Lurie KG, Lindner KH. Pressor with promise. Using vasopressin in cardiac arrest. *Circulation* 1997;96:2453–2454.
10. The American Heart Association in collaboration with the International Liaison Committee on Resuscitation (ILCOR). Guidelines 2000 for cardiopulmonary resuscitation and emergency cardiovascular care. Part 6: advanced cardiovascular life support, section 6: pharmacology II: agents to optimize cardiac output and blood pressure. *Circulation* 2000; 102: I-129–I-35.
11. Butterworth JF IV, Prielipp RC, Royster RL, et al. Dobutamine increases heart rate more than epinephrine in patients recovering from aortocoronary bypass surgery. *J Cardiothorac Vasc Anesth* 1992;6:535–541.
12. Brooker RF, Butterworth JF IV, Kitzman DW, et al. Treatment of hypotension after hyperbaric tetracaine spinal anesthesia: a randomized, double-blind, cross-over comparison of phenylephrine and epinephrine. *Anesthesiology* 1997;86:797–805.
13. Butterworth JF IV, Hines RL, Royster RL, et al. A pharmacokinetic and pharmacodynamic evaluation of milrinone in adults undergoing cardiac surgery. *Anesth Analg* 1995;81:783–792.
14. Zaloga GP, Strickland RA, Butterworth JF IV, et al. Calcium attenuates epinephrine's beta-adrenergic effects in postoperative heart surgery patients. *Circulation* 1990;81: 196–200.
15. Figgitt DP, Gillies PS, Goa KL. Levosimendan. *Drugs* 2001;61:613–627.
16. Friederich JA, Butterworth JF IV. Sodium nitroprusside: twenty years and counting. *Anesth Analg* 1995;81:152–162.
17. **Balser JR. Pharmacologic management of arrhythmias. In: Estafanous FG, Barash PG, Reves JG, eds. *Cardiac anesthesia: principles and clinical practice,* 2nd ed. Philadelphia: Lippincott Williams & Wilkins, 2001:103–116.**
18. Task Force of the Working Group on Arrhythmias of the European Society of Cardiology. Sicilian Gambit: a new approach to the classification of antiarrhythmic drugs based on their actions on arrhythmogenic mechanisms. *Circulation* 1992;84:1831–1851.
19. Priori SG, Barhanin J, Hauer RN, et al. Genetic and molecular basis of cardiac arrhythmias: impact on clinical management, parts I and II. *Circulation* 1999;99:518–528.
20. O'Kelly B, Browner WS, Massie B, et al. Ventricular arrhythmias in patients undergoing noncardiac surgery. *JAMA* 1992;268:217–221.
21. **The American Heart Association in collaboration with the International Liaison Committee on Resuscitation (ILCOR). Guidelines 2000 for cardiopulmonary resuscitation and emergency cardiovascular care. Part 6: advanced cardiovascular life support: section 5: pharmacology I: agents for arrhythmias. *Circulation* 2000;102:I-112–I-128.**
22. Kudenchuk PJ, Cobb LA, Copass MK, et al. Amiodarone for resuscitation after out-of-hospital cardiac arrest due to ventricular fibrillation. *N Engl J Med* 1999;341:871–878.
23. Larach DR, Solina AR. Cardiovascular drugs. In: Hensley FA, Martin DE, eds. *A practical approach to cardiac anesthesia,* 2nd ed. Boston: Little, Brown and Company; 1995: 32–95.
24. **Roden DM. Antiarrhythmic drugs. In: Hardman JG, Limbird LE, eds. *Goodman and Gilman's: the pharmacological basis of therapeutics,* 9th ed. New York: McGraw-Hill, 1996:839–874.**
25. Balser JR, Clarke AW, Winters BD, et al. Beta blockade is superior to calcium channel blockade for conversion of postoperative SVT. *Anesthesiology* 1998;89:1052–1059.
26. Balser J. Pro: all patients should receive pharmacologic prophylaxis for atrial fibrillation following cardiac surgery. *J Cardiothorac Vasc Anesth* 1998;13:1–3.

3. MONITORING THE CARDIAC SURGICAL PATIENT

Thomas M. Skeehan and Michael Jopling

Patients presenting for cardiac surgery require extensive monitoring because of (a) severe, often unstable cardiovascular disease; (b) coexisting multisystemic diseases; (c) the unphysiologic conditions associated with cardiopulmonary bypass (CPB); and (d) special considerations for minimally invasive cardiac surgery. Monitoring techniques have been developed to provide early warning of conditions that may lead to potentially life-threatening complications. This chapter provides a system-by-system discussion of the indications, applications, and techniques of currently available monitoring modalities as well as their advantages, disadvantages, and complications.

I. Cardiovascular monitors

A. Electrocardiogram. The intraoperative use of the electrocardiogram (ECG) has increased during the last several decades. Originally, this monitor was used during anesthesia for the detection of dysrhythmias only in high-risk patients. However, its importance as a standard monitor has been recognized, and its use during any anesthetic now is recommended. Its usefulness for the intraoperative diagnosis of myocardial ischemia now is well established.

1. Indications

a. Diagnosis of dysrhythmias

b. Diagnosis of ischemia (see Chapter 11). In the anesthetized patient, the detection of ischemia by ECG becomes more important because the usual symptom, angina, cannot be elicited (see Fig. 11.5) (for characteristic patterns of ECG detection of ischemia).

c. Diagnosis of conduction defects

d. Diagnosis of electrolyte disturbances

2. Techniques

a. The three-electrode system. This system utilizes electrodes only on the right arm, left arm, and left leg. The potential difference between two of the electrodes is recorded, while the third electrode serves as a ground. One pair of electrodes can be selected for monitoring at one time; therefore, three ECG leads (I, II, III) can be examined.

The three-lead system has been expanded to include the augmented leads. It identifies one of the three leads as the exploring electrode and couples the remaining two at a central terminal with zero potential. This creates leads in three more axes (aVR, aVL, aVF) in the frontal plane (Fig. 3.1). Leads II, III, and aVF are most useful for monitoring the inferior wall, and leads I and aVL for the lateral wall; however, the anterior wall cannot be monitored using these leads.

b. The modified three-electrode system. Numerous modifications of the standard bipolar limb lead system have been developed (Table 3.1). Modified leads can be used to maximize P-wave height for the diagnosis of atrial dysrhythmias or to increase the sensitivity of the three-lead ECG for the detection of anterior myocardial ischemia. In clinical studies, these modified three-electrode systems have been shown to be as sensitive as the standard V_5 lead system for the intraoperative diagnosis of ischemia. However, the use of only three electrodes limits the areas (anterior, inferior, or lateral walls) that can be simultaneously monitored; thus, modified leads are not routinely used in the cardiac operating room.

c. The five-electrode system. Use of five electrodes (one lead on each extremity and one precordial lead) allows the simultaneous recording of the six standard frontal limb leads as well as one precordial unipolar lead. All limb leads act as a common ground for the precordial unipolar lead. The unipolar lead usually is placed in the V_5 position, along the anterior axillary line in the fifth intercostal space, to best monitor the left ventricle (LV). The precordial lead also can be placed on the right precordium to monitor the right ventricle (RV; V_{4R} lead).

(1) Advantages. With the addition of only two electrodes to the ECG system, seven different leads can be monitored simultaneously. More important, all but the posterior wall of the myocardium can be monitored for ischemia. In patients with coronary artery disease, it has

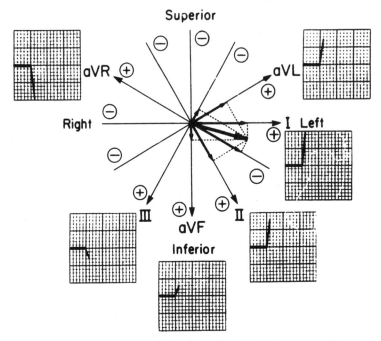

FIG. 3.1 The six frontal plane axes that are available from three leads (right arm, left arm, and left leg) are shown. I, II, and III are bipolar leads, meaning that the potential between two electrodes (one positive, one negative) is monitored. The augmented leads (*aVR, aVL,* and *aVF*) are unipolar leads; one lead is the exploring electrode (the positive terminal), and the other two are connected and set at zero potential (indifferent, or neutral). The potential difference is then the absolute difference between the exploring and zero terminals. Connecting the two indifferent leads together produces the augmented lead axes that are between the bipolar lead axes. A sample electrical vector is shown (*heavy arrow*), with its projections to the six frontal axes. The direction of the electrical vector, then, is dictated by the direction of the deflection seen on the axis of each particular lead of the surface ECG. (From Thys DM, Kaplan JA. *The ECG in anesthesia and critical care.* New York: Churchill Livingstone, 1987:5, with permission.)

been shown that the unipolar V_5 lead is the best single lead in diagnosing myocardial ischemia [1]; moreover, 90% of ischemic episodes will be detected by ECG if leads II and V_5 are analyzed simultaneously [2]. Therefore, a correctly placed V_5 lead in conjunction with limb leads should enhance the diagnosis of the vast majority of intraoperative ischemic events. Multiple ECG leads also are useful in the diagnosis of atrial and ventricular dysrhythmias.

(2) **Disadvantage.** The V_5 electrode should not interfere with the operative field for a median sternotomy, although it certainly will interfere with a left thoracotomy incision. The four limb leads should be placed on the back of the shoulders and hips, where they will be disturbed the least during median sternotomy. The V_5 lead, as well as the two leg leads, should be well protected with waterproof tape, as surgical preparation solutions will loosen electrode patches and interfere with the electrical signal.

Table 3.1 Bipolar and augmented leads for use with three electrodes

Lead identifier	Right arm electrode	Left arm electrode	Left leg electrode	Lead select	Useful for diagnosing
Standard					
I	Right arm	Left arm	Ground	I	Lateral ischemia
II	Right arm	Ground	Left leg	II	Dysrhythmias (maximal P wave and QRS height); inferior ischemia
III	Ground	Left arm	Left leg	III	Inferior ischemia
Augmented					
aVR	Right arm	Common ground	Common ground	aVR	Lateral ischemia
aVL	Common ground	Left arm	Common ground	aVL	Lateral ischemia
aVF	Common ground	Common ground	Left leg	aVF	Inferior ischemia
Special					
MCL$_1$	Ground	Under left clavicle	V$_1$ position	III	Dysrhythmias (maximal P wave and QRS height)
CS$_5$	Under right clavicle	V$_5$ position	Ground	I	Anterior ischemia
CM$_5$	Manubrium sternum	V$_5$ position	Ground	I	Anterior ischemia
CB$_5$	Center of right scapula	V$_5$ position	Ground	I	Anterior ischemia; dysrhythmia (maximal P wave)
CC$_5$	Right anterior axillary line	V$_5$ position	Ground	I	Global ischemia

Modified from Griffin RM, Kaplan JA. ECG lead systems. In: Thys D, Kaplan J, eds. *The ECG in anesthesia and critical care.* New York: Churchill Livingstone, 1987:20.

d. Invasive ECG

(1) Esophageal. Esophageal leads can be incorporated into the esophageal stethoscope and are very useful for the diagnosis of atrial dysrhythmias. The relative ease and safety of the esophageal ECG lead have been demonstrated. In addition, the esophageal lead is sensitive for the detection of posterior wall ischemia.

(2) Endotracheal. ECG leads have been incorporated into the endotracheal tube and may be useful in pediatric cardiac patients for the diagnosis of atrial dysrhythmias.

(3) Multipurpose pulmonary artery (PA) catheter. The multipurpose PA catheter has all the features of a standard PA catheter (see Section **F**). In addition, three atrial and two ventricular electrodes have been incorporated into the catheter. These electrodes allow not only recording of intracavitary ECGs but also atrial or atrioventricular (AV) pacing. A selective ECG can be recorded to diagnose atrial, ventricular, or AV nodal dysrhythmias or conduction blocks.

(4) Epicardial electrodes. Cardiac surgeons routinely place ventricular and/or atrial epicardial pacing wires before weaning the patient from CPB or before sternal closure. Although the primary intent of these wires is to allow AV pacing in the postbypass period, they also can be utilized to record atrial and ventricular epicardial ECGs. These leads are most useful in the postoperative diagnosis of complex conduction problems and dysrhythmias (see Chapter 10).

3. Recording and interpretation. To utilize fully the capabilities of ECG monitoring, particular attention must be paid to the elimination of major sources of artifact and error.

a. Patient–electrode interface. The electrical signal generated by the heart and monitored by the ECG is very weak, amounting to only 0.5 to 2.0 mV at the skin surface. It is imperative that the skin be prepared optimally to avoid signal loss at the skin–electrode interface. The skin should be clean and free of all dirt, and it is best to abrade the skin lightly to remove part of the stratum corneum, which can be a source of high resistance. Skin resistance can be as great as 1,000,000 Ω (ohms). To avoid the problem of muscle artifact, electrodes should not be placed over large muscle masses whenever possible.

b. Electrodes. Electrodes should all be of the silver chloride type to avoid a resistance mismatch between various kinds of electrodes. Needle electrodes should be avoided at all times because of the risk of thermal injury related to cautery use.

c. Leads and connecting cables

(1) Insulation. The main source of artifact from ECG leads is loss of integrity of the insulation on leads and connecting cables.

(2) Motion artifact. Lead movement will lead to artifact, which can be minimized by twisting the leads on themselves.

(3) Crossing cables. Crossing other monitoring cables (especially the pulse oximeter cable, which transmits an amplified signal) over the ECG leads may cause significant interference.

d. Electronic filtering system. Modern ECG monitors have electronic filters to decrease environmental artifacts. They usually can operate in two modes, each with a different frequency response:

(1) The monitoring mode (0.5 to 40.0 Hz) eliminates both low- and high-frequency artifacts such as wandering baseline but also distorts the height of the QRS complex and the degree of ST-segment depression or elevation.

(2) The diagnostic mode (0.05 to 100.00 Hz) does not filter the higher-frequency signals but is more subject to artifact. The ECG in diagnostic mode will reflect abnormal (i.e., ischemic) changes accurately.

e. Display. ECG displays are commonly of the cathode ray, oscilloscope type, although newer flat screen monitors are becoming popular because of their narrow profile. Calibration of the trace with the 1-mV calibration signal is necessary to interpret ST-segment changes properly. A calibrated strip chart recording of the ECG should be available so that a more careful analysis of dysrhythmias and ST-segment abnormalities can be performed.

    f. Computer-assisted ECG interpretation. Computer programs for on-line analysis of dysrhythmias and ischemia currently are available, but the accuracy of this technology in the cardiac operating room has not been completely validated. One study demonstrated a 60% to 78% sensitivity in detecting ischemia compared with the Holter monitor; the authors suggested that relying solely on automated ST-segment trend data was not warranted [3].

4. Risks associated with ECG. Patient risk with skin electrodes should be minimal as long as needle electrodes are not utilized. Even the more invasive forms of ECG monitoring, such as esophageal, endotracheal, and intracavitary recordings, are safe provided the patient is protected from microshock, as discussed later in this chapter.

5. Recommendations for ECG monitoring. It is recommended that for cardiac surgical anesthesia, a five-electrode surface ECG monitor be used in the diagnostic mode. Ideally, this monitor should be able to display at least two leads simultaneously. Use of two simultaneous leads to monitor two different areas of myocardium supplied by two different coronary arteries facilitates the diagnosis of dysrhythmias and increases the ability to detect ischemia. None of the standard ECG leads can detect posterior wall ischemia. Likewise, RV ischemia usually is undetected unless a right-sided precordial lead is used, but this should be reserved for individual cases. If a more detailed ECG is required postoperatively, the epicardial atrial and ventricular wires can be used. If these wires are not available, other methods of invasive ECG monitoring should be considered. A hard copy of ECG patterns should be available for more accurate diagnoses.

B. Noninvasive blood pressure monitors

1. Indications in the cardiac patient. Usually, noninvasive methods for measuring blood pressure (BP) are not adequate for monitoring hemodynamic parameters during a cardiac surgical procedure, especially one that involves CPB. Because of the following limitations, they often are used merely as adjuncts to invasive BP monitoring.

    a. Inaccuracy. Inaccurate measurements occur, especially at extremes of hypertension or hypotension.

    b. Intermittent data. BP measurements are provided only every 1 to 2 minutes.

    c. Requirement for pulsatile flow. These methods cannot be used during nonpulsatile CPB.

2. Techniques. Noninvasive BP detection relies on the principle of pulsatile flow. If a cuff is applied to a limb and inflated to a pressure greater than systolic, flow to the arteries distal to the occlusion is reduced to zero. As the cuff pressure is released slowly through the systolic and then diastolic pressure, characteristic changes occur in pressure or flow distal to the cuff. These changes can be detected by one of four methods: (i) auscultation of the classic Korotkoff sounds; (ii) microprocessor-assisted interpretation of the oscillations within the cuff (Fig. 3.2); (iii) measurement of shifts in frequency of an ultrasonic beam directed at the brachial artery; and (iv) changes in the plethysmographic signal of the finger with a small occluding cuff. Of these methods, the oscillometric is the most commonly used in clinical practice.

3. Risks of noninvasive BP measurement. In addition to compression-related injuries from noninvasive BP measurements, another potential risk to the patient lies in the clinician's aggressive treatment of an inaccurate BP reading. All noninvasive BP methods are prone to artifacts that should be checked before they are accepted.

4. Recommendations for noninvasive BP measurement. The availability of an indirect BP measurement is desirable during all cardiac surgical procedures.

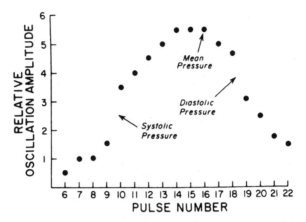

FIG. 3.2 The noninvasive oscillatory blood pressure technique measures the amplitude of oscillation in the cuff pressure itself during the time the cuff is cycling. The cuff first is inflated to suprasystolic pressures; during this time, only weak pressure fluctuations in the proximal portion of the cuff are sensed from the proximal, nonoccluded segment of the artery. As the pressure is decreased, oscillations in cuff pressure increase in amplitude as distal portions of the artery begin to pulse. A sudden, large increase in the oscillation amplitude has been correlated with systolic pressure. As mean arterial pressure is reached, the oscillation amplitude reaches a peak and thereafter declines. As the pressure on the cuff is decreased, a sudden decrease in oscillation amplitude occurs, which correlates with diastolic pressure. This system can be microprocessor controlled and automated and can function in a noisy environment. (Modified from Apple HP. Automatic noninvasive blood pressure monitors: what is available? In: Gravenstein JS, et al., eds. *Essential noninvasive monitoring in anesthesia.* New York: Grune & Stratton, 1980:11.)

It can serve as a backup for the intraarterial system and may prove very useful before invasive monitoring is established and in the immediate postbypass period when the direct **radial** arterial pressure measurement may be falsely low. In order *not* to interfere with a direct form of measurement, noninvasive BP should be obtained in the contralateral limb.

  C. **Intravascular pressure measurements.** In cardiac anesthesia, it is very common to measure pressures within blood vessels directly. Arterial pressure often is measured by placing a catheter in a peripheral artery, while other catheters are placed within the central circulation to measure the central venous or intracardiac pressures. The components of a system of intravascular pressure measurement are the intravascular catheter, fluid-filled connector tubing, a transducer, and an electronic analyzer and display system.

    1. **Characteristics of a pressure waveform.** Pressure waves in the cardiovascular system can be characterized as complex periodic sine waves. These complex waves are a summation of a series of simple sine waves of differing amplitudes and frequencies, which represent the natural harmonics of a fundamental frequency. The first harmonic, or fundamental frequency, is equal to the heart rate (Fig. 3.3), and the first ten harmonics of the fundamental frequency will contribute significantly to the waveform.

    2. **Properties of a monitoring system**

      a. **Frequency response** (or **amplitude ratio**) is the ratio of the measured amplitude versus the input amplitude of a signal at a specific frequency. In a good monitoring system, the frequency response should be constant over the desired range of input frequencies—that is, the signal is not dis-

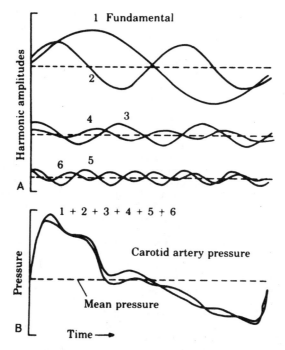

FIG. 3.3 A: Generation of the harmonic waveforms from the fundamental frequency (heart rate) by Fourier analysis. **B:** The first six harmonics are shown. The addition of the six harmonics reproduces an actual blood pressure wave. The first six harmonics are superimposed, showing a likeness to, but not a faithful reproduction of, the original wave. The first ten harmonics of a pressure wave must be sensed by a catheter–transducer system, if that system is to provide an accurate reproduction of the wave. (From Welch JP, D'Ambra MN. Hemodynamic monitoring. In: Kofke WA, Levy JH, eds. *Postoperative critical care procedures of the Massachusetts General Hospital.* Boston: Little, Brown and Company, 1986:146, with permission.)

torted (amplified or diminished). The ideal amplitude ratio is close to 1. The signal frequency range of an intravascular pressure wave response is determined by the heart rate. For example, if a patient's heart rate is 120 beats/min, the fundamental frequency is 2 Hz. Because the first ten harmonics contribute to the arterial waveform, frequencies up to 20 Hz will contribute to the morphology of an arterial waveform at this heart rate.

   b. Natural frequency (or **resonant frequency),** a property of all matter, refers to the frequency at which a monitoring system itself resonates and amplifies the signal. The natural frequency (f_n) of a monitoring system is directly proportional to the catheter lumen diameter *(D),* inversely proportional to the square root of the tubing connection length *(L),* inversely proportional to the square root of the system compliance **($\Delta V/\Delta P$),** and inversely proportional to the square root of the density of fluid contained in the system **(δ).** This is expressed as follows:

$$f_n \propto D \cdot L^{-1/2} \cdot (\Delta V/\Delta P)^{-1/2} \cdot \delta^{-1/2}$$

To increase f_n and thereby reduce distortion, it is imperative that a pressure-sensing system be composed of short, low-compliance tubing of reasonable diameter, filled with a low-density fluid (such as water).

Ideally, the natural frequency of the measuring system should be at least ten times the fundamental frequency to reproduce the first ten harmonics of the pressure wave without distortion. In clinical practice, the natural frequency of most measuring systems is in the range from 10 to 20 Hz. If the input frequency is close to the system's natural frequency (which is usually the case in clinical situations), the system's response will be amplified (Fig. 3.4). Therefore, these systems require the correct amount of **damping** to minimize distortion.

   c. The **damping coefficient** reflects the rate of dissipation of the energy of a pressure wave. This property can be altered to decrease the erroneous amplification of an underdamped system or increase the frequency response of an overdamped system. Figure 3.5 shows the relationship among frequency response, natural frequency, and damping coefficient.

When a pressure-monitoring system with a certain natural frequency duplicates a complex waveform with any one of the first ten harmonics close to the natural frequency of the system, amplification will result if correct damping of the catheter–transducer unit is not performed. The problem is compounded when the heart rate is fast (as in a child or a patient with a rapid atrial rhythm), which increases the demands of the system by increasing the input frequency (Fig. 3.6). **Correct damping of a pressure-monitoring system should not affect the natural frequency of the system.**

Both the natural frequency and the damping coefficient of a system can be estimated using an adaptation of the square wave method known as the "pop" test. The natural frequency is estimated by measuring the time period

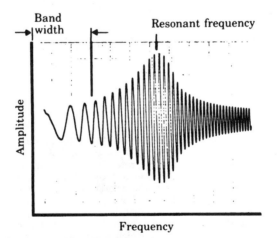

FIG. 3.4 Pressure recording from a pressure generator simulator, which emits a sine wave at increasing frequencies (*horizontal axis*). The frequency response (ratio of signal amplitude$_{OUT}$ to signal amplitude$_{IN}$) is plotted on the vertical axis for a typical catheter–transducer system. The useful band width (range of frequency producing a "flat" response) and the amplification of the signal in the frequency range near the natural frequency of the system are shown. (From Welch JP, D'Ambra MN. Hemodynamic monitoring. In: Kofke WA, Levy JH, eds. *Postoperative critical care procedures of the Massachusetts General Hospital*. Boston: Little, Brown and Company, 1986:148, with permission.)

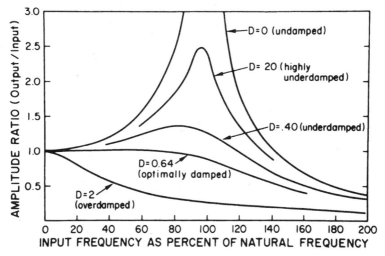

FIG. 3.5 Amplitude ratio (or frequency response) on the vertical axis is plotted as a function of the input frequency as a percentage of the natural frequency (rather than as absolute values). In the undamped or underdamped system, the signal output is amplified in the region of the natural frequency of the transducer system; in the overdamped system, a reduction in amplitude ratio for most input frequencies is seen. This plot exhibits several important points. (i) If a catheter–transducer system has a high natural frequency, less damping will be required to produce a flat response in the clinically relevant range of input frequencies (10 to 30 Hz). (ii) For systems with a natural frequency in the clinically relevant range (usual case), a level of "critical" (optimal) damping exists that will maintain a flat frequency response. (From Grossman W. *Cardiac catheterization,* 3rd ed. Philadelphia: Lea & Febiger, 1985:122, with permission.)

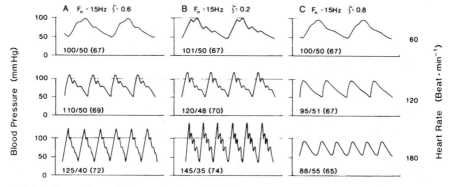

FIG. 3.6 Comparison of three catheter–transducer systems with the same natural frequency (15 Hz) under different conditions of heart rate. Pressures are displayed as systolic-diastolic (mean). The reference blood pressure for all panels is 100/50. **A:** A critically damped system ($\zeta = 0.6$) provides an accurate reproduction until higher heart rates (greater than 150) are reached. **B:** An underdamped system ($\zeta = 0.2$) shows distortion at lower rates, leading to overestimation of systolic and underestimation of diastolic pressures. **C:** An overdamped system ($\zeta = 0.8$) demonstrates underestimation of systolic pressure and overestimation of diastolic pressure. Note also that diastolic and mean pressures are affected less by the inadequate monitoring systems. f_n, natural frequency; ζ, damping coefficient.

of one oscillation as the system settles to baseline after a high-pressure flush. The damping coefficient is calculated by measuring the amplitude ratio of two successive peaks (Fig. 3.7).

After a rapid pressure change, an underdamped system will continue to oscillate for a long period of time. In terms of pressure monitoring, this translates to an overestimation of systolic BP and an underestimation of diastolic BP. An overdamped system will not oscillate at all but will settle to baseline slowly, thus underestimating systolic and overestimating diastolic pressures. A critically damped system will settle to baseline after only one or two oscillations and will reproduce systolic pressures accurately. An optimally or *critically* damped system will exhibit a constant (or *flat*) frequency response in the range of frequencies up to the f_n of the system (Fig. 3.5). If a given system does not meet this criterion, components should be checked, especially for air, or the system replaced. Even an optimally damped system will begin to distort the waveform at higher heart rates because the tenth harmonic exceeds the system's natural frequency (Fig. 3.6).

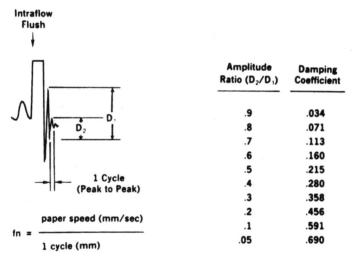

FIG. 3.7 The "pop" test allows one to derive f_n and ζ of a catheter–transducer system. The test should be done with the catheter in the artery in order to test the system in its entirety, as all components contribute to the harmonics of the system. The test involves a rapid flush (with the high-pressure flush system used commonly), followed by a sudden release. This produces a rapid decrease from the flush bag pressure and, owing to the inertia of the system, an overshoot of the baseline. The subsequent oscillations about the baseline are used to calculate f_n and ζ. For example, the arterial pulse at the far left of the figure is followed by a fast flush and sudden release. The resulting oscillations have a definite period, or cycle, measured in millimeters. The natural frequency f_n is the paper speed divided by this period, expressed in cycles per second, or Hertz. If the period were 2 mm and the paper speed 25 mm/sec, $f_n =$ 12.5 Hz. For determining f_n, a faster paper speed will give better reliability. The ratio of the amplitude of one induced resonant wave to the next, D_2/D_1, is used to calculate damping coefficients **(right column).** A damping coefficient of 0.2 to 0.4 describes an underdamped system, 0.4 to 0.6 an optimally damped system, and 0.6 to 0.8 an overdamped system. (From Bedford RF. Invasive blood pressure monitoring. In: Blitt CD, ed. *Monitoring in anesthesia and critical care medicine.* New York: Churchill Livingstone, 1985:59, with permission.)

3. **Strain gauges.** The pressure-monitoring transducer can be described as a variable-resistance transducer. A critical part of the transducer is the diaphragm, which acts to link the fluid wave to the electrical input. When the diaphragm of a transducer is distorted by a change in pressure, voltages are altered across the variable resistor of a Wheatstone bridge contained in the transducer. This in turn produces a change in current, which is electronically converted and displayed.

4. **Sources of error in intravascular pressure measurement**

    a. **Low-frequency transducer response.** Low-frequency response refers to a low-frequency range over which the ratio of output-to-input amplitude is constant (i.e., no distortion). If the natural frequency of the system is low, its frequency response also will be low. **Most transducer systems used in clinical anesthesia can be described as underdamped systems with a low natural frequency.** Thus, any condition that further decreases f_n response should be avoided. **Air within a catheter–transducer causes most monitoring errors.** Because of its compressibility, air not only decreases the response of the system but also leads to overdamping of the system. Therefore, the commonly held belief that an air bubble placed in the pressure tubing decreases artifact by increasing the damping coefficient is incorrect. A second common cause of diminution of frequency response is the formation of a partially obstructing clot in the catheter due to depressurization of the flush device.

    b. **Catheter whip.** Catheter "whip" is a phenomenon in which the motion of the catheter tip itself produces a noticeable pressure swing. This artifact usually is not observed with peripheral arterial catheters but is more common with PA or LV catheters.

    c. **Resonance in peripheral vessels.** The systolic pressure measured in a radial arterial catheter may be up to 20 to 50 mm Hg higher than the pressure measured in the central aorta. This is due to many complex interactions of the blood as it is ejected from the LV into the aorta. The characteristics of the pressure wave as it travels down the arterial tree are modified as a result of narrowing of the arteries, the decrease of elastic tissue in distal vessels, and the addition of reflected waves to the arterial waveform as it progresses distally in the arterial system (Fig. 3.8).

    d. **Changes in electrical properties of the transducer.** *Electrical balance,* or *electrical zero,* refers to the adjustment of the Wheatstone bridge within the transducer so that zero current flows to the detector at zero pressure. Transducers should be electronically balanced periodically during a procedure because the zero point may drift, for instance, if the room temperature changes. This drift can be due to a membrane–dome coupling phenomenon or to a drift in the pressure amplifier circuitry. In the presence of baseline drift in a transducer system, the pressure waveform may not change, and aggressive treatment conceivably could be started on the basis of erroneous values.

    e. **Transducer position errors.** By convention, the reference position for hemodynamic monitoring is the right atrium (RA). With the patient supine, the RA lies at the level of the midaxillary line. Once its zero level has been established, the transducer must be maintained at the same level as the RA. If the transducer position changes, falsely high or low-pressure values will result. This is less of a concern when measuring relatively high arterial pressures but can be significant when monitoring lower pressure, such as central venous pressure (CVP), PA pressure, or pulmonary capillary wedge pressure (PCWP).

5. **Transducer-tipped catheters.** Catheters are available with miniature transducers in their tip. These catheters reduce artifacts and errors related to the many linkages in the fluid-filled transducer systems (stopcocks, tubing, air bubbles, clots). With a flat frequency response of up to 40 Hz, they provide extremely accurate BP measurements. The major drawback of these transducers is their expense and relative fragility. Another transducer-tipped catheter

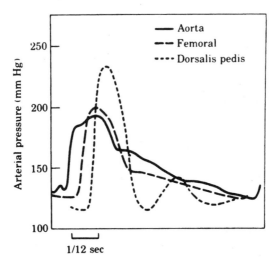

FIG. 3.8 Change of pulse pressure in different arteries. The central aortic waveform is more rounded and has a definite dicrotic notch. The dorsalis pedis and, to a lesser extent, the femoral artery show a delay in pulse transmission, sharper initial upstrokes (and thus higher systolic pressure), and slurring (femoral) and loss (dorsalis) of the dicrotic notch. The dicrotic notch is better maintained in the upper-extremity pressure wave (not shown). The small second "hump" in the dorsalis wave probably is due to a reflected wave from the arterial–arteriolar impedance mismatching. (From Welch JP, D'Ambra MN. Hemodynamic monitoring. In: Kofke WA, Levy JH, eds. *Postoperative critical care procedures of the Massachusetts General Hospital.* Boston: Little, Brown and Company, 1986:144, with permission.)

that uses fiberoptic rather than electrical transduction of the pressure signal may reduce the cost of the catheters to the point that they can be manufactured for single use at a competitive price.

D. Arterial catheterization

    1. Indications. For several reasons, arterial catheterization has become standard in the monitoring of the cardiac surgical patient:

        a. Direct arterial pressure measurement is possible during nonpulsatile extracorporeal circulation.

        b. Cardiac surgical patients usually are hemodynamically unstable in the perioperative period.

        c. Close surveillance of arterial blood gases and other blood chemistries is indicated in these patients.

    2. Sites of cannulation. Several sites used for cannulation of the arterial tree can be used:

        a. Radial artery. This site is used most commonly for arterial catheterization because catheter insertion is easy and the radial artery provides a reasonably accurate estimation of the true aortic pressure.

            (1) Technique. Table 3.2 summarizes the steps used for radial arterial cannulation. One technique, that of transfixing the radial artery for catheter insertion, is shown in Figure 3.9.

            (2) Contraindications. Inadequate collateral flow to the hand is a relative contraindication to the use of a radial artery catheter. The **modified Allen's test** screens for patients with inadequate palmar collateralization from the ulnar artery. Originally described by Allen in 1927 and modified by Bedford, it is performed as follows. Apply firm pressure over both radial and ulnar arteries simultaneously and ask

Table 3.2 Steps for arterial catheter placement

Steps	Rationale and possible complications
1. Immobilize and dorsiflex at wrist	Too much dorsiflexion or tape too tight—occludes artery
2. Immobilize thumb with tape	Stabilize the artery against the radial head
3. Palpate artery 3–4 cm along its course	Increases the likelihood of a central puncture
4. a. Make small skin wheal with 0.5% lidocaine after sterile preparation	Keep volume small for this and deeper infiltration to avoid altering anatomy
b. Infiltrate deeper planes on either side of artery	Decreases the incidence of spasm
5. Make skin nick with 18-gauge needle	Facilitates maneuvering of the catheter
6. Introduce 20-gauge, 2-inch catheter-over-needle unit	Larger bore possibly associated with increased thrombogenesis
7. Advance in rapid, short, 1-mm increments until flashback is seen. Three options available:	Rapid advance increases chance of arterial wall puncture. These three methods are not mutually exclusive but describe three different depths of needle and catheter tip placement:
a. Advance unit 0.5 mm; slide catheter off needle into artery	a. Placement in the arterial **lumen**
b. Advance unit until flashback stops, then withdraw needle (holding catheter stationary); when flashback returns, advance catheter into artery	b. Placement in the **back wall** of the artery (catheter tip will remain in lumen with this method)
c. Advance unit several millimeters, remove needle completely, back catheter until good flow returns, advance catheter into artery either directly or after passing flexible wire	c. Placement of needle and catheter **through** back wall—also termed *transfixing* the artery. Wire should be advanced through lumen of catheter only if pulsatile flow via catheter is present; forcing wire may result in arterial dissection
8. Remove air from tubing	Prevents arterial air emboli

the patient to squeeze his or her hand several times to promote exsanguination. Then release the pressure on the ulnar artery, keeping the radial artery compressed, and measure the time needed to refill the nail bed capillaries. If refill time is greater than 15 seconds, the test result is considered **positive,** suggesting **inadequate collateral flow** from the ulnar artery. Although there is debate as to whether a positive result on Allen's test correlates with any significant morbidity, it is prudent to consider other catheter sites before cannulating the radial artery in patients with peripheral vascular disease.

   (3) Radial artery harvest. If a coronary bypass that will utilize the radial artery as a free graft is planned, an alternative site must be used.

   b. Femoral artery. The femoral artery offers two advantages over the radial site. First, the artery is not only superficial but also allows excellent access to the central arterial tree. Second, the femoral artery catheter provides appropriate access should placement of an intraaortic balloon pump become necessary during the surgical procedure. Placement of a femoral artery catheter as an additional catheter site should be considered in any patient in whom difficulty in weaning from CPB is expected (e.g., those with depressed ejection fraction, severe wall-motion abnormalities, or significant coronary disease).

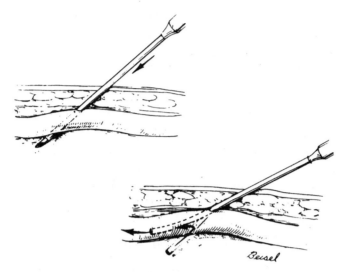

FIG. 3.9 One technique used for radial artery cannulation. The needle–catheter unit is advanced through the artery, as shown in the **upper drawing.** The **lower drawing** shows the needle removed and the catheter withdrawn until pulsatile flow is obtained (indicating that the catheter tip is in the lumen). The catheter then is advanced into the artery. (From Freis ES. Vascular cannulation. In: Kofke WA, Levy JH, eds. *Postoperative critical care procedures of the Massachusetts General Hospital.* Boston: Little, Brown and Company, 1986:137, with permission.)

      (1) **Technique.** The femoral artery is entered most easily using a Seldinger technique after sterile preparation and draping.

      (2) **Contraindications.** Cannulation of the femoral artery should be avoided in any patient who had prior vascular surgery involving the femoral arteries or who has a skin infection of the groin.

   c. Aortic root. Aortic root cannulation is not an option at the beginning of a cardiac case but should always be considered in the patient whose chest is open and in whom difficulties are encountered in obtaining a reliable BP. Pressure tubing can be handed to the anesthesiologist from the sterile field after a needle or catheter is inserted in the aortic root by the surgeon.

   d. Axillary artery. The axillary artery, like the femoral artery, provides the anesthesiologist with a superficial, large artery that has good access to the central arterial tree.

      (1) **Technique.** The axillary artery is most easily entered using a Seldinger technique. Placement of the axillary catheter in the left axilla somewhat reduces the likelihood that any air or debris flushed from the catheter could cause an embolus in a cerebral vessel.

      (2) **Contraindications.** Cannulation of the axillary artery should be avoided in the presence of any localized skin irritation in the axilla. The increased risk of cerebral embolus of air or debris must be recognized.

   e. Brachial artery. The brachial artery is an easily accessible artery located medially in the antecubital fossa.

      (1) **Brachial artery** cannulation is similar to that described for the radial artery. A 20-gauge catheter can easily be placed in the brachial artery. The elbow must be immobilized with a long arm board for stability.

(2) **Contraindications.** Because the brachial artery is an end artery, its cannulation is relatively contraindicated. In prospective studies, however, the incidence of brachial artery thromboembolism with an 18-gauge or smaller catheter was low, and this incidence can be minimized by using the shortest and smallest gauge catheter possible.

f. **Ulnar artery.** The ulnar artery can be used in those rare circumstances when the radial artery cannot be entered easily. Before insertion of an ulnar artery catheter, Allen's test should be repeated as described previously, except that pressure over the radial artery should be released to check for adequate radial artery collateral flow.

g. **Dorsalis pedis and posterior tibialis arteries.** In general, these two sites of cannulation are not recommended because they present difficult management problems in the postoperative period. Further, the distal location increases distortion of the arterial wave (Fig. 3.8).

3. **Interpretation of arterial tracings.** The arterial pressure waveform contains a great deal of hemodynamic information.

a. **Heart rate and rhythm.** The heart rate can be determined from the arterial pressure wave. This is especially helpful if the patient is being paced or if electrocautery is being used because pacer spikes or cautery interference can distort the ECG. In the presence of numerous atrial or ventricular ectopic beats, the arterial trace can provide useful information on the hemodynamic consequences of these dysrhythmias (i.e., if an ectopic beat is perfusing).

b. **Pulse pressure.** The difference between the systolic and diastolic pressures provides useful information about fluid status and valvular competence. Pericardial tamponade and hypovolemia are accompanied by a narrow pulse pressure on the arterial waveform. A sudden increase in pulse pressure may be a sign of worsening aortic valvular insufficiency.

c. **Respiratory variation and volume status.** Hypovolemia is suggested by a decrease in arterial systolic pressure with positive-pressure ventilation. Positive intrathoracic pressure impedes venous return to the heart and will have a more pronounced effect in the hypovolemic patient. Because this finding is not uniformly seen in patients with hypovolemia, correlation with other findings can help make the diagnosis.

d. **Qualitative estimates of hemodynamic indices.** As long as the pressure transducer system is of reasonable quality (adequate natural frequency, properly damped), some inferences can be made about contractility, stroke volume, and vascular resistance. Contractility can be grossly judged by the rate of pressure rise during systole, keeping in mind that heart rate, preload, and afterload can affect this parameter. Stroke volume can be estimated from the area under the aortic pressure wave from the onset of systole to the dicrotic notch. Finally, the position of the dicrotic notch correlates with the systemic resistance. A notch appearing high on the downslope of the pressure trace suggests a high vascular resistance, whereas a low resistance tends to cause a dicrotic notch that is lower on the diastolic portion of the pressure trace.

4. **Complications of arterial catheterization**

a. **Ischemia.** The incidence of ischemic damage after radial artery cannulation is reported low. A study by Slogoff et al. [4], in which the Allen's test was not performed, showed that although abnormal flow patterns were present in up to 25% of patients between 1 and 7 days after radial artery catheterization, there were no adverse signs of ischemia with these findings. Nonetheless, the possible complication of distal ischemia should always be considered, especially in the presence of abnormal results from the Allen's test. If the radial artery is cannulated under these conditions, the hand should be monitored carefully for signs of ischemia.

b. **Thrombosis.** Although the incidence of thrombosis from radial artery catheterization is high, studies have not demonstrated adverse sequelae, and recanalization of the radial artery occurs in a majority of cases. Patients with significant morbidity from radial cannulation include those with diabetes or severe peripheral vascular disease; in these patients, arterial cannulation should be avoided if results of the Allen's test are positive.

   c. **Infection.** With proper sterile technique, the risk of infection from cannulation of the radial artery should be minimal. In the series of 1,700 cases reported by Slogoff et al. [4], no catheter site was overtly infected. Other studies demonstrate a higher infection rate among femoral arterial lines.

   d. **Bleeding.** Although transfixing the artery will put a hole in its back wall, the layers of the muscular media will seal. In the patient with a bleeding diathesis, however, there is a greater tendency to bleed. Unlike central venous catheters, arterial catheters are not heparin bonded.

   e. **False lowering of radial artery pressure immediately after CPB.** In a large number of patients (up to 72% in one series), the radial artery pressure was significantly lower than the aortic pressure at the completion of CPB [5]. Vasoconstriction was not found to be the primary reason for this phenomenon in this series. Forearm vasodilation secondary to rewarming may lead to arteriovenous AV shunting, resulting in a steal phenomenon 5 to 30 minutes or longer in duration. Other studies have suggested that the inaccuracy of radial pressure is due to hypovolemia and vasoconstriction [6]. Whatever the mechanism, if suspicion arises that a peripheral arterial trace is dampened (owing to slow upstroke or loss of the dicrotic notch, for example), a direct pressure measurement should be obtained from a central site.

5. **Recommendations for BP monitoring.** Under most circumstances, the radial arterial pressure measurement will be accurate before and after CPB. In the patient with poor LV function, addition of a femoral arterial catheter before CPB is warranted, not only to obtain a second comparable BP but also to ensure arterial access should intraaortic balloon counterpulsation become necessary. If an internal mammary artery (IMA) is dissected to be used as one of the coronary bypass vessels, the radial artery catheter should be placed in the side opposite the IMA harvest, because retraction of the chest wall and compression of the subclavian artery can dampen or obliterate the radial artery traces. If bilateral IMA grafts are planned, a femoral artery catheter may be helpful.

E. **Central venous pressure.** CVP measures RA pressure and is affected by one or all of the following: (a) circulating blood volume, (b) venous tone, and (c) RV function.

   1. **Indications**

      a. **Monitoring.** Monitoring of ventricular preload, and at least CVP, is indicated for any cardiac patient requiring CPB; for surgery in which large blood losses or large volume shifts are expected; or for patients in whom preexisting hypovolemia is suspected.

      b. **Fluid and drug therapy.** CVP can be used to infuse fluid or blood products; as a port for administering vasoactive drugs; and for postoperative hyperalimentation.

      c. **Special uses.** One may elect to place a CVP catheter in a patient who ordinarily would require a PA catheter when the latter cannot be placed either easily or safely. Placement of a PA catheter can be difficult in patients with numerous congenital cardiac disorders, in those with anatomic distortion of the right-sided venous circulation, or in those requiring surgical procedures of the right heart or implantation of a right heart mechanical assist device.

   2. **Techniques.** There are numerous routes by which a catheter can be placed in the central circulation.

      a. **Internal jugular.** The internal jugular vein is the most common access route for the cardiac anesthesiologist.

         (1) **Techniques.** Cannulation of the internal jugular vein is relatively safe and convenient and various approaches exist for its cannulation (Table 3.3, Fig. 3.10). The process of cannulation, regardless of the approach, involves the steps outlined in Table 3.4.

Table 3.3 Sites for internal jugular cannulation

Approaches	Landmarks	Complications
Central	Apex of triangle formed by lateral (clavicular) and medial (sternal) head of SCM. Aim needle caudally and laterally toward ipsilateral nipple	Low incidence of pneumothorax; hemothorax; medial direction has higher incidence of carotid puncture
Posterior	Intersection of lateral border of lateral (clavicular) head of SCM and line drawn laterally from cricoid ring. Aim needle caudally and ventrally (anteriorly) toward sternal notch	Higher incidence of carotid puncture; low incidence of pneumothorax; hemothorax
Anterior	Medial border of medial head, 5 cm above clavicle. Direct needle toward ipsilateral nipple	Carotid puncture more likely unless retracted medially; hemothorax
Supraclavicular	Interscalene groove 2 cm above clavicle. Direct needle caudally and medially	Higher chance of pneumothorax and subclavian artery puncture; hemothorax

SCM, sternocleidomastoid muscle.

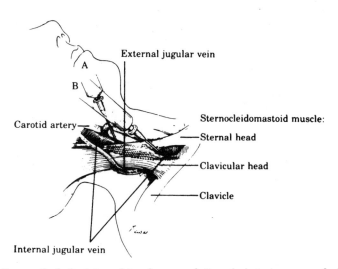

FIG. 3.10 Two methods for internal jugular cannulation. *A,* Anterior approach. *B,* Central approach (see text for further details). (From Freis ES. Vascular cannulation. In: Kofke WA, Levy JH, eds. *Postoperative critical care procedures of the Massachusetts General Hospital.* Boston: Little, Brown and Company, 1986:130, with permission.)

Table 3.4 Steps for right internal jugular cannulation

Steps	Rationale and possible problems
1. Verify functioning ECG	Critical for monitoring dysrhythmias
2. Remove pillow, rotate head completely to left. Ask patient to raise head off bed and note position of tensed sternocleidomastoid muscle	Optimizes visualization of landmarks
3. Place patient in Trendelenburg position	Distends IJ and reduces risk of air embolism; may worsen symptoms due to congestive or right ventricular failure
4. Perform careful sterile preparation and drape	Mandatory for central venous cannulation; full glove and gown should be used
5. Recheck landmarks, skin wheal, and, in awake patients, deeper infiltration with 1% lidocaine	IJ often is superficial and may be found during infiltration; withdraw on syringe before injecting local anesthetic
6. Remove local anesthetic from syringe, replace infiltration needle with 19- or 21-gauge 1½-inch "finder" needle	Not necessary if vein has been found previously; presence of local anesthetic will make aspirated blood appear bright red
7. Once vein has been located:	
a. Leave finder needle in place *or*	Serves as reminder of vein location
b. Remove finder, remember direction	Finder needle may interfere with subsequent cannulation
8. Insert 18-gauge 1¾-inch catheter over needle unit into IJ, following same line	Constant aspiration as unit is advanced is required to see flashback
9. When flashback is seen, advance unit ≈1 mm, then advance catheter over needle into vein	Once IV placement is established, end of catheter is capped with finger or syringe to avoid air embolism
10. If blood is not aspirated freely:	Catheter is probably through back wall
a. Remove needle	Patient may be hypovolemic, and IV fluid bolus will increase success
b. Replace syringe and aspirate	Increased head-down position may be needed
c. Withdraw catheter until free flow of blood occurs	
d. Advance catheter slowly into vein, or insert a wire through catheter	
11. Confirm IV placement by	
a. Check for lack of pulsatile flow	If arterial cannulation is diagnosed, remove catheter and hold pressure for at least 5 min to avoid hematoma formation
b. Measure pressure in the 18-gauge catheter and simultaneous arterial pressure, comparing absolute values and pressure waveforms	
c. Compare IJ and arterial blood samples, visually or by oximetry	
12. Pass flexible wire through catheter, remove catheter	ECG should be monitored because arrhythmias can result
13. Place central venous pressure catheter over wire or dilator-introducer assembly (pulmonary artery catheter)	Skin nick needed if larger introducer will be placed
14. Place sterile dressing	

ECG, electrocardiogram; IJ, internal jugular; IV, intravenous.

(2) **Contraindications and recommendations.** Internal jugular vein cannulation is recommended over other approaches to the central circulation in the absence of relative contraindications such as:

    (a) Presence of carotid disease.

    (b) Recent cannulation of the internal jugular vein (with the concomitant risk of thrombosis).

    (c) Contralateral diaphragmatic dysfunction.

    (d) Thyromegaly or prior neck surgery.

      In these cases, the internal jugular vein on the contralateral side should be considered. It should be remembered that the thoracic duct lies in close proximity to the left internal jugular vein and that laceration of the left brachiocephalic vein or superior vena cava by the catheter is more likely with the left-sided approach. This risk is due to the more acute angle between the left internal jugular and innominate veins.

(3) **Sonographic guidance.** Although still not available in many centers, commercially available hand-held ultrasound units (Site Rite, Dymax Corp., Pittsburgh, PA, U.S.A.) can be used to identify the internal jugular vein, especially in difficult circumstances. In a recent study, up to 30% of "normal" patients had some abnormality of the jugular vein, and all were successfully cannulated using this technique [7].

b. **External jugular.** The external jugular vein courses superficially across the sternocleidomastoid muscle to join the subclavian vein close to the junction of the internal jugular and subclavian veins. Its course is more tortuous, and the presence of valves makes central access via the external jugular more difficult.

  (1) **Techniques.** The head-down position is needed to distend the vein. Traction also is necessary to introduce an 18-gauge catheter into the external jugular vein. A flexible J-guidewire is used to negotiate the tortuous course of the vessel. Central passage of the catheter usually is easier from the left jugular vein. The remainder of the insertion is similar to that described for the internal jugular.

  (2) **Advantages and disadvantages.** The external jugular provides safe access to the central circulation and can be cannulated in a patient receiving heparin or in whom internal jugular cannulation is unsuccessful or contraindicated. The central circulation was successfully cannulated in 75% to 90% of patients in some reports.

      The tip of the external jugular catheter can pass into the subclavian vein or up the internal jugular on the same side or may cross over to the contralateral side. Although drug infusions can be given through a catheter so placed, monitoring of the CVP under these conditions will lead to incorrect values. The position of the catheter should be confirmed by chest x-ray film before drug therapy based on a CVP reading from an external jugular catheter is instituted.

c. **Subclavian.** The subclavian vein is readily accessible and thus has been popular for use during cardiopulmonary resuscitation.

  (1) **Techniques.** The patient is placed in a head-down position to distend the vein. Optimal positioning can be obtained by placing a roll vertically under the patient's spine to move the clavicle out of the way during cannulation.

  (2) **Advantages.** The main advantage to subclavian vein cannulation is its relative ease and the stability of the catheter during long-term cannulation.

  (3) **Disadvantages**

    (a) Subclavian vein cannulation carries the highest rate of pneumothorax of any approach. **If subclavian vein cannulation is unsuccessful on one side, an attempt on the contralateral side is contraindicated without first obtaining a chest x-ray film.** Bilateral pneumothoraces can be lethal.

        (b) The subclavian artery is entered easily instead of the vein.

        (c) In a left-sided cannulation, the thoracic duct may be lacerated.

        (d) The left subclavian approach may make threading the catheter into the RA difficult because an acute angle must be made by the catheter in order to enter the innominate vein.

   d. Arm vein

     (1) Techniques. Central access can be obtained through the veins of the antecubital fossa. The basilic vein, which is located more medially than the cephalic vein, provides the most direct venous route to the central circulation. The best approach for this type of insertion is to place a short 14-gauge intravenous catheter into the basilic vein and then insert a 16-gauge, 30-cm CVP catheter through the lumen of the 14-gauge catheter. This approach not only allows threading of a CVP catheter but also, in the event the CVP catheter **cannot** be threaded, ensures the existence of a large-bore catheter for IV access. Alternatively, prepackaged peripheral CVP kits are available.

     (2) Advantages. The main advantage of placing a CVP catheter through the peripheral veins is that bleeding can be well controlled in the anticoagulated patient.

     (3) Disadvantages. The disadvantage of this route is the low rate of success in gaining reliable access to the central circulation. Maneuvers that can aid in placing the catheter are the following:

        (a) Rapid advancement of the catheter so that venous spasm will not halt its placement.

        (b) Traction on the arm as the catheter is threaded.

        (c) Abduction of the arm at the shoulder while threading.

        (d) Rotation of the head toward the arm that is being cannulated.

3. Complications. The site-specific complications of CVP catheter insertion are listed in Table 3.5. The most severe complications of CVP insertion usually are preventable.

4. Interpretation

   a. Normal waves. The normal CVP trace contains three positive deflections, termed the *A, C,* and *V* waves, and two negative deflections termed the *X* and *Y* descents (Fig. 3.11).

   b. Abnormal waves. A common abnormality in the CVP trace occurs in the presence of AV dissociation, when RA contraction occurs against a closed tricuspid valve. This produces a large "cannon A wave" that is virtually diagnostic of this condition. Abnormal V waves can occur with tricuspid valve insufficiency, in which retrograde flow through the incompetent valve produces an increase in RA pressure during systole.

   c. RV function. CVP offers direct measurement of RV filling pressure.

   d. LV filling pressures. CVP is a reasonable indicator of LV filling in the presence of good LV function and in the absence of pulmonary hypertension or mitral valvular disease. In patients with coronary artery disease but good ventricular function (ejection fraction greater than 40% and no regional wall-motion abnormalities), CVP correlates well with PCWP. However, because the RV is a thinner walled chamber, the compliance of the RV is higher than that of the LV. Therefore, for any given preload, CVP will be lower than either PA diastolic pressure or PCWP.

F. PA catheter

   1. Parameters measured

     a. PA pressure reflects RV function, pulmonary vascular resistance, and left atrial (LA) filling pressure.

     b. PCWP is a more direct measure of LA filling pressure. With the balloon inflated and "wedged" in a distal branch PA, a valveless hydrostatic column exists between the distal port and the LA at end-diastole (Fig 3.12).

     c. CVP. A sampling port of the PA catheter is located in the RA and allows measurement of the CVP.

Table 3.5 Complications of central venous cannulation

Complication	Internal jugular	Subclavian	Femoral	External jugular
Infection	x	x	x	x
Air embolism	x	x	x	x
Catheter shearing and embolization	x	x	x	x
Thrombophlebitis	x	x	x	x
Local extravasation of fluid and drugs	x	x	x	x
Pneumothorax	x	x		
Hemothorax	x	x		
Pericardial tamponade	x	x		
Tissue trauma				
Nerve	Brachial plexus	Brachial plexus	Femoral	
Artery	Carotid Subclavian	Subclavian	Femoral	
Vein	SVC	SVC	Inferior vena cava	SVC
Other	Thoracic duct (L) Cervical nerve roots	Thoracic duct (L)		
Sites of fluid infusion with malpositioned catheter	Mediastinum, pericardium, pleural cavity	Pleural cavity, mediastinum	Retroperitoneum, peritoneal cavity	Retrograde up ipsilateral or contralateral internal jugular

SVC, superior vena cava; L, Left side.

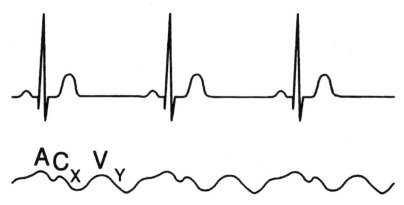

FIG. 3.11 Relationship between the electrocardiogram **(top)** and central venous pressure (CVP) **(bottom).** The normal CVP trace contains three positive deflections, known as the *A, C,* and *V waves,* and two negative deflections, the *X* and *Y* descents. The *A* wave occurs in conjunction with the P wave on the ECG and represents atrial contraction. The *C* wave occurs in conjunction with the QRS wave and represents the bulging of the tricuspid valve into the right atrium with right ventricular contraction. The *X* descent occurs next as the tricuspid valve is pulled downward during the latter stages of ventricular systole. The final positive wave, the *V* wave, occurs after the T wave on the ECG and represents right atrial filling before opening of the tricuspid valve. The *Y* descent occurs after the *V* wave when the tricuspid valve opens and the atrium empties into the ventricle. (Modified from Reich DL, Moskowitz DM, Kaplan JA. Hemodynamic monitoring. In: Kaplan JA, ed. *Cardiac anesthesia,* 4th ed. Philadelphia: WB Saunders, 1999:330.)

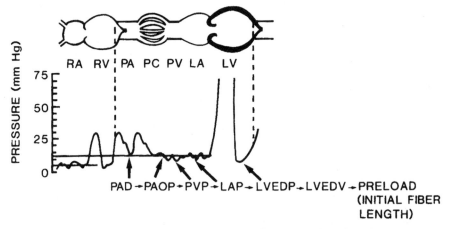

FIG. 3.12 The cardiopulmonary circulation. **Top:** Valveless conduit from the pulmonary artery (PA) to left ventricle (LV) is depicted with the mitral valve open at end-diastole. **Bottom:** Typical pressure waveforms corresponding to each chamber or vessel, with *horizontal lines* drawn at values for right ventricular and left ventricular preload. *LA,* left atrium; *LVEDP,* LV end-diastolic pressure; *LVEDV,* LV end-diastolic volume; *PC,* pulmonary capillary bed; *PV,* pulmonary vein; *RA,* right atrium; *RV,* right ventricle. Note that during diastole, the pulmonic valve is closed, which explains why the PA diastolic pressure, LA pressure, and LVEDP (equal to 12 mmHg) are greater than the RA pressure and RV end-diastolic pressure (not labeled, but equal to 5 mmHg). (From Tuman KJ, Carroll GC, Ivankovich AD. Pitfalls in interpretation of pulmonary artery catheter data. *J Cardiothorac Anesth* 1989;3:626, with permission.)

   d. Cardiac output. A thermistor located at the tip of the PA catheter allows measurement of the output of the RV by the thermodilution technique. In the absence of intracardiac shunts, this measurement equals LV output.

   e. Blood temperature. The thermistor can provide a constant measurement of blood temperature, which is an accurate reflection of core temperature.

   f. Derived parameters. Several indices of ventricular performance and cardiovascular status can be derived from parameters measured by the PA catheter. Their formulas, physiologic significance, and normal values are listed in Table 3.6.

2. Indications for PA catheterization. In some institutions, cardiac surgery with CPB represents a universal indication for PA pressure monitoring in adults. Particular indications are listed in Table 3.7. Many of the indications for use of the PA catheter for cardiac procedures reflect the necessity to monitor the LV separately from the RV, as in many cardiac patients pressures measured on the right side (i.e., CVP) do not adequately reflect those on the left side [8]. The benefits of PA monitoring in these patients include:

   a. Assessing volume status. In many patients with differences in RV and LV function, volume status is difficult to determine because of the large disparity between right (CVP) and left (PCWP) ventricular filling pressures. Knowing both of these values can aid in the diagnosis of hypovolemia or hypervolemia.

   b. Diagnosing RV failure. The RV is a thin-walled, highly compliant chamber that can fail during cardiac surgery either because of a primary disease process (inferior myocardial infarction) or as a result of the surgical procedure (inadequate myocardial protection). RV failure presents as an increase in CVP, a decrease in the CVP to mean PA gradient, and a low cardiac output.

   c. Diagnosing LV failure. Knowledge of PA and wedge pressures can aid in the diagnosis of left-sided heart failure if other causes (ischemia, mitral valve disease) are eliminated. Simultaneous readings of high PA pressures and wedge pressure in the presence of systemic hypotension and low cardiac output are hallmarks of LV failure.

   d. Diagnosing pulmonary hypertension. With normal pulmonary vascular resistance, the PA diastolic and wedge pressure agree closely with one another. A disparity in these parameters, characterized by a higher PA diastolic pressure, suggests the presence of pulmonary hypertension.

   e. Assessing valvular disease

      (1) Tricuspid and pulmonary valve stenosis can be diagnosed by means of a PA catheter by measuring pressure gradients across these valves (**tricuspid:** CVP-to-RV end-diastolic pressure (RVEDP) gradient; **pulmonic:** RV systolic-to-PA systolic pressure gradient). These measurements can be accomplished by the "pullback" method, measuring gradients with the distal port, or by using a Paceport (Baxter Edwards Critical Care, Irvine, CA, USA) PA catheter with an RV port (see Section 5 following for types of catheters).

      (2) Mitral valvular disease is reflected in the wedge pressure tracing. Mitral insufficiency appears as an abnormal V wave, representing an increase in pulmonary venous pressure from the regurgitant flow into the LA. This abnormal wave appears slightly out of phase from the arterial pulse pressure; the delay is due to slower transit of the regurgitant pulse pressure in the highly compliant pulmonary circuit (see Chapter 12). V waves also appear in other conditions, including myocardial ischemia, ventricular pacing, and presence of a ventricular septal defect. The presence and degree of V-wave abnormalities also depend on the compliance of the LA. In patients with chronic mitral valve insufficiency, for example, the LA has a high compliance, and a large regurgitant volume will not always result in a dramatic V wave. Measuring a valvular gradient in mitral stenosis requires

Table 3.6 Derived hemodynamic indices

Parameter	Physiologic significance	Formula	Normal value
Systemic vascular resistance (SVR)	Reflects impedance of the systemic vascular tree; assumes laminar flow of homogeneous fluid	80·(MAP–CVP)/CO	700–1,600 dyne·s·cm^{-5}
Pulmonary vascular resistance (PVR)	Reflects impedance of pulmonary circuit	80·(PAM–PCWP)/CO	20–130 dyne·s·cm^{-5}
Cardiac index (CI)	Index flows to body surface area (BSA), allows for meaningful comparison between patients	CO/BSA	2.5–4.2 L·min^{-1}·m^{-2}
Stroke volume index (SVI)	Reflects fluid status and ventricular performance	CI/HR·1,000	40–60 mL·beat^{-1}·m^{-2}
Left ventricular stroke work index (LVSWI)	Estimates work of left ventricle, reflects contractile state	(MAP–PCWP)·SVI·0.0136	45–60 g·m·m^{-2}
Right ventricular stroke work index (RVSWI)	Estimates work done by right ventricle and RV performance	(PAM–CVP)·SVI·0.0136	5–10 g·m·m^{-2}

CO, cardiac output; CVP, central venous pressure; HR, heart rate; MAP, mean arterial pressure; PAM, pulmonary artery mean pressure; PCWP, pulmonary capillary wedge pressure.
Modified from Kaplan JA. Hemodynamic monitoring. In: Kaplan JA, ed. Cardiac anesthesia, 2nd ed. Philadelphia: WB Saunders, 1987:203.

Table 3.7 Indications for using the pulmonary artery catheter in cardiac surgery

---

Patients for coronary artery bypass graft with
  Poor LV function (ejection fraction <0.40; LV end-diastolic pressure >18 mm Hg)
  LV wall-motion abnormalities
  Recent MI (<6 mo) or complication of MI
  Severe angina
  Significant (>75% stenosis) left main coronary disease
Patient with valvular disease
Presence of pulmonary hypertension
Combined coronary stenoses and valvular disease
Complex cardiac lesions
Patient age >65 yr
Patients with other systemic disease

LV, left ventricular; MI, myocardial infarction.
Modified from Kaplan JA. Hemodynamic monitoring. In: Kaplan JA, ed. *Cardiac anesthesia,* 2nd ed.
Philadelphia: WB Saunders, 1987:193.

simultaneous measurement of LV end-diastolic pressure (LVEDP), which is not routinely performed in the operating room.

  f. Early diagnosis of ischemia. Although the ECG is the cornerstone for diagnosis of ischemia, it is not always sensitive, particularly in the case of subendocardial ischemia. Alterations in wall motion during systole, measured by the transesophageal echocardiogram (TEE), have been shown to be a more sensitive indicator of myocardial ischemia than either the ECG or PA pressure. Usually, significant ischemia (transmural or subendocardial) is associated with a decrease in ventricular compliance, which is reflected in either an increase in PA pressure or an increase in PCWP. In addition, the development of pathologic V waves may occur secondary to ischemia of the papillary muscle (Fig. 3.13).

3. Interpretation of PA pressure data

  a. Effects of ventilation. The effects of ventilation on PA pressure readings can be significant in the low-pressure system of the right-sided circulation because airway or transpleural pressure is transmitted to the pulmonary vasculature.

  (1) When a patient breathes spontaneously, the negative intrapleural pressure that results from inspiration can be transmitted to the intravascular pressure. Thus, "negative" PA diastolic, wedge, and central venous pressures may occur with spontaneous ventilation.

  (2) Positive airway pressures can be transmitted to the vasculature during positive-pressure ventilation, leading to elevations in pulmonary pressures with controlled ventilation.

  (3) The established convention is to read pulmonary pressures at **end-expiration.** This is best done by reading the data directly from a calibrated screen or from a hard copy of the trace. The digital monitor numerical readout may give incorrect information because these numbers reflect the absolute highest (systolic), lowest (diastolic), and mean (area under pressure curve) values for **several seconds,** which may include one or more breaths.

  b. Location of catheter tip. PA pressure measurements depend on where the tip of the catheter resides in the pulmonary vascular tree. In areas of the lung that are well ventilated but poorly perfused (West zone I), the readings will be more affected by changes in airway pressure. Likewise, even when the tip is in a good location in the middle or lower lung fields, large amounts of positive end-expiratory pressure (greater than 10 mm Hg) will affect PA values.

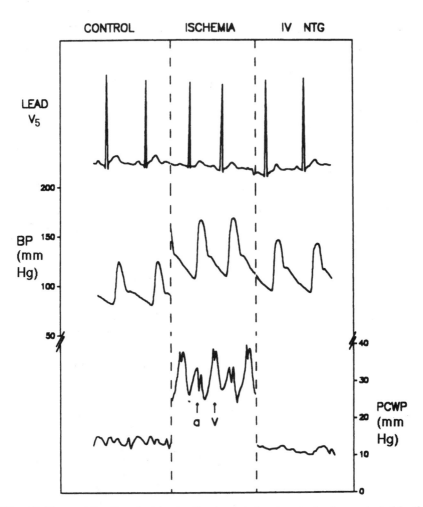

FIG. 3.13 Hypertension from incision leading to an ischemic episode, demonstrated by the appearance of significant *A, C,* and *V* waves in the pulmonary capillary wedge pressure (*PCWP*) trace. These resolve with the institution of intravenous nitroglycerin. Note the lack of significant changes on the electrocardiogram (*V5*) during this episode. *BP,* blood pressure. (Modified From Kaplan JA, Wells PH. Early diagnosis of myocardial ischemia using the pulmonary arterial catheter. *Anesth Analg* 1981;60:792.)

   4. **Timing of placement.** A debate exists regarding whether PA catheter insertion before induction is indicated in adult patients with good LV function. Opponents to preinduction insertion argue that the discomfort associated with PA catheter placement may cause deleterious hemodynamic changes. Another argument against preinduction insertion is that, in the vast majority of patients, recent hemodynamic information based on the cardiac catheterization data is available; therefore, additional preoperative information is not necessary. In the appropriately medicated patient, however, placement of a PA catheter is not associated with any significant hemodynamic changes [9]. Also,

the hemodynamic data collected in the catheterization laboratory may not accurately reflect the current hemodynamic status, especially if the patient was sedated to a different level or was experiencing discomfort during the catheterization. The patient also may have had episodes of myocardial ischemia during the catheterization or may be experiencing ischemia when entering the operating room. If a patient is not sufficiently sedated, the deleterious effects of the anxiety related to the placement of the catheter should be weighed against the benefits expected from its placement. Proper sedation can be achieved in most adult patients so that preinduction insertion can be performed safely.

5. **Types of PA catheters.** A variety of PA catheters currently are available for clinical use. The thermodilution catheter has a PA port for pressure monitoring and a thermistor for cardiac output measurements at its tip, an RA port for CVP monitoring and for injection of cold saline 30 cm from the tip, and a lumen for inflation of the balloon (Fig. 3.13). In addition, PA catheters are available that provide the following:

   a. **A venous infusion port.** This catheter supplies a third port 1 cm proximal to the CVP (31 cm from the tip), for infusion of drugs and fluids.

   b. **Pacing.** Some PA catheters have the capacity to provide intracardiac pacing in one of three ways.
      (1) PA catheters with permanently installed atrial and ventricular bipolar pacing electrodes can be used to establish atrial or ventricular pacing or to perform electrophysiologic studies of atrial, ventricular, and AV nodal electrical activity.
      (2) In other PA catheters, a lumen terminates 19 cm from the catheter tip. When the catheter tip lies in the PA with a normal-sized heart, this port is positioned in the RV. A separate sterile, prepackaged pacing wire can be placed through this port to contact the RV endocardium for RV pacing.
      (3) Swan–Ganz thermodilution using an AV Paceport provides atrial or AV pacing with two separate bipolar pacing probes. This catheter has been shown to provide stable pacing before and after CPB [10].

   c. **Mixed venous oxygen saturation.** Special fiberoptic PA catheters can be used to monitor mixed venous oxygen saturation (S_vO_2) continuously during surgery by the principle of absorption and reflectance of light through blood. The normal S_vO_2 is 75%, with a 5% to 10% increase or decrease considered significant. A significant decrease in S_vO_2 may have several causes.
      (1) Decrease in perfusion (cardiac output), with a higher O_2 extraction ratio
      (2) Increase in metabolic rate (increased O_2 extraction)
      (3) Decrease in arterial oxygen saturation (S_aO_2) from a decreased O_2 supply.
         Changes in saturation usually precede hemodynamic changes by a significant period of time, making this a useful adjunct to other monitors in the cardiac operating room.

   d. **Ejection fraction catheter.** PA catheters with faster thermistor response times can be used to determine RV ejection fraction in addition to the cardiac output. The thermistor responds rapidly enough that the exponential decay that normally results from a thermodilution cardiac output [see Section **H.1.b(2)**] has end-diastolic "plateaus" with each cardiac cycle. From the differences in temperature of each succeeding plateau, the residual fraction of blood left in the RV after each contraction is calculated, as is RV stroke volume, end-diastolic volume, and end-systolic volume. Monitoring these parameters can be helpful in patients with RV dysfunction secondary to pulmonary hypertension, infarction, or reactive pulmonary disease.

   e. **Transthoracic.** PA catheters are available that can be placed surgically. These are useful in patients with difficult IV access and in emergency situations when time does not allow placement of a transvenous PA line. They are available as two separate catheters. The first has a thermistor probe at the tip and a lumen that ends at the tip for PA pressure monitoring. This catheter is placed directly into the RV outflow tract and is guided into the PA. This probe **is not** balloon tipped and therefore cannot be wedged. The second catheter is placed in the RA and is used for injecting the thermal indicator. An existing CVP line can be used to inject the indicator as well.

   f. Continuous cardiac output. PA catheter that uses low power thermal filaments to impart small temperature changes to RV blood have been developed (**Intellicath,** Baxter Edwards; and **Opti-Q,** Abbott Critical Care Systems, Mountain View, CA, USA). Fast-response thermistors in the PA allow for semicontinuous (every 30 to 60 seconds) cardiac output determinations. Due to the problems with continual temperature changes before, during, and after bypass, their use probably is more suited to the critical care setting.

  6. Techniques of insertion. Certain general guidelines should be followed when placing a PA catheter. The steps are outlined in Table 3.8. The introducer is placed in a manner similar to that described for CVP insertion. However, special care should be observed with PA catheter placement, noting especially the following points:

   a. Sedation. As mentioned previously, proper sedation is an important part of PA catheter insertion. Because the patient is under a large drape for a longer period of time, he or she should be asked questions periodically to check for oversedation. A clear drape allows visual inspection of the patient's color and may produce a less suffocating feeling.

   b. ECG monitoring during placement. It is essential to monitor the ECG during placement of the catheter because dysrhythmias are the most common complication associated with this procedure.

   c. Pulse oximetry. This simple form of monitoring is essential when the patient is under the sterile drapes (where the color of the mucous membranes cannot be observed) and in a head-down position, which renders breathing more difficult. Pulse oximetry also gives the anesthesiologist an **audible** signal of rhythm and may alert him or her to an abnormal rhythm.

   d. Preferred approach. The right internal jugular vein approach offers the most direct route to the RA and thus results in the highest rate of successful PA cannulation.

   e. Balloon inflation. Air may be used for balloon inflation, although CO_2 is safer because it is 20 times more soluble in blood and will be resorbed faster in the event of balloon rupture. If any suspicion exists about balloon competency, no gas injections should be made through the balloon port.

   f. Waveform. PA catheter placement can be accomplished without the use of fluoroscopy if the pressure at the distal tip of the catheter is measured as it passes from the RA to RV to PA to PCWP position. Representative waveforms are shown in Figure 3.14.

  7. Complications. Complications can be divided into vascular access, catheter placement, and monitoring problems. Complications associated with PA monitoring are listed in Table 3.9.

  8. Conclusions. PA catheters provide a wealth of information about the right and left sides of the circulation. For this reason, they are used for every cardiac surgical procedure in some institutions because their benefits are perceived to outweigh the risks. Studies that show low morbidity rates with PA catheter use support this viewpoint. In other institutions, however, clinicians are more selective about which patients require PA catheters, because use of PA monitoring has not been demonstrated to incontrovertibly improve outcomes of cardiac surgery.

G. LA pressure. In some patients, direct LA pressure can be measured after surgical insertion of a LA catheter via the LA appendage. LA catheters also are used in corrective surgery for congenital lesions when PA catheter insertion is not possible.

Table 3.8 Steps for pulmonary artery catheter insertion

Steps	Rationale and comments
1. Establish monitoring: blood pressure cuff, electrocardiogram, pulse oximetry	Monitor for ischemia, hypoxemia, arrhythmia
2. Place nasal cannula	Avoids hypoxemia in sedated patient in head-down position
3. Cannulate central circulation, place dilator-introducer	See Table 3.4
4. Remove catheter from package. Place sheath over catheter	Exercise care so as to not damage balloon
5. Hand off proximal end to assistant. Flush appropriate ports of catheter with heparinized saline. Monitor at least the distal port	Placing a PA catheter requires nonsterile assistant, to connect ports to transducer tubing
6. Check balloon for competence	Should be done after sheath is placed over catheter
7. While watching monitor and holding 30-cm mark fixed, raise the distal tip from horizontal to vertical position	Ensures that the correct monitor channel is connected to the distal port. **Only** the pressure channel for the distal port should reflect a rise in pressure
8. Insert PA catheter to 20 cm with balloon **down**	Puts balloon past end of introducer; inflation before this point may damage balloon
9. Inflate balloon with 1.5 cc of air or CO_2	Do not force air into balloon; there is a small amount of resistance before the opening pressure is reached
10. Advance slowly, monitoring the distal port	Look for progressive pressure changes from right atrium to RV, PA, and PCWP (Fig. 3.14)
11. When RV reached, advance more rapidly	Avoids arrhythmia but advancing slowly may be required to reach the pulmonary outflow tract
12. If RV or PA is difficult to enter:	
a. Have patient take deep breath	Increases pulmonary blood flow
b. Place in head-up position or tilt table to left or right	Places the RV or PA outflow at highest point, where balloon will float
c. Flush PA port with 1–2 mL cold sterile saline	Stiffens catheter, making threading easier
13. When PA entered, advance slowly	Look for phase shift of V wave or damping of phasic pulse, or both
14. Release balloon	PA trace should return
15. "Size" the PA by inserting gas in 0.5-cc increments, watching PA trace	If PCWP is seen before full 1.5 cc is inserted, the catheter should be pulled back 3–4 cm to avoid PA rupture
16. Do not withdraw the catheter at any time with the balloon inflated	Avoids rupture of pulmonic or tricuspid valves

The LA pressure tracing is comparable to the CVP tracing, with A, C, and V waves occurring at identical points in the cardiac cycle. LA catheters are used to monitor valvular function (after mitral valve replacement or mitral valvuloplasty) or to monitor LV filling pressures, whether or not a PA catheter is available. LA pressure measured directly is more accurate than that measured with a PA catheter because the effects of airway pressure on the pulmonary vasculature are removed. However, LA pressure does not necessarily reflect LVEDP in the presence of mitral valvular disease. Air should be meticulously removed from LA flush systems to avoid catastrophic air emboli.

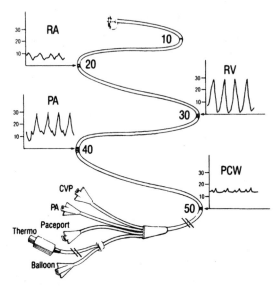

FIG. 3.14 Pressure waves that will be encountered as a pulmonary artery (*PA*) catheter is inserted into the wedged position from the right internal jugular vein. Distances on the catheter correspond to insertion distances read at the diaphragm of the introducer and are approximate. Actual distances may vary by ±5 cm. PA catheters should not be advanced more than 60 cm from this approach because this increases the risk of PA rupture or catheter knotting. *CVP*, central venous pressure; *PCW*, pulmonary capillary wedge; *RA*, right atrium; *RV*, right ventricle; *Thermo*, thermistor connection for cardiac output determination.

H. Cardiac output
1. Methods
a. Fick method.
In the classic application of the Fick principle, O_2 is used as the "indicator," using the formula:

$$Q = 10 \times [\dot{V}O_2/(a - v)\, O_2]$$

The arterial-to-venous difference $(a - v)$ in O_2 content can be estimated closely by using the O_2 content of arterial blood minus the O_2 content of mixed venous blood. O_2 consumption can be calculated from the inspired and expired O_2 concentrations and the volume of a sample of expired gas. This method, however, does not lend itself to easy application in the operating room.

b. Indicator dilution method.
In this method, an indicator that is not metabolized is injected into the central circulation.

(1) Dye dilution.
A nontoxic dye such as indocyanine green or methylene blue is used. After total mixing in the pulmonary circuit, the dye is carried to the arterial circuit, where blood is sampled continually for the dye and its concentration is measured. For most indicators, such as indocyanine green or methylene blue, the concentration is calculated by using spectrophotometric analysis of blood as it is drawn past an infrared light source. The usefulness of this method is limited by the inability to repeat the measurement frequently owing to the increasing background dye concentration.

Table 3.9 Complications associated with pulmonary artery monitoring

Vascular access complications
  Inability to gain access
  Hemorrhage
  Damage to the vessel or associated structure(s)
  Pneumothorax, hemothorax
Catheter placement complications
  Dysrhythmias
  Catheter coiling, knotting
  Damage to the tricuspid or pulmonary valve(s)
  Endocarditis, sepsis
  Cardiac perforation
  Intracardiac thrombus formation, pulmonary embolus
  Paradoxical (systemic arterial) embolus
  Pulmonary artery rupture
  Pulmonary infarction
  Balloon rupture
  Thrombocytopenia
Monitoring complications
  Incorrect data collection
  Data misinterpretation or misapplication
  "Mesmerism" by pulmonary artery catheter data to the exclusion of other monitoring
  data or clinical factors
  Expense

Modified from Schwartz AJ, Conahan TJ III. Pulmonary artery catheters: there are still concerns with their routine use. *J Cardiothorac Anesth* 1987;1:7–9.

(2) **Thermodilution with cold injectate.** This method is the most commonly utilized cardiac output technique because of its ease of use. The indicator is an aliquot of saline, which is at a lower temperature than the temperature of blood, injected into the RA. The change in temperature produced by injection of this indicator is measured in the PA by a thermistor and is integrated over time to generate a value for RV output, which is equal to systemic cardiac output if no intracardiac shunts are present. This method requires no withdrawal of blood and no arterial line, uses an inexpensive indicator, and is not greatly affected by recirculation.

(3) **Continuous thermodilution.** This is discussed in Section **F.5.f.**

(4) **RV ejection fraction.** As discussed in Section **F.5.d.,** the stroke volume of the RV is measured with this catheter, and because heart rate is also measured, the RV cardiac output is obtained. However, because vascular resistance in the pulmonary beds occurs separately from the systemic arterial tree, changes in RV output do not always reflect similar alterations in LV function.

c. **Doppler ultrasound.** Using the change in frequency of an ultrasonic beam as it reflects off a moving object (Doppler shift), blood flow velocity can be measured. These methods have the advantage of providing continuous measurements. To achieve accurate measurements, at least three conditions must be met: (i) the cross-sectional area of the vessel must be known; (ii) the ultrasound beam must be directed parallel to the flow of blood; and (iii) the beam direction cannot move to any great degree between measurements. Variations from these conditions lead to inaccuracies. Clinical use of these techniques has produced problems with accuracy and precision.

Two methods that use ultrasound are:

(1) **Transtracheal.** Aortic flow is determined with a transducer bonded to the distal portion of the endotracheal tube, designed to ensure contact of the transducer with the wall of the trachea.

(2) **Transesophageal and suprasternal.** Again, flow in the aorta is measured using a transducer placed in the esophagus. Initial measurements of the aortic cross-sectional area are provided with a suprasternal transducer.

   d. **Echocardiography.** End-diastolic and end-systolic dimensions measured by echocardiography can be converted to volumes, allowing stroke volume and cardiac output to be determined. More details about this technique are provided in Chapter 4.

   e. **Bioimpedance.** Electrical impedance can be measured in the thorax by sending an alternating current that is sensed by two sets of electrodes placed at the neck and the xiphoid process. Ventilation and pulsatile blood flow in the thorax will change bioimpedance, and, if the ventilatory component is factored out, stroke volume can be assessed. Unfortunately, **this method is limited by the need for specific lead placement, which may interfere with the surgical field;** therefore, bioimpedance is best suited for the intensive care unit.

2. **Accuracy and precision.** Accuracy refers to the capability of a measurement to reflect the true cardiac output. This means that a measurement is compared to a "gold standard" method. Comparisons among various cardiac output methods, however, have used different gold standards, making accuracy data difficult to interpret. *Precision* indicates the reproducibility of a measurement and refers to the variability between determinations. The methods used clinically are summarized in terms of accuracy and precision in Table 3.10.

For the thermodilution method, studies of precision have involved probability analyses of large numbers of cardiac output determinations. Using this approach, it was found that with two injections, there was only a 50% chance

Table 3.10 Accuracy and precision of cardiac output measurements

Method	"Gold-standard" comparison	Accuracy	Precision
O_2 consumption (Fick method)	Rotameter or electromagnetic flow probe placed in pulmonary artery	Good	Good
Thermodilution	Fick method	Overestimates output by as much as 10%	Poor; repeat measurements needed
Dye dilution	Fick method Thermodilution	Yields lower values compared to both methods	Good
Doppler ultrasound	Thermodilution	Good, if initial estimate of vessel diameter is accurate	Poor; probe can move easily
Transesophageal echocardiography	Ventricular angiography	Good, if ventricular asynergy is not present	Good

that the numbers obtained were within 5% of the true cardiac output [11]. If three injections yield results that are within 10% of one another, there is a 90% probability that the average value is within 10% of the true cardiac output. Although the precision of thermodilution is not great, variability can be minimized by knowing which factors lead to an increase in errors.

3. **Assumptions and errors.** Certain assumptions made when the Fick and indicator dilution methods are used may or may not be true. These are outlined in Table 3.11, along with sources of errors in the various measurements. Some specific errors in cardiac output determination are detailed here.

   a. **Thermodilution method**

      (1) **Volume of injectate.** Because the output computer will base its calculations on a particular volume, an injectate volume less than that for which the computer is set will cause a falsely high value and vice versa.

Table 3.11 Possible sources of errors in cardiac output determinations

Thermodilution	Dye dilution	Fick method
Assumptions		
Flow is constant	Same as for thermodilution	Steady state exists for the
Blood volume is constant		duration of the study
No significant venous pooling		
Indicator flow represents total flow		
O_2 uptake by tissues equals uptake by lungs		
Disadvantages (sources of errors)		
Volume of injectate must be correct	Affected by:	Subject to gas sampling errors
Temperature of injectate must be accurate	1. Intracardiac shunts	Mixed venous sample will
Affected by:	2. Volume of dye injected	be misleading if catheter
1. Intracardiac shunts	3. Speed of injection	is wedged
2. Coadministration of intravenous fluids		
3. Phase of respiratory cycle		
4. Differences in computer algorithms		
5. Patient position		
6. Position of catheter in pulmonary artery		
7. Speed of injection		
Comments		
Rapid; easy to use	Arterial line required	More time consuming;
Repetitive measurements possible	Dye must be prepared same day	repeat measurements not practical
No arterial line required	Repeated measurements not possible	Cumbersome to perform in operating room
	Not affected by respiratory cycle	More equipment required

(2) **Temperature of injectate.** The controversy over iced versus room-temperature injectate centers around the concept that a larger difference between the temperature of the injectate and blood temperatures should increase the accuracy of the cardiac output determination. Some studies have not supported this hypothesis, and the extra inconvenience of keeping syringes on ice, together with the increased risk of infection (nonsterile water surrounding the Luer tip), make the iced saline method a less attractive alternative. If the injectate temperature factor is set incorrectly, errors can occur. For example, an increase of 1°C will cause a 3% overestimation of cardiac output.

(3) **Shunts.** Intracardiac shunts will cause erroneous values for thermodilution cardiac output values. This technique should not be used if a communication exists between the pulmonary and systemic circulations. A shunt should always be suspected when thermodilution cardiac output values do not fit the clinical findings.

(4) **Timing with the respiratory cycle.** As much as a 10% difference in cardiac output will result, depending on when injection occurs during the respiratory cycle. These changes are most likely due to actual changes in pulmonary blood flow during respiration.

(5) **Catheter position.** The tip of the pulmonary catheter must be in the PA; otherwise, nonsensical curves are obtained.

   b. **Dye dilution method**

   (1) **Shunts.** The normal dye dilution curve appears as a quick upstroke in dye concentration, followed by a smooth, exponential decay. A smaller recirculation peak occurs late in the curve. A left-to-right shunt causes what is known as an *early recirculation,* which appears as a "hump" in the downstroke of the exponential phase. A right-to-left shunt will cause a small amount of dye to reach the arterial circulation without passing through the lungs, yielding an early small peak during the initial upstroke. The presence of these aberrant peaks can be used to diagnose congenital lesions and to test the adequacy of a repair.

   (2) **Repeat measurements.** Buildup of dye in the bloodstream prohibits repeated measurements because the background concentration will cause errors in accuracy.

   c. **Oxygen consumption (Fick) method**

   (1) **Sampling errors.** Gas sampling errors can occur, for instance, when a true expired sample is not obtained or when the volume of the exhaled gas is not accurate. Sampling of arterial rather than mixed venous blood occurs if the catheter tip is out too far in the PA, resulting in withdrawal of capillary blood.

   (2) **Oxygen consumption.** Because O_2 consumption by the lungs rather than the tissues is quantified by this method, significant error can be introduced if lung volumes change (as with the ventilation mode or the presence of atelectasis or lung collapse).

I. **Echocardiography.** Echocardiography, and especially **TEE,** has gained widespread use in the cardiac operating room. Indications for intraoperative TEE are listed in Table 3.12. For a complete discussion of TEE, see Chapter 4.

II. **Pulmonary system**

A. **Pulse oximetry**

1. **Indications**

   a. **Preoperative uses.** Pulse oximetry can help in the general preoperative assessment of a patient and can be easily used during the preoperative visit. Baseline O_2 saturation before premedication can alert the clinician to possible intraoperative or postoperative respiratory problems. In the patient with preexisting pulmonary hypertension, preoperative oximetry will alert one to the need for supplemental O_2 if premedication is given.

   b. **Assessment of oxygenation intraoperatively.** Continuous oximetry will rapidly diagnose airway or pulmonary complication. This capability is

Table 3.12 Indications for intraoperative transesophageal echocardiography

Judge adequacy of valvuloplasty procedures
   Mitral or tricuspid valve repair
   Mitral commissurotomy
Judge adequacy of valve replacement
   Rule out perivalvular leak
   Rule out malfunctioning prosthesis
Judge adequacy of repair of congenital heart disease
   Atrial or ventricular septal defect closure
   Flow through an intracardiac baffle
   Flow postarterioplasty (e.g., repair of pulmonary branch stenosis)
   Flow through a pulmonary-to-systemic shunt
Assessment of left or right ventricular function
   Global performance
   Wall-motion abnormalities
   Specific systolic and diastolic functional indices
Evaluation of myotomy or myomectomy in hypertrophic obstructive cardiomyopathy
Evaluation of retained intracardiac air

of special importance in cardiac patients because hypoxia will lower myocardial O_2 supply and may contribute to myocardial ischemia.

    c. Assessment of perfusion. The pulse oximeter utilizes plethysmography as a part of its basic operation. Thus, adequacy of perfusion is likely when the oximeter shows a saturation reading.

    d. Pulse rate. In the patient with a dysrhythmia, not every beat will lead to adequate perfusion, and this will be sensed by the pulse oximeter. An audible monitor of the heart rhythm is available.

  2. Advantages and disadvantages are listed in Table 3.13. Of note, cardiac surgery was found to be an independent predictor of pulse oximetry failure in one study that detected a better than 9% intraoperative oximetry failure rate of at least a 10-minute period [12].

B. Capnography

  1. Indications

    a. All patients. End-tidal capnography offers evidence of endotracheal intubation on an immediate, noninvasive basis and now is considered to be part

Table 3.13 Pulse oximetry in cardiac procedures

Advantages	Disadvantages
Ease of use	Poor perfusion states (shock, hypothermia) make the saturation unobtainable
Continuous monitor	Some dyes (methylene blue) interfere with the light absorbance
Noninvasive	Electrocautery causes interference
Most models have a variable pitch that correlates with the degree of saturation (obviates the need to view the screen)	Despite shielding, the oximeter cable can cause interference on other monitors if wires cross
Accuracy	Requires pulsatile flow to operate
	Extraneous lights (e.g., older Pilling operating room lights) cause interference

of the minimum standard of anesthetic care. It also provides continuous monitoring of the expired CO_2.

    b. Patients with lung disease. The capnograph provides evidence of the severity of small airway obstruction. Obstructive disease causes an up-sloping rather than a plateau or constant level of alveolar CO_2.

    c. Patients with pulmonary hypertension or reactive pulmonary vasculature. These patients often are asked to hyperventilate voluntarily just before induction (to prevent a deleterious rise in arterial CO_2 and worsening PA pressures). A capnograph can provide noninvasive evidence that an acceptable level of arterial P_{CO_2} has been attained. It also will guide the anesthesiologist in providing an effective, safe level of relative hyperventilation, which is essential in the management of these patients upon weaning from CPB.

  2. Types

    a. In-line models. An infrared sensor detects CO_2 in the respiratory gas passing through the endotracheal tube.

    b. Sampling models. These models continuously withdraw gas from the circuit and analyze it in a remote apparatus.

III. Temperature

  A. Indications

    1. Assessment of evenness of cooling and rewarming

    2. Diagnosing hazardous hypothermia or hyperthermia. Below 32°C, the myocardium is irritable and subject to complex arrhythmias, especially ventricular tachycardia and fibrillation. Likewise, significant enzyme desaturation and cell damage can occur with temperatures much higher than 41°C.

  B. Types of measuring devices

    1. Thermistor. Commonly used because of their accuracy, thermistors use thermal-sensitive semiconductors. Resistance through the conductor changes with changes in temperature. Thermistors are used in PA catheters and nasal probes to sense temperature.

    2. Thermocoupling. Thermocoupled probes are made by joining two strips of metal with different specific heats. As temperature changes in the strips, the metals expand or contract to different degrees, producing an electromotive force that is compared to a reference junction in a remote unit. Thermocoupling is used commonly in tympanic membrane probes.

  C. Sites of measurement. Considering the numerous possible sites in which to measure temperature, the question immediately arises as to which is the most accurate. The answer depends on which compartment one desires to measure, the core or the shell.

    1. Core temperature

      a. General. The core temperature represents the temperature of the vital organs. The term *core temperature* used here is perhaps a misnomer because gradients exist even within this vessel-rich group during rapid changes in blood temperature.

      b. PA catheter thermistor. This is the best estimate of the core temperature when pulmonary blood flow is present (i.e., before and after CPB). Most cardiac output monitors will display the thermistor temperature.

      c. Nasopharyngeal temperature. Nasopharyngeal temperature provides an accurate reflection of brain temperature during CPB, although there may be a lag between it and the actual brain temperature. The probe should be inserted into the nasopharynx to a distance equivalent to the distance from the naris to the tip of the earlobe.

      d. Tympanic membrane temperature. This temperature will reflect brain temperature, with the same limitations of lagging behind the actual brain temperature.

      e. Bladder temperature. This modality has been used to measure core temperature, although it may be inaccurate in instances when renal blood flow and urine production are decreased.

      f. Esophageal temperature. Because the esophagus is a mediastinal structure, it will be greatly affected by the temperature of the blood returning from the extracorporeal pump and should not be used routinely for cases involving CPB.

      g. CPB arterial line temperature. This is the temperature of the heat exchanger (i.e., the lowest temperature during active cooling and the highest temperature during active rewarming). During either of these phases, a gradient always exists between the arterial line temperature and any other temperature.

      h. CPB venous line temperature. This is the "return" temperature to the oxygenator and probably best reflects core temperature during CPB when no active warming or cooling is occurring.

  2. Shell

      a. General. The shell compartment represents the majority of the body (muscle, fat, bone), which receives a smaller proportion of the blood flow, thus acting as an energy sink that can significantly affect temperature fluxes. Shell temperatures will react more slowly than core temperatures. Shell temperature lags behind core temperature during cooling and rewarming. At the point of bypass separation, the core temperature will be significantly higher than shell temperature. The final equilibrium temperature with thermal redistribution probably will be closer to the shell temperature than the core temperature measured initially.

      b. Rectal temperature. Although traditionally thought of as a core temperature, during CPB procedures the rectal temperature most accurately reflects muscle mass temperature. If the tip of the probe rests in stool, a significant lag will exist with changing temperatures.

      c. Skin temperature. Skin temperature is affected by local factors (warming blanket, topical cooling device) and will lead to errors in gauging temperature.

D. Risks of bleeding. If the nasal mucosa is disrupted during probe placement, nasal bleeding can result, especially when the patient has been given heparin. Similar problems have been reported after placement of probes in the external ear canal. Otherwise, the risks of temperature monitoring are minimal.

E. Recommendations for temperature monitoring. Monitoring temperature at two sites is recommended, one at a core site and one at a shell site. Arterial and venous line temperatures are available directly from the CPB apparatus. Nasal temperature monitoring is recommended for core temperature because it will most rapidly reflect changes in the arterial blood temperature. Because rectal temperature monitoring is simple to establish, this is recommended for monitoring shell temperature.

IV. Renal function

A. Indications for monitoring

  1. Incidence of renal failure after CPB. Acute renal failure is a recognized complication of CPB, occurring in 2.5% to 31% of cases. Acute renal failure is related to preoperative renal function as well as to the presence of coexisting disease. CPB also may affect renal function adversely because the unphysiologic state of nonpulsatile flow may upset the normal autoregulatory mechanisms of renal blood flow.

  2. Use of diuretics in CPB prime. Mannitol is used routinely during CPB for two reasons:

      a. Hemolysis occurs during CPB, and serum hemoglobin levels rise. Urine output should be maintained to avoid damage to renal tubules.

      b. Deliberate hemodilution is induced with the onset of hypothermic CPB. Maintenance of good urine output during and after CPB allows removal of excess free water.

B. Urinary catheter. This monitor is the single most important monitor of renal function during surgical cases involving CPB. Establishing a urinary catheter should be a priority in emergencies.

1. **Anuria on bypass.** Not uncommonly, little urine will be made while the patient is on CPB. Hypothermia and the reduction of arterial flow will cause a diminution in renal function. Therefore, anuria should not usually be treated aggressively with additional diuretic therapy, especially while the patient is hypothermic.
2. **How much urine is adequate?** After CPB, adequacy of urine output depends on several factors, all of which should be optimized:
    a. Volume status
    b. Cardiac output
    c. Hematocrit
    d. Amount of surgical bleeding
C. **Electrolytes.** Serum electrolytes, especially potassium, should be checked toward the end of CPB and after bypass. Cardiac patients receive large amounts of potassium if cardioplegia is used, and elimination of this agent depends in part on satisfactory urine output. A low serum ionized calcium level may be the cause of diminished pump function and can be checked easily before separation from bypass.

V. Neurologic function

A. **General considerations.** The cardiac surgical patient is at increased risk of having an adverse neurologic event during surgery because of the unphysiologic state created by CPB (core cooling, alterations in blood flow) and because of the potential to introduce emboli (air, atheromatous material, thrombus). Advances in processing capability have made available new devices to monitor neurologic function during surgery. Monitoring the central nervous system is done for three primary reasons: (i) to diagnose cerebral ischemia, (ii) to assess the depth of anesthesia and prevent intraoperative awareness, and (iii) to assess the effectiveness of medications given for brain or spinal cord protection. The indications and types of neurologic monitors are outlined briefly here; for in depth applications, see Chapter 23.

B. **Indications for monitoring neurologic function**
    1. Associated carotid disease
    2. Diagnosis of embolic phenomenon
    3. Diagnosis of aortic cannula malposition
    4. Diagnosis of inadequate arterial flow on CPB
    5. Confirmation of adequate cooling
    6. Hypothermic circulatory arrest, in an adult or a child (see Chapter 23)

C. **Monitors of CNS electrical activity**
    1. **Electroencephalogram** (see Chapter 23). The electroencephalogram (EEG) measures the electrical currents generated by the postsynaptic potentials in the pyramidal cell layer of the cerebral cortex. The basic principle of clinical EEG monitoring is that cerebral ischemia causes slowing of the electrical activity of the brain, as well as a decrease in signal amplitude. An experienced electroencephalographer can interpret raw EEG data from four or eight channels, but would be hard pressed to also administer an anesthetic and monitor other organ systems.
    2. **Processed EEG.** To increase its intraoperative utility, the EEG data are processed by fast Fourier analysis into a single power versus time **spectral array** that is more easily interpreted. Examples of power spectrum analysis include **compressed spectral array, density spectral array,** and **bispectral index (BIS).** The BIS monitor analyzes the phase relationships between different frequency components over time, and the result is reduced via a proprietary method to a single number scaled between 0 (electrical silence) and 100 (alert wakefulness). The BIS may be a useful indicator of the depth of anesthesia for many procedures, but its significance in cardiac anesthesia has not been determined. Studies of BIS values as a predictor of anesthetic depth during intravenous anesthesia (narcotic plus benzodiazepine) are conflicting. One study found a positive correlation between the BIS and arousal or hemodynamic responses [13], whereas another study found no such correlation between the BIS value and plasma concentrations of fentanyl and midazolam [14].
    3. **Evoked potentials**
        a. **Somatosensory evoked potentials (SSEP).** SSEP can be used to monitor the integrity of the spinal cord. It is most useful in operations such as

surgery for a thoracic aneurysm, in which the blood flow to the spinal cord may be compromised. A stimulus is applied to a peripheral nerve (usually the tibial nerve), and the resultant brainstem and brain activity is quantified. Specific uses are discussed further in Chapter 24.

  b. **Visual evoked response and brainstem audio evoked responses.** These techniques do not have routine clinical application in cardiac surgical procedures and are not discussed here.

  c. **Motor evoked potentials (MEP).** MEPs are useful to monitor the spinal cord during surgery of the descending aorta and are discussed in more detail in Chapter 24.

D. **Monitors of cerebral metabolic function**

  1. **Jugular bulb venous oximetry.** Measuring the oxygen saturation of the cerebral jugular bulb with a fiberoptic catheter is akin to measuring the mixed venous oxygen saturation in the PA. Cerebral oxygen consumption is the product of cerebral blood flow (**CBF**) and the oxygen extraction by the brain. If CBF decreases, oxygen extraction would increase and the jugular O_2 saturation would decrease. Owing to a significant interpatient variability, trend monitoring yields more information than individual measurements. For applications of this technology, see Chapter 23.

  2. **Near-infrared spectroscopy (NIRS).** NIRS is a noninvasive method to monitor cerebral metabolic function. A near-infrared light is emitted from a scalp sensor and penetrates the scalp, skull, cerebrospinal fluid, and brain. The light is reflected by tissue but differentially absorbed by hemoglobin-containing moieties. The amount of absorption correlates with the oxygenation state of the hemoglobin in the tissue. Again, trend monitoring is possible because NIRS data are updated continuously.

E. **Monitors of CNS hemodynamics.**

  1. **Transcranial doppler ultrasonography (TCD).** The Doppler technology in TCD monitoring is similar to that used in echocardiography (see Chapter 4 for details). One difference is the signal attenuation caused by the skull, which is a source of artifact. Nonetheless, this technology is useful in detecting emboli in the cerebral circulation (see Chapter 23).

VI. **Electrical safety in the cardiac operating room**

A. **Electrical hazards.** The major hazards can be classified as macroshock, microshock, and thermal burns. Some general electrical terms are listed in Table 3.14. Our discussion will focus on microshock hazard.

  1. **Macroshock.** *Macroshock* is an uncommon occurrence in the operating room because of (i) isolation transformers, (ii) isolation of electrical equipment, (iii) patient isolation from ground, (iv) proper grounding of equipment, and (v) line isolation monitoring.

Table 3.14 Electrical terms

Ampere (amp or A)	Unit of electron flow, or current (I). One amp = 6.24×10^{18} electrons per second passing a point. Amount of current in a circuit will depend on voltage and resistance
Volt (V)	Potential difference that produces a current of 1 amp in a substance with a resistance of 1 Ω
Resistance (Ω)	Analogous to flow resistance. Related to current and voltage by: Resistance (Ω) = potential (V)/current (I)
Hertz (Hz)	For alternating current, refers to the frequency with which the current changes polarity each second
Macroshock	Current >1 mA, which is the perception threshold
Microshock	Current <1 mA, which bypasses skin resistance to cause hazard
Electrical burn	Thermal injury resulting from the dissipation of electrical energy in the form of injurious heat

2. **Microshock.** The term *microshock* applies to very small amounts of current (i.e., 1 mA). Significant morbidity has resulted from currents as low as 20 μA and often takes the form of cardiac dysrhythmias. Standard operating room isolation transformers provide no protection against currents of this magnitude. **Microshock cannot occur unless the skin resistance has been bypassed.** Because cardiac patients often have indwelling catheters that lead directly to the heart, as well as intracavitary or epicardial pacemaker wires, these patients are more susceptible to microshock hazard from these low-resistance pathways.

3. **Burns.** Electricity is a form of energy, and dissipation of energy takes the form of heat. *Burns* usually are a complication secondary to use of the electrocautery unit. Improper patient grounding is the usual cause.

B. **Determinants of electrical hazard**

1. **Current density.** The disruption of physiologic function produced by a given electrical current is inversely proportional to the area over which this current is applied. In the case of a small-bore central venous catheter in the RA, the amount of current needed to produce a significant arrhythmia is small.

2. **Current duration.** Cardiac muscle can recover quickly from a direct current that is applied for only microseconds but may become depolarized if the current is applied for 1 or more seconds.

3. **Type of current. Direct** current (DC) is the unidirectional, nonoscillating current that results when a constant voltage is applied across a resistor. When DC passes through skeletal or cardiac muscle, a sustained contraction can result. **Alternating** current (AC) is current that changes polarity at a specified rate. It is the rate, or **frequency,** of the change in polarity that determines the magnitude of the hazard. Low-frequency alternating currents, such as the standard 60 Hz, can cause significant tetanic contraction of skeletal muscles as well as ventricular fibrillation with small currents.

4. **Skin resistance.** Resistance across intact skin can be as large as 1 million Ω when the skin is dry. This amount can drop by a factor of 1,000 when skin is wet. A centrally placed fluid-filled catheter that punctures the skin lowers resistance to 500 Ω and places the patient at a higher risk of sustaining a microshock injury.

5. **Current threshold (AC).** *Current threshold* is a term used by some to quantify that amount of current at 60 Hz needed to cause ventricular fibrillation. Several studies have determined the value to be anywhere between 50 and 1,000 μA (microshock range). One group found that as catheter size decreases (resulting in an increased current density), the total amount of current needed to produce fibrillation also decreases (Fig. 3.15).

C. **Results of microshock**

1. **Ventricular fibrillation.** Several reviews of accidents occurring in humans have established the current threshold to be approximately 100 μA, but this amount depends on the size of the catheter and other factors.

2. **Dysrhythmias.** It is noteworthy that in many animal studies, rhythm disturbances occur before reaching currents needed to produce ventricular fibrillation. It is important to note that these rhythm disturbances can cause severe hypotension and mortality similar to that associated with ventricular fibrillation. Pump failure produced by rhythm disturbances occurs at approximately half the current threshold needed to produce ventricular fibrillation (Fig. 3.15).

D. **Mechanisms of microshock.** Electrical hazard is possible when there is a path by which electrical current can flow from an electronic device through a patient to ground *and* there is some fault in the electrical grounding of the apparatus. These conditions must be present simultaneously in order for a shock hazard to exist. If the circuit includes an intracardiac monitor such as a CVP line, the leakage current can be transmitted directly to the heart, creating a microshock hazard.

E. **Prevention of electrical hazard**

1. **Macroshock.** The combined use of isolation transformers and line isolation monitors will provide some protection against macroshock, although if the conditions for electrical hazard exist (i.e., a faulty electrical grounding), electrical safety is not necessarily guaranteed.

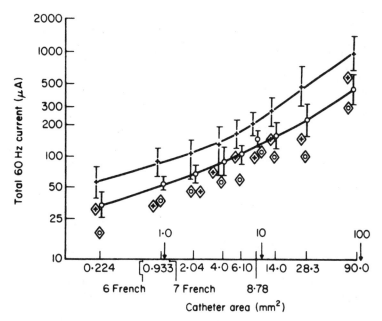

FIG. 3.15 Current thresholds for ventricular fibrillation and pump failure (caused by dysrhythmias) in anesthetized dogs as a function of catheter size. + and ◈, average and lowest fibrillation thresholds; 0 and ⬦, average and lowest pump failure thresholds. (Modified from Roy OZ, Scott JR, Park GC. 60-Hz ventricular fibrillation and pump failure thresholds versus electrode area. *IEEE Trans Biomed Eng* 1976;23:47.)

2. Microshock. Avoidance of the conditions that lead to an AC path will prevent microshock hazard. Good equipment design and maintenance are essential. Equipment that incorporates infrared coupling between patient connections and the internal circuitry effectively will eliminate any possible current flow through a patient. Isolation of the monitoring equipment–patient connection from the internal circuitry by an isolation transformer reduces the risk of microshock hazard. In addition, any equipment that bypasses skin resistance (central fluid-filled catheters, epicardial pacemakers) should be handled with care to avoid any leakage current reaching the patient. (For example, the caregiver could touch a faulty piece of equipment and then touch a CVP catheter simultaneously.)

3. There is no substitute for vigilance in preventing electrical hazards (macroshock or microshock). Situations in which measuring or recording systems display excess noise in the form of humming or drifting in the baseline may represent a problem with the electronic circuitry. If the line-isolation monitor is used in the operating room and this alarm demonstrates a low resistance between the isolated power lines and ground, it cannot be ignored. The offending piece of equipment should be identified and sent for repair.

References
1. London MJ, Hollenberg M, Wong MG, et al. Intraoperative myocardial ischemia: localization by continuous 12-lead electrocardiography. *Anesthesiology* 1988;62:232–241.
2. Kaplan JA, King SB. The precordial electrocardiographic lead (V5) in patients w o have coronary artery disease. *Anesthesiology* 1976;45:570–574.

3. **Leung JM, Voskanian A, Bellows WH, et al. Automated electrocardiograph ST segment trending monitors: accuracy in detecting myocardial ischemia.** *Anesth Analg* **1998;87:4–10.**
4. Slogoff S, Keats AS, Arlund C. On the safety of radial artery cannulation. *Anesthesiology* 1983;59:42–47.
5. Stern DH, Gerson JI, Allen FB, et al. Can we trust the direct radial artery pressure immediately following cardiopulmonary bypass? *Anesthesiology* 1985;62:557–561.
6. Mohr R, Lavee J, Goor DA. Inaccuracy of radial artery pressure measurement after cardiac operations. *J Thorac Cardiovasc Surg* 1987;94:286–290.
7. Caridi JG, Hawkins IF Jr, Wiechmann BN, et al. Sonographic guidance when using the right internal jugular vein for central venous access. *Am J Roentgenol* 1988;171:1259–1263.
8. **Tuman, KJ, Carroll GC, Ivankovich AD. Pitfalls in interpretation of pulmonary artery catheter data.** *J Cardiothorac Anesth* **1989;3:626–641.**
9. Waller JL, Zaidan JR, Kaplan JA, et al. Hemodynamic responses to preoperative vascular cannulation in patients with coronary artery disease. *Anesthesiology* 1982;56:219–221.
10. Trankina MF, White RD. Perioperative cardiac pacing using an atrioventricular pacing pulmonary artery catheter. *J Cardiothorac Anesth* 1989;3:154–162.
11. Hoel BL. Some aspects of the clinical use of thermodilution in measuring cardiac output. *Scand J Clin Lab Invest* 1978;38:383–388.
12. Reich DK, Timcenko A, Bodian CA, et al. Predictors of pulse oximetry data failure. *Anesthesiology* 1996;84:859–864.
13. Heck M, Kumle B, Boldt J, et al. Electroencephalogram bispectral index predicts hemodynamic and arousal reactions during induction of anesthesia in patients undergoing cardiac surgery. *J Cardiothorac Vasc Anesth* 2000;14:693–697.
14. **Barr G, Anderson RE, Samuelsson S, et al. Fentanyl and midazolam anaesthesia for coronary bypass surgery: a clinical study of bispectral electroencephalogram analysis, drug concentrations and recall.** *Br J Anaesth* **2000;84:749–752.**

4. TRANSESOPHAGEAL ECHOCARDIOGRAPHY

Jack S. Shanewise, Robert Savage, Solomon Aronson, and Daniel M. Thys

I. Basic principles of ultrasound imaging

Medical ultrasound is produced by a piezoelectric crystal that vibrates in response to a high frequency, alternating electrical current. The same crystal is deformed by returning echoes producing an electrical signal that is detected by the instrument. Ultrasound transmitted from the transducer into the patient interacts with the tissues in four ways: (i) reflection, (ii) refraction, (iii) scattering, and (iv) attenuation. Ultrasound is reflected when it encounters the interface between tissues of different acoustic impedance, primarily a function of tissue density, and the timing, intensity, and phase of these echoes are processed to form the image. The velocity of transmission of ultrasound through soft tissues is relatively constant (1,540 m/s), and the time it takes the waves to travel to an object, be reflected, and return is determined by its distance from the transducer. Selecting the frequency of an ultrasound transducer is a trade-off between image resolution and depth of penetration. Higher frequencies have better resolution than lower frequencies, but they do not penetrate as far into tissue. The frequency of the ultrasound used in transesophageal echocardiography (TEE) typically ranges from 3.5 to 7.0 million cycles per second (MHz).

II. Basic principles of Doppler echocardiography

A. Doppler echocardiography uses ultrasound scattered from blood cells to measure the velocity and direction of blood flow. The Doppler effect increases the frequency of waves scattered from cells moving toward the transducer and decreases the frequency of waves from cells moving away. This change in the transmitted frequency (F_T) and the scattered frequency (F_S) is called the Doppler shift ($F_S - F_T$) and is related to the velocity of blood flow (V) by the Doppler equation:

$$V = c(F_S - F_T)/2F_T \text{ (cos } \theta)$$

where c is the speed of sound in blood (1,540 m/s) and θ is the angle between the direction of blood flow and the ultrasound beam. The 2 in the denominator corrects for the time it takes the ultrasound to travel to and from the blood cells. In order to get a reasonably accurate (less than 6% error) measurement of blood velocity with Doppler echocardiography, the angle between the flow and the ultrasound beam (θ) should be less than 20 degrees.

B. The Bernoulli equation describes the relationship between flow velocity through a stenosis and the pressure gradient across the stenosis. It is a complex relationship that includes factors for convective acceleration, flow acceleration, and viscous resistance. In certain clinical applications, such as aortic and mitral stenosis, a simplified form may be used. The **simplified Bernoulli equation** is:

$$\Delta P = 4V^2$$

where ΔP is pressure gradient in millimeters of mercury (mm Hg) and v is velocity in meters per second (m/s). The simplified Bernoulli equation should only be used in applications validated against another gold standard.

III. Modes of cardiac ultrasound imaging

A. **M-mode echocardiography** was the primary imaging mode for echocardiography for many years before the development of two-dimensional (2D) imaging in the late 1970s. It directs pulses of a single, linear beam of ultrasound into the tissues and displays the distance from the transducer of the returning echoes on the y-axis of a graph with signal strength indicated by brightness. The x-axis of the graph shows time, and motion of the structures is seen as curved lines. M-mode is useful for precisely timing events within the cardiac cycle. Its other advantage is very high temporal resolution, making thousands of images per second, which allows high-frequency oscillating motion, such as vibrating vegetations, to be detected.

B. **Two-dimensional echocardiography** is made by very rapidly moving the ultrasound beam through a plane, creating multiple scan lines that are displayed simultaneously to construct a 2D tomographic image. Mechanical transducers accomplish this by physically rotating or oscillating the crystal. However, TEE probes usually have phased-array transducers, which consist of an array of many (64 to 128) small crystals that are electrically activated in sequence to move the beam through the imaging plane. The number of 2D images that can be formed each second is called the frame rate (temporal resolution), which is determined by the width (number of scan lines per image) and depth (time for each pulse to return) of the imaging sector. Typical frame rates for 2D echocardiography are 30 to 60 frames per second, which is fast enough to accurately reflect most motion in the heart.

C. **Pulsed-wave Doppler** measures the velocity and direction of blood flow in a specific location, called the sample volume, which can be placed by the user in the area of interest of a 2D image. The velocity of flow is displayed through time on the x-axis with velocity toward the transducer above the baseline on the y-axis and velocity away below. Pulsed-wave Doppler (PWD) uses one transducer to both send and receive signals, determining the depth of the sample volume from the transducer by listening at a predetermined interval after transmission. This limits the maximum rate at which pulses can be sent (pulse repetition frequency), which in turn limits the maximum Doppler shift (**Nyquist limit**) and blood velocity that can be measured with PWD. The farther the sample volume is from the transducer, the lower the maximum velocity that can be measured. Typically, velocities more than 1.5 to 2.0 m/s cannot be measured with PWD.

D. **Continuous-wave Doppler** measures the velocity and direction of blood flow along the line of sight of the ultrasound beam. The information is displayed with time on the x-axis and velocity on the y-axis, as with PWD. Continuous-wave Doppler (CWD) uses two transducers: one to continuously transmit and the other to continuously receive. As a result, CWD cannot determine the depth from the transducer from which a returning signal originated (range ambiguity), only its direction. But, unlike PWD, CWD has no limit on the maximum velocity measured. CWD is used to measure blood velocity too high for PWD, such as aortic stenosis (AS), and to determine the maximum velocity of a flow profile, such as with mitral stenosis.

E. **Color-flow Doppler** is a form of PWD that superimposes the velocity information onto the simultaneously created 2D image of the heart, allowing the location and timing of flow disturbances to be easily seen. Flow toward the transducer usually is mapped as red and away as blue. Some color-flow Doppler (CFD) maps, called **variance maps,** add green to indicate turbulence in the flow. Because it is a form of PWD, CFD cannot accurately measure higher flow velocities, such as mitral regurgitation (MR) and AS, and these flows appear as a mixture of red and blue, called a mosaic pattern. Also, as the flow velocity passes the limit of the CFD velocity scale (Nyquist limit), the color will alias, or change from red to blue or from blue to red, depending on the direction of flow. The aliasing velocity or Nyquist limit for CFD varies with the depth of the color sector, but typically is less than 100 cm/s. Because the instrument must develop both the 2D and Doppler images, the frame rate is lower with CFD than with 2D imaging alone, typically in the range from 12 to 24 frames per second. At frame rates below 15 frames per second, the image becomes noticeably jerky as the eye can discern the individual images. Decreasing the width and depth of the 2D image and the CFD sector within it will maximize frame rate.

IV. **Indications for TEE during cardiac surgery**

TEE can be used as a diagnostic tool during cardiac surgery to direct the surgical procedure and diagnose unanticipated problems and complications. TEE also is useful to the cardiac anesthesiologist as a monitor of cardiac function. Often, TEE is used for both purposes during heart surgery. The American Society of Anesthesiologists and the Society of Cardiovascular Anesthesiologists (ASA/SCA) practice guidelines for perioperative TEE state that the need for TEE is determined by (i) the characteristics of the patient, (ii) the nature of the procedure to be performed, and (iii) the setting in which the procedure will occur, i.e., the availability of equipment and expertise. The guidelines place the indications for TEE into three categories. Category one includes those for which there is the strongest evidence that TEE is helpful, such as valve repair, congenital heart defects, hypertrophic obstructive cardiomyopathy, aortic dissection, infective endocarditis, and unstable, life-threatening hemodynamics. Category two includes indications supported by weaker evidence than category one but for which TEE may be of benefit, such as monitoring for myocardial ischemia, valve

Table 4.1 Relative contraindications to transesophageal echocardiography

---

History
  Dysphagia
  Odynophagia
  Mediastinal radiation
  Recent upper gastrointestinal surgery
  Recent upper gastrointestinal bleeding
Esophageal pathology
  Stricture
  Tumor
  Diverticulum
  Varices
  Esophagitis
  Recent chest trauma

---

replacement, cardiac aneurysms, and intracardiac tumors. Category three includes indications for which there is little support in the literature, such as assessment of myocardial perfusion, monitoring for emboli during orthopedic procedures, and placement of intraaortic balloon pumps and pulmonary artery catheters.

  V. Safety, contraindications, and risk of TEE

    A. Preoperative screening for esophageal disease should be completed before proceeding with TEE. The patient should be interviewed when possible and asked about a history of esophageal disease, dysphagia, and hematemesis. The medical record should be reviewed as well. Relative contraindications to TEE are listed in Table 4.1. The presence of a relative contraindication requires balancing the risk with the importance of TEE to the procedure. In patients with distal esophageal or gastric pathology, it often is possible to obtain the information needed with TEE without advancing into the distal esophagus. Preoperative esophagoscopy is another option to consider when the need for TEE is important and the risk is unclear.

    B. TEE probe insertion and manipulation should be performed gently. The probe must never be forced through a resistance, and excessive force must never be applied to the control wheels.

    C. Complications of TEE are uncommon in properly screened patients, but they may be serious [2]. Complications of TEE are listed in Table 4.2. Serious injuries may not be apparent at the time of the procedure [3].

  VI. Intraoperative TEE examination

    A. Probe insertion is performed after the patient is anesthetized and the endotracheal tube secured. An orogastric tube is inserted and the contents of the stomach and esophagus suctioned. As the mandible is displaced anteriorly, the probe is gently placed into the posterior pharynx in the midline and inserted into the esophagus. A laryngoscope may be used to displace the mandible and better visualize the

Table 4.2 Complications of transesophageal echocardiography

Dental and oral trauma (usually minor)
Laryngeal dysfunction
  Postoperative aspiration
Endotracheal tube displacement
Bronchial compression in infants
Aortic compression in infants
Upper gastrointestinal bleeding (mucosal injury)
Pharyngeal perforation (rare)
Esophageal perforation (rare)

---

esophageal opening if necessary. As the probe is advanced into the thoracic esophagus (approximately 30 cm), the heart should come into view. On rare occasions, the probe cannot be placed in the esophagus, in which case the TEE is abandoned.

B. **Probe manipulation** is accomplished by advancing and withdrawing the probe within the esophagus, rotating the probe to the patient's left or right, flexing the tip anteriorly and posteriorly with the large control wheel, and flexing the tip to the patient's right and left with the small control wheel. With a multiplane TEE probe, the angle of the transducer is rotated axially from 0 degrees (horizontal plane), through 90 degrees (vertical plane), to 180 degrees (mirror image of 0 degrees horizontal plane) (Fig. 4.1).

C. **Machine settings** are adjusted to optimize the TEE image. These settings are continuously adjusted by the user as the examination proceeds.

   1. **Transducer frequency** is adjusted to the highest frequency that provides adequate depth of penetration to the structure being examined.

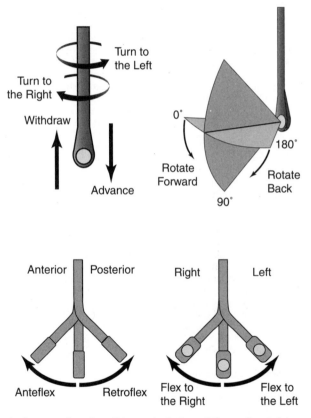

FIG. 4.1 Terminology used to describe manipulation of the probe and transducer during image acquisition. (From Shanewise JS, Cheung AT, Aronson S, et al. ASE/SCA guidelines for performing a comprehensive intraoperative multiplane transesophageal echocardiography examination: recommendations of the American Society of Echocardiography Council for Intraoperative Echocardiography and the Society of Cardiovascular Anesthesiologists Task Force for Certification in Perioperative Transesophageal Echocardiography. *Anesth Analg* 1999;89:870–884, with permission.)

2. **Image depth** is adjusted to center the structure being examined in the display.
3. **Overall image gain** and **dynamic range** (compression) are adjusted so that the blood in the chambers appears nearly black and is distinct from the shades of gray representing tissue.
4. **Time gain compensation** controls are adjusted so that there is uniform brightness from the near field to the far field of the image.
5. **CFD gain** is adjusted to a threshold that just eliminates any background noise within the color sector.

D. TEE views

The American Society of Echocardiography/Society of Cardiovascular Anesthesiologists (ASE/SCA) guidelines for performing a comprehensive intraoperative multiplane TEE examination [4] define 20 views that comprise a comprehensive TEE examination (Table 4.3). These 20 views are shown in Figure 4.2. The views are named for the location of the transducer (echocardiographic window), a descriptive term of the imaging plane [e.g., short axis (SAX) or long axis (LAX)], and the major anatomic structure in the view. All of these views can be developed in most patients. Additional views may be needed to completely examine a patient with a particular form of pathology. The sequence in which these views are obtained will vary from examiner to examiner, but it is generally most efficient to develop the midesophageal (ME) views and then the transgastric (TG) views.

1. **ME views** are developed with the TEE transducer posterior to the left atrium (LA). With a multiplane TEE probe, detailed examinations of cardiac chambers and valves can be completed in most patients from this window alone.
2. **TG views** are obtained by passing the transducer into the stomach and directing the imaging plane superiorly through the diaphragm to the heart. Images of the left ventricle (LV) and right ventricle (RV) and the mitral valve (MV) and tricuspid valve (TV) are made from this window. Views to align the Doppler beam parallel to flow through the left ventricular outflow tract (LVOT) and aortic valve (AV) can be developed from the TG window.
3. **Upper esophageal (UE) views** are made with the transducer at the level of the aortic arch, which is examined in LAX and SAX. In many patients, images of the main pulmonary artery and pulmonic valve also may be developed, allowing alignment of the Doppler beam parallel to flow in these structures.

E. Examination of specific structures

1. **Left ventricle.** The LV is examined with the ME four-chamber, ME two-chamber, ME LAX, TG mid-SAX, and TG two-chamber views.
   a. **LV size** is assessed by measuring the inside diameter at the junction of the basal and mid thirds at end diastole. Normal is less than 5.5 cm. Normal thickness of the LV wall at this level is 1.2 cm or less at end diastole.
   b. **LV global function** may be assessed quantitatively or qualitatively. Fractional area change (FAC) is a 2D TEE equivalent of ejection fraction (EF) and is obtained by measuring the LV chamber area in the TG mid-SAX view by tracing the endocardial border to measure the end diastolic area (EDA) and the end systolic area (ESA) and using the formula: FAC = (EDA − ESA)/EDA. Normal FAC is greater than 0.50. This method is not as accurate when wall-motion abnormalities are present in the apex or the base of the LV. Qualitative assessment of LV function is performed by considering all views of the LV and estimating the ejection fraction (EEF) as normal (EEF >55%), mildly decreased (EEF 45% to 54%), moderately decreased (EEF 35% to 44%), moderately severely decreased (EEF 25% to 34%), or severely decreased (EEF <25%). EEF by experienced echocardiographers correlates with nonechocardiographic measures of EF as well or better than quantitative echocardiographic measurements of EF [5].
   c. **Assessment of regional LV function.** The LV is divided into 16 regions or segments (Fig. 4.3). Each segment is rated qualitatively for thickening during systole using the following scale: 1 = normal (>30% thickening), 2 = mild hypokinesis (10% to 30% thickening), 3 = severe hypokinesis (<10% thickening), 4 = akinesis (no thickening), and 5 = dyskinesis (thinning and paradoxical motion during systole). An increase in scale of 2 or

Table 4.3 Recommended transesophageal echocardiographic cross sections

Window (depth from incisors)	Cross section (panel in Fig. 4.3)	Multiplane angle range	Structures imaged
Upper esophageal (20–25 cm)	Aortic arch long axis (s)	0°	Aortic arch, left brachiocephalic vein
	Aortic arch short axis (t)	90°	Aortic arch, PA, PV, left brachiocephalic vein
Mid esophageal (30–40 cm)	Four chamber (a)	0°–20°	LV, LA, RV, RA, MV, TV, IAS
	Mitral commissural (g)	60°–70°	MV, LV, LA
	Two chamber (b)	80°–100°	LV, LA, LAA, MV, CS
	Long axis (c)	120°–160°	LV, LA, AV, LVOT, MV, asc aorta
	RV inflow-outflow (m)	60°–90°	RV, RA, TV, RVOT, PV, PA
	AV short axis (h)	30°–60°	AV, IAS, coronary ostia, LVOT, PV
	AV long axis (i)	120°–160°	AV, LVOT, prox asc aorta, right PA
	Bicaval (l)	80°–110°	RA, SVC, IVC, IAS, LA
	Asc aortic short axis (o)	0°–60°	Asc aorta, SVC, PA, right PA
	Asc aortic long axis (p)	100°–150°	Asc aorta, right PA
	Desc aorta short axis (q)	0°	Desc thoracic aorta, left pleural space
	Desc aorta long axis (r)	90°–110°	Desc thoracic aorta, left pleural space
Transgastric (40–45 cm)	Basal short axis (f)	0°–20°	LV, MV, RV, TV
	Mid short axis (d)	0°–20°	LV, RV, papillary muscles
	Two chamber (e)	80°–100°	LV, MV, chordae, papillary muscles, CS, LA
	Long axis (j)	90°–120°	LVOT, AV, MV
	RV inflow (n)	100°–120°	RV, TV, RA, TV chordae, papillary muscles
Deep transgastric (45–50 cm)	Long axis (k)	0°–20° (anteflexion)	LVOT, AV, asc aorta, arch

asc, ascending; AV, aortic valve; CS, coronary sinus; desc, descending; IAS, interatrial septum; IVC, inferior vena cava; LA, left atrium; LAA, left atrial appendage; LV, left ventricle; LVOT, left ventricular outflow tract; MV, mitral valve; PA, pulmonary artery; prox, proximal; PV, pulmonic valve; RA, right atrium; RV, right ventricle; RVOT, right ventricular outflow tract; SVC, superior vena cava; TV, tricuspid valve.

more in a region should be considered significant and suggestive of myocardial ischemia [6].

  d. **Assessment of diastolic LV function** can be made by examining with PWD the transmitral inflow velocity profile during diastole. The normal pattern has an E wave corresponding to early passive filling of the LV, followed by a period of diastasis, and finally an A wave corresponding to atrial contraction in late diastole (Fig. 4.4A). Milder forms of diastolic dysfunction result in the **impaired relaxation pattern** with decreased peak E-to-A velocity ratio and prolonged E-wave deceleration time (Fig. 4.4B).

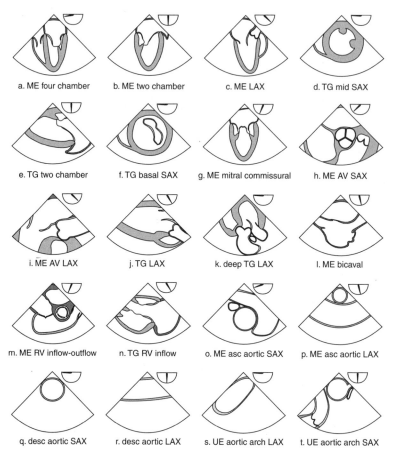

FIG. 4.2 Twenty cross-sectional views composing the recommended comprehensive transesophageal echocardiographic examination. Approximate multiplane angle is indicated by the icon adjacent to each view. *asc,* ascending; *AV,* aortic valve; *desc,* descending; *LAX,* long axis; *ME,* midesophageal; *RV,* right ventricle; *SAX,* short axis; *TG,* transgastric; *UE,* upper esophageal. (From Shanewise JS, Cheung AT, Aronson S, et al. ASE/SCA guidelines for performing a comprehensive intraoperative multiplane transesophageal echocardiography examination: recommendations of the American Society of Echocardiography Council for Intraoperative Echocardiography and the Society of Cardiovascular Anesthesiologists Task Force for Certification in Perioperative Transesophageal Echocardiography. *Anesth Analg* 1999;89:870–884, with permission.)

Advanced diastolic dysfunction causes the **restrictive pattern** with increased peak E-to-A velocity ratio and decreased E-wave deceleration time (Fig. 4.4C). As diastolic dysfunction progresses from mild to severe over a number of years, the transmitral flow pattern may pass through a period in which it appears normal, a condition termed **pseudonormal pattern.** Normal may be distinguished from pseudonormal by examination of the

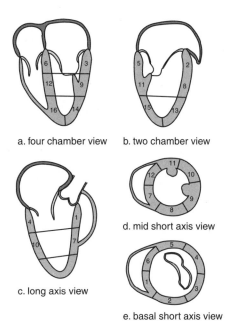

a. four chamber view   b. two chamber view

d. mid short axis view

c. long axis view

e. basal short axis view

FIG. 4.3 Sixteen-segment model of the left ventricle. **A:** Four-chamber views show the three septal and three lateral segments. **B:** Two-chamber views show the three anterior and three inferior segments. **C:** Long-axis views show the two anteroseptal and two posterior segments. **D:** Mid short-axis views show all six segments at the mid level. **E:** Basal short-axis views show all six segments at the basal level. Basal segments: *1,* basal anteroseptal; *2,* basal anterior; *3,* basal lateral; *4,* basal posterior; *5,* basal inferior; *6,* basal septal. Mid segments: *7,* mid anteroseptal; *8,* mid anterior; *9,* mid lateral; *10,* mid posterior; *11,* mid inferior; *12,* mid septal. Apical segments. *13,* apical anterior; *14,* apical lateral; *15,* apical inferior; *16,* apical septal. (From Shanewise JS, Cheung AT, Aronson S, et al. ASE/SCA guidelines for performing a comprehensive intraoperative multiplane transesophageal echocardiography examination: recommendations of the American Society of Echocardiography Council for Intraoperative Echocardiography and the Society of Cardiovascular Anesthesiologists Task Force for Certification in Perioperative Transesophageal Echocardiography. *Anesth Analg* 1999;89: 870–884, with permission.)

pulmonary venous inflow velocity profile, which normally has positive inflow waves during systole (S wave) and diastole (D wave) and a small, negative wave corresponding to atrial contraction (A wave) (Fig. 4.5A). The pseudonormal pattern has prolongation of the A wave and attenuation of the S wave compared to the normal pattern (Fig. 4.5B). Age and preload also affect the transmitral and pulmonary venous inflow velocity patterns.

2. **Mitral valve.** The MV is examined with the ME four chamber, ME mitral commissural, ME LAX, and TG basal SAX views, with and without CFD. It consists of an anterior leaflet and a posterior leaflet joined at two commissures, the anterolateral and the posteromedial. There is a papillary muscle corresponding to each commissure. The posterior leaflet is divided into three scallops and the anterior leaflet into thirds for purposes of describing the location of lesions (Fig. 4.6). Prolapse of the MV is present when a portion of the leaflet

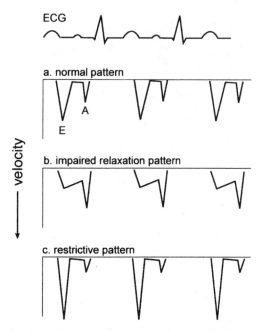

FIG. 4.4 Transmitral inflow velocity profiles measured with pulsed-wave Doppler by placing the sample volume between the open tips of the mitral leaflets. **A:** Normal pattern. The pseudonormal pattern has a similar appearance. **B:** Impaired relaxation pattern indicative of mild diastolic dysfunction. The peak E wave velocity is less than the A wave (E-to-A reversal) and the deceleration time of the E wave is prolonged. **C:** Restrictive pattern indicative of advanced diastolic dysfunction. The peak E wave velocity is increased and the E wave deceleration time is decreased. *A,* atrial filling wave; *E,* early filling wave.

moves to the atrial side of the annulus during systole. Flail is said to be present when a chordae tendineae is ruptured and the corresponding segment of the valve leaflet is seen oscillating in the LA during systole.

a. Mitral regurgitation

Judging severity of MR with TEE is based on several factors. The structure of the valve leaflets is examined with 2D echocardiography, looking for defects of coaptation. CFD is used to detect retrograde flow through the valve into the LA. The width of the jet as it passes through the valve and its size in the LA are noted. Eccentric jets of MR tend to be more severe than central jets of a similar size. CFD also can detect flow convergence proximal to the regurgitant orifice, indicating more significant MR. Pulmonary venous inflow velocity profile is examined with PWD for systolic flow reversal, a specific but not very sensitive sign of severe MR. Severity is graded on a semiquantitative scale of 1+ (mild) to 4+ (severe). Most patients have at least trace amounts of MR detected with TEE.

Functional MR is due to dilation of the MV annulus or displacement of the papillary muscles causing a decrease in the surface of coaptation of the MV leaflets. The structure of the valve leaflets is normal. Functional

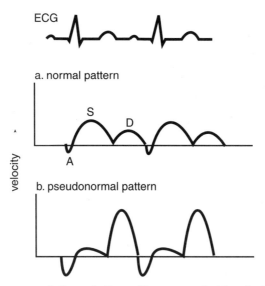

FIG. 4.5 Pulmonary venous inflow velocity profiles measured with pulsed-wave Doppler by placing the sample volume in the left upper pulmonary vein. **A:** Profile seen with normal diastolic function and transmitral inflow. The S wave is larger than the D wave and a small A reversal is present. **B:** Pattern seen with diastolic dysfunction and pseudonormal transmitral inflow. The S wave is attenuated and smaller than the D wave and an enlarged A wave is present. *A*, atrial reversal wave; *D*, diastolic wave, *S*, systolic wave.

MR can be very dynamic and is markedly affected by loading conditions. The most common causes of functional MR are regional wall motion abnormalities (RWMAs) from coronary artery disease and generalized dilation of the LV.

Myxomatous degeneration of the MV is a common cause of MR requiring surgery. The leaflets are elongated and redundant, prolapsing into the LA during systole. Rupture of a chordae is common in this condition and causes a flail segment of the involved leaflet. TEE can be used to locate the portion of the MV involved and is helpful in guiding surgical therapy. Prolapse and flail of the middle scallop of the posterior leaflet is the most common form and most amenable to repair by resection of the involved portion and reinforcement of the annulus with an annuloplasty ring.

Rheumatic MR is caused by thickening and shortening of the MV leaflets and chordae restricting motion and closure during systole. This type of MR typically is difficult to repair and usually requires prosthetic valve replacement.

b. Mitral stenosis

Significant mitral stenosis almost always is due to rheumatic heart disease. Mitral annular calcification is a rare cause of significant stenosis. Two-dimensional images show thickening of the leaflets with fusion at the

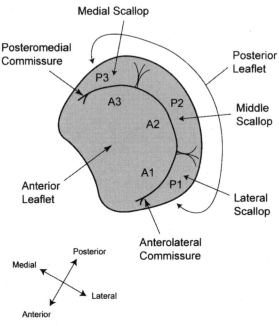

FIG. 4.6 Anatomy of the mitral valve. *A1,* lateral third of the anterior leaflet; *A2,* middle third of the anterior leaflet; *A3,* medial third of the anterior leaflet; *P1,* lateral scallop of the posterior leaflet; *P2,* middle scallop of the posterior leaflet; *P3,* medial scallop of the posterior leaflet. (From Shanewise JS, Cheung AT, Aronson S, et al. ASE/SCA guidelines for performing a comprehensive intraoperative multiplane transesophageal echocardiography examination: recommendations of the American Society of Echocardiography Council for Intraoperative Echocardiography and the Society of Cardiovascular Anesthesiologists Task Force for Certification in Perioperative Transesophageal Echocardiography. *Anesth Analg* 1999;89:870–884, with permission.)

commissures and restricted opening during diastole. Doppler velocity measurements of the transmitral inflow shows increased peak and mean velocities, which can be used to calculate peak and mean transvalvular gradients ($\Delta P = 4V^2$).

TEE can be used measure valve area in mitral stenosis by the following methods:

(1) Planimetry. Images of the stenotic orifice may be directly measured from the TG basal SAX view. The imaging plane is moved above and below the valve until the minimal orifice is seen, then the image is frozen in diastole and the orifice traced. Calcification of the annulus or leaflets may create acoustic shadowing limiting the ability to accurately image the orifice in many patients.

(2) Pressure half-time. The rate at which the pressure gradient decreases across a stenotic MV during diastole is directly related to the severity of the stenosis. A measure of this rate is the pressure half-time, which can be measured from the transmitral inflow velocity profile. An empirically derived formula gives the mitral valve area (MVA) in square centimeters as:

MVA = 220/PHT

where PHT is the pressure half-time in milliseconds. This formula has been validated only for patients with rheumatic mitral stenosis. It cannot be used if there is more than mild aortic regurgitation (AR) or immediately after a mitral commissurotomy.

3. **Aortic valve.** The AV is examined in the ME AV SAX and ME LAX views, with and without CFD. Doppler measurements of flow velocity through the AV are made from the TG LAX and deep TG LAX views, which allow the ultrasound beam to be directed parallel to AV flow. The AV is a semilunar valve that has three cusps: the right coronary cusp, which is most anterior; the noncoronary cusp, which is adjacent to the atrial septum; and the left coronary cusp.

   a. **Aortic regurgitation**

   The severity of AR is assessed with TEE primarily by the size of the regurgitant jet on CFD and the depth to which it extends into the LV. The valve cusps also should be examined with 2D echocardiography, looking for perforations and defects in coaptation. Other signs of severe AR include holodiastolic flow reversal in the descending thoracic aorta, pressure half-time of AR less than 300 msec as measured from the AR velocity profile, presystolic closure of the MV, and presystolic MR.

   b. **Aortic stenosis**

   Evaluation of AS with TEE is based on the appearance of the valve on 2D images and Doppler velocity measurements of the flow through the stenotic valve. In AS, the valve leaflets are thickened with markedly restricted opening during systole. Calcification of the cusps and the annulus may cause acoustic shadowing. TEE may be used to quantify the severity of AS by three methods:

   (1) **Transaortic gradients** may be calculated with the simplified Bernoulli equation ($\Delta P = 4V^2$) by using CWD to measure the flow velocity in meters per second through a stenotic AV from the TG LAX or deep TG LAX views. For example, if the peak AV outflow velocity is 5 m/s, the peak instantaneous gradient would be 100 mm Hg. Peak velocities greater than 4 m/s (peak gradient >64 mm Hg) are consistent with severe AS, but severe AS may be present with lower velocities if stroke volume (SV) is low due to poor ventricular function.

   (2) AV area (AVA) is a better means of assessing severity of AS than gradients and may be measured by **planimetry** from the ME AV SAX view. The 2D image is frozen during systole at the level of the free edge of the leaflets, scrolled to identify the maximum systolic orifice, which then is traced using the caliper function. Acoustic shadowing from calcification may obscure the image in many patients and make planimetry difficult. AVA less than 1.0 cm^2 is considered significant.

   (3) **AVA may be calculated using the continuity equation,** which states that the same amount of flow passes through the AV and the LVOT with each stroke. Flow rate is equal to the velocity of the flow multiplied by the area through which the flow occurs (Flow = V * A) and by the continuity equation is the same at the AV and the LVOT. Thus,

   $$\mathrm{Flow_{AV} = Flow_{LVOT}}$$

   $$\mathrm{V_{AV} * A_{AV} = V_{LVOT} * A_{LVOT}};$$

   rearranging, we obtain

   $$\mathrm{A_{AV} = (V_{LVOT} * A_{LVOT})/V_{AV}}.$$

The area of the LVOT is obtained from the ME LAX view of the AV by measuring its diameter during systole and applying the formula for the area of a circle:

$$A_{CIRCLE} = IIr^2 = II(D/2)^2 = (II/4) * D^2 = 0.785 * D^2.$$

V_{LVOT} is measured with PWD by placing the sample volume just proximal to the AV in the LVOT and V_{AV} by directing the CWD through the stenotic valve. It is most convenient to use units of centimeters per second and centimeters in order to obtain the AVA in units per square centimeter. Common pitfalls in using the continuity equation to measure AVA are underestimation of the LVOT diameter, an error that is squared in the calculation, and underestimating the peak AV velocity due to a large angle between the direction of the flow and the Doppler beam.

4. **Right ventricle.** The RV is examined in the ME four-chamber, ME RV inflow outflow view, and TG RV inflow view, assessing size and global function. The RV appears to be somewhat smaller than the LV in most views and does not normally share the apex with the LV. Pressure and/or volume overload will cause RV enlargement. Global function usually is based on qualitative assessment of decrease in chamber size during systole. It is rated as normal function or as mild, moderate, or severe decrease in function.

5. **Tricuspid valve.** The TV lies between the RV and the right atrium (RA) and has three leaflets: anterior, posterior, and septal. It is examined with the ME four-chamber, ME RV inflow outflow view, and TG RV inflow view, with and without CFD. Some tricuspid regurgitation (TR) usually is detected. Severity of TR is graded on a semiquantitative scale of 1+ (mild) to 4+ (severe) based primarily on the size of the regurgitant jet. Significant TR usually is due to annular dilation secondary to right heart failure. Tricuspid stenosis is uncommon and usually due to rheumatic heart disease. On TEE it causes high-velocity, turbulent flow across the TV detected with CFD, PWD, and CWD.

6. **Pulmonic valve.** The pulmonic valve is located anterior and to the left of the AV and is examined with the ME RV inflow outflow view and UE aortic arch SAX view with and without CFD. PWD and CWD measurements of flow across the pulmonic valve are made with the UE aortic arch SAX view because the Doppler beam is parallel to the flow in this view. Trace pulmonic regurgitation usually is seen and normal. Pulmonic stenosis usually is congenital and rare in adults. It causes high-velocity, turbulent flow across the valve seen with CFD, PWD, and CWD.

7. **Left atrium.** The LA is examined in the ME four-chamber and ME two-chamber views for size and the presence of masses. It normally is less than 5 cm in its anteroposterior and mediolateral dimensions. Thrombus usually is associated with atrial fibrillation and LA enlargement and is most commonly in the LA appendage, seen at the superior lateral aspect of the body of the atrium.

8. **Right atrium.** The RA is examined in the ME four-chamber and ME bicaval views for size and masses. A variably sized fold of tissue at the junction of the inferior vena cava and the RA, the **Eustachian valve,** is seen frequently. Fine, filamentous mobile strands may be seen in this region as well and are termed the **Chiari network.** Both are normal structures.

9. **Interatrial septum.** The interatrial septum (IAS) is examined in the ME four-chamber, ME LAX, and ME bicaval views. Two portions usually are seen, the thinner fossa ovalis centrally and a thicker region anteriorly and posteriorly. Atrial septal defects are seen with 2D echocardiography and interatrial shunts with CFD. Atrial septal aneurysms cause redundancy and hypermobility of the IAS. Agitated saline contrast may be injected into the RA following release of positive airway pressure to look for the appearance of contrast in the LA. This indicates the presence of a patent foramen ovale, which may predispose patients to right-to-left interatrial shunting in the presence of right heart failure causing hypoxia and/or paradoxical systemic embolization.

10. Thoracic aorta. Although most of the thoracic aorta lies close to the esophagus and can be easily seen with TEE, the trachea may come between the esophagus, the distal ascending aorta, and the proximal aortic arch, obscuring TEE images of these parts of the aorta.

   a. Ascending aorta

   The ascending aorta is examined with the ME ascending aortic SAX and ME ascending aortic LAX views by withdrawing the TEE probe superior to the LA from the ME AV views. The distal third may be obscured by the trachea and not well seen with TEE. The inside diameter is normally less than 3.5 cm at the mid level (anterior to the right pulmonary artery). A more complete and detailed examination of the ascending aorta may be performed after sternotomy with **epiaortic echocardiography,** in which an echocardiographic transducer is covered by a sterile sheath and placed directly on the aorta in the surgical field by the surgeon.

   b. Aortic arch

   The aortic arch is examined with the UE aortic arch LAX and UE aortic arch SAX views. The distal arch is easily seen in most patients, but the mid and proximal arch may be obscured by the trachea. The inside diameter normally is less than 3.0 cm. The great vessels often are seen coursing toward the head to the right of the image in the UE aortic arch SAX view.

   c. Descending thoracic aorta

   The descending thoracic aorta is examined in SAX (approximately 0 degrees multiplane angle) and LAX (approximately 90 degrees angle) from the arch to the diaphragm. The inside diameter normally is less than 3.0 cm. The proximal descending thoracic aorta is lateral to the esophagus and the distal portion is posterior, so the probe must be rotated as different levels are examined to keep the aorta centered in the image. It often is possible to see the proximal abdominal aorta by advancing the probe past the diaphragm.

   d. Aortic diseases. Three common abnormalities of the aorta are detected with TEE:

   (1) Atherosclerosis

   Atherosclerosis causes thickening and irregularity of the intimal layer of the aorta that is easily seen with TEE. The normal intima is smooth and less than 2 mm thick. Severity of atherosclerosis is graded on a five-point scale: grade 1 for normal or minimal disease (intima <2 mm thick), grade 2 for mild disease (intima 2 to 3 mm thick), grade 3 for moderate or sessile disease (intima 3 to 5 mm thick), grade 4 for severe or protruding disease (intima >5 mm thick), and grade 5 for mobile lesions. The location and extent of the lesions also are noted.

   (2) Aneurysm

   Aneurysmal dilations of the aorta are classified by their location and shape as either diffuse or saccular. They often are associated with atherosclerotic changes and/or mural thrombus, which are easily seen with TEE. Aneurysms with inside diameter 4 cm or less are considered mild and those greater than 6 cm are considered severe.

   (3) Dissection

   An aortic dissection is the separation of the intimal layer from the rest of the aorta through the media. With TEE, a mobile membrane is seen within the aorta dividing the vessel into a true and a false lumen. CFD is applied to the aorta to characterize the flow in the true and false lumens. Dissections are classified into type A, which involve the ascending aorta and are a surgical emergency, and type B, which do not involve the ascending aorta and usually are treated without surgery. TEE findings that may be associated with aortic dissections include aneurysmal dilation of the aorta, hemopericardium and tamponade, left hemothorax, AR, and RWMAs due to coronary artery involvement.

VII. TEE for specific types of surgery

A. Coronary artery bypass grafting

TEE for coronary artery bypass graft (CABG) surgery focuses on global and regional LV function. Baseline examination of all 16 segments of the LV is performed and recorded for later comparison. A baseline RWMA may represent previously infarcted, nonviable myocardium; chronically ischemic hibernating myocardium; or acutely ischemic myocardium. Examination of the LV is repeated after grafting. The appearance of a new RWMA before or after bypass grafting should be considered to be due to acute ischemia. A new RWMA seen immediately after CPB may indicate stunned myocardium, i.e., viable muscle that is perfused but transiently not functioning due to inadequate cardioplegia during CPB. RV infarction causes dilation and hypokinesis of the RV on TEE, often associated with significant TR. Complications of coronary artery disease, such as ischemic MR, LV thrombus, LV aneurysm, ruptured papillary muscle, and postinfarction ventricular septal defect, may be detected with TEE. TEE also is important in detecting atherosclerosis in the aorta, which may increase the risk of stroke during CABG surgery.

B. Valve repair surgery

Intraoperative TEE is very helpful during valve repair surgery. Detailed baseline examination of the diseased valve can provide the surgeon with information about the mechanism and etiology of the lesion, indicating the feasibility of repair and the type of repair needed. Assessment of the repair after CPB is done so that any problems can be detected and immediately addressed. MV repairs are assessed with TEE for three potential problems:

1. **Residual regurgitation.** Residual MR is assessed with CFD after MV repair. Ideally there is no or only trace MR. Mild (1+) MR probably is acceptable. Moderate (2+) or more MR should lead to consideration of revision of the repair or valve replacement.

2. **Systolic anterior motion of the MV.** Repair of myxomatous MVs with redundant leaflets can cause mitral systolic anterior motion (SAM), which is easily diagnosed with TEE. There is abnormal anterior motion of the excessive leaflet tissue toward the ventricular septum during systole. This leads to dynamic LVOT obstruction and MR. SAM can be managed successfully in some cases by increasing intravascular volume, administering pure α-agonist drugs, and stopping positive inotropic drugs. In severe cases that do not respond to appropriate treatment, revision of the repair or valve replacement is needed.

3. **Stenosis.** Excessive narrowing of the mitral orifice by valve repair creating stenosis is possible but very uncommon. This is seen on TEE by limited opening of the leaflets and high peak transmitral inflow velocity (>2 m/s).

C. Valve replacement surgery.

After valve replacement surgery, the prosthesis is evaluated with TEE. CFD is used to examine the valve annulus for paravalvular leaks. Trace, insignificant paravalvular leaks often are seen after CPB and are not a cause for concern. Moderate (2+) or more regurgitation may need to be addressed surgically. Different types of prosthetic valves have characteristic, normal patterns of regurgitation seen with CFD that should not be confused with pathologic regurgitation. Bileaflet mechanical valve prostheses may have a leaflet immobilized, usually in the closed position, by impinging tissue, so TEE evaluation of these valves should document that both leaflets move freely. An immobile leaflet should be corrected immediately with surgical intervention. Stentless aortic bioprostheses and aortic homograft prostheses may develop significant AR if they are not inserted properly. This can be detected with CFD. Moderate (2+) or more AR usually warrants further surgical intervention.

D. Surgery for congenital heart disease.

TEE can confirm the diagnosis before CPB and occasionally finds previously undiagnosed lesions in patients with complex congenital heart disease. Septal defect closure and adequacy of flow through prosthetic conduits and intracardiac baffles can be assessed intraoperatively with TEE using CFD, PWD, and CWD, allowing immediate correction of inadequate repairs.

E. Surgery for infective endocarditis.

TEE is helpful in confirming the location and extent of infection and assessing the severity of associate lesions such as valvular regurgitation and fistulae. Intraoperative TEE often detects progression of the infection since the preoperative studies, guiding the surgical intervention. TEE examination after CPB confirms the adequacy of the resection of infected tissue and repair of hemodynamic lesions.

F. **Surgery for hypertrophic obstructive cardiomyopathy.** TEE is used before CPB to measure the thickness of the ventricular septum and the location of contact of the MV with the septum to guide the surgeon in sizing the myectomy. The adequacy of the myectomy can be assessed with TEE after CPB by looking for residual SAM, measuring residual gradients across the LVOT, and assessing severity of residual MR. Moderate (2+) or more MR and a peak LVOT gradient greater than 50 mm Hg indicates that a more extensive myectomy is needed. A ventricular septal defect created by an excessive myectomy can be detected with CFD.

VIII. **Monitoring applications of TEE**

A. **Assessing preload**

The most direct measurement of preload is LV end-diastolic volume. TEE provides 2D images of the LV, so LV end-diastolic area (EDA) of the TG mid-SAX view has been used as an estimation of end-diastolic volume. Studies have shown that decreases in blood volume as little as 1.5% can be detected by this technique [7] and that correlation between EDA and cardiac output is better than that between pulmonary artery occlusion pressure and cardiac output [8].

B. **Measuring intracardiac pressures**

Measuring flow velocities with Doppler echocardiography and applying the modified Bernoulli equation allow calculation of gradients between chambers of the heart at various locations. If the absolute pressure of one of these chambers is known, the pressure of the other chamber can be calculated. Thus, by measuring the peak velocity of TR with CWD, one can estimate the peak RV systolic pressure as the RV to RA gradient ($\Delta P = 4V_{TR}^2$) plus the RA pressure. This is equal to the PA systolic pressure if there is no pulmonic stenosis. Similar logic can be used to measure LA, PA diastolic, and LV end-diastolic pressures by measuring the velocities of MR, PR, and AR jets and knowing the LV systolic (same as systolic BP), RV diastolic (same as CVP), and aortic diastolic (same as diastolic BP) pressures.

C. **Measuring cardiac output**

Calculating SV with TEE requires making two measurements: (i) the velocity profile of flow with PWD or CWD; and (ii) the area through which the flow occurs with 2D echocardiography. These measurements can be made with TEE in several locations: AV, LVOT, MV, and PA. The accuracy of this technique depends on both the velocity and area measurements being made **in the same location and at the same time in the cardiac cycle.** The velocity profile of the flow is traced and integrated through time to yield a value called the **time velocity integral** (TVI), which is in units of length, usually centimeters. Then the area A through which the flow passes is measured with 2D echocardiography to give a value in units of length squared, usually square centimeters. The product of TVI and A yields the SV in units of volume, usually cubic centimeters or milliliters. SV times the heart rate gives the cardiac output. The best validated technique for intraoperative TEE uses CWD across the AV from the TG LAX or deep TG LAX views [9]. The area of the valve then is calculated from the ME AV SAX view by measuring the intercommissural distance S and applying the formula for the area of an equilateral triangle: $A_\Delta = 0.433 * S^2$.

D. **Monitoring for myocardial ischemia**

Appearance of a new RWMA on TEE during surgery has been shown to be a more sensitive indicator of myocardial ischemia than electrocardiographic changes and a better predictor of progression to myocardial infarction [10]. After complete baseline examination of all 16 LV segments is recorded for comparison, the TG mid-SAX view is monitored because it simultaneously shows regions supplied by all three major coronary arteries. A decrease in the wall motion score of two or more grades in a segment suggests acute ischemia. Severe hypovolemia also may produce wall-motion abnormalities without ischemia [11]. TEE is not a true monitor for ischemia unless it is continuously observed during surgery and is more often checked at crucial points of the operation, such as aortic cross clamping, or when another monitor suggests ischemia, such as electrocardiographic or hemodynamic changes.

E. Intracardiac air

Air in the heart is easily seen with TEE as hyperdense or white areas within the chambers. In a supine patient, air in the LA accumulates along the IAS and adjacent to the right upper pulmonary vein. Air in the LV accumulates along the apical septum. Tiny white spots seen floating within the chambers are microscopic bubbles and are not of great concern. Large bubbles have air–fluid levels visible on TEE as straight lines perpendicular to the direction of gravity that wobble as the heart beats. They typically have a shimmering artifact extending from the air–fluid level away from the transducer. Large bubbles should be evacuated before discontinuing CPB.

IX. Future directions

A. Myocardial contrast echocardiography

Echocardiographic contrast agents that transit the pulmonary circulation have been developed that theoretically could increase the video intensity of perfused myocardium over unperfused myocardium after intravenous injection. Such a technique would allow the differentiation of stunned from ischemic myocardium in the operating room or the intensive care unit. The initial hope and enthusiasm has waned over the past few years as the complexities of myocardial perfusion physiology and the detection and quantification of myocardial contrast echocardiographic effect have become more apparent. A practical, clinically relevant application of contrast echocardiography to measure myocardial perfusion with TEE requires additional study.

B. Three-dimensional echocardiography

Three-dimensional (3D) reconstruction of echocardiographic images from a series of 2D images has been in clinical use for several years. This technique has been most helpful in imaging complex congenital heart defects, but its practical application to intraoperative use has been limited by the time required to acquire the multiple images and render the 3D reconstruction with a high-powered computer. Transducers that acquire echocardiographic data from a volume of space and create a 3D image in real time are in a fairly advanced stage of development, but currently they are too large for TEE. Undoubtedly, as the technology evolves and becomes practical, 3D imaging will revolutionize echocardiography in the same way 2D imaging did in the late 1970s.

References

1. **Practice guidelines for perioperative transesophageal echocardiography. A report by the American Society of Anesthesiologists and the Society of Cardiovascular Anesthesiologists Task Force on Transesophageal Echocardiography. *Anesthesiology* 1996;84:986–1006.**
2. Kallmeyer IJ, Collard CD, Fox JA, et al. The safety of intraoperative transesophageal echocardiography: a case series of 7200 cardiac surgical patients. *Anesth Analg* 2001;92:1126–1130.
3. Brinkman WT, Shanewise JS, Clements SD, et al. Transesophageal echocardiography: not an innocuous procedure. *Ann Thorac Surg* 2001;72:1725–1726.
4. **Shanewise JS, Cheung AT, Aronson S, et al. ASE/SCA guidelines for performing a comprehensive intraoperative multiplane transesophageal echocardiography examination: recommendations of the American Society of Echocardiography Council for Intraoperative Echocardiography and the Society of Cardiovascular Anesthesiologists Task Force for Certification in Perioperative Transesophageal Echocardiography. *Anesth Analg* 1999;89:870–884.**
5. Stamm RB, Carabello BA, Mayers DL, et al. Two-dimensional echocardiographic measurement of left ventricular ejection fraction: prospective analysis of what constitutes an adequate determination. *Am Heart J* 1982;104:136–144.
6. **Smith JS, Cahalan MK, Benefiel DJ, et al. Intraoperative detection of myocardial ischemia in high-risk patients: electrocardiography versus two-dimensional transesophageal echocardiography. *Circulation* 1985;72:1015–1021.**
7. Cheung AT, Savino JS, Weiss SJ, et al. Echocardiographic and hemodynamic indexes of left ventricular preload in patients with normal and abnormal ventricular function. *Anesthesiology* 1994;81:376–387.

8. Thys DM, Hillel Z, Goldman ME, et al. A comparison of hemodynamic indices derived by invasive monitoring and two-dimensional echocardiography. *Anesthesiology* 1987;67: 630–634.

9. Darmon PL, Hillel Z, Mogtader A, et al. Cardiac output by transesophageal echocardiography using continuous-wave Doppler across the aortic valve. *Anesthesiology* 1994; 80: 796–805.

10. Leung JM, O'Kelly B, Browner WS, et al. Prognostic importance of postbypass regional wall-motion abnormalities in patients undergoing coronary artery bypass graft surgery. SPI Research Group. *Anesthesiology* 1989;71:16–25.

11. Seeberger MD, Cahalan MK, Rouine-Rapp K, et al. Acute hypovolemia may cause segmental wall motion abnormalities in the absence of myocardial ischemia. *Anesth Analg* 1997;85:1252–1257.

5. INDUCTION OF ANESTHESIA

Michael B. Howie and Glenn P. Gravlee

Induction of anesthesia in a cardiac patient is not a simple technique creating a rapid transition from an awake to a stabilized anesthetic state. Consideration of all aspects of the patient's cardiac condition allows selection of an anesthetic that best accommodates current cardiac status and medications the patient is taking. No single agent or technique can guarantee hemodynamic stability. Hemodynamic change with induction can be attributed to the patient's pathophysiology and to a reduction in sympathetic tone potentially causing vasodilation, cardiac depression, and relative hypovolemia.

I. Premedication

A. Just as the patient's chronic medications can mostly be used to advantage, so can premedication be an integral component of the anesthetic technique.

B. With rare exception, chronic cardiac medications should be administered preoperatively on the day of surgery with as little water as possible.

II. Preinduction period.

Unstable patients probably should not be premedicated before they reach an area that permits continuous observation by an anesthesia caregiver. Examples include patients with heart failure or symptomatic aortic stenosis. Some examples of premedication regimens are shown in Table 5.1. Monitoring catheters, such as arterial and central venous "lines," ideally should be placed under the influence of premedication such as intravenous midazolam.

A. Basic monitors and supplemental oxygen are important to initiate before giving supplemental sedation (if needed) and placing invasive monitors.

    1. Electrocardiogram

    2. Noninvasive blood pressure (BP)

    3. Pulse oximeter

B. Invasive monitors are useful during induction [1], so many clinicians choose to place them before induction. Some clinicians prefer to defer central line placement until after anesthetic induction.

    1. In emergency situations, it may be necessary to proceed with anesthetic induction before placing invasive monitors. Examples include:

        a. Ruptured or rupturing thoracic aortic aneurysm

        b. Cardiac tamponade

        c. Ventricular rupture

    2. In these situations, if a large-bore intravenous catheter is already present, opening the chest is far more important than pulmonary artery (PA) or central venous pressure catheter measurements.

Table 5.1 Anesthetic premedication for cardiac surgical patients

Poorly compensated patients	Lorazepam or midazolam 1–2 mg intravenously (approximately 15–20 µg/kg)
Compensated patients	1. Midazolam 3–8 mg (0.05–0.1 mg/kg) intravenously, titrated to effect with or without intravenous morphine 2–5 mg (0.03–0.07 mg/kg), hydromorphone 1–2 mg (15–30 µg/kg), or fentanyl 50–100 µg (0.5–1 µg/kg) intravenously after arrival in the preinduction area or the operating room 2. Morphine 3–10 mg (0.05–0.15 mg/kg) with or without scopolamine 0.3–0.4 mg (40–50 µg/kg), both given intramuscularly 30–60 min before transport to operating room area 3. Lorazepam 2–4 mg (30–40 µg/kg) by mouth with or without an orally (e.g., methadone 5–10 mg, or 0.1 mg/kg) or intramuscularly (e.g., morphine 0.1 mg/kg) administered narcotic 30–60 min before arrival in operating room area

C. Clinical tips in preparing for cardiac anesthesia
    1. Emergency drugs that may be needed can be prepared as dilute bolus doses in syringes or as intravenous or syringe infusion pumps attached to a port of the PA (or some other central venous) catheter via a manifold.
    2. The drugs selected for anesthesia depend on the patient's condition and the preferences of the anesthesiologist.
        a. Commonly, fentanyl, sufentanil, or remifentanil are selected as opioids.
        b. Among the potent inhalational agents, isoflurane probably should be selected for economy, desflurane for rapid titratibility, and sevoflurane for an airway that is suspected to be difficult.
        c. Amnestics may include lorazepam, midazolam, or the seldom used, but sometimes appropriate, scopolamine [approximately 5 µg/kg intravenously (IV)].
        d. Muscle relaxants suggested would be succinylcholine (or no muscle relaxant) for a suspect airway; pancuronium for economy and low heart rates (HRs); vecuronium, rocuronium, or cisatracurium for hemodynamic blandness; and cisatracurium in the case of liver or renal failure.
    3. Specific cardiovascular medications to have available (asterisk indicates probable need to have the drug drawn up and ready for administration) before surgery:
        a. Anticholinergic: atropine*
        b. Inotrope*: Epinephrine, dobutamine, or dopamine as infusions; epinephrine also in a syringe for bolus administration
        c. Phosphodiesterase III inhibitor: milrinone or amrinone
        d. Calcium chloride
        e. Ephedrine* as a bolus (mixed vasopressor/inotrope)
        f. Vasopressors
            (1) Phenylephrine as a 50- to 100-µg bolus, or as an infusion, or norepinephrine*
            (2) Vasopressin (for vascular collapse and resuscitation, especially after left ventricular assist device placement)
        g. Vasodilators: nitroglycerin*, nitroprusside, or nicardipine
        h. Antiarrhythmics
            (1) Adenosine
            (2) Diltiazem or verapamil
            (3) Lidocaine
            (4) Procainamide
            (5) Amiodarone
            (6) Magnesium
        i. Anticoagulation and its reversal
            (1) Heparin*
            (2) Protamine
        j. To be most prepared, at least one inotrope, one vasopressor, and one vasodilator (probably nitroglycerin) should be set up and connected in a pump that is preprogrammed and ready to use. Similarly, syringes should be prepared for bolus administration of at least one vasopressor, inotrope, and vasodilator.
        k. A custom-built IV pole with a built-in electrical outlet and the capability for attachment of multiple pumps ideally should be available.
D. Last-minute checks: Immediately before anesthetic induction, the following points should be considered:
    1. Assessment of the patient's overall cardiopulmonary status
    2. Availability of blood for transfusion
    3. Proximity of a surgeon or a senior resident or fellow
    4. Any special endotracheal tube needs (double-lumen, bronchial blocker)
    5. Immediate availability of emergency cardiac drugs
III. Induction. The cardiac anesthesiologist must induce a patient who under normal circumstances would not receive a general anesthetic. Objectives include:
    A. Attenuation of hemodynamic responses to laryngoscopy and surgery without undue hypotension

  1. Conservative drug amounts, as the anesthetic requirement rapidly becomes relatively minor with surgical preparation and draping (exception: high-dose opioid induction technique) (Table 5.2)
  2. Use drug onset time and interactions to advantage
  3. Adapt induction drug doses to physical status of patient
B. **Guiding principles** for anesthetic induction include:
  1. Modifications of techniques as new knowledge is gained. For example, trace the history of sufentanil as used during anesthetic induction.
      a. In the 1980s, the recommended dose of sufentanil was as high as 25 µg/kg.
      b. In the 1990s, recommendations changed to 6 to 10 µg/kg.
      c. In 2000, as little as 1 µg/kg is commonly used and sometimes even less.
      d. Combinations of sufentanil or fentanyl with etomidate and muscle relaxants exemplify efficient induction techniques.
  2. Physiologic issues
      a. Hypovolemia, which often is difficult to assess, frequently is caused by diuretics and prolonged NPO (nothing by mouth) status.
          (1) It is difficult to assess in part because of the absence of preoperative urine output documentation or left ventricular preload assessment.
          (2) Most cardiac patients do not tolerate more than 10% depletion of intravascular volume without hemodynamic compromise.
          (3) Tachycardia and vasoconstriction, which are useful compensatory mechanisms in normal individuals, may be deleterious in cardiac patients.
          (4) Anesthetic drugs may impair appropriate hemodynamic responses.

          • Thiopental reduces BP by inducing venodilation with peripheral pooling of blood, decreasing sympathetic tone to decrease systemic vascular resistance (SVR), and depressing myocardial contractility.
          • In decreasing order of circulatory depression:

          Propofol is most depressant
          Midazolam and thiopental are intermediate
          Etomidate is least depressant

          (5) The most physiologically efficient method of combating hypovolemia is to augment intravascular volume in the preinduction period using balanced salt solutions, being careful not to overdo this in patients with mitral valve lesions or congestive heart failure.

Table 5.2 Recommended induction doses

Hypnotics	Propofol 1–1.5 mg/kg
	Thiopental 3–4 mg/kg
	Etomidate 0.2–0.3 mg/kg
Opioids	Fentanyl 3–10 µg/kg
	Sufentanil 0.5–1 µg/kg
	Remifentanil 0.1–0.75 µg/kg/min or bolus 1 µg/kg
Muscle relaxants	Cisatracurium 70–100 µg/kg
	Vecuronium 70–100 µg/kg
	Pancuronium 70–100 µg/kg
	Succinylcholine 1–2 mg/kg
Maintenance of anesthesia in critically ill patients	Lorazepam 2–4 mg (25–50 µg/kg)
	Midazolam 0.25–0.5 µg/kg/min
	plus
	An opioid infusion
	0.1 µg/kg/min remifentanil
	0.05–0.1 µg/kg/min fentanyl
	0.01 µg/kg/min sufentanil

3. Pharmacodynamic issues. **With the exception of ketamine, which can stimulate the cardiovascular system, all anesthetics decrease BP by some combination of removing sympathetic tone, directly decreasing SVR, depressing the myocardium, increasing venous pooling (reducing venous return), or inducing bradycardia.**
   Important individual drug characteristics to be considered:
   a. In critically ill patients, ketamine can decrease BP because depletion of catecholamines may lead to an inability of indirect central nervous system–mediated sympathomimetic effects to counterbalance its direct negative inotropic and vasodilatory effects.
   b. The conflict between the need to attenuate the hemodynamic response to intubation and other noxious stimuli without overdosing can be illustrated by propofol.
      (1) Propofol may induce hypotension if used for induction, yet a small dose may not suppress the hypertensive response to laryngoscopy.
      (2) In combination with other drugs: After an induction dose of propofol, systolic BP fell an average of 28 mmHg when no fentanyl was administered, whereas it fell 53 mmHg when 2 μg/kg of fentanyl was administered. However, the hemodynamic response to intubation was decreased in proportion to the preinduction dose of fentanyl [2].
      (3) Propofol can be given in small increments (0.5 to 1 mg/kg) judging from the patient's physical status and can be used with a small well-timed dose of opioid (e.g., 1 to 3 μg/kg of fentanyl 1 to 2 minutes preceding propofol).
   c. The principle of using the relationship between the plasma drug concentration and the bioeffector site onset (biophase or Ke_0) must be considered, such that the maximal effects of both the opioid and hypnotic are used to best advantage.
      (1) The mean onset time for peak effect of propofol is 2.9 minutes and for fentanyl is 6.4 minutes. Ideally, endotracheal intubation should be performed at the peak concentration of both drugs and after optimal muscle relaxation has been achieved. This may require a second dose or a continuous infusion of ultrashort-acting agents such as propofol, thiopental, and methohexital, because the muscle relaxant onset time may occur after the peak effect of the bolus dose has dissipated as a result of rapid redistribution.
   d. **Increasing the opioid dose beyond 4 to 8 μg/kg of fentanyl, 0.75 μg/kg of sufentanil, or 1.2 μg/kg/min of remifentanil does not further attenuate the stress response (increased BP and HR) to intubation.**
   e. Depth of anesthesia provided by propofol or other sedative–hypnotic agents does not determine the degree of stress–response suppression; rather, the central nervous system level of opioid analgesia tends to do so.
   f. Reducing the doses of anesthetic drugs is often the safest way to induce critically ill patients.
   g. For a hemodynamically stable patient, one might prefer a hemodynamically bland muscle relaxant except for patients with a baseline HR less than 50 beats/min or with valvular regurgitation, where pancuronium is still useful.
   h. Induction drugs are administered most efficiently through a central venous catheter, such as the side-port introducer, or an infusion port in a PA catheter.
   i. **Muscle relaxants are given early in the sequence. Onset time is important to consider.** This can be defined for most agents in the context of ED_{95}, or the average dose required to induce 95% suppression of the twitch response. For most nondepolarizing neuromuscular blockers, the time to achieve maximum twitch suppression at a dose of $1 \times ED_{95}$ is 3 to 7 minutes. Use of $2 \times$ or $3 \times ED_{95}$ reduces onset time to 1.5 to 3 minutes, and to as low as 1 to 1.5 minutes for $3 \times ED_{95}$ with rocuronium.

(1) Succinylcholine (1 to 2 mg/kg) can be used to reduce onset time of neuromuscular blockade to 1 to 1.5 minutes.

j. An example of a drug combination that combines rapid onset (intubating conditions in 1 to 2 minutes) and good suppression of the stress response to laryngoscopy is remifentanil 1 μg/kg, etomidate 0.2 mg/kg, and succinylcholine 1.5 mg/kg, all administered as a simultaneous bolus.

k. High-dose opioid induction techniques:

(1) Achieved popularity in the 1970s with morphine (1 to 2 mg/kg) or fentanyl (50 to 100 μg/kg) because of the combination of excellent stress–response suppression and hemodynamic stability.

(2) Sufentanil (10 to 25 μg/kg) rose to popularity for the same reasons in the 1980s.

(3) This technique lost favor in the 1990s because of long postoperative intubation times, but it still is potentially useful for high-risk patients who will require overnight mechanical ventilation regardless of the anesthetic technique chosen.

(4) Because of marked vagotonic effects, pancuronium nicely complements high-dose opioids and should be given early in the induction sequence to minimize chest wall rigidity.

(5) These doses of fentanyl and sufentanil can be given as a bolus or over 3 to 5 minutes. Morphine must be given slowly (5 to 10 mg/min) to avoid hypotension.

(6) Beware of hypotension if hypnotics are given simultaneously and of inadequate amnesia if they are not.

IV. Opioids

A. There are two basic structures:

1. Rigid interlocked molecules of the morphine group known as pentacyclides, and

2. Flexible molecules of phenylpiperidine rings such as fentanyl.

3. There are three opioid receptors (μ, κ, and δ) with subgroups.

   a. Opioid receptors are γ-protein–coupled receptors.

B. Properties of opioids. **Analgesia is more than the relief of pain or of the conscious perception of a nociceptive stimulus.** A noxious stimulus can affect an unconscious (and unparalyzed) person as demonstrated by withdrawal of the stimulated part (withdrawal reflex). The stimulus can produce increased autonomic activity. Narcotics in general are poor hypnotics and cannot be counted upon to induce amnesia.

C. Induction pharmacokinetics:

1. Pharmacokinetics are similar among three modern synthetic opioids (fentanyl, sufentanil, and alfentanil) with a few differences [3].

   a. All have a three-compartment model.

   b. **Ninety-eight percent of fentanyl is redistributed from the plasma in the first hour.**

   c. Brain levels parallel plasma levels with a lag of 5 minutes.

   d. Fentanyl has a large volume of distribution, which can limit hepatic access. However, the liver will clear all the fentanyl it gets.

   e. Sufentanil is seven to ten times more potent than fentanyl. It has a higher pK$_a$ and only 20% is ionized.

   f. Sufentanil is half as lipid soluble as fentanyl and is more tightly bound to receptors. It has a lower volume of distribution and a faster recovery time.

2. Remifentanil pharmacokinetics:

   a. Remifentanil has a unique pharmacokinetic profile, as it is subject to widespread extrahepatic hydrolysis by nonspecific tissue and blood esterases.

   b. It has an onset time of 1 minute and a recovery time of 9 to 20 minutes. These properties make it very advantageous when there is variation of surgical stimulus or a desire for early postoperative extubation. The anesthesiologist can give as much as he or she feels is needed without impeding rapid recovery.

   c. Careful provision of postoperative pain control is essential, as remifentanil-induced analgesia dissipates rapidly after the infusion is terminated.

V. Other intravenous anesthetic agents
  A. Etomidate
    1. Etomidate is very useful and potent; it is 25 times more potent than thiopental.
    2. It is reliable at achieving hypnosis when combined with a small amount of an opioid. Administering the primary dose just after giving an opioid may attenuate myoclonus, which sometimes occurs as a result of subcortical disinhibition.
    3. Etomidate reaches the brain in 1 minute.
    4. There may be an increased incidence of epileptiform activity in patients with known epileptic seizure disorders.
    5. A dose of etomidate typically produces a 10% to 15% decrease in mean arterial pressure and SVR and a 3% to 4 % increase in HR and cardiac output.
    6. Importantly, stroke volume, left ventricular end-diastolic pressure, and contractility remain unchanged in normovolemic patients.
    7. Etomidate can be used to anesthetize heart transplant patients, because it preserves myocardial contractility better than any induction technique other than a high-dose opioid induction [4].
    8. Although traditional induction doses of etomidate and opioids given individually most often preserve hemodynamics, when they are given together hypotension may ensue.
  B. Thiopental
    1. Thiopental has a rapid onset and can be used safely in hemodynamically stable patients.
    2. Rapid redistribution to highly perfused tissues causes cessation of thiopental's effects.
    3. Cardiovascular effects
      a. Predominantly venous pooling and resultant decreased cardiac preload.
      b. Myocardial depressant above 2 mg/kg.
      c. Increases HR by activating baroreceptor reflex.
      d. In patients who have low cardiac output, a greater proportion of the drug dose goes to the brain and myocardium; thus, a smaller amount of thiopental has a larger effect.
      e. Overall, there is a dose-related negative inotropic effect from a decrease in calcium influx.
  C. Propofol
    1. A normal induction dose of 2 mg/kg will drop BP 15% to 40%.
    2. Because propofol resets the baroceptor reflex, lower BP does not increase HR.
    3. There are significant reductions in SVR, cardiac index, stroke volume, and left ventricular stroke work index.
    4. There is direct myocardial depression at doses above 0.75 mg/kg.
    5. Propofol should be titrated according to the patient's age, weight, and individual need and ideally injected into a central vein, thereby allowing the smallest dose to be used effectively.
    6. Propofol's metabolic clearance is ten times faster than that of thiopental.
    7. There is extensive redistribution and movement from the central compartment to a peripheral one, which enables rapid recovery.
    8. Unless one wishes to decrease BP, use of propofol for induction does not have an advantage over etomidate. Because it has direct myocardial depressant effects and easily induces hypotension, propofol should be used with caution or reserved for use in hemodynamically stable cardiac patients with good ventricular function.
  D. Midazolam
    1. Midazolam is a good premedicant but is difficult to titrate to a minimum effective dose for induction because of a large variation in the required dose and a relatively slow onset time of 2 to 3 minutes.
    2. It is an effective amnestic, and this constitutes its appeal.
    3. The hypotensive effect from an induction dose is similar to or less than that for thiopental, and it is dose related.

4. In patients who have high cardiac filling pressures, midazolam seems to mimic low-dose nitroglycerin by reducing filling pressures.
5. The addition of opioids produces a supra-additive hypotensive effect.

E. Lorazepam
1. Lorazepam is a very potent benzodiazepine.
2. Because of its potency, it produces anxiolytic, sedative, and amnestic effects in lower doses and with fewer side effects than midazolam.
3. It is very useful in sick cardiac patients when only small amounts of drugs are desired.
4. If rapid recovery is expected, as in minimally invasive direct coronary artery bypass surgery, lorazepam is a poor choice because of its relatively long clinical action (typically several hours).

F. Ketamine
1. Ketamine produces a unique cataleptic trance known as disassociative anesthesia.
2. It is extensively redistributed and eliminated.
3. Bioavailability on intravenous injection is 97% and 2 mg/kg produces unconsciousness in 20 to 60 seconds.
4. **Ketamine induces significant increases in HR, mean arterial pressure, and plasma epinephrine levels.** This sympathetic nervous system stimulation is centrally mediated.
5. Ketamine may be advantageous in hypovolemia, major hemorrhage, or cardiac tamponade.
6. It allows humane obtundation of the hemodynamically unstable patient, giving the surgeon an opportunity to get to the problem. In these situations, skin preparation should be performed before induction.
7. **The hemodynamic stimulatory effect with ketamine depends on the presence of a robust myocardium and sympathetic reserve. In the absence of either, hypotension may ensue from myocardial depression** [5].
8. Coronary blood flow may not be sufficient to meet the increased oxygen demands induced by sympathetic stimulation.
9. Ketamine should be avoided in patients with elevated intracranial pressure.
10. The S+ isomer produces much longer periods of hypnosis and analgesia, and less postanesthetic stimulation. This compound, currently available in some European countries, may become available in the United States.
11. Ketamine is very useful for patients who have experienced severe acute blood loss.

VI. Inhalational agents
A. Hemodynamic effects. Similar levels of myocardial depression occur with all three popular inhalational agents, **isoflurane, desflurane,** and **sevoflurane.** Serious consequences may occur in patients with congestive heart failure, as a narrow range of anesthetic concentrations may be tolerated by the compromised myocardium. **The predominant hemodynamic effect of these three agents is dose-dependent vasodilation,** hence reducing BP and SVR [5]. All three agents also induce a dose-dependent reflex tachycardia that can be attenuated or prevented by β-blockers or opioids.
B. Desflurane has unique titratability for induction of anesthesia because of its rapid onset and offset, but because of its pungent aroma it is poorly tolerated unless it is preceded by an intravenous induction. **Sevoflurane** has a much more pleasant aroma, offers hemodynamic stability in most induction situations, and has an onset time only slightly slower than that of desflurane.
C. Isoflurane, like desflurane, has a pungent aroma, and it is best introduced after an intravenous induction.
D. Halothane, a potent myocardial depressant, is seldom used for anesthetic induction in adult cardiac surgical patients.
E. Nitrous oxide is seldom used during anesthetic induction in cardiac surgical patients, but it is generally safe to use with the probable exception of patients with markedly increased pulmonary vascular resistance.

F. Clinical use. Whereas clinically significant brain concentrations [≥1.0 × minimal anesthetic concentration (MAC)] can be attained with desflurane and sevoflurane in 2 to 4 minutes, generally lower concentrations are achieved over the same time frame with isoflurane. Consequently, **desflurane and sevoflurane are more likely to reach concentrations consistent with stress–response suppression (generally 1.3 to 1.5 times MAC) during a customary induction period than is isoflurane.** One potential drawback to desflurane is sympathetic stimulation when the inspired concentration is increased rapidly, perhaps owing to its airway irritant effects. Any of these inhalation agents can be used during induction as a complement to an intravenous induction. Desflurane is useful in cardiac anesthesia not because of its rapid offset but because of its rapid onset.

VII. Muscle relaxants
   A. A suspected difficult intubation precludes giving the patient a nondepolarizing neuromuscular blocker before achieving intubation.
   B. Succinylcholine still has the fastest onset and offset of all muscle relaxants.
   C. Significant β-adrenergic blockade and high-dose opioid induction are potential indications for **pancuronium,** as its vagolytic effects tend to counter bradycardia.
   D. Intermediate-duration agents: Cisatracurium, rocuronium, and vecuronium are hemodynamically bland.
      1. If hepatic or renal failure exists, cisatracurium appears to be the wisest choice.
   E. Timing of the administration of the muscle relaxant is important.
      1. Laryngoscopy should await optimal relaxation (see Section **I.B.3.i**). Early administration obviates opioid-induced truncal rigidity, which may impair mask ventilation and result in systemic oxygen desaturation.

VIII. Immediate postinduction period. After induction and intubation, several different techniques may be used for maintenance of anesthesia. First priorities, however, are to assess the airway (confirm endotracheal tube location via end-tidal CO_2 and auscultation), assess hemodynamic stability, and respond appropriately to any problems identified.
   A. A low-dose continuous infusion of the opioid used for induction or of remifentanil (0.1 µg/kg/min) can be implemented.
   B. Consider using an inhalational agent.
   C. Continuous infusion or intermittent bolus doses of a sedative–hypnotic agent (e.g., midazolam) can be initiated if no potent inhalational agent is used.
   D. A propofol infusion may be useful in hemodynamically robust patients.
   E. A simple technique used daily and varied in dosage according to the physical status of the patient probably provides the most consistent results for most clinicians.

References
   1. Reich DL, Kaplan JA. Hemodynamic monitoring. In: Kaplan JA, ed. *Cardiac anesthesia,* 3rd ed. Philadelphia: WB Saunders, 1993:261–298.
   2. Billard V, Moulla F, Bourgain JL, et al. Hemodynamic response to induction and intubation: propofol/fentanyl interaction. *Anesthesiology* 1994; 81:1384–1393.
   3. **Bovill JG. Opioids. In: Bovill JG, Howie MB, eds. *Clinical pharmacology for anaesthetists.* London: WB Saunders, 1999:87–102.**
   4. Schuttler J, Zsigmond EK, White PF. Ketamine and its isomers. In: White PF, ed. *Textbook of intravenous anesthesia.* Philadelphia: Williams & Wilkins 1997:171–188.
   5. **Pagel PS, Warltier DC. Anesthetics and left ventricular function. In: *Ventricular function,* a Society of Cardiovascular Anesthesiologists monograph. Baltimore: Williams & Wilkins, 1995:213–252.**

6. ANESTHETIC MANAGEMENT IN THE PRECARDIOPULMONARY BYPASS PERIOD

Michael G. Licina and Mark E. Romanoff

The period of time between induction of anesthesia and institution of cardiopulmonary bypass (CPB) is characterized by widely varying surgical stimuli. Anesthetic management during this high-risk period must strive to:

1. Optimize the myocardial O_2 supply/demand ratio and monitor for myocardial ischemia. The incidence of ischemia during this period has been reported to be 7% to 56% [1].
2. Optimize the ventricular pressure/volume relationship in patients with valvular dysfunction. Manipulation of myocardial preload and afterload may be necessary to compensate for valvular lesions.
3. Maintain adequate ventricular contractility and cardiac output in patients with impaired ventricular function.
4. Optimize systemic vascular resistance (SVR) and pulmonary vascular resistance (PVR) in patients with congenital heart disease to avoid worsening of intravascular and intracardiac shunts.
5. Optimize heart rate and rhythm and avoid dysrhythmias.
6. Manage "fast track" patients with short-acting agents.

Adverse hemodynamic changes increase the risk of developing ischemia, heart failure, hypoxemia, or dysrhythmias. These complications may alter surgical management, leading to urgent institution of CPB or failure to perform internal mammary artery (IMA) or radial artery dissection, along with an increased risk of bleeding.

A few simple rules may assist in the management of cardiac patients before CPB:

1. **"Keep them where they live"**

    Check the preoperative vital signs and stress test records of heart rate and blood pressure for each patient. If the patient was comfortable and had no ischemia with these vital signs, then use these values as a gauge in maintaining the patient's hemodynamics during the pre-CPB period.
2. **"The enemy of good is better."**

    If the patient's blood pressure and heart rate are acceptable, does it matter if the cardiac index is 1.8 L/min/M²? When a patient is anesthestized, oxygen consumption decreases, so a lower cardiac index may be adequate. Trying to increase it to "normal" may lead to other problems, such as dysrhythmias or myocardial ischemia.
3. **"Do no harm."**

    These patients frequently are very ill. If you are having problems managing the patient, ask for help.

I. **Management of events before cardiopulmonary bypass**
   A. **Stages of the precardiopulmonary bypass period.** The pre-CPB period can be subdivided into stages based on the level of surgical stimulation.
       1. **High levels of stimulation** include incision, sternal split, sternal spread, sympathetic nerve dissection, and aortic cannulation. Inadequate anesthesia or sympathetic activation at these times leads to increased catecholamine levels, possibly resulting in hypertension, dysrhythmias, tachycardia, ischemia, or heart failure (Table 6.1).
       2. **Low-level stimulation** occurs during preincision, radial artery harvesting, internal mammary (thoracic) artery dissection, and CPB venous cannulation. Risks during these periods include hypotension, bradycardia, dysrhythmias, and ischemia (Table 6.1).
   B. **Preincision.** The duration of this period, including surgical preparation and draping, usually is 5 to 20 minutes. Several parameters should be checked during this time:
       1. **Confirm bilateral breath sounds** after final patient positioning.
       2. **Check pressure points.** Ischemia, secondary to compression and compounded by decreases in temperature and perfusion pressure during CPB, may cause peripheral neuropathy or damage to soft tissues.
           a. **Brachial plexus injury** can occur if the arms are hyperextended or if chest retraction is excessive (e.g., occult rib fracture using a sternal retractor) [2]. Excessive chest retraction can occur not only with the sternal spreader but also during IMA dissection even if the arms are tucked to the

Table 6.1 Typical hemodynamic responses to surgical stimulation before cardiopulmonary bypass

	Preincision	Sternotomy and sternal spread		Sympathetic dissection	IMA dissection	Cannulation
		Incision				
Surgical stimulation						
Heart rate	↓↓	— or ↑	↑	↑↑	— or →	— or ↓ᵃ
Blood pressure	↓↓	↑	↑↑↑	↑↑	↑ or ↑↑	— or →
Preload	— or →	— or ↑	↑↑	— or ↑	— or ↑	— or →
Afterload	— or →	↑↑	↑↑ or ↑↑↑	↑↑ or ↑↑↑	↑ or ↑↑	— or →
Myocardial O₂ demand	→	— or ↑	↑↑ or ↑↑↑	↑↑ or ↑↑↑	↑ or ↑↑	→

All values are compared to control (preinduction) values.

ᵃ Dysrhythmias secondary to mechanical stimulation of the heart are likely.

IMA, internal mammary artery; ↑, slightly increased; ↑↑, moderately increased; ↑↑↑, markedly increased; ↓, slightly decreased; ↓↓, moderately decreased; —, unchanged.

sides. If the arms are placed on arm boards, obtain the proper position by minimizing pectoralis major muscle tension. Do not extend arms more than 90 degrees from the body to avoid stretching the brachial plexus.

   b. Ulnar nerve injury can occur from compression of the olecranon against the metal edge of the operating room table. To obtain the proper position, provide adequate padding under the olecranon. Do not allow the arm to contact the metal edge of the operating room table.

   c. Radial nerve injury can occur from compression of the upper arm against the "ether screen" or the support post of the chest wall sternal retractors used in IMA dissection.

   d. Finger injury can occur secondary to pressure from members of the operating team leaning against the operating table if the fingers are positioned improperly. To obtain the proper position, hands should be next to the body, with fingers in a neutral position away from the metal edge of the table. One method to prevent upper extremity injury is to have the patient position himself or herself. The patient can grasp a surgical towel in each hand to ensure that the fingers are in a comfortable and protected position.

   e. Occipital alopecia can occur 3 weeks after the operation secondary to ischemia of the scalp, particularly during hypothermia. To obtain the proper position, pad the head and reposition the head frequently during the operation.

   f. Heel skin ischemia and tissue necrosis are possible. Heels should be well padded in such a way as to redistribute weight away from the heel to the lower leg.

   g. The eyes should be closed, taped, and free from any pressure.

3. Adjust fresh gas flow.

   a. Use of 100% O_2 maximizes inspired O_2 tension. Inclusion of a small amount of nitrogen (air) will not decrease arterial O_2 content significantly and may prevent absorption atelectasis and reduce the risk of O_2 toxicity if the patient is exposed to high inspired oxygen concentrations over the next several days. The inspired oxygen concentration can be titrated based on pulse oximeter readings.

   b. Nitrous oxide can be used during the pre-CPB period in stable patients. It will, however:

   (1) Decrease the concentration of inspired oxygen (FIO_2).

   (2) Increase PVR in adults.

   (3) Increase catecholamine release.

   (4) Possibly induce ventricular dysfunction.

   (5) Evidence **suggests** that nitrous oxide should not be used in patients with an evolving myocardial infarct or in patients with ongoing ischemia because the decrease in FIO_2 and potential catecholamine release theoretically can increase the risk of ischemia and infarct size. This point remains controversial.

4. Check all monitors and lines after final patient position is achieved.

   a. Intravenous (IV) infusions should flow freely, and the arterial pressure waveform should be assessed for dampening or hyperresonance.

   b. IV injection ports should be accessible.

   c. All IV and arterial line connections (stopcocks) should be taped or secured to prevent their movement and minimize the risk of blood loss from an open connection.

   d. Confirm electrical and patient reference "zero" of all transducers (see Chapter 3).

5. Check hemodynamic status.

   a. Cardiac index, ventricular filling pressures, mixed venous oxygen saturation (S_vO_2), and cardiac work indices should be evaluated after intubation.

   b. If transesophageal echocardiography (TEE) is used, check and document the status of the probe with regard to dental and oropharyngeal injury.

Make sure the TEE probe is not in a locked position, as this may lead to pressure necrosis in the gastrointestinal tract.

c. Baseline TEE examination should be performed at this time. Ejection fraction, wall-motion abnormalities, valvular function, and shunts can be identified (see Chapter 4). The TEE probe should be placed before heparinization to avoid excessive bleeding.

6. **Check blood chemistry.**

a. Once a stable anesthetic level is achieved and ventilation and FIO_2 have been constant for 10 minutes, an arterial blood gas (ABG) measurement should be determined to confirm adequate ventilation and to correlate with noninvasive measurements (pulse oximetry and end-tidal CO_2 concentration). Maintain a near-normal P_aCO_2, as hypercapnia may increase PVR.

b. Mixed venous hemoglobin O_2 saturation can be measured at this time, if necessary, to calibrate a continuous mixed venous PA catheter.

c. Electrolytes, calcium, and glucose levels should be determined as clinically indicated. High glucose levels should be treated to minimize neurologic injury and to decrease postoperative infection rates.

d. A blood sample to determine a baseline activated clotting time (ACT) before heparinization may be drawn at the same time as the sample for ABG. The blood can be taken from the arterial line after withdrawal of 5 mL of blood to clear the line of residual heparin from the flush solution. The perfusionist may require a blood sample to perform a heparin dose–response curve, which in some institutions is used to determine the initial heparin dosage.

e. Before any manipulation of the arterial line (zeroing, blood sample withdrawal), it is important to announce your intentions. This avoids alarming your colleagues, who may notice the loss of the arterial waveform.

7. **Antibiotics** often are administered at this time and should be timed not to coincide with the administration of other medications, should an allergic reaction occur. Precautions include slow infusion of vancomycin to avoid hypotension and attention to potential allergic reactions associated with cephalosporin use in penicillin-allergic patients.

8. If **aprotonin** is being used, a test dose should be given at this time. Wait at least 5 minutes after any previous medication exposure to prevent confusion if an allergic reaction does occur.

9. Preparing **for saphenous vein excision** involves lifting the legs above the level of the heart. Increased venous return raises the myocardial preload. This change is desirable in patients with low filling pressures and normal ventricular function but may be harmful in someone with borderline ventricular reserve. Gradual elevation of the legs may be useful in attenuating the hemodynamic changes. The reverse occurs when the legs are returned to the neutral position.

10. **Maintenance of body temperature** is not a concern during the pre-CPB time period unless the patient may be an OP-CAB (off pump) candidate. It is preferable to allow the temperature to drift down slowly, as this allows for more homogeneous hypothermia at institution of CPB. Before CPB, increasing the room temperature, humidifying anesthetic gases, warming IV solutions, and using a warming blanket are not necessary. These measures must be available for post-CPB management. The physiologic changes of mild hypothermia (34°C to 36°C) include the following:

a. Decrease in O_2 consumption and CO_2 production (8% to 10% for each degree Celsius)

b. Increase in SVR and PVR

c. Increase in blood viscosity

d. Decrease in central nervous system (CNS) function [amnesia, decrease in cerebral metabolic rate of O_2 consumption ($CMRO_2$), decrease in cerebral blood flow]

e. Decrease in anesthetic requirement [minimum alveolar concentration (MAC) decreases 5% for each degree Celsius]

f. Decrease in renal blood flow and urine output

g. Decrease in hepatic blood flow

      h. Minimal increase in catecholamines
- **11. Maintain other organ system function.**
  - **a.** Renal system [3]
    - **(1)** Inadequate urine output must be addressed immediately:
      - **(a)** Rule out technical problems (kinked urinary catheter tubing or disconnected tubing).
      - **(b)** Optimize and maintain an adequate intravascular volume and cardiac output (using CVP, PA, or TEE information)
      - **(c)** Avoid or treat hypotension.
      - **(d)** Maintain adequate oxygenation.
      - **(e)** Mannitol (0.25 g/kg IV) may be used to redistribute renal blood flow to the cortex and to maintain renal tubular flow.
      - **(f)** Dopamine (2.5 to 5.0 µg/kg/min) infusion may be given to increase renal blood flow by renal vascular dilation. Currently, there is no evidence that "renal" dose dopamine will prevent perioperative renal dysfunction. Its use may increase the incidence of perioperative atrial dysrhythmias.
      - **(g)** Diuretics (furosemide, 10 to 40 mg; bumetanide, 0.25 to 1.00 mg) can be given to maintain renal tubular flow if other measures are ineffective or if the patient had taken preoperative diuretics.
      - **(h)** Newer agents such as atrial natriuretic hormone and more specific dopamine agonists may be appropriate at this time.
    - **(2)** Patients undergoing emergent surgery may have received a large radiocontrast dye load at angiography. Avoiding acute tubular necrosis from the dye, utilizing the techniques mentioned earlier, is crucial. Volume loading may be the most important maneuver described.
  - **b.** Central nervous system
    - **(1)** Adequate cerebral perfusion pressure must be maintained.
      - **(a)** The patient's lowest and highest mean arterial pressures on the ward should be the limits accepted in the operating room to avoid cerebral ischemia. Remember "keep them where they live."
      - **(b)** Elderly patients have a decreased cerebral reserve and are more sensitive to changes in cerebral perfusion pressure.
    - **(2)** Patients at risk for an adverse cerebral event include those with known carotid artery disease, peripheral vascular disease, or a known embolic focus. Management considerations for these patients are discussed in Chapter 23.
  - **c.** Pulmonary system
    - **(1)** Maintain normal pH, P_aCO_2, and adequate P_aO_2.
    - **(2)** Treatment of systemic hypertension with a vasodilator may induce hypoxemia secondary to inhibition of hypoxic pulmonary vasoconstriction. FIO_2 may have to be increased.
    - **(3)** Use of an air–oxygen mixture may prevent absorption atelectasis.
- **12. Prepare for incision.**
  - **a.** Ensure adequate depth of anesthesia using clinical signs. If available, a bispectral index (BIS) monitor may be helpful. A small dose of a narcotic or hypnotic or increased concentration of inhaled agent may be necessary.
  - **b.** Ensure adequate muscle relaxation to avoid movement with incision and sternotomy. If movement occurs, make sure the patient is anesthetized as you are paralyzing the patient.
- **C. Incision**
  - **1.** An adequate depth of anesthesia is necessary but may not be sufficient to avoid tachycardia and hypertension in response to the stimulus of incision. If hemodynamic changes occur, they are usually short lived, so medications with a brief duration of action are recommended.
    - **a.** Treatment can include:
      - **(1)** Vasodilators
        - **(a)** Nitroglycerin (20- to 80-µg bolus) or infusion
        - **(b)** Sodium nitroprusside infusion

       (2) β-Blockers

          (a) Esmolol (0.25 to 1.0 mg/kg)

2. Observe the surgical field for patient movement and blood color. Despite an abundance of monitors, the presence of bright red blood remains one of the best ways to assess oxygenation and perfusion.

3. If the patient responds clinically to the incision (tachycardia, hypertension, other signs of "light" anesthesia, or BIS monitor changes), then the level of anesthesia must be deepened before sternotomy. **Do not** allow sternal split until the patient is anesthetized adequately and hemodynamics are controlled.

D. Sternal split

1. A very high level of stimulation accompanies sternal split. The incidence of hypertension has been reported to be as high as 88% during a narcotic-based anesthetic. A cumulative dose of fentanyl, 50 to 70 μg/kg, before sternal split should decrease the incidence of hypertension to less than 50%. However, fentanyl doses greater than 150 μg/kg are necessary for further reduction in the incidence of hypertension [4]. This high a dose of fentanyl, however, will prevent the patient from being ready for early extubation. Hypertension and tachycardia, if they occur, should be treated as described for skin incision.

   Bradycardia secondary to vagal discharge can occur. It usually is self-limiting, but if it is persistent and causes hemodynamic compromise then a dose of atropine or ephedrine may be necessary.

2. A reciprocating power saw often is used to open the sternum. The lungs should be "deflated" during opening of the internal table of the sternum to avoid damage to the lung parenchyma.

3. The patient should have adequate muscle relaxation during sternotomy to avoid an air embolism. If the patient gasps as the right atrium is cut, air can be entrained owing to the negative intrapleural pressure.

4. This is the most common time period for awareness and recall due to the intense stimulation.

   a. Awareness has been reported with fentanyl dosages as large as 150 μg/kg and with lower fentanyl doses supplemented with amnestic agents. Awareness usually, but not always, is associated with other symptoms of light anesthesia (movement, sweating, increased pupil size, hypertension, or tachycardia). A BIS monitor may be helpful, but recall has occurred in patients with an "adequate" BIS reading.

   b. If an amnestic agent has not been administered previously, it should be considered before sternotomy because these agents decrease the incidence of recall but **will not** produce retrograde amnesia. Amnestic supplements do not always protect against the hypertension and tachycardia associated with awareness. However, amnestic supplements may cause hypotension. The most common amnestic agents, their dosages, and side effects include:

      (1) Benzodiazepines (midazolam, 2.5 to 20.0 mg; diazepam, 5 to 15 mg; lorazepam, 1 to 4 mg) in divided doses usually are well tolerated but can decrease SVR and contractility in patients with poor ventricular function, especially when the drugs are added to a narcotic-based anesthetic.

      (2) Scopolamine, 0.2 to 0.4 mg IV, may cause tachycardia if it is administered rapidly. It may prolong emergence in a "fast track" patient and it will cause pupillary dilation.

      (3) Nitrous oxide may lead to catecholamine release, left ventricular dysfunction, increased PVR, and increased risk of hypoxia.

      (4) Inhalation agents can cause myocardial depression, bradycardia, tachycardia, dysrhythmias, or decreases in SVR, but they are effective in low concentrations and have become a standard part of the anesthetic technique to "fast track" the patient.

      (5) Droperidol (0.0625 to 2.5 mg) may cause hypotension by blocking α_1-receptors. This effect may last several hours.

      (6) Ketamine (5 to 100 mg) can cause sympathetic stimulation unless the patient is pretreated with a narcotic or benzodiazepine.

(7) Propofol (10 to 50 mg) can cause decreased blood pressure and cardiac output.

(8) Sodium thiopental (25 to 150 mg) can cause decreased blood pressure and cardiac output.

5. **Concerns with cardiac reoperation ("redo heart").** The heart, or a previous graft, may be adherent to the sternum and can be torn or cut with sternotomy. Looking at the lateral chest x-ray film may provide a clue as to potential problems, especially if there is no space between the heart and internal border of the sternum. An oscillating saw is used to decrease the likelihood of damage to soft tissue. This takes longer than a routine sternotomy, so ventilation should continue.

   a. The femoral vessels should **always** be identified, prepared, and draped. Femoral artery cannulation should be considered before sternal split.

   b. If a graft is cut, the patient may develop profound ischemia. Nitroglycerin may be helpful, but if significant myocardial dysfunction or hypotension occurs, the ultimate treatment is prompt institution of CPB.

   c. If the right atrium, right ventricle, or great vessels are cut, a surgeon or assistant will put a "finger in the dike" while the tear is fixed or a decision is made to go emergently on CPB. CPB can be initiated using:

      (1) "Sucker bypass" with a femoral artery cannula or aortic cannula and the cardiotomy suckers used as the venous return line if the right atrium cannot be cannulated.

      (2) Complete femoral vein–femoral artery bypass.

   d. The prolonged surgical dissection increases the risk of dysrhythmias.

      (1) The availability of external defibrillator pads or sterile external paddles should be considered. Defibrillation may be necessary before complete exposure of the heart, rendering internal paddles ineffective.

      (2) Many institutions use a defibrillation pad that adheres to the back and is placed before induction. This allows for use of an internal paddle even if the heart is not totally exposed, as current will flow in an anteroposterior fashion through the heart.

   e. Volume replacement (crystalloid, colloid, blood) may be necessary to provide adequate preload if hemorrhage is brisk during the dissection.

      (1) Have at least 2 units of blood available in case it is necessary to transfuse the patient.

      (2) After the patient is heparinized, the surgical team should use the CPB suckers to help salvage blood.

6. **Concerns with urgent or emergent cardiac operation**

   a. Indications include:

      (1) Cardiac catheterization complications (failed angioplasty with persistent chest pain, coronary artery dissection) [5]

      (2) Persistent ischemia with or without chest pain that is refractory to medical therapy or an intraaortic balloon pump (IABP)

      (3) Left main coronary artery disease or left main equivalent

      (4) Acute aortic dissection

      (5) Fulminant infective endocarditis

      (6) Multiple high-grade lesions with significant myocardium at risk

   b. Aggressively treat ischemia and dysrhythmias that may be present.

   c. Continue heparin infusion until sternotomy. This will increase operative bleeding but will decrease the risk of worsening coronary thrombosis.

   d. Consider heparin resistance and increase the initial heparin dose to avoid delays in starting CPB because the ACT is too low.

   e. Continue antianginal therapy, particularly the nitroglycerin infusion, during an acute myocardial ischemic event.

   f. **Maintain coronary perfusion pressure.** Phenylephrine or norepinephrine boluses and/or infusions may be necessary. An IABP may be in use or required. Maintain IABP triggers.

   g. Continue blood pressure, pulse oximeter, and electrocardiographic (ECG) monitoring during transport and preparation.

h. In these cases, time is of the essence. Decisions must be made regarding the risks and benefits of additional monitoring (arterial line and PA catheter) relative to the delay required for catheter insertion. Access to the central circulation and some form of direct blood pressure monitoring are required before surgery can begin.

(1) If all lines are placed before induction at your institution, then the decision involves how to proceed while the patient is awake. If the patient has resolution of chest pain and ECG changes, then proceed cautiously with monitoring line insertion. It often is necessary to replace a femoral PA line with one that is closer to the patient's head for accessibility. Keep the femoral catheter in place for monitoring until just before floating the new PA catheter, at which time it should be pulled back to avoid complications.

(2) If ischemia is still present while the patient is awake, proceed to the induction of anesthesia with the monitors you have. Often, after anesthesia is induced, the reduction in myocardial O_2 demand will significantly improve the ischemia and correct hemodynamic changes. In this case, insertion of further monitoring would be appropriate.

(3) If the patient continues to have significant hemodynamic and ischemic changes after induction that are unresponsive to treatment, proceed to CPB urgently.

(4) In an arrest situation, go directly to CPB. The surgeon can hand off central venous and PA lines before weaning the patient from CPB. TEE is a fast alternative to obtain much of the information derived from a PA catheter.

i. Urgency of initiating CPB does not supersede obtaining adequate heparinization documented by ACT, or adequate anesthetic levels. In a cardiac arrest situation, double or triple the usual dose of heparin to ensure adequate heparinization. The surgeon may give the heparin directly into the heart if access is not available.

j. If a "bailout" (coronary perfusion) catheter has been placed across a coronary dissection, it should not be disturbed. It can be withdrawn from the femoral arterial sheath just before application of the aortic cross-clamp.

k. Fibrinolytic or antiplatelet agents may have been given in the catheterization laboratory. These drugs will increase bleeding before and after CPB.

E. Sternal spread

1. Very high level of stimulation can be expected.
2. Visually confirm equal inflation of the lungs after the chest is open.
3. PA catheter malfunction with sternal spread has been reported. Most occurrences are with external jugular or subclavian approaches and involve kinking of the PA catheter as it exits the introducer sheath. A reinforced introducer can decrease the incidence of kinking. The surgeon could decrease the amount of sternal retraction.

   Sheath withdrawal may rectify the problem but can lead to the following:
   a. Loss of the IV line
   b. Bleeding
   c. Contamination of the access site
4. Innominate vein rupture, as well as brachial plexus injury, is possible after aggressive sternal spread.

F. Internal mammary artery and radial artery dissection

1. This is a period of low-level stimulation.
2. The chest is retracted to one side using the chest wall retractor, and the table is elevated and rotated away from the surgeon. The left IMA (LIMA) is most commonly grafted to the left anterior descending artery.
   a. This procedure can cause difficulties in blood pressure measurement.
      (1) Left-sided radial arterial lines may not function during LIMA dissection owing to compression of the left subclavian artery with sternal retraction. The same may be true with a right-sided catheter and a

right IMA (RIMA) dissection. An axillary, brachial, or femoral artery catheter may be used.

(2) Transducers must be kept level with the right atrium.

b. Extubation may occur with patient movement during retraction.

c. Radial nerve injury due to compression by the support post of the Favaloro retractor is possible.

3. **Bleeding** may be extensive but hidden from view in the chest cavity (consider volume replacement to treat hypotension).

4. **Heparin,** 5,000 units, may be given during the vessel dissection process.

5. Papaverine may be injected into the IMA for dilation and to prevent spasm. Systemic effects may include hypotension or anaphylaxis.

6. IMA blood flow usually should be more than 100 mL/min (25 mL collected in 15 seconds) to be considered acceptable for grafting.

7. If the radial artery is being harvested as a conduit, the arterial line should be placed on the other side.

G. **Sympathetic nerve dissection**

1. After the pericardium is opened, the postganglionic sympathetic nerves are dissected from the aorta to allow insertion of the aortic cannula.

2. This is the most overlooked period of high-level stimulation due to sympathetic discharge. Treatment of hemodynamic changes are explained in Section **I.C.**

II. Perioperative stress response

A. **Afferent loop**

1. The body responds to stress with a catabolic response and an increase in substrate mobilization. This response is mediated primarily through the hypothalamic-pituitary-adrenal axis.

2. Stimuli that can trigger this response include the following:

a. **Psychologic**

(1) Preoperative anxiety

(2) Light anesthesia, awareness

b. **Physiologic**

(1) Pain associated with invasive monitor placement

(2) Intubation

(3) Surgical stimulation

(4) Changes in blood pressure (hypotension or hypertension)

(5) Hypoxia

(6) Hypercapnia

(7) CPB

(8) Aortic cross-clamp removal

B. **Humoral mediators** involved in the stress response:

1. **Antidiuretic hormone (ADH):** Increased levels are associated with surgery and positive-pressure ventilation

2. **Adrenocorticotropic hormone (ACTH):** Increased; causes increase in cortisol levels

3. **Cortisol:** Increased; leads to an increase in glucose level

4. **Catecholamines:** Epinephrine, norepinephrine, dopamine; increased owing to adrenal medulla stimulation

5. **Insulin:** Decreased inappropriately for level of glucose

6. **Glucagon:** Increased; causes increased glucose level and contractility of the heart

7. **Growth hormone (GH):** Increased; causes increased rate of protein synthesis

8. **Renin:** Increased; converts angiotensinogen to angiotensin I, causing vasoconstriction and hypertension

9. **Prolactin:** Increased levels, possibly due to increased levels of endorphins

10. **Endorphins:** Increased

C. **Efferent loop:** Organ system responses to humoral mediators

1. **Cardiovascular effects**

a. **Catecholamines**

(1) Hypertension

(2) Tachycardia

(3) Dysrhythmias

(4) Myocardial O_2 supply/demand ratio affected adversely

b. Renin, angiotensin, ADH

(1) Increased blood volume (preload)

(2) Increased SVR (afterload)

c. Glucagon: Increased inotropy

2. Renal effects

a. Increased aldosterone levels

b. Decreased urine output (ADH)

c. Decreased plasma potassium and increased plasma sodium secondary to aldosterone

d. Decreased renal blood flow

3. Metabolic effects

a. Increased myocardial O_2 consumption

b. Increased cerebral metabolic rate

c. Increased lactate and pyruvate levels

d. Increased blood glucose level (CNS dysfunction, increased infection rate)

e. Decreased liver and renal blood flow, which may decrease clearance and increase the duration of action of medications

f. Increased free fatty acid levels

4. Neurologic effects

a. Decreased MAC of anesthetic agents from endorphin production

5. Pulmonary effects

a. Increased conversion of angiotensin I to angiotensin II

b. Bronchodilation and increased dead space

D. Modification of the stress response

1. Systemic opioids (high-dose)

a. Fentanyl (50 to 150 µg/kg) blunts almost all responses except for prolactin increase and an occasional increase in myocardial lactate production before CPB.

b. Sufentanil (10 to 30 µg/kg) is similar to fentanyl, but some studies have shown increased norepinephrine levels with sternotomy. Free fatty acid levels increase with cannulation but may be associated with heparin.

c. Complications. High-dose narcotics will lead to prolonged mechanical ventilation and delayed extubation. They also do not ensure amnesia.

2. Inhalation anesthetics

a. MAC that blocks adrenergic response in 50% of patients (MAC BAR)

(1) MAC BAR is approximately equal to 1.5 MAC.

(2) Cortisol and GH levels will increase with this depth of anesthesia.

(3) To reduce catecholamine responses in 95% of patients, 2.0 MAC is needed.

(4) MAC BAR is associated with myocardial depression, decreased blood pressure, and increased pulmonary capillary wedge pressure.

3. Systemic medications that decrease catecholamine effects

a. β-Blockers

(1) β-Blockers attenuate increases in heart rate and myocardial O_2 demand.

(2) Adverse effects include the following:

(a) Decreased myocardial contractility

(b) Bronchospasm

b. Centrally acting α_2-adrenergic agonists (clonidine, dexmedetomidine) [6]

(1) Both agents decrease peripheral efferent sympathetic activity.

(2) They cause a decrease in all catecholamine levels (reduced norepinephrine levels are most prominent) and enhance cardiovascular stability.

(3) They can decrease heart rate, blood pressure, and SVR in the perioperative period.

(4) Some attenuation of adrenergic response during or after CPB is seen with preoperative dosing.

(5) They may cause bradycardia and hypotension, especially when combined with angiotensin-converting enzyme (ACE) inhibitors or vasodilators. Paradoxically, high doses may cause increases in PVR, hypertension, and decreases in cardiac index.

(6) Dexmedetomidine will produce analgesia and sedation. Infusions often are used after CPB for "fast track" anesthesia.

c. Vasodilators

(1) Vasodilators are used as treatment for increases in SVR, often secondary to elevated norepinephrine levels.

(2) Adverse effects include the following:

(a) Reflex increase in catecholamines

(b) Reflex increase in heart rate

(c) Inhibition of hypoxic pulmonary vasoconstriction

4. Regional (epidural or subarachnoid) anesthetic techniques [7]

a. Local anesthetics

(1) These drugs decrease GH, ACTH, ADH, and catecholamine responses to lower abdominal procedures.

(2) Thoracic epidural anesthesia is inconsistent in blocking the stress response to thoracic surgery, possibly due to insufficient somatic or sympathetic blockade or from unblocked pelvic afferents.

(3) Adverse effects include decreased SVR, bradycardia, decreased inotropy from sympathectomy, and risk of epidural hemorrhage after heparinization.

b. Narcotics

(1) Peridural narcotics poorly block the stress response to surgery.

(2) They provide postoperative analgesia.

III. **Treatment of hemodynamic changes.** Pressor and vasodilator treatment of any hemodynamic change ideally should involve the use of agents with a very short half-life, for the following reasons. (i) The surgical stimuli and the patient response usually are short lived (after sternotomy the duration of patient response usually is limited to 5 to 15 minutes). (ii) Many agents (β-blockers, calcium channel blockers, vasodilators, ACE inhibitors, phosphodiesterase inhibitors) will affect hemodynamic parameters for longer than 15 minutes and have half-lives of several hours. Their actions could affect weaning from CPB. For these reasons, the use of short-acting agents (esmolol, nitroglycerin, sodium nitroprusside, phenylephrine, and ephedrine) should be encouraged.

A. **Hypotension**

1. Causes

a. Mechanical causes must first be ruled out before treatment. Among these are:

(1) Surgical compression of the heart

(2) Technical problems with invasive blood pressure measurement (kinked catheter, wrist position, air bubbles)

b. The most common cause of hypotension is hypovolemia (Table 6.2).

c. Myocardial ischemia is another potentially treatable cause of hypotension.

2. Treatment is outlined in Figure 6.1.

B. **Hypertension**

1. Hypertension is less common in patients with left ventricular dysfunction than in patients with normal contractility, but it still occurs.

2. **The most likely cause of hypertension is sympathetic discharge.** This is seen most often in younger patients and in those with preoperative hypertension (Table 6.3).

3. Treatment is outlined in Figure 6.2.

C. **Sinus bradycardia**

1. The most common cause of sinus bradycardia is vagal stimulation, which often results from the vagotonic effects of narcotics (Table 6.4).

2. Treatment

a. Treatment is indicated for:

Table 6.2 Differential diagnosis of hypotension

1. Hypovolemia
2. Deep anesthetic plane for level of stimulation
3. Decreased venous return
   a. Mechanical compression of the heart or great vessels
   b. Increased airway pressure
   c. Tension pneumothorax
4. Impaired myocardial contractility
5. Ischemia
6. Dysrhythmia
   a. Bradycardia
   b. Tachycardia (decrease in diastolic filling time)
   c. Dysrhythmia leading to loss of atrial contraction and its contribution to ventricular filling
7. Decrease in systemic vascular resistance
8. Constrictive pericarditis in reoperation cases
9. Steroid depletion with chronic steroid administration

Causes of hypotension are listed in order of frequency of occurrence.

        (1) Any heart rate decrease associated with a significant decrease in blood pressure.

        (2) Heart rate less than 40 beats/min, even without decrease in blood pressure, if it is associated with a nodal or ventricular escape rhythm.

    b. The underlying cause should be treated.

    c. Atropine, 0.2 to 0.4 mg IV, can cause an unpredictable response.

        (1) It may cause uncontrolled tachycardia and ischemia.

        (2) It often is ineffective.

        (3) Glycopyrrolate (0.1 to 0.2 mg IV), another vagolytic agent, may induce less increase in heart rate, but it is unpredictable and has a longer half-life than atropine.

    d. Pancuronium, 2 to 4 mg IV, often is effective owing to its sympathomimetic activity, but it can be unpredictable.

    e. Ephedrine, 2.5 to 25.0 mg IV, is indicated if bradycardia is associated with hypotension. The response may be unpredictable.

    f. PA catheters with pacing capabilities and esophageal atrial pacing may provide safe and predictable, although expensive, means of increasing the heart rate.

    g. Atropine and pacing can be used for life-threatening bradycardia. For minimally invasive procedures, placement of external patches may be needed to provide pacing.

D. Sinus tachycardia

    1. Sinus tachycardia appears to be the most significant risk factor for intraoperative ischemia. Sinus tachycardia greater than 100 beats/min has been associated with a 40% incidence of ischemia. Heart rate greater than 110 beats/min was associated with a 32% to 63% incidence of ischemia [8]. The most likely cause is light anesthesia (sympathetic stimulation) (Table 6.5).

    2. Treatment

        a. Rule out ventilation abnormalities and correct them if present.

        b. Increase anesthetic level if other signs of light anesthesia or BIS monitor changes are seen. An empiric small dose of narcotic often is used.

        c. Treat the underlying cause.

            (1) Give volume infusion if low preload is evident.

            (2) Address the other causes of tachycardia listed in Table 6.5.

            (3) β-Blockade with esmolol can be used, particularly if ischemia is noted.

E. Dysrhythmias

    1. The most likely cause of dysrhythmia in the prebypass period is surgical manipulation of the heart (Table 6.6).

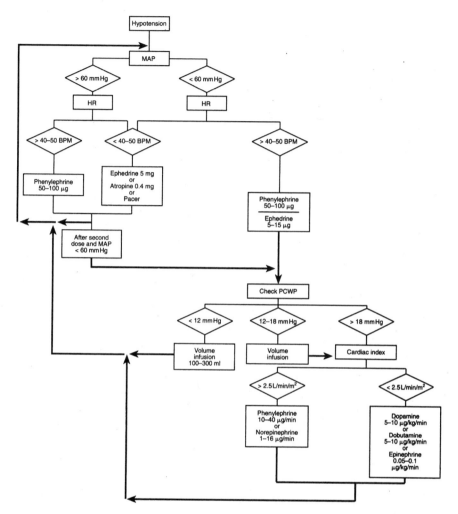

FIG. 6.1 Treatment of hypotension in the prebypass period. Once hypotension is identified: (i) supply 100% O_2; (ii) check end-tidal carbon dioxide level ($ETco_2$) and blood gas; (iii) decrease inhalation agent concentration; and (iv) rule out dysrhythmias and technical or mechanical factors. Treat per algorithm. *HR*, heart rate; *MAP*, mean arterial pressure; *PCWP*, pulmonary capillary wedge pressure.

2. Treatment
   a. **Treatment of the underlying cause.** Potassium replacement in the pre-CPB period should be limited to treatment for symptomatic hypokalemia because the cardioplegic solution used during CPB may increase the serum potassium level significantly. Magnesium replacement has been useful in patients who have dysrhythmias and are hypomagnesemic.
   b. **Dysrhythmias causing minor hemodynamic disturbances**
      (1) Supraventricular tachycardia (including acute atrial fibrillation or flutter)

Table 6.3 Differential diagnosis of hypertension

1. Light anesthesia (increased narcotic requirements are noted in patients with chronic tobacco, alcohol, or caffeine use)
2. Dissection of sympathetic nerves from the aorta in preparation for aortic cannulation
3. Hypoxia
4. Hypercapnia
5. Hypervolemia
6. Withdrawal syndromes
   a. β-Blockers
   b. Clonidine
   c. Alcohol } Rare
7. Thyroid storm
8. Malignant hyperpyrexia
9. Pheochromocytoma

Causes of hypertension are listed in order of frequency of occurrence.

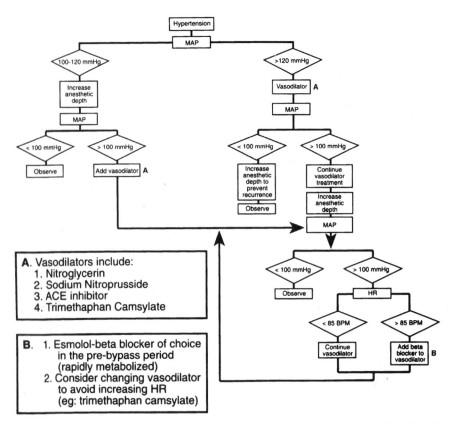

FIG. 6.2 Treatment of hypertension in the prebypass period. First, rule out technical problems and airway difficulties. *HR,* heart rate; *MAP,* mean arterial pressure.

Table 6.4 Differential diagnosis of sinus bradycardia

---

1. Vagal stimulation
   a. Vagotonic effects of narcotics
   b. Intense surgical stimulation with light plane of anesthesia (e.g., during sternotomy)
      i. Sufentanil more effective than fentanyl, which is more effective than morphine
      ii. Associated with rapid administration
      iii. Associated with initial dose (less bradycardia occurs with subsequent narcotic doses)
      iv. More pronounced when nitrous oxide is not present (nitrous oxide may increase sympathetic tone)
      v. More pronounced with vecuronium, atracurium, or metocurine compared with pancuronium
   c. Vagotonic effects of halothane
2. Deep anesthetic levels
3. Hypoxia
4. β-Blockade
5. Calcium channel blockers (verapamil and diltiazem produce greater effects than nifedipine)
6. Ischemia
7. Sick sinus syndrome
8. Reflex bradycardia secondary to:
   a. Hypervolemia
   b. Hypertension
      i. Secondary to vasoconstrictor use
      ii. Secondary to other causes of hypertension (see Table 6.3)

Causes of sinus bradycardia are listed in order of frequency of occurrence.

Table 6.5 Differential diagnosis of sinus tachycardia

---

1. Light anesthesia insufficient for level of surgical stimulation
2. Medications
   a. Pancuronium
   b. Scopolamine
   c. Inotropic agents
   d. Isoflurane
   e. Aminophylline preparations
   f. β-Agonists
   g. Monoamine oxidase inhibitors or tricyclic antidepressants
3. Hypovolemia
4. Ischemia
5. Hypoxia
6. Hypercapnia
7. Congestive heart failure
8. Withdrawal syndromes ⎤
   a. β-Blockers |
   b. Clonidine |
   c. Alcohol   ⎬ Rare
9. Thyroid storm |
10. Malignant hyperpyrexia |
11. Pheochromocytoma   ⎦

Causes of sinus tachycardia are listed in order of frequency of occurrence.

Table 6.6 Common causes of dysrhythmias

1. Mechanical stimulation of the heart (e.g., placement of pursestring sutures, cannulation, vent placement, and lifting the heart to study coronary anatomy)
2. Preexisting dysrhythmias
3. Increase in catecholamine levels
   a. Light anesthesia
   b. Hypercapnia
   c. Nitrous oxide
   d. Halothane (sensitization of myocardium to catecholamines)
4. Direct and indirect autonomic stimulants
   a. Pancuronium
   b. Inotropic agents
   c. Aminophylline preparations
   d. β-Agonists
   e. Monoamine oxidase inhibitors and tricyclic antidepressants
5. Electrolyte abnormalities including hypokalemia
6. Hypertension
7. Hypotension
8. Ischemia[a]
9. Hypoxemia

Causes of dysrhythmias listed in order of frequency of occurrence.
[a] More frequent in patients with severe coronary disease.

(a) Stop mechanical irritation.
(b) Use vagal maneuvers, adenosine, digoxin, calcium channel blockers, β-blockers, Neo-Synephrine, or edrophonium.
(2) Premature ventricular contractions
   (a) Stop mechanical irritation.
   (b) Treat with lidocaine, procainamide, β-blockers, amiodarone
c. **Dysrhythmias causing major hemodynamic compromise.** Continue chemical resuscitation as in Section **b** above, concurrent with:
   (1) Cardioversion or defibrillation for atrial dysrhythmias, ventricular tachycardia, or ventricular fibrillation
      (a) Internal cardioversion
         (i) Small paddles are applied directly to the heart when the chest is open.
         (ii) Low energy levels (10 to 25 J) are needed for cardioversion (skin impedance is bypassed).
         (iii) Synchronization capabilities are desirable for atrial dysrhythmias and ventricular tachycardia. This may require additional cables or equipment.
         (iv) Defibrillation requires similar energy levels in a nonsynchronized mode.
      (b) External cardioversion
         (i) Usual paddle size is used with the chest closed.
         (ii) Energy levels of 25 to 300 J are needed.
         (iii) Sterile external paddles are desirable (see Section **I.D.5.d**).
         (iv) Defibrillation should be initiated with 300 J.
IV. **Preparation for cardiopulmonary bypass**
   A. **Heparinization** [9].
      1. Unfractionated heparin is the preferred agent for anticoagulation. It is a water-soluble mucopolysaccharide with an average molecular weight of 15,000 daltons.
         a. Mechanism of action
            (1) Binds to antithrombin III (AT III), a protease inhibitor.
            (2) Increases the speed of the reaction between AT III and several activated clotting factors (II, IX, X, XI, XII, XIII).

   b. Onset time: Immediate.
   c. Half-life: Approximately 2.5 hours at usual cardiac surgery dose.
   d. Metabolism
      (1) 50% by liver (heparinase) or reticuloendothelial system
      (2) 50% unchanged by renal elimination
   e. Potency of different preparations may differ markedly.
      (1) Potency is measured in units (not milligrams).
      (2) Heparin solutions usually contain at least 120 to 140 units/mg, depending on the lot or manufacturer.
   f. Protamine sulfate rapidly reverses heparin activity by combining with heparin to form an inactive compound.
   g. Dosage
      (1) The initial dosage of heparin for anticoagulation before CPB is 300 units/kg. This initial dose has been established by many investigators. However, some patients may remain inadequately anticoagulated using this dose, so adequate anticoagulation must be established on an individual basis according to the ACT (see Section **3** below).
      (2) Some institutions use a heparin dose–response titration to establish an initial dose.
2. Routes of administration. Heparin must be administered directly into a central vein or into the right atrium, with documentation that heparin is being administered into the intravascular space (aspiration to confirm blood return).
3. ACT technique
   a. The ACT monitors the effect of heparin on coagulation. Two milliliters of blood is placed in a tube that contains diatomite (clay), which causes contact activation of the coagulation cascade. The tube is heated to 37°C, and the solution is mixed continuously. The time from introduction of blood into the tube until the first clot is formed is the ACT. This measurement now is automated.
   b. Normal automated ACT is 105 to 167 seconds.
   c. An ACT of at least 300 seconds is safe for initiating CPB, provided the ACT is rechecked immediately after starting CPB and heparin (3,000 to 5,000 units) is included in the pump prime.
   d. An ACT greater than 400 seconds is known to prevent fibrin monomer appearance during CPB. Some institutions require an ACT of 480 seconds before CPB.
4. Inadequate ACT
   a. Causes of inadequate ACT are listed in Table 6.7.
   b. Treatment of inadequate ACT
      (1) Check ACT before and after heparin administration.
      (2) If ACT is less than 300 seconds, **do not begin CPB.**
      (3) Give more heparin in 5,000- to 10,000-unit increments (from different vials or different lots).
      (4) Recheck ACT.
      (5) AT III concentrates as well as recombinant AT III can be given empirically for treatment of presumed AT III deficiency if ACT less than 300 seconds persists despite administration of large doses of heparin (800 to 1,000 units/kg) and if other causes of inadequate ACT are ruled out (Table 6.7).
         (a) If available, a heparin dose–response curve can indicate heparin resistance early in this process.
         (b) If AT III is not available, 2 to 3 units of fresh frozen plasma (FFP) should be given to increase the levels of AT III that presumably are depleted.
         (c) Recheck ACT after AT III or FFP is given.
B. Cannulation (Fig. 6.3)
   1. A pericardial sling is created before cannulation to increase working space and to provide a dam for external cooling fluid and ice slush solution. The sling may lift the heart, which can decrease venous return and lead to hypotension.

Table 6.7 Causes of inadequate activated clotting time before initiation
of cardiopulmonary bypass

Technical causes
  Mislabeled syringe
  Heparin not injected intravascularly (extravasation, not injected into right atrium,
    line disconnection)
  Heparin having low activity (old or nonrefrigerated vials)
  Type of heparin (bovine vs. porcine)
  Source of heparin (intestinal vs. lung)
Heparin resistance (most causes related to low antithrombin III levels)
  Previous heparin use or ongoing infusion
  Nitroglycerin infusion
  Hemodilution
  Pregnancy or oral contraceptives
  Intraaortic balloon pump
  Shock
  Streptokinase
  Hereditary antithrombin III deficiency
  Low-grade disseminated intravascular coagulation
  Infective endocarditis
  Intracardiac thrombus
  Elderly patient

Modified from Anderson EF. Heparin resistance prior to cardiopulmonary bypass. *Anesthesiology* 1986;
64:505.

2. Pursestring sutures are used to keep the aortic and venous cannulae in place
during surgery and to close the incisions after decannulation.
3. Nitrous oxide is discontinued to avoid enlargement of air emboli.
4. Heparin is **always** given before cannulation.
5. The aortic cannula is inserted first to allow infusion of volume in case of hemorrhage associated with venous cannulation. Systolic blood pressure should
be decreased to 90 to 100 mm Hg to reduce the risk of aortic dissection and to
facilitate cannulation. If necessary, emergency CPB can be instituted using
cardiotomy suckers to deliver venous return (so-called "sucker bypass") if
necessary.
6. The surgical and anesthesia teams both should check the aortic cannula for
air bubbles as it is filled with saline and connected to CPB tubing. A test transfusion of 100 mL should be performed to ensure proper placement and functioning of the cannula.
7. If you request an infusion of volume before CPB, make sure the surgical team
or the perfusionist does not have any clamps on the tubing.
8. Positive end-expiratory pressure may be applied to increase intracardiac pressures to avoid air entrainment during cannulation of the right atrium and left
ventricle (vent insertion).
9. Complications of cannulation
    a. Aortic cannulation
        (1) Embolic phenomena from air or atherosclerotic plaque dislodgment
        can occur. Epiaortic echocardiography sometimes is used to identify
        intimal plaque and to find a "safe" location for the cannula.
        (2) Hypotension
            (a) Hypotension usually is secondary to hypovolemia (blood loss).
            (b) It may result from mechanical compression of the heart.
            (c) A partial occlusion clamp used for cannulation may narrow the
                aortic lumen (more common in children). Check the aortic pres-
                sure immediately when the clamp is applied.

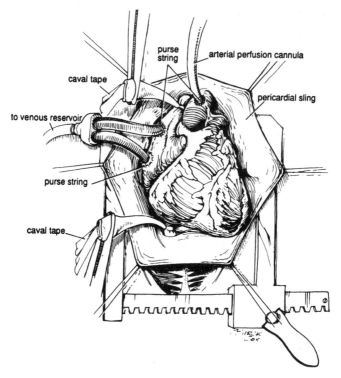

FIG. 6.3 View of an open chest with formation of a pericardial sling (see text). Note arterial and venous cannulation sites. Caval tapes, placed around the superior and inferior vena cava, are tightened to institute complete CPB (see Chapter 7 for a discussion of complete and partial CPB).

      (3) Dysrhythmias are most likely due to surgical manipulation.

      (4) Aortic dissection can occur due to cannula misplacement. A pulsatile pressure from the aortic cannula that correlates with the radial mean arterial blood pressure effectively rules out dissection (see Chapter 7).

      (5) Bleeding

          (a) Minor bleeding is not uncommon with cannulation.

          (b) Major bleeding may occur if the aorta is torn.

          (c) Treatment consists of infusion of volume as needed or initiation of CPB.

      (6) Rarely, air entrainment around the cannulae occurs, with resultant systemic embolization.

   b. Venous cannulation

      (1) Hypotension

          (a) If hypotension is due to hypovolemia, give volume in 100-mL increments for adults and 10 to 25 mL for pediatric patients through the aortic line as needed.

          (b) Mechanical compression of the heart may cause hypotension, especially during inferior vena caval cannulation.

(2) Bleeding
  (a) Bleeding can occur from a tear of the right atrium or the superior or inferior vena cava.
  (b) Treatment is accomplished by infusing volume or initiating emergency CPB.
(3) Dysrhythmias
  (a) Dysrhythmias usually result from surgical manipulation.
  (b) No treatment is required if they do not cause hemodynamic deterioration.
  (c) Cessation or limitation of mechanical stimulation may be all that is necessary.
  (d) Treatment consists of medications, cardioversion, or initiating CPB (see Section **II.D**).
(4) Air entrainment
  (a) Air entrainment from around the cannula with subsequent signs of pulmonary embolization is possible.

C. **Autologous blood removal**
  1. **Sequestration of platelets and clotting factors.** Autologous blood may be removed to sequester platelets and clotting factors from damage during CPB, with return at the conclusion of CPB. Some centers believe this practice enhances coagulation after CPB and decreases the need for transfusion of homologous blood and blood products during this period. Sequestration of platelets and clotting factors can be accomplished in a variety of ways.
  2. **Techniques**
     a. Blood, 500 to 1,000 mL, can be withdrawn in the pre-CPB period and stored in a citrate phosphate dextrose (CPD) solution, similar to banked blood.
     b. Before initiation of bypass, 500 to 1,000 mL of heparinized blood can be removed from the venous bypass drainage line and saved for later infusion.
     c. Plateletpheresis cell salvage equipment can be used in the prebypass period to remove blood, if necessary, from a central venous catheter. After centrifugation, the red cells are returned to maintain hemoglobin levels and O_2 transport. The platelet-poor fraction may be returned to maintain intravascular volume or reserved along with the platelet-rich fraction for later infusion after bypass.
  3. **Risks**
     a. Hypotension secondary to hypovolemia. Treat with vasopressors and decrease the withdrawal rate while increasing the infusion rate.
     b. Decreased O_2-carrying capacity, as evidenced by a decreased mixed venous oxygenation saturation. Treat with 100% FIO_2, halt blood removal, return red cells as needed, and begin CPB as soon as possible.
     c. **Infection.** Maintain sterile technique for removal and return of blood.
     d. **Relative contraindications**
        (1) Left main coronary disease or equivalent
        (2) Left ventricular dysfunction
        (3) Anemia with hemoglobin less than 12 g/dL
        (4) Emergent surgery

References

1. O'Connor JP, Ramsey JG, Wynands JE, et al. The incidence of myocardial ischemia during anesthesia for coronary artery bypass surgery in patients receiving pancuronium or vecuronium. *Anesthesiology* 1989;70:230–236.
2. Sharma AD, Parmley CL, Sreeram G, et al. Peripheral nerve injuries during cardiac surgery: risk factors, diagnosis, prognosis, and prevention. *Anesth Analg* 2000;91: 1358–1369.
3. Aronson S, Blumenthal R. Perioperative renal dysfunction and cardiovascular anesthesia: concerns and controversies. *J Cardiothorac Vasc Anesth* 1998;12:567–586.
4. **Bovill JG, Sebel PS, Stanley TH. Opioid analgesics in anesthesia: with special reference to their use in cardiovascular anesthesia. *Anesthesiology* 1984;61:731–755.**

5. **Bates ER. Ischemic complications after percutaneous transluminal coronary angioplasty.** *Am J Med* **2000;108:309–316.**
6. Kamibayashi T, Maze M. Clinical Uses of [alpha]2-adrenergic agonists. *Anesthesiology* 2000;93:1345–1349.
7. Liu S, Carpenter RL, Neal JM. Epidural anesthesia and analgesia: their role in postoperative outcome. *Anesthesiology* 1995;82:1474–1506.
8. Slogoff S, Keats AS. Randomized trial of primary anesthetic agents on outcome of coronary artery bypass operations. *Anesthesiology* 1989;70:179–188.
9. Despotis GJ, Gravlee G, Kriton F, et al. Anticoagulation monitoring during cardiac surgery: a review of current and emerging techniques. *Anesthesiology* 1999;91:1122–1129.

7. ANESTHETIC MANAGEMENT DURING CARDIOPULMONARY BYPASS

David R. Larach and Neville M. Gibbs

I. Preparations for cardiopulmonary bypass
A. The cardiopulmonary bypass circuit (Fig. 7.1)

1. **Function.** Cardiopulmonary bypass (CPB) permits blood to bypass the heart and lungs, draining instead by gravity from the central veins through an artificial lung (oxygenator) and an external pump that injects oxygenated blood at arterial pressure into one of the great arteries. Thus, CPB sustains systemic blood flow, oxygenation, and ventilation during periods of time when (a) the heart is asystolic or not ejecting a normal cardiac output and (b) the lungs are unable to perform physiologic gas exchange because of inadequate perfusion.

   Even though CPB can provide a normal cardiac output, a number of important differences exist between the natural and artificial circulations, including nonpulsatile flow, bypass of the lung's endocrine function, and trauma to blood elements. See Chapter 20 for a discussion of the pathophysiology of CPB.

2. **Circuit design.** The **venous conduit** (Fig. 7.1) drains systemic venous blood to the CPB machine; most commonly, a single cannula is inserted in the right

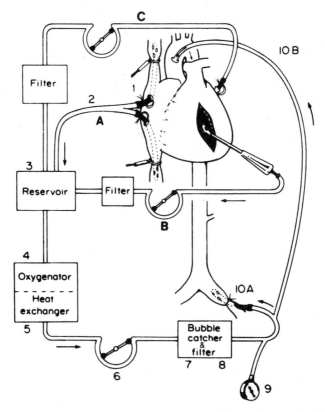

FIG. 7.1 Cardiopulmonary bypass circuit (example). Blood drains by gravity (A) from venae cavae (1) through venous cannula (2) into venous reservoir (3). Blood from surgical field suction and from vent is pumped (B,C) into cardiotomy reservoir (not shown) and then drains into venous reservoir (3). Venous blood is oxygenated (4), temperature adjusted (5), raised to arterial pressure (6), filtered (7,8), and injected into either aorta (10B) or femoral artery (10A). Arterial line pressure is monitored (9). Note that items 3, 4, and 5 often are single integral units. (Modified from Nose Y. The oxygenator. St. Louis: Mosby, 1973:53.)

atrium, with openings to admit right atrial and inferior vena caval (IVC) blood, or separate cannulas are inserted in the superior and inferior venae cavae. The **arterial cannula** returns oxygenated blood from the pump to the aorta, usually inserting either in the ascending aorta or in a femoral artery. See Chapter 19 for complete details of bypass circuit and design.

3. **Circuit components.** Most commonly, a roller pump is used (Fig. 7.1). For longer or more complex procedures, a centrifugal pump or heparin-coated circuit may be advantageous. Centrifugal pumps reduce trauma to blood components, and heparin-coated circuits reduce activation of coagulation factors. A leuco-depleting filter in the arterial circuit may reduce the inflammatory response to CPB. See Chapter 19 for a discussion of circuit components.

4. **Total versus partial CPB. Total (or complete) CPB** occurs when **all** venous blood draining toward the heart is diverted into the pump oxygenator. **Partial CPB** occurs when only a **portion** of systemic venous blood drains to the pump oxygenator while the remainder passes through the right heart and lungs and is ejected by the left ventricle (LV). Partial CPB can occur only when the aorta is not cross-clamped, but simply removing the aortic cross-clamp does not necessarily mean that total CPB will cease. That depends on whether the heart is filled and is capable of ejecting blood.

B. **Preparing the CPB pump for bypass**

1. **Composition of bypass perfusate.** In consultation with the anesthesiologist and surgeon, the perfusionist determines the composition of the **pump priming solution.** Generally, this consists of a mixture of electrolytes, colloid, buffer, mannitol, and heparin. If the use of a "clear" (i.e., blood-free) prime would result in excessive hemodilution, e.g., hemoglobin concentration [Hb] less than 5 to 7 g/dL, given the patient's size and hematocrit, then blood or packed red blood cells (RBCs) are added to the priming solution. See Chapter 19 for a detailed discussion of priming the bypass pump.

2. **Perfusionist's prebypass checklist.** When setting up the CPB pump apparatus and circuit, safe clinical practice requires that the perfusionist take particular care to ensure that at least the following conditions are met: (a) All gas bubbles are expelled from the tubing to prevent arterial air embolism or venous air lock; (b) All tubing is connected to the pumps for antegrade flow because retrograde flow can cause arterial air injection and lack of perfusion; (c) O_2 is being supplied to the oxygenator; (d) all safety alarms and automatic shutdown sensors are functional and are engaged; and (e) when the arterial perfusion cannula is inserted in the aorta, its transduced pressure shows a **pulsatile** waveform that **correlates** with radial arterial pressure (this helps rule out aortic dissection). A prebypass checklist and a written perfusion record are recommended.

C. **Anesthesiologist's pre-CPB checklist.** Preparation for CPB by the anesthesiologist begins with a thorough understanding of the proposed sites of cannulation and the bypass procedures to be used. Will the heart be arrested? What degree of hypothermia is anticipated? Will total circulatory arrest be used? Will special efforts be necessary to provide protection for the heart or other vital organs from ischemia? The pre-CPB checklist includes the following (Table 7.1):

1. **Anticoagulation.** Has heparin been given (by the anesthesiologist or surgeon)? Does the patient show **signs** of adequate heparinization? Just because heparin was administered does not guarantee that the patient is anticoagulated! Generally, adequate heparinization requires an activated clotting time (ACT) of **more than 480 seconds.** A higher ACT (greater than 750 seconds) is required if aprotinin is used, because aprotinin prolongs the celite-activated ACT [1]. Alternatively, a kaolin-activated ACT cartridge (which is less affected by aprotinin) should be used. The ACT may be accurately measured within 2 minutes of heparin administration [2]. However, when the CPB prime contains additional heparin (e.g., 5,000 units), CPB frequently is initiated when the ACT exceeds 300 seconds.

2. **Anesthesia.** Is the patient adequately anesthetized and is adequate muscle relaxation present? Because concentrations of drugs in the blood are diluted

Table 7.1 Prebypass checklist

Anticoagulation—adequate?
Anesthesia—adequate?
Cannulation—proper and patent?
Drips turned off
Monitoring in place and checked
  Pressure transducers
  Temperatures
  Foley catheter
Pupils inspected

---

by the prime when CPB begins, it may be necessary to give supplemental doses of intravenous (IV) anesthetics and muscle relaxants immediately before CPB.

3. **Cannulation.** Is the aortic cannula positioned within the true lumen of the aorta? This placement is documented by examining the pressure waveform within the arterial cannula (measured by the perfusionist). The aortic pressure should be **pulsatile** and should **correlate** with the radial arterial pressure after correcting for the vertical height difference between the pump's pressure transducer and the right atrium (1 mm Hg = 1.3 cm H_2O). Are any bubbles evident within the cannula? Check for equality of both **carotid pulses** or the presence of a carotid thrill, because the cannula may be obstructing carotid flow (especially if a straight or unflanged aortic cannula is used; see Section **III.A**).

4. **Drips.** Once the patient is heparinized, all IV lines should be closed to prevent unnecessary hemodilution. Hypovolemia usually can be managed by infusing priming solution from the CPB pump intermittently in 100-mL boluses (in adults) once the arterial cannula has been inserted, debubbled, and unclamped. Be aware that pump priming boluses may induce myocardial ischemia or dysrhythmias because the fluid injected into the aortic root enters the coronary arteries without much dilution and initially may be cold and unoxygenated.

   Antiischemia drugs (e.g., nitroglycerin) often are continued until aortic clamping. If the surgeon has cannulated the descending aorta via the ductus arteriosus (due to a hypoplastic aortic arch), then prostaglandin E may be discontinued at this time.

   If anesthetic or other drugs (e.g., propofol) are infused through a central catheter, it is important to ensure that the catheter tip is proximal to the superior vena cava (SVC) cannula snare. Alternatively, the infusions may be transferred to the CPB circuit.

5. **Monitoring**
   a. Check the zero and calibration of the arterial pressure transducer.
   b. Insert a nasopharyngeal temperature probe **before** heparinization.
   c. Empty the Foley catheter drainage bag or urometer device because it is important to determine fresh urine output during CPB.
   d. If present, a Swan–Ganz catheter should be withdrawn a few centimeters before institution of CPB to reduce the risk of pulmonary artery (PA) rupture. Similarly, a **Paceport** Swan–Ganz pacing wire should be withdrawn from the right ventricle (RV) before the surgeon lifts the heart to prevent ventricular perforation.
   e. The transesophageal echocardiography (TEE) probe, if present, should be returned to a nonflexed position within the esophagus during CPB.
6. **Pupils.** Both of the patient's eyes should be examined before CPB so that acute **changes** in pupil size or conjunctival chemosis (edema), which may occur upon commencing CPB, can be properly interpreted.

II. **Practical aspects of anesthetic management**
   A. **Initial bypass checklist.** During the first 30 to 60 seconds after initiation of CPB, the anesthesiologist should investigate carefully the items listed in Table 7.2.

Table 7.2 Initial cardiopulmonary bypass checklist

Face: Examine for color, temperature, plethora, edema, symmetry
Eyes: Examine pupils for size and symmetry and conjunctiva for chemosis (edema) and injection
Pump lines: Arteriovenous color difference should be visible.
Arterial blood pressure: Normally 30–60 mm Hg initially
Pulmonary artery pressure: If monitored, should be <15 mm Hg mean.
Central venous pressure: Should be <5 mm Hg.
Examine the heart: Distention, contractility
Stop ventilation when aortic ejection by the heart ceases

  B. **The CPB sequence**
   1. **Typical coronary artery bypass graft operation.** A typical coronary artery bypass graft operation (CABG) proceeds as follows. Total CPB is initiated and mild-to-moderate hypothermia is induced (30°C to 32°C). The aorta is cross-clamped and cardioplegic solution is infused antegrade through the aortic root and retrograde via the coronary sinus to arrest the heart. The distal saphenous vein grafts are placed on the most severely diseased coronary arteries first, to facilitate administration of additional cardioplegic solution (via the vein graft) distal to the stenoses. The internal mammary artery anastomosis (if used) is constructed last because of its fragility and short length. Rewarming begins when the final distal anastomosis is started. The aorta is unclamped and a partial aortic clamp is applied, permitting construction of proximal vein graft anastomoses during rewarming while cardioplegic solution is being washed out of the heart. When it is sufficiently warm, the heart is defibrillated if necessary, and the surgeon continues completing the proximal grafts. Alternatively, the proximal anastomoses are completed with the aortic clamp in place, in order to reduce instrumentation of the aorta (with the risk of dislodging of atheroma). Total CPB continues until the heart is reperfused from its new blood supply. Finally, when the patient is adequately rewarmed and the coronary artery grafts are completed, epicardial pacing wires are placed, and CPB then is terminated.
   2. **Typical aortic valve replacement or repair operation.** After initiation of CPB and application of the aortic cross-clamp, the aortic root is opened, and cardioplegic solution is infused into each coronary ostium under direct vision (to prevent retrograde filling of the LV with cardioplegic solution through an insufficient aortic valve). More commonly, cardioplegia is administered retrograde via the coronary sinus. The valve is repaired or replaced. Rewarming commences during valve replacement. The heart is irrigated to remove air or tissue debris, and the aortotomy is closed except for a vent. The patient then is placed in steep head-down position, the aortic cross-clamp is removed, and the heart is defibrillated if necessary. Final de-airing occurs as venous drainage to the pump is retarded, the heart fills and begins to eject (partial CPB), and air is aspirated through the aortic vent, an LV vent, or a needle placed in the apex of the heart. During de-airing, the lungs are ventilated vigorously to help flush bubbles out of pulmonary veins and the heart chambers.
   3. **Typical mitral valve replacement or repair operation.** This operation is similar to aortic valve surgery (see **2** above), except that the left atrium is opened instead of the aorta and the cardioplegic infusion can take place through the aortic root and the coronary sinus. The valve is replaced or repaired, and a large vent tube is passed through the mitral valve into the LV to prevent ejection of blood into the aorta until de-airing is completed. After thorough irrigation of the field and closure of the atriotomy except for the LV vent, the patient is placed in a steep head-down position, and the cross-clamp is removed. The heart is defibrillated if necessary, and de-airing occurs as described previously. Finally, the LV vent is removed, and de-airing is completed.

4. **Typical combined valve–CABG operation.** Usually the distal vein–graft anastomoses are created first, to permit cardioplegia of the myocardium distal to severe coronary stenoses. Also, lifting the heart to access the posterior wall vessels can disrupt myocardium if an artificial valve has been inserted. Next, the valve is operated on, and the operation proceeds as already described.
C. **Maintenance of bypass: checklist.** During CPB, the following items should be evaluated intermittently.
   1. **Anticoagulation.** The ACT or a similar rapid test of anticoagulation (e.g., Hepcon) must periodically confirm adequate anticoagulation (e.g., ACT greater than approximately 480 seconds; see also Section **1.C.1**). The ACT should be checked after initiating CPB and every 30 to 60 minutes thereafter. During periods of **normothermia,** heparin elimination is faster, so prolonged periods of normothermic CPB are much more likely to require heparin supplementation. Additional heparin usually is given in 5,000- to 10,000-unit increments, and the ACT is repeated to confirm the response. Use of heparin-coated circuits does not eliminate the need for heparin; an ACT of 250 seconds or greater is recommended [3].
   2. **Blood gas and acid–base status** should be checked soon after initiation of CPB and at least every 30 to 60 minutes thereafter. Continuous monitoring of S_aO_2 in the arterial cannula and S_vO_2 in the venous cannula is recommended. A continuous blood gas monitoring system, if used, should be correlated initially with standard blood gas electrodes during CPB. Arterial oxygen tension (P_aO_2) usually is maintained between 100 and 300 mm Hg by adjusting F_iO_2 to the membrane oxygenator, and desired mixed venous oxygen tension (P_vO_2) values are kept greater than 30 to 40 mm Hg (measured at 37°C) by adjusting pump flow and [Hb]. For discussion of alpha-stat and pH-stat acid–base management, see Chapter 20.
      Arterial carbon dioxide tensions usually are maintained between 35 and 40 mm Hg (alpha-stat) by adjusting the gas flow rate to the oxygenator. If continuous blood gas monitoring is not available, trends in CO_2 levels can be obtained by monitoring CO_2 in the oxygenator exhaust gas. This can be achieved by connecting the end-tidal gas sampling line end to side to the oxygenator exhaust during CPB [4].
   3. **Serum electrolytes, blood glucose, and hemoglobin** should be checked with each blood gas sample. Potassium levels may be affected by cardioplegia solution or renal function (see Sections **VII.D and VII.E**). Lactate levels provide an index of anaerobic metabolism (see Section **IV.B.3**). Glucose tolerance often is impaired during CPB, and hyperglycemia may exacerbate neuronal injury (see Chapter 23). Hemoglobin levels should be monitored frequently to avoid excessive hemodilution.
   4. **Anesthetic depth** should be sufficient (a) to prevent awareness (as assessed ideally by periodic tests of responsiveness, e.g., requesting patient to open eyes), (b) to prevent spontaneous movement including breathing, and (c) to suppress hypertensive or tachycardic responses to surgical stimuli. Potent anesthetics (e.g., isoflurane, enflurane) may he administered by connecting a vaporizer to the oxygenator gas inlet. Nitrous oxide is never used immediately before or during CPB because air emboli would enlarge rapidly. IV agents (e.g., propofol, opioids, benzodiazepines, barbiturates, scopolamine), either by bolus or infusion, are best administered into the venous blood reservoir. Because hypothermia itself reduces minimal alveolar concentration and neuronal activity, additional anesthetic drugs are most commonly required during **warm** periods at the beginning and end of CPB. If warm CPB is used or if the degree of hypothermia is mild or moderate, additional anesthetic drugs are required throughout CPB.
   5. **Ventilation** of the lungs should cease when total CPB begins. This is identified by loss of LV and RV ejection (flat arterial and PA pressure waveforms). Application of continuous positive airway pressure (2 to 5 cm H_2O) during total CPB is advocated by some to keep the lungs expanded but probably has little effect. Anesthetic **vaporizers** on the anesthesia machine should be turned off. During **partial** bypass (with ejection), occasional ventilation with 100% O_2 may

be needed to ensure that blood traversing the lung is oxygenated, although all of the body's CO_2 elimination continues to be performed by the artificial lung. A **pulse oximeter** during partial CPB or pulsatile perfusion can be helpful to identify pulmonary shunting or oxygenator difficulties because arterial blood gases measured at the CPB pump will **not** identify arterial desaturation caused by pulmonary shunt in the patient during partial CPB!

6. **Paralysis** should be sufficient to prevent (a) gross movement; (b) spontaneous ventilation (with risk of air entrainment by negative pulmonary venous pressure if cardiac structures are open); and (c) shivering (which increases the body's O_2 consumption). However, some advocate retention of a small degree of neuromuscular function sufficient to permit eye opening when testing for intraoperative awareness.

7. **Electrocardiogram. Ventricular fibrillation** may occur during CPB, particularly during cooling and rewarming of the heart. Ventricular fibrillation during cooling is less common if the aortic clamp is placed and cardioplegia is administered, soon after commencing CPB. The onset of ventricular fibrillation should be identified promptly and the surgeon informed. When ventricular fibrillation occurs during cooling, the aortic cross-clamp usually is applied and cardioplegia administered, but sometimes defibrillation is performed to keep the heart beating until an intracardiac vent can be placed. During periods of myocardial arrest, the appearance of electrical activity should be communicated to the surgeon, because additional cardioplegia may be indicated. Ventricular fibrillation during rewarming often is short lived and resolves spontaneously. If it is persistent, it should be treated with defibrillation, with or without lidocaine administration, because fibrillation depletes myocardial energy stores more quickly than does a spontaneous cardiac rhythm in the empty heart. Atrial and ventricular **ectopic beats** occur frequently with cardiac manipulation. Significant ectopy requires therapy only if it persists during unstimulated periods and it is not due to metabolic abnormalities.

8. **Urine production** should be identified and quantified as a sign of adequate renal perfusion and to assist in appropriate fluid management by the perfusionist. Urine flow rates of 300 to 1,000 mL/hour are commonly seen in hemodilution, especially if mannitol is present in the priming solution. Oliguria (less than 1 mL/kg/hour) should prompt an investigation because it may indicate inadequate renal perfusion (see Section **IV.C.I.b**). However, some hypothermic patients demonstrate oliguria without an apparent cause.

9. **Temperature** is monitored in at least two locations during CPB.
   a. **Core temperature** monitors the well-perfused organs. Nasopharyngeal or tympanic membrane probes reflect brain temperature. The bladder probe reflects renal temperature **only** if urine flow is adequate and should not be relied on during CPB. Slowed nasopharyngeal cooling could signify impaired cerebral blood flow (so long as the probe is correctly placed; see Section **IV.A.6**).
   b. **Shell temperature** monitors the relatively poorly perfused muscle–fat tissues that constitute most of the body's mass and thermal inertia. During rapid cooling and warming on CPB, the shell temperature lags behind the core temperature. A rectal probe or skeletal muscle needle sensor measures shell temperature. Because hypothermia induces vasoconstriction in peripheral beds, cooling and rewarming tend to be nonuniform during CPB. Thus, large gradients (8°C to 10°C or more) often develop between core and shell temperature during cooling.
   c. **Esophageal and PA temperature.** A PA thermistor receives little blood flow during total CPB, and esophageal temperature is affected by ice in the pericardial space, making these ineffective sites of temperature monitoring during CPB.
   d. Temperature during initial CPB cooling should decrease faster in the core (i.e., nasopharyngeal temperature) than in the shell (i.e., rectal temperature).
   e. **Rewarming** usually is associated with large gradients between shell and core temperatures due to rapid distribution of warm blood to the

well-perfused core organs and reduced flow to peripheral areas owing to vasoconstriction. Administration of vasodilator drugs, such as nitroprusside or phentolamine, often can hasten rewarming. The perfusionist must not warm the arterial blood too quickly because O_2 becomes less soluble in blood as temperature increases. Thus, rapid rewarming (greater than 10°C gradient between heat exchanger and blood) can cause gas bubble formation.

D. De-airing of the heart before weaning from CPB. Intracardiac air often is present during open chamber procedures (e.g., valve surgery). Temporarily raising the venous pressure and inflating the lungs will fill the LV and permit easier surgical aspiration of air. The presence of air and the efficacy of de-airing procedures can be monitored using TEE [5]. Flushing the surgical field with CO_2 gas before chamber closure may reduce residual air [4].

E. Port access CPB is similar to conventional CPB but requires additional instrumentation and monitoring [6]. Arterial and venous CPB cannulas are inserted peripherally (e.g., femoral artery and vein). An aortic occlusion catheter is placed in the ascending aorta under fluoroscopic or TEE guidance. An endocoronary sinus catheter is inserted for delivery of retrograde cardioplegia, and a PA vent catheter is inserted to decompress the heart through the left atrium. Correct position of the inflated aortic occlusion catheter balloon should be checked regularly using TEE. Loss of the right radial arterial pressure trace may indicate cephalad migration of the balloon. Greater interaction among surgeon, perfusionist, and anesthesiologist is required for a successful outcome (see Chapter 13).

III. Potential bypass catastrophes

The safe conduct of perfusion requires vigilance on the part of the anesthesiologist, working in conjunction with the cardiac surgeon and perfusionist, to ensure that perfusion-related problems are diagnosed early and managed quickly. The following complications must be actively sought during initiation of CPB. They may, however, occur at any time during CPB.

A. Malposition of arterial (*"return"*) cannula

The CPB pump may be expelling blood into undesired locations. Some examples follow.

1. Aortic dissection
    a. Etiology. The cannula orifice is situated within the arterial wall, not in the true lumen, possibly because a dissection was created during the cannulation process.
    b. Prevention is primarily surgical. However, the degree of damage can be markedly reduced if bypass is not initiated into an aortic false lumen. Thus, the arterial cannula pressure waveform should always be transduced, and one should ensure that it is **pulsatile** and that pressure **correlates** with the radial or femoral arterial monitoring line (after correcting for the height difference between the CPB pump and patient) before starting CPB.
    c. Diagnosis
        (1) Occlusion of the arterial true lumen may cause low or zero blood pressure to be measured by the radial or femoral arterial monitoring catheter depending on the site of the dissection.
        (2) Inappropriately high arterial "line" pressure may be detected. Ischemia or aortic insufficiency may occur.
        (3) Organ hypoperfusion (oliguria, pupil asymmetry) may be evident.
        (4) Visual inspection or palpation of the aorta may reveal the diagnosis.
        (5) If TEE is utilized, detection of a dissection is possible.
    d. Management
        (1) Discontinue CPB.
        (2) The surgeon must reposition or replace the arterial cannula.
        (3) Surgical repair of an aortic dissection may be necessary, especially if the origin of a critical artery is occluded (e.g., coronary).

2. **Carotid or innominate artery hyperperfusion**
    a. Etiology. Most or all of the pump outflow can be directed into a carotid artery, usually on the right side (Fig. 7.2). Similar effects may be seen if a

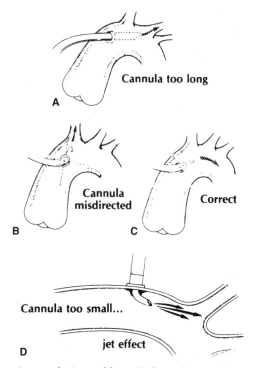

FIG. 7.2 Potential aortic cannulation problems. **A:** Cannula extends into carotid owing to excessive length, causing excessive carotid flow. **B:** Angle of cannula insertion is improper, which also causes carotid hypoperfusion. **C:** Correct placement. **D:** Cannula diameter is too small; high-velocity jet of blood may damage intima and occlude a vessel. (From Moores WY. Cardiopulmonary bypass strategies in patients with severe aortic disease. In: Utley JR, ed. *Pathophysiology and techniques of cardiopulmonary bypass, vol. 2.* Baltimore: Williams & Wilkins, 1983:190, with permission.)

jet of blood is directed into a carotid artery. Deleterious effects include cerebral edema or arterial rupture due to high perfusion pressure or creation of an intimal flap that obstructs arterial flow.
   b. Prevention. The surgeon's vigilance, the anesthesiologist's checking for bilateral carotid pulses without thrills after cannulation, and use of a short aortic cannula with a flange may help prevent this complication.
   c. Diagnosis
       (1) Ipsilateral blanching of face (transient; not seen if blood is present in CPB priming solution)
       (2) Ipsilateral pupillary dilation
       (3) Ipsilateral conjunctival chemosis (edema)
       (4) Low blood pressure measured by left radial or femoral arterial catheter (a right radial catheter may show **hypertension** due to innominate artery hyperperfusion)
   d. Management
       (1) Surgeon must reposition the arterial cannula.
       (2) Consider measures to reduce cerebral edema (e.g., mannitol, head-up position)

B. Reversed cannulation

1. **Etiology.** The pump circuit's venous drainage tubing is accidentally connected to the aorta, and the arterial return pump line is attached to the right atrium or vena cava.

   Blood is drained out of the aorta, causing arterial hypotension, and is infused into the vena cava at high pressures. High venous pressures and low aortic pressures may allow some organs to be perfused retrograde, but high pressures may rupture veins. The greatest risk is bubble formation within the aorta causing air embolization when antegrade perfusion is established.

2. **Prevention.** It is critical that the arterial cannula show pulsatile pressure that correlates with the pressure monitoring line. Pump lines should be traced onto the field. The tubing should be checked for proper connection to the pump and the roller head checked to ensure that it is not set for "reverse" rotation.

3. **Diagnosis**
   a. Arterial hypotension, which may be extreme
   b. Facial edema and conjunctival chemosis, which usually is severe
   c. High central venous pressure (CVP) (depending on exact position of CVP line and pump cannulas)
   d. In infants, tense bulging fontanelle
   e. Flaccid aorta and tense vena cava by palpation

4. **Management**
   a. Discontinue CPB.
   b. Place patient in steep head-down position.
   c. Disconnect and carefully inspect cannulas for air; if air is found, execute gas embolism protocol (Table 7.3).
   d. After de-airing the aorta and arterial cannula, reverse the tubing connections and resume CPB. Set the blender to deliver 100% O_2.
   e. Consider taking steps to reduce cerebral damage (mannitol, steroids, barbiturates).

C. Obstruction to venous return

1. **Etiology.** There is reduced blood flow draining into the pump.
   a. **Air lock.** The presence of large air bubbles within the venous ("drainage") cannula or tubing prevents blood flow due to surface tension and the low pressure gradient.
   b. **Mechanical.** Lifting of the heart within the chest by the surgeon often impedes venous drainage. The venous cannulas may be too small. Also, a kinked or malpositioned cannula or the presence of a thrombus or tumor mass will diminish venous blood flow.
   c. **Consequences.** CPB pump outflow must be reduced immediately to avoid emptying the reservoir. Elevated venous pressure will decrease perfusion to the affected organs by reducing the arteriovenous pressure gradient. This causes organ ischemia. The brain, liver, and kidneys are particularly vulnerable.

2. **Prevention.** Look for large bubbles in the venous pump line and for high regional venous pressures in patient. Always maintain adequate heparinization.

3. **Diagnosis**
   a. **Decreasing venous blood reservoir volume.** If the perfusionist does not reduce the pump flow rate **immediately,** the reservoir may empty, presenting a risk of massive arterial air embolism. Large volumes of fluid often are added to the blood volume until the diagnosis is made.
   b. **Increased CVP.** The surgeon may have placed separate SVC and IVC cannulas and may tighten the "caval tapes," thereby preventing vena caval blood from entering the right atrium (total CPB). In this case, a CVP monitoring catheter with its orifice within the right atrium will show a **low** CVP even if poor venous drainage conditions exist.

      Routine monitoring of pressures in the more cephalad portions of the jugular system is advocated. This is facilitated by attaching the side port of the PA catheter introducer cannula (if used) to a transducer. Pressures

Table 7.3 Massive gas embolism emergency protocol

1. **Stop CPB** immediately.
2. Place patient in steep **head-down** position.
3. Remove aortic cannula; **vent air** from aortic cannulation site.
4. **De-air** arterial cannula and pump line.
5. Institute hypothermic **retrograde SVC perfusion** by connecting arterial pump line to the SVC cannula with caval tape tightened. Blood at 20°–24°C is injected into the SVC at 1–2 L/min or more, and air plus blood is drained from the aortic root cannulation site to the pump (Fig. 7.3). Ensure that retrograde perfusion pressure does not exceed 30 mm Hg.
6. **Carotid compression** is performed intermittently during retrograde SVC perfusion to allow retrograde purging of air from the **vertebral** arteries (Fig. 7.4).
7. Maintain retrograde SVC perfusion for at least 1–2 min. Continue for an additional 1–2 min if air continues to exit from aorta.
8. In **extensive** systemic air injection accidents in which emboli to splanchnic, renal, or femoral circulation are suspected, **retrograde IVC perfusion** may be performed **after** head de-airing procedures are completed. This is performed while the **carotid arteries are clamped** and the patient is in **head-up position** to facilitate removal of air through the aortic root vent but prevent reembolization of the brain.
9. When no additional air can be expelled, **resume anterograde CPB,** maintaining hypothermia at 20°C for at least 40–45 min. Lowering patient temperature is important because increased gas solubility helps to reabsorb bubbles and because decreased metabolic demands may limit ischemic damage prior to bubble resorption. Set blender to deliver **100% O_2.**
10. Induce **hypertension** with vasoconstrictor drugs. Hydrostatic pressure shrinks bubbles; also, bubbles occluding arterial bifurcations are pushed into one vessel, opening the other branch.
11. Express coronary air by massage and needle venting.
12. **Steroids** may be administered, although this is controversial. The usual dose of methylprednisolone is 30 mg/kg.
13. **Barbiturate coma** should be considered if the embolism occurred during warm CPB and if the myocardium will be able to tolerate the significant negative inotropy. Thiopental, 10 mg/kg loading dose plus infusion at 1–3 mg/kg/hr, may be used empirically. If EEG monitoring is available, titration of barbiturate to an EEG burst-suppression (1 burst/min) pattern is preferable.
14. Patient is weaned from CPB.
15. Continue ventilating the patient with **100% O_2** for at least 6 hr to maximize the blood–alveolar gradient for elimination of N_2.
16. A **hyperbaric chamber** (if locally available) can accelerate resorption of residual bubbles. However, the risk of moving a critically ill patient must be weighed against the potential benefits.

This protocol should be reviewed together by all members of the cardiac team every 3 months.
CPB, cardiopulmonary bypass; EEG, electroencephalogram; IVC, inferior vena cava; SVC, superior vena cava.
Modified from Mills NL, Ochsner JL. Massive air embolism during cardiopulmonary bypass: Causes, prevention, and management. *J Thorac Cardiovasc Surg* 1980;80:712.

should be less than 5 to 10 mm Hg after correcting for changes in operating room table position.
  c. **Oliguria, conjunctival chemosis,** or injection, facial plethora, bulging fontanelle. High venous pressures are seen upstream from the obstruction, which can cause organ ischemia by reducing the arteriovenous perfusion pressure. Obstruction may be **regional** (i.e., affecting only the SVC flow) or **global.** It is very difficult to diagnose isolated IVC flow obstruction, so a high index of suspicion must be maintained, and causes for oliguria must be sought.

4. Management
   a. Reduce pump flow or suspend CPB until cause is found.
   b. Air lock. The surgeon can propel air through the tubing by progressively raising and tapping the tubing downstream to the bubble. Search for the source of venous air (is a CVP catheter open to air?).

D. Massive gas embolism. Most massive (macroscopic) gas emboli [7,8] consist of air, although oxygen emboli can be generated by a defective or clotted oxygenator. (For further discussion of this and CPB safety devices, see Chapter 19.) Use of a vented arterial line filter on the pump is an important safety device that can help prevent gas embolization; its routine use is strongly recommended. Because of the high risk of stroke, myocardial infarction, or death after massive gas embolism, **prevention is of utmost importance.**

1. Etiology
   a. Inattention to oxygenator reservoir level. Air may be pumped from an empty reservoir. Vortexing can permit air embolism when the blood level is very low but not empty. This is **the most important cause of bypass catastrophes** when utilizing a closed reservoir system. Use of a membrane oxygenator may decrease but not exclude the risk.
   b. Ejection of blood from heart before de-airing procedures; opening a beating heart.
   c. Reversed roller pump flow in vent line or arterial cannula.
   d. Leak or kink in the negative side of the arterial tubing (before or upstream from roller pump). Negative (suction) pressure at this site may cavitate gas out of solution or entrain room air.
   e. Clotted oxygenator.
   f. Pressurized cardiotomy reservoir (causing retrograde flow of air through nonocclusive vent line roller head into heart or aorta).
   g. Runaway pump head (switch inoperative; must unplug pump and crank by hand).
   h. Disconnection, breakage, or detachment of oxygenator (bubble) or lines during CPB.
   i. Suction deep in PA branch entrains air from other branches, and air enters left atrium. Aortic line not clamped at end of CPB: if the pump head is accidentally restarted, inadvertent air infusion might occur.

2. Other etiologies not isolated to CPB
   a. Improper flushing technique for arterial or left atrial pressure monitoring lines.
   b. Paradoxical transfer of venous air across atrial or ventricular septal defect.
   c. Occasionally, a persistent left SVC communicates with the left atrium. IV air from a left-sided IV may enter the systemic circulation.

3. Prevention. Vigilance is required. Safety devices must be **turned on.**

4. Diagnosis. Embolism is diagnosed by visual inspection, signs of myocardial or other organ ischemia, and withdrawal of air from arterial pressure monitoring lines.

5. Management. See Table 7.3 and Figures 7.3 and 7.4.

E. Failure of oxygen supply
   1. Etiology. Inadequate gas flow or hypoxic mixture.
   2. Prevention. Vigilance; use of pump arterial line O_2 saturation or Po_2 analyzer; use of an O_2 analyzer on pump gas inflow line.
   3. Diagnosis. Dark blood in arterial cannula (same color as venous cannula blood); blood gas analysis.
   4. Management. Restore O_2 supply immediately. Connect a portable O_2 tank to the oxygenator if necessary. If a delay is anticipated, cool patient maximally until O_2 supply is restored. Ventilation with **room air** is preferable to no ventilation at all, if immediate restoration of O_2 supply is not possible.

F. Pump or oxygenator failure
   1. Etiology.
      a. Pump failure may be due to electrical or mechanical failure, tubing rupture or disconnection, or automatic shutoff by the bubble or low reservoir

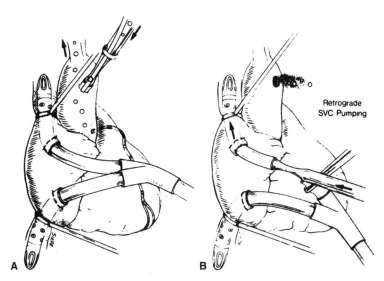

Retrograde SVC Pumping

A   **B**

FIG. 7.3 Retrograde perfusion in the treatment of massive air embolism. **A:** Massive arterial gas embolism has occurred. **B:** Bubbles in the arterial tree are flushed out by performing retrograde body perfusion into the superior vena cava (SVC) by connecting the de-aired arterial pump line to the SVC cannula (and tightening caval tapes). Blood and bubbles exit the aorta from the cannulation wound. (From Mills NL, Ochsner JL. Massive air embolism during cardiopulmonary bypass: causes, prevention, and management. *J Thorac Cardiovasc Surg* 1980;80:713, with permission.)

detector. A runaway pump head may raise the pump flow to maximum inappropriately, and the pump control switch will be inoperable. For systems designed to be used with an electromagnetic or ultrasonic transducer, failure of the sensor can prevent one from knowing the actual pump flow rate.

If the occlusion of a roller pump is improperly set, excessive regurgitation occurs (causing hemolysis), and the forward flow is reduced (leading to hypotension and metabolic acidosis).

   b. **Oxygenator failure** may be due to manufacturing defect, clogging due to clot (see Section **G** below), disruption of shell (trauma, spill of volatile liquid anesthetic), leakage of water from heat exchanger into blood, or depletion of defoamer.
2. **Prevention.** Vigilance, availability of backup equipment, adequate heparinization.
3. **Diagnosis.** Blood gas abnormality, acidosis, hypotension, blood leak, excessive hemolysis, high premembrane pressures
4. **Management.** If body perfusion will be low or absent for more than 1 or 2 minutes and if the patient cannot be immediately weaned from CPB, then hypothermia to 18°C to 20°C should be induced and consideration given to brain, myocardial, and renal protection, including packing the head and heart in ice. Open cardiac massage may be necessary, depending on the stage of the operation.
   a. **Pump failure.** CPB pumps can be hand cranked until a replacement is obtained or tubing is replaced. In case of a runaway pump head, the CPB machine must be unplugged and the tubing switched to a different roller head.
   b. **Oxygenator failure.** For severe failure, the oxygenator must be r placed. A protocol should be in place for rapid oxygenator replacement.

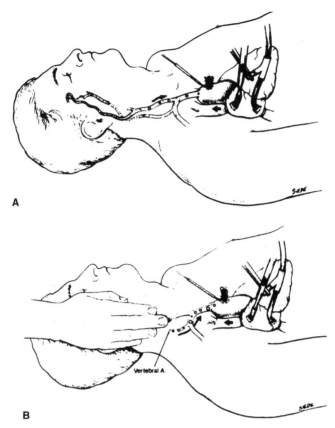

FIG. 7.4 Carotid (**A**) and vertebral (**B**) artery de-airing during retrograde perfusion. In the management of massive arterial gas embolism, steep head-down position helps to flush bubbles out of the *carotid arteries*. Application of intermittent pressure to the carotid arteries increases retrograde *vertebral artery* flow, which helps to evacuate bubbles. (From Mills NL, Ochsner JL. Massive air embolism during cardiopulmonary bypass: causes, prevention, and management. *J Thorac Cardiovasc Surg* 1980;80:713, with permission.)

G. Clotted oxygenator or circuit. This serious event can interfere with gas exchange, prevent CPB flow, or cause massive gas embolus.
  1. **Etiology**
     a. **Inadequate heparinization** (heparin must be exerting adequate effect regardless of dose or plasma concentration)
     b. **Direct administration of fresh frozen plasma** to the CPB reservoir during CPB (this may present less risk with a bubble oxygenator). Fresh frozen plasma increases anti-thrombin III levels but may reduce heparin levels due to increased plasma protein binding.
  2. **Prevention.** This lethal catastrophe should never occur if the patient's coagulation status is assessed before initiating CPB and at frequent intervals thereafter. It can be diagnosed by visual inspection of the clot, observation of air exiting from the bubble oxygenator, or high arterial cannula pressure

(evidence of partially clotted arterial line filter). **Fresh frozen plasma** should be heparinized in the bag (1,000 units per 250-mL bag) **before** administering it into the venous reservoir.

3. **Management**
   a. Stop CPB.
   b. If the patient is not cold, perform open cardiopulmonary resuscitation and apply topical hypothermia.
   c. Reheparinize the patient using a different lot of heparin.
   d. Replace the oxygenator and CPB circuit.
   e. Follow the massive gas embolization emergency protocol if necessary (Table 7.3).

IV. **Differential diagnosis of abnormalities during CPB**
   A. **Cardiovascular abnormalities**
      1. **Hypotension.** During CPB, systemic vascular resistance (SVR) may be calculated in the usual fashion.

$$\text{SVR (dynes} \cdot \sec \cdot \text{cm}^{-5}) = \frac{[(\text{MAP} - \text{CVP}) \times 80]}{F}$$

where F = pump flow rate in liters per minute (L/min), and MAP = mean arterial pressure in millimeters of mercury (mm Hg).

Normally during CPB without venous obstruction, CVP = 0, and this term can be ignored. Always check with the perfusionist before assuming that hypotension is due to a low SVR. The flow rate may have been decreased for some reason!

   a. **Low SVR** may be caused by vasodilation due to drugs, anesthetics, metabolic factors, or hyperthermia. Low blood viscosity due to hemodilution will decrease the effective SVR even though blood vessel caliber is unchanged. (This often is the cause of the immediate decrease in blood pressure seen on commencing CPB with hemodilution.)
   b. **Low perfusion flow rate** may be due to an arterial cannula that is clamped or kinked, inadequate roller pump head occlusion causing regurgitation, error in pump flowmeter calibration, error in calculated flow based on temperature and body size, or low *effective* pump flow rate due to excessive venting (through arterial filter), shunting, or cardiotomy suction.
   c. **Cannula disaster** may be due to aortic dissection, carotid or innominate cannulation, or reversed cannulation.
   d. **Measurement error** may be due to transducer zero drift, calibration error, a clot in the monitoring line or transducer, or tubing disconnection. (**Note:** A bubble in the monitoring line should not change the **mean** pressure.)

      2. **Hypertension**
         a. **High SVR.** Causes include vasoconstriction due to release of catecholamines or other vasoconstrictor hormones, hypothermia after initiation of CPB and after rewarming begins, light plane of anesthesia, awareness, drugs, hypothermia, and metabolic factors (hyperoxia).
         b. **Excessive perfusion flow rate** (see Section **A.1.b** above).
         c. **Innominate artery cannulation** with right radial arterial pressure monitoring.
         d. **Measurement error** (see Section **A.1.d** above).

      3. **High pressure in arterial pump line.** Normally, line pressure is up to three times the patient pressure due to high resistance in the tubing and arterial cannula.
         a. **Occlusion** may be due to a kinked, clamped, or occluded arterial cannula; carotid or innominate artery cannulation; or aortic dissection.
         b. **Clotted arterial filter.** Arterial filters should always have a bypass loop for use after restoring adequate anticoagulation.
         c. **High SVR in the patient**
         d. **Measurement error** (see Section **A.I.d** above).

      4. **High pressure in PA or left atrium.** Whenever there is doubt about the reason for high PA pressure during CPB, ask the surgeon to palpate the LV because

LV distention is the most serious cause of PA hypertension during CPB. Causes include the following:
  a. **Distention of the LV** with retrograde transmission of pressure to the lung vasculature.
      (1) **Consequences** of LV distention
          (a) Myocardial ischemia and subendocardial necrosis due to compression by fluid in the LV under pressure, which lowers the coronary perfusion pressure to as low as zero (occurring when the LV pressure equals the aortic root pressure)
          (b) Warming of the myocardium despite cardioplegia
          (c) Myocardial damage due to stretching
          (d) Pulmonary edema
      (2) **Etiology** of LV distention
          (a) Inadequate venous drainage (blood traversing lungs)
          (b) Aortic insufficiency with fluid entering LV retrograde across aortic valve (before aortic cross-clamping or during cardioplegic solution infusion into aortic root)
          (c) Blood entering LV through bronchial arterial flow, septal defects, pulmonary–systemic shunts, thebesian drainage, coronary sinus effluent, pericardial collateral vessels, or persistent left SVC with left atrial connection
      (3) **Management** of LV distention. Improve venous drainage, insert vent in LV or PA, or infuse cardioplegic solution into individual coronary ostia. In certain cases, deliberate hypotension or total circulatory arrest may be necessary (e.g., for excessive systemic-to-pulmonary collaterals). In the latter situation, collateral flow can steal flow away from the brain during CPB.
  b. **Collapse of nonperfused lung** around the tip of the PA catheter during total CPB may produce an "overwedge" pressure tracing. This is the **most common** etiology of a high PA pressure during CPB.
      (1) **Diagnosis.** Inability to withdraw blood from catheter on **gentle** aspiration or palpation of a flaccid LV.
      (2) **Management.** Withdraw PA catheter several centimeters or until pressure approaches zero. Prophylactic withdrawal of all PA catheters by approximately 5 cm is advocated on commencing CPB.
  c. **Kinked or compressed PA catheter.** The PA catheter may be compressed against the clavicle by a sternal retractor (especially if the catheter is introduced through the subclavian or external jugular route). It may not be possible to withdraw blood from the catheter.
5. **High CVP** may be caused by the following:
  a. Poor venous drainage (see Section **III.C**)
  b. Artifact caused by the surgeon tightening the caval tape around the CVP catheter orifice. This is diagnosed by an inability to withdraw blood from the catheter.
6. **Slowed nasopharyngeal or tympanic cooling** may indicate impaired brain cooling. Causes include the following:
  a. Temperature sensor displaced or calibration error
  b. Inadequate carotid artery perfusion due to
      (1) Improper cannulation
      (2) Carotid occlusions
      (3) Increased intracranial pressure (hematoma?)
      (4) Increased SVC pressure impeding venous drainage and lowering perfusion pressure gradient
      (5) Low pump flow
7. **Slowed body rewarming** may be caused by
  a. Temperature sensor displaced or calibration error
  b. Inadequate pump flow rate
  c. Excessive vasoconstriction (use vasodilator drugs to treat this)
  d. Failure of heat exchanger

B. Respiratory and metabolic abnormalities. For a detailed discussion of oxygenation assessment during CPB, see Chapter 20.

1. **Hypoxemia of arterial blood.** Possible causes include

   a. **Transpulmonary shunt.** During **partial CPB,** desaturated blood may be ejected from the LV unless the patient's lungs are ventilated. Systemic arterial hypoxemia may be missed unless the blood sample is drawn from the **patient** instead of from the bypass pump or unless a pulse oximeter is in use.

   b. **Gas supply to artificial lung.** An hypoxic gas mixture or inadequate flow rate may be present.

   c. **Dysfunction of artificial lung.** For bubble oxygenators, excessive filling of the blood reservoir reduces the amount of oxygenation that normally takes place in the debubbling section.

   d. **Note:** During hypothermia, the diagnosis of hypoxemia should be made using the P_{O_2} calculated for the patient's actual temperature, as this value will be **lower** than the value measured at 37°C by the blood gas analyzer.

2. **Hypoxemia of mixed venous blood** indicates an imbalance between total body O_2 supply and demand. Maintenance of P_vO_2 at greater than 35 mm Hg is associated with a lower incidence of lactic acidosis. Causes of venous hypoxemia include

   a. **Decreased O_2 delivery, causing increased O_2 extraction from blood by tissues.** Possible causes include

      (1) Hypoxemia of **arterial** blood
      (2) Low pump flow rate (see Section **IV.A.1.b**).
      (3) Regional hypoperfusion
      (4) Excessive hemodilution
      (5) Increased oxygen–hemoglobin affinity, reducing O_2 release to tissues. (S_vO_2 may be normal.)

   b. **Increased body O_2 consumption rate.** Causes include

      (1) Hyperthermia
      (2) Shivering (may be subclinical)
      (3) Malignant hyperthermia
      (4) Thyrotoxicosis

3. **Lactic acidosis** may be due to

   a. Decreased O_2 delivery to tissues, causing anaerobic metabolism of glucose.

   b. Improved perfusion of previously ischemic tissue. Tissues receiving little perfusion may accumulate large quantities of lactic acid that is not washed out into the circulation until regional perfusion improves at a later time.

4. **Hypercapnia** may be due to

   a. Inadequate fresh gas inflow rate to artificial lung
   b. Use of CO_2-containing gas mixture (pH-stat control)
   c. Increased body CO_2 production rate
   d. Bicarbonate administration. (In the buffering process, CO_2 is produced.)
   e. Flooding of wound with CO_2 gas during open chamber procedures [4].

5. **Spontaneous respiratory effort** may be due to

   a. Hypercapnia
   b. Inadequate narcosis
   c. Inadequate paralysis
   d. Awareness

C. Renal abnormalities

1. **Oliguria** may result from

   a. **Postrenal problems.** These must be ruled out first. Kinked Foley tubing is the most common etiology; ureteral, bladder outlet, urethral, or other Foley tubing obstruction (e.g., blood clots) may be involved.

   b. **Decreased renal perfusion with reduced glomerular filtration rate.** This situation may result from

      (1) Inadequate pump flow rate
      (2) Relative arterial hypotension due to low SVR (urine output may increase with phenylephrine-induced pressor effect)

(3) Nonpulsatile perfusion

(4) Renal artery vasoconstriction by drugs

(5) Increased IVC pressure

c. Hormone-induced free water retention

d. Renal failure

e. Hypothermia

2. **Renal protection.** It may be possible to reduce the risk of development of acute renal failure through the use of drugs to increase renal blood flow and urine production. Mannitol, low-dose dopamine, furosemide, prostaglandin E, and, more recently, fenoldapam have been advocated for use in high-risk patients during CPB, particularly if oliguria is present.

3. **Hemoglobinuria or hematuria.** Whenever pink or red urine is noted, a test should be performed to distinguish **hemoglobinuria** (free hemoglobin in urine) from **hematuria** (RBCs in urine). A laboratory urinalysis can achieve this, or a sample can be quickly centrifuged and the supernatant examined. Clear supernatant implies hematuria; pink supernatant defines hemoglobinuria.

A quick screening test for red or pink urine may be less accurate: **cloudy** urine usually is hematuria, and **clear** urine usually is hemoglobinuria.

a. Hemoglobinuria may be caused by

(1) Hemolysis due to pump sucker trauma or the CPB pump (most common)

(2) Blood transfusion reaction

(3) Hyperoxia

(4) Water leak from heat exchanger into blood (hyponatremia also present)

b. Management of hemoglobinuria

(1) Promote a diuresis using mannitol, loop diuretics, dopamine, vasodilators, or vasoconstrictors. Consider elevating pump flow.

(2) Measure urine pH and administer systemic sodium bicarbonate or induce hypocapnia to maintain an alkaline urine pH (avoids acid hematin formation).

c. Hematuria may be due to urinary tract hemorrhage. To manage it, irrigate the Foley catheter tubing.

V. **Blood pressure control during CPB**

A. **Desired blood pressure during various phases of CPB.** Blood pressure management during CPB is controversial. At one extreme, some believe that pressure is irrelevant during CPB as long as the pump provides adequate flow. Others believe, however, that blood pressure should be kept within a certain range by administering vasodilators or vasoconstrictor drugs. This section is written from the viewpoint that, provided pump flow is adequate, blood pressure is less important in determining **global** perfusion during CPB, but may be significant for providing certain **regional** vascular beds with adequate perfusion. Blood pressure control may be especially important during certain periods of CPB.

1. **Phase of initial total bypass: warm, aorta not clamped**

a. **Rationale for regulating MAP: altered regional blood flow autoregulation**

(1) **Critical organ stenosis.** In this phase of CPB, the heart still is beating and still is being perfused from the aorta, but it is collapsed with low LV systolic wall tension. Although the O_2 consumption of a beating empty heart is less than that of a beating filled heart, myocardial ischemia still may develop given the proper pathology. Thus, if critical coronary stenoses are present, coronary autoregulation may **not** be able to maintain flow to the distal myocardium during hypotension because the distal bed will be maximally vasodilated already. Thus, flow will be pressure dependent. The same mechanism would be active if cerebrovascular or renovascular stenoses were present.

(2) **Chronic hypertension** tends to shift toward higher blood pressures the range of pressures over which blood flow is autoregulated. At pressures lower than these, regional blood flow will become pressure dependent at a value less than the autoregulated flow. This me-

chanism is particularly important in determining brain and kidney perfusion.

   (3) **Myocardial hypertrophy** increases O_2 demand, but muscle growth often advances faster than development of the blood supply, thus altering the ability of coronary artery autoregulation to provide adequate flow at low pressures.

b. **Management**

   (1) **Lower limit of MAP.** Patients with impaired organ flow autoregulation should not be permitted to develop hypotension below a certain critical limit during this phase of CPB. However, it usually is not possible to determine precisely what this lower limit should be.

   (2) **Individualization based on cardiac pathology.** Factors to be considered when determining an individual's lower pressure limit include severity and location of stenoses, collateral flow sources, range of asymptomatic blood pressures preoperatively, extent of hemodilution, heart rate, presence of myocardial hypertrophy, presence of aortic regurgitation, and adequacy of LV drainage.

   (3) **Hypothesis testing.** Once an initial value is selected, it should be constantly subjected to hypothesis testing by looking for signs of inadequate regional perfusion at that MAP. Examples include ischemic electrocardiographic changes, loss of urine output, change in the electroencephalogram, and pupil asymmetry.

c. **Practical guidelines.** In the patient without altered flow autoregulation, perfusion generally is maintained at a MAP higher than 50 mm Hg. Usually, pediatric patients are permitted to develop an even lower MAP without evidence of organ ischemia. However, if evidence of altered flow autoregulation exists (as discussed in Section **1.b** above), then MAP usually is maintained at approximately 70 and 90 mm Hg during this phase of CPB.

2. **Phase of hypothermic bypass, aorta cross-clamped**

a. **Rationale for regulating MAP.** Because the heart and coronary vasculature now are disconnected from the circulation by the aortic clamp, maintenance of perfusion to other vital organs (brain, kidney) assumes primary importance. **Higher** pressures (MAP greater than 70 mm Hg) often are avoided because of **noncoronary collateral** blood flow into the heart through the pericardium and pulmonary venous drainage. Such collateral flow of relatively warm blood tends to wash the colder cardioplegic solution out of the heart and reduces protection against myocardial ischemia.

b. **Practical guidelines.** During **mild-to-moderate hypothermia** (30°C to 32°C) the MAP is generally maintained at 50 to 70 mm Hg. If colder bypass is used, patients **without** altered flow autoregulation may tolerate a MAP as low as 30 to 40 mm Hg, so long as flow is adequate. The presence of **urine production** is a reassuring sign of renal perfusion, although low or absent urine does not necessarily imply ischemia. If a patient is oliguric at very low perfusion pressures, raising pressure with a vasoconstrictor often will induce a diuresis, presumably as renal perfusion reenters the autoregulatory range. Commonly, **pediatric** patients are permitted to be perfused at pressures as low as 15 to 20 mm Hg.

3. **Phase of rewarming, aortic side-biting clamp in place**

a. **Rationale for regulating MAP.** A heart with coronary artery disease is **not** receiving any **new** sources of blood during this phase because saphenous vein grafts are not yet connected to the aorta, but flow through the native coronary vasculature has been reestablished. Thus, this situation parallels that of the warm prearrest bypass phase (see Section **1** above), and the heart is at risk for ischemia unless an adequate coronary perfusion pressure is supplied. An exception might be patients in whom an internal mammary–coronary connection was created; this connection does not require a proximal anastomosis and provides flow to one coronary artery (and its collateral-linked beds) immediately. Avoidance of high aortic pressures during early reperfusion of arrested myocardium may help limit reperfusion damage (see Chapter 22).

    b. Practical guidelines. As soon as the aortic cross-clamp is removed, transient hypotension often occurs (probably due to reopening of the vasodilated coronary bed and washout of metabolites), but this usually is not treated unless it persists for more than several minutes. For patients with significant coronary stenoses not supplied by a patent internal mammary graft or for those with other organs with abnormal flow autoregulation, the MAP during this phase of CPB often is controlled in the range from 70 to 90 mm Hg.

  4. Phase of warm bypass, aorta not clamped, heart revascularized

    a. Rationale for regulating MAP. The SVR during warm CPB usually is similar to the SVR in the patient after termination of CPB. Therefore, during this preweaning stage, it may be useful to adjust the SVR pharmacologically into the normal range. In this way, very low or high blood pressures can be avoided immediately after CPB termination.

    b. Practical guidelines. During this phase of CPB, the MAP often is adjusted so that it is similar to or slightly lower than values desired after CPB, common adult values being 50 to 80 mm Hg. Remember that once the heart begins to eject blood before weaning, the MAP will rise in relation to the height of the systolic pressure above the bypass-generated mean pressure.

B. Methods of adjusting blood pressure during CPB

  1. Varying pump flow rate. Although it is possible to vary the pump flow rate as necessary to keep blood pressure at desired levels, this rarely is appropriate. Increasing pump flow rate to compensate for low SVR usually is **not** performed because it involves added trauma to blood elements. Decreasing pump flow to compensate for high SVR is not the best form of management because tissue perfusion will suffer and metabolic acidosis will ensue. However, in cases of acute severe vasoconstriction causing MAPs in excess of 100 mm Hg, it may be useful to reduce pump flow **transiently** until vasodilation can be achieved pharmacologically.

  2. Increasing SVR is the primary means of increasing blood pressure when necessary during CPB. **α-Adrenergic agonists** are the drugs most commonly used to raise SVR during CPB. **Phenylephrine** (Neo-Synephrine) is used in 100- to 200-µg bolus doses injected into the oxygenator reservoir and repeated or increased as necessary to achieve the target blood pressure. Rare patients refractory to vasoconstrictor drugs may require 1- to 5-mg boluses to achieve only small rises in SVR. **Methoxamine** (Vasoxyl) and **norepinephrine** (Levophed) also are used occasionally during CPB, although the β_1 cardiac actions of norepinephrine may be detrimental. See Chapter 2 for further details on this and other vasoconstrictor drugs.

  3. Decreasing SVR is the primary means of lowering blood pressure during bypass.

    a. Anesthetics commonly are used to reduce SVR during bypass, even during times when unconsciousness has been ensured by other drugs and hypothermia. **Opioids** (e.g., fentanyl) and volatile anesthetics (e.g., isoflurane) both will achieve vasodilation. However, fentanyl displays tachyphylaxis in its ability to lower SVR; once approximately 100 µg/kg (total dose) has been administered, little or no further effect is produced. Usual adult IV bolus doses during CPB are 250 to 500 µg. Sufentanil is more effective than fentanyl in lowering SVR; the usual incremental bolus doses during CPB are 2 to 3 µg/kg, with a total dose of 15–20 µg/kg for the entire case. If total IV anesthesia is used (e.g., propofol), the target concentration or infusion rate can be increased.

    b. Volatile anesthetics such as isoflurane produce a reliable dose-dependent vasodilation that is probably a combination of sympatholysis and direct vasodilation. They are administered by calibrated vaporizer in the oxygenator gas inlet line. Usual isoflurane vaporizer settings are 0.5 to 2.0 vol%. Usually, volatile anesthetics are not administered after aortic cross-clamp removal, to ensure adequate time for washout.

c. **Direct vasodilators** such as nitroprusside are useful in controlling SVR and improving perfusion to vasoconstricted peripheral vascular beds. **Nitroprusside sodium** (Nipride) usually is administered by infusion into the pump reservoir or via the SVC during bypass. Hypothermia may retard the conversion of cyanide ion to thiocyanate [9], although production of clinical cyanide toxicity during CPB rarely is seen. Care must be taken to infuse drugs into the bloodstream during CPB and not into the stagnant blood within a cardiac chamber or distal to a caval tape. For example, a drug infused into the RV port of a Paceport catheter will not enter the circulation during total CPB. Usual CPB nitroprusside doses are 1 to 5 µg/kg/min (see Chapter 2).

d. **α-Adrenergic antagonists** will lower SVR and may allow more uniform cooling and rewarming. Phentolamine (Regitine) often is used at initiation of pediatric CPB in a bolus dose of 0.1 to 0.5 mg/kg.

e. **Other drugs.** Calcium channel blockers (verapamil IV, diltiazem IV, or nifedipine sublingual) will cause vasodilation, although the first two drugs cause cardiac depression. Benzodiazepines (diazepam, midazolam) given IV are especially useful in managing hypertensive episodes when awareness cannot be ruled out.

VI. Pharmacology of drugs used during CPB

A. Use of potent anesthetics via pump oxygenator

1. **Administration.** Potent inhalation anesthetics (e.g., isoflurane) may be administered during CPB using a temperature- and flow-compensating vaporizer placed in the gas inlet line to the oxygenator. Factors affecting the uptake of anesthetic include the gas and blood flow rates, temperature (solubility increases with cold), oxygenator efficiency, and distribution of blood flow. Nitrous oxide should never be used during CPB (due to bubble enlargement).

2. **Filling vaporizers.** Care must be used to avoid spilling liquid anesthetic on the plastic oxygenator shell. Rapid dissolution and destruction of the oxygenator have been reported to result from such spillage.

3. **Anesthetic washout.** In the near-normothermic patient, anesthetic will wash out of the body rapidly because of the relatively high fresh gas flow and blood flow rates. Only 5 to 15 minutes usually is required to eliminate clinically important anesthetic concentrations unless body stores are unusually large. However, when low gas flow rates are being used (i.e., with membrane oxygenators), the onset and offset of these agents may be slowed [10].

B. Pharmacology of IV drugs during CPB

1. **Pharmacokinetics.** The plasma drug concentrations of numerous drugs can be affected by CPB. CPB factors that are involved include the following:

   a. **Dilution.** The enlarged circulating blood volume at the initiation of CPB dilutes both drugs and plasma proteins and enlarges the volume of distribution. Despite marked decreases in **total** drug concentrations, the pharmacologically active **nonprotein-bound** drug concentration may remain relatively constant because of a decrease in the protein-bound fraction (e.g., propofol) [11]. Moreover, the decrease often is transient, because the increased volume of distribution due to CPB is minor compared to the total volume of distribution of most lipid-soluble drugs.

   b. **Altered elimination.** Due to changes in hepatic, renal, and pulmonary blood flow and enzymatic function, clearance of drugs may be impaired during CPB, especially with hypothermia.

   c. **Extracorporeal absorption.** Drugs (e.g., fentanyl, nitroglycerin) may be absorbed onto the foreign surfaces comprising the oxygenator and CPB circuit.

   d. **Lung isolation.** During total CPB, the lung is not perfused, making it unavailable for drug or hormonal metabolism. Basic drugs administered during partial CPB (e.g., propranolol, fentanyl) may be sequestered in the lung when CPB becomes total. With resumption of pulmonary blood flow at the end of CPB, sudden increases in plasma drug concentrations may occur.

   e. **Tissue sequestration.** As blood flow is redistributed during CPB, peripheral tissues binding the drug (e.g., skeletal muscle) become relatively poorly perfused owing to hypothermia. Drugs administered pre-CPB may become "trapped" within tissues and are not released until the peripheral tissues become fully rewarmed. Thus, for drugs given pre-CPB, plasma drug concentrations may decrease, causing the apparent volume of distribution during CPB to rise. Possible examples are dantrolene and digoxin.
   2. **Pharmacodynamics.** The **responsiveness** of tissues to a given plasma concentration of a drug may be altered by CPB. Potential causes include hypothermia, electrolyte shifts, and an altered hormonal state. For example, the myocardium may be more sensitive to digoxin after CPB.
   3. **Practical considerations.** The pharmacology of most drugs during CPB has not been evaluated sufficiently because knowledge of the nonprotein-bound drug concentrations and their tissue effects is required. Also, there is variability of responses between drugs and for the same drug at different times during CPB. Therefore, the principle of **titrating** drug dosage to achieve a certain endpoint is especially important during CPB.
VII. **Fluid management during CPB**
   A. **Benefits of hemodilution**
       1. Hemodilution is defined as a reduction in [Hb] caused by addition of non-hemoglobin-containing fluids to the circulating blood volume.
       2. **Blood viscosity** normally increases with cold, causing reduced microcirculatory flow at a constant perfusion pressure during hypothermia. This effect may promote sludging of RBCs and could cause organ ischemia.
       3. **Hemodilution** lowers **blood viscosity,** counteracting the deleterious viscosity changes caused by hypothermia. Organ blood flow is improved during hypothermia when [Hb] is kept below approximately 10 g/dL.
       4. Blood is not required in the priming solution, avoiding the risks of blood transfusion.
   B. **Risks of hemodilution**
       1. **Blood pressure decreases** when CPB commences, in part because dilution markedly reduces blood viscosity.
       2. **Lowered colloid oncotic pressure** due to dilution of plasma proteins leads to increased fluid administration requirements and development of tissue edema.
       3. **Hemoglobin oxygen saturation** of arterial blood (S_aO_2) must be kept near 100% during hemodilution to prevent a further decline in blood O_2 transport (O_2 transport = O_2 content × blood flow, where O_2 content = 1.34 × [Hb] × S_aO_2 plus a dissolved O_2 term).
       4. **Excessive hemodilution** occurs when blood flow cannot increase further to compensate for the reduction in blood O_2 content; ischemia of critical organs then appears, and signs of anaerobic metabolism may develop. Note that blood O_2 transport should match or exceed the normal body oxygen consumption rate (VO_2).
       5. **Increased blood flow.** If [Hb] is reduced by 50% below normal, blood flow must **double** if O_2 transport is to be maintained unchanged. Such a marked rise in flow is not feasible during CPB, hence the importance of combining hemodilution with hypothermia.
       6. **Importance of cold.** With hypothermia, body VO_2 decreases. This means that less O_2 is needed to match body O_2 supply to O_2 demand. Once normal body temperature is restored, O_2 transport also must rise, but this may be difficult to achieve when [Hb] is too low, causing mixed venous PO_2 to decrease.
       7. **Cold CPB versus warm CPB and post-CPB hemodilution.** Rewarming usually dilates the capacitance vessels in the body, increasing fluid requirements. Often a decision must be made whether to administer additional fluid as blood or blood-free solution. Hemodilution, which is advantageous during hypothermic CPB, may be undesirable during the later normothermic phases of CPB or after termination of CPB (see Section **C.5** below). However, despite these concerns, adult patients infrequently receive blood transfusion during CPB.

8. The **limits of hemodilution** cannot be predicted with certainty. Most patients with good overall physical status can tolerate hemodilution to [Hb] approximately 7 to 9 g/dL. Factors that tend to reduce the body's ability to tolerate marked reductions include

   a. **Stenosis** of arteries feeding critical organs. This will prevent blood flow from increasing adequately as [Hb] declines, although the reduction in viscosity accompanying hemodilution helps to increase blood flow past a stenosis.

   b. **Cardiac pump failure** that cannot provide the increased cardiac output necessary to maintain adequate O_2 delivery after CPB.

   c. **Left-shifted oxyhemoglobin dissociation curve** (increased binding of O_2 by hemoglobin). This reduces O_2 release in peripheral tissues. Factors contributing to this effect include alkalosis, hypothermia, and decreased 2,3-diphosphoglycerate levels.

   d. **Lung disease** that may prevent attainment of 100% S_aO_2 following CPB.

C. **Practical fluid management**

   1. **"Clear" pump priming solution.** Usually a clear (i.e., nonblood-containing) priming solution is utilized. Typically, this is composed of a buffered electrolyte solution with optional addition of mannitol, heparin, or colloid.

   2. **Autotransfusion.** If [Hb] is sufficiently high, 0.5 to 1.0 L of blood may be slowly removed from the patient while the pump prime is being infused to maintain arterial pressure before initiating CPB. This anticoagulated autologous blood may be reinfused after CPB, saving platelets and clotting factors. For more details, see Chapter 6.

   3. **Blood prime.** Addition of whole blood or packed RBCs to the priming solution is indicated only if use of a clear prime would result in excessive hemodilution as would be the case, for example, in adults with severe anemia pre-CPB or in pediatric patients in whom the pump prime represents a large fraction of the patient's blood volume. For infants receiving a heparinized blood prime, calcium chloride often is added to prevent citrate-induced hypocalcemia on initiating CPB.

   4. **Time course of hemodilution.** Hemodilution usually is most severe at the beginning of CPB. As bypass proceeds, free water and electrolytes are filtered by the kidneys and are redistributed by diffusion into interstitial tissue spaces as edema. These effects cause a progressive **rise in [Hb]** and loss of circulating blood volume. This hemoglobin time course is fortuitous because as O_2 consumption rises with increasing temperature, increasing [Hb] will allow a concomitant rise in O_2 transport.

   5. **Fluid replacement.** Selection of the type of fluid to administer when additional circulating blood volume is required during CPB is based on the following considerations:

      a. **Hemoglobin.** If [Hb] is less than 4 to 5 g/dL, it usually is necessary to add RBCs because urinary hemoconcentration is unlikely to raise [Hb] sufficiently by the end of CPB.

      b. **Decreased reserve for hemodilution.** Incomplete myocardial revascularization during coronary artery bypass (CAB) surgery increases the need for adequate [Hb] post-CPB. In this condition, it may be desirable to maintain [Hb] at greater than 9 to 10 g/dL after CPB.

      c. **General medical condition.** Patients who are expected to have difficulty mobilizing edema fluid postoperatively (e.g., those with renal or heart failure) may benefit from colloid (albumin, hetastarch) instead of crystalloid administration, although this concept remains controversial.

   6. **Contracting the blood volume.** When excessive volume is present within the CPB circuit and is not due to venous constriction (cold, vasoconstrictor drugs), then it may be desirable to remove fluid from the patient. Fluid can be removed by one of the following methods.

      a. **Diuresis.** Volume contraction is best accomplished through the kidneys. If urine output is inadequate, administration of 12.5 to 25.0 g of mannitol or 2.5 to 5.0 mg of furosemide to an adult patient not receiving chronic diuretic therapy usually is effective and avoids the marked and prolonged diuresis with hypokalemia caused by larger doses. In patients receiving chronic diuretic therapy, the furosemide dose should be 20 to 40 mg initially, increased as necessary. If necessary, another diuretic may be added to increase urine output, such as ethacrynic acid (50 mg IV), chlorothiazide (500 mg IV), or bumetanide (1 to 5 mg).

   b. Ultrafiltration. If adequate diuresis cannot be produced, an ultrafiltration device may be added to the CPB circuit to remove excess water and small ions without significantly affecting plasma electrolyte, blood urea nitrogen (BUN), and protein concentrations. Using a microporous membrane, these devices often can remove 1 to 2 L/hour. Because **heparin may be removed** by this method, anticoagulation must be monitored frequently.

   c. Hemodialysis. In the presence of renal failure, a hemodialyzer machine can be connected to the CPB pump [12]. The composition of the dialysate is adjusted according to the individual conditions present, and reductions in potassium, BUN, and creatinine concentrations can be achieved.

D. Systemic effects of cardioplegia

   1. Potassium load. Cardioplegic solution is designed to produce diastolic cardiac arrest using a combination of high K^+ concentration ($[K^+]$) and profound hypothermia. During the most common adult CPB cases (CAB, aortic valve replacement), the right atrium usually is not opened. Therefore, cardioplegic solution drains from the coronary sinus into the venous cannula, enters the circulating blood volume, and raises the plasma $[K^+]$. Hyperkalemia can cause heart block, negative cardiac inotropy, arrhythmias, and vasoconstriction.

   2. Avoiding systemic K^+ administration. In patients with impaired renal function or preexisting hyperkalemia and in children, added K^+ should be avoided. During antegrade cardioplegia administration, this is accomplished best by cannulating the venae cavae separately, opening the right atrium, and removing the coronary sinus effluent to the wall suction (not recirculated). Alternatively, retrograde cardioplegia can be used, with the aortic root effluent being discarded.

   3. Treatment of hyperkalemia is accomplished by increasing elimination of K^+ from the body with diuretics or hemodialysis; shifting plasma K^+ into cells by inducing alkalosis with hyperventilation or bicarbonate, or with use of glucose-insulin; or reducing the cardiac effects of hyperkalemia by administering calcium salts. For more details see Chapter 2.

E. Treatment of hypokalemia. If a patient is hypokalemic, initiating K^+ replacement during CPB is much safer than waiting until after bypass, thus avoiding hypokalemic dysrhythmias during CPB weaning and cardiac arrest during rapid K^+ replacement. K^+ may be administered in bolus doses as large as 8 mEq directed into the venous reservoir without apparent hemodynamic effects; the dose can be repeated as necessary. Larger doses may cause an initial vasodilation followed by vasoconstriction.

VIII. Intraoperative awareness

A. Etiology

   Dilution of IV anesthetics by the priming solution, absorption of drugs such as fentanyl onto the pump circuit, and a desire to avoid the negative inotropic effects of volatile and IV anesthetics with cardiac depressant actions all may contribute to the return of consciousness during CPB. Because hypothermia itself (below approximately 30°C) induces unconsciousness, the high-risk periods are when the patient is warm. However, many procedures now are performed with mild-to-moderate hypothermia (greater than 30°C), which increases the risk of awareness. During rewarming, the risk of awareness increases further because the brain and body core warm much faster than the body shell. Patients may be able to recall specific events, conversations and, rarely, pain during and after CPB. It is wise to inform patients of this risk preoperatively.

B. Prevention and diagnosis. Due to interindividual differences in responses to anesthetic and hypnotic drugs, there is no way to guarantee that a patient is unconscious except by avoiding total paralysis, regularly asking the patient by name to respond to a command purposefully (e.g., open eyes), and observing the response. If total paralysis is not maintained, it is necessary to ensure that the depth of anesthesia is adequate to prevent gross movement or spontaneous ventilation. If total paralysis is maintained during warm bypass or mild-to-moderate hypothermia (greater than 30°C) it is necessary to administer sufficient **opioid, sedative-hypnotic,** or **volatile agent** to prevent awareness. In addition, it is prudent to prophylactically administer additional **opioid and sedative-hypnotic drugs** on initiation of rewarming. Typical doses are the equivalent of fentanyl 500 μg and midazolam 2 to 5 mg. This is particularly important if volatile agents are allowed to wash out before separation from CPB. If total IV anesthesia is used (e.g., propofol, remifentanil), the infusion rates or target concentrations should be returned to pre-CPB levels on initiation of rewarming. The risk of awareness can be reduced by monitoring the bispectral index (BIS) and maintaining BIS less than 50 [13].

C. **Treatment.** If a patient is found to respond to stimuli, adequate doses of **opioid, sedative-hypnotic,** or **anesthetic drugs** must be administered before additional muscle relaxant. Reassurance should be given. During the postoperative interview, all cardiac surgical patients should be asked to describe (a) the last event before loss of consciousness and (b) the next event. In this fashion, intraoperative awareness can be assessed without prompting. If awareness has occurred, question the patient to make sure operating room and not intensive care unit events are being remembered. Frank discussion of the real nature of intraoperative memories is important to prevent the potential development of neurosis. In certain cases, psychiatric consultation may be indicated.

IX. **Total circulatory arrest during bypass**

It is necessary to stop CPB and remove the perfusion cannulas during certain surgical procedures, including repairs of the aortic arch, vena cava, and certain congenital heart lesions. Because all organs are rendered totally ischemic, steps must be taken to preserve vital organs. These include the following procedures (in addition to cardioplegia for the heart).

A. **Profound hypothermia** (often to 15°C) is the most important factor in preservation because of its ability to reduce the metabolic rate vastly. Cooling is best performed **during CPB,** when the cold can be supplied to all organs directly through the vasculature (core cooling). α-Adrenergic blockade with phentolamine (0.1 to 0.5 mg/kg for infants) often is used to speed cooling and make it more uniform. Alternatively, cold can be applied to the skin, but such surface cooling is slower and less even. Commonly, surface cooling is added to core cooling (cooling blanket plus ice around the head) to prevent heat gain from the environment during circulatory arrest.

B. **Brain preservation.** Frequently, other modalities are added to the effects of cold in an attempt to render the brain less susceptible to ischemic damage [14]. These empirical therapies include **barbiturates** (thiopental titrated to EEG suppression of 1 burst/min or approximately 9 to 10 mg/kg), **corticosteroids** (e.g., methylprednisolone 30 mg/kg), and **mannitol** (0.25 g/kg, also may provide renal protection). Glucose administration often is avoided to help reduce intracellular acidosis during ischemia. (See Chapter 23 for an in-depth discussion of this subject.)

C. **Anesthetic management.** Large doses of a nondepolarizing muscle relaxant should be given immediately before circulatory arrest because cerebrospinal fluid acidosis can stimulate ventilation, and it is not possible to administer drugs during circulatory arrest. Spontaneous ventilation may cause dangerous vascular air entrainment when the heart is open.

X. **Management of relevant rare diseases affecting bypass**

A. **Heparin resistance.** This is a term used to describe the inability to achieve adequate heparinization despite conventional doses of heparin [15]. It may be due to a variety of causes, but it is most common in patients who have received heparin therapy for several days preoperatively. Most cases will respond to **increased doses of heparin.** However, if ACT greater than 400 seconds cannot be achieved despite heparin greater than 600 units/kg, consideration should be given to administering **supplemental antithrombin III** (AT-III). A dose of 1,000 units of AT-III concentrate will increase the AT-III level in an adult by about 30%. Fresh frozen plasma 2 to 4 units is a less expensive alternative, but it is less specific and carries the risk of infective complications (see Chapter 18).

B. Heparin-induced thrombocytopenia (HIT). A mild, reversible, and self-limiting degree of thrombocytopenia may develop during heparin therapy. This is known as heparin induced thrombocytopenia (HIT) **Type 1** and is of little clinical significance. In contrast, during prolonged heparin therapy, usually of 5 or more days' duration, immunoglobulin G (IgG) antibodies may develop to heparin-platelet factor 4 complexes on the surface of platelets and endothelial cells [15]. The binding of antibody to these complexes results in complement activation, endothelial cell injury, and **platelet aggregation.** The clinical syndrome, known as HIT **Type 2,** consists of thrombocytopenia, tachyphylaxis to heparin, and, in 20% of cases, **venous or arterial thrombosis.** Clinical signs include unusual bleeding or thrombosis despite heparin. Development of thrombotic complications is associated with a high morbidity and mortality. The syndrome is rare, but may occur in up to 3% of patients who receive IV heparin for 14 days or more. The diagnosis is confirmed by the demonstration of **in vitro heparin-induced platelet aggregation** or serotonin release.

   Management of HIT Type 2 requires immediate discontinuation of heparin and pharmacologic inhibition of platelet aggregation (with aspirin, dipyridamole, or prostacyclin derivatives). The antibody levels usually fall within 4 to 8 weeks but may persist for 12 months. For patients who require cardiac surgery, the alternatives include delaying surgery for 4 to 8 weeks (or until in vitro heparin-induced platelet aggregation can no longer be demonstrated), plasmapheresis to remove the abnormal antibody, or choosing another anticoagulant drug (see Chapter 18). Consultation with a hematologist is advised.

C. AT-III deficiency. See Chapters 6 and 18.

D. Sickle cell disease or trait [16–18]

   The congenital presence of abnormal hemoglobin S allows RBCs to undergo sickle transformation and occlude the microvasculature or lyse. RBC sickling may be induced by exposure to hypoxia, vascular stasis, hyperosmolarity, or acidosis. Hypothermia produces sickling only by causing vasoconstriction and stasis. Although anesthesia for noncardiac surgery usually is well tolerated in sickle trait patients, the situation is different for operations requiring CPB. CPB may induce sickling by redistributing blood flow, causing stasis, and reducing venous O_2 tensions [18]. **Sickle trait** (heterozygous) patients are at low risk for RBC sickling unless the O_2 saturation is below 40%. Recent experience suggests that CPB with moderate hypothermia can be performed safely in sickle trait patients without the need for routine preoperative partial exchange transfusion. In contrast, **sickle disease** (homozygous) patients develop RBC sickling at O_2 saturations less than 85% and are at risk for developing potentially fatal thromboses during CPB unless appropriate measures are taken. CPB and hypothermia should be avoided if alternative treatment options are available (e.g., off-pump surgery).

   1. **Diagnosis. All black patients should undergo hemoglobin S evaluation** before surgery with CPB, as sickle trait may be completely asymptomatic. The rapid "sickle-dex" test or "sickle-prep" is appropriate for screening, whereas Hb electrophoresis yields important quantitative information if the result of a screening test is positive. Expert preoperative hematologic consultation is advised for sickle trait as well as sickle disease patients before CPB.

   2. **Management.** Hypoxia, acidosis, and conditions leading to vascular stasis should be avoided or minimized in all patients with **sickle trait or disease.** In addition, patients with **sickle disease** may require dilution of Hb-S RBCs with donor Hb-A RBCs. This can be achieved preoperatively or intraoperatively.

      a. **Preoperative transfusion** is required to correct severe anemia only. Increasing the hematocrit improves O_2 carriage, dilutes Hb-S, and suppresses erythropoiesis, but also it increases viscosity, which may promote sickling.

      b. **Preoperative partial exchange transfusion** with Hb-A donor blood is required for **sickle disease** patients undergoing hypothermic CPB. Patients with **sickle trait** are unlikely to require partial exchange transfusion unless deep hypothermia is planned. Heiner and colleagues [16] recommended that the proportion of Hb-S–containing RBCs *(RBC$_s$)* be reduced from 100% to less than 33% as follows:

(1) Measure the percentage of all **hemoglobin** that is Hb-S by Hb electrophoresis (call this $Hb\text{-}S_{pre}$).

(2) Perform the partial exchange transfusion and repeat the Hb electrophoresis to obtain $Hb\text{-}S_{post}$.

(3) Calculate

$$RBC_s \text{ (percentage of body RBCs that contain Hb-S)} = (Hb\text{-}S_{post})/(Hb\text{-}S_{pre}) \times 100.$$

(4) RBC_s should be decreased below approximately 33% as a result of the exchange transfusion (and will be reduced further with initiation of CPB if a blood-containing prime is used). For patients with severe disease with recent crises, RBC_s during CPB should be less than 5% [17].

c. **Intraoperative exchange transfusion** has an advantage because invasive monitoring may be used to guide transfusion and volume replacement. Donor Hb-A can be used to prime the CPB circuit. Upon commencement of CPB, the patient's venous blood can be diverted into a separate reservoir. The diverted blood can be replaced by further donor Hb-A transfusion and volume replacement, resulting in an Hb-S fraction during CPB of less than 5%. Another advantage of this approach is the ability to sequester platelets and plasma from the diverted blood and return these to the patient, while discarding the patient's Hb-S RBCs [17].

d. If **cold cardioplegia** is required, crystalloid cardioplegia can be used to flush out Hb-S from the coronary circulation. If blood cardioplegia is used, it should have less than 5% Hb-S.

e. Avoid arterial or venous hypoxemia, acidosis, dehydration, and hyperosmolarity. Higher-than-usual pump flow rates theoretically may raise P_vO_2 and reduce sickling.

f. If hypothermia is used, vasodilator therapy may prevent vascular stasis. Shivering or other factors that increase O_2 consumption when systemic O_2 transport cannot increase will reduce venous PO_2 saturation and induce sickling.

E. **Cold hemagglutinin disease** [19]

1. **Pathophysiology**

a. Autoantibodies against RBCs in patients with cold hemagglutinin disease are activated by even transient cold exposure. At temperatures below the **critical temperature** for an individual patient, hemagglutination will occur, resulting in **vascular occlusion** with organ ischemia or infarction. Hemagglutination also can fix complement, leading to **hemolysis** on RBC rewarming.

b. In modern cardiac surgery, the organ at greatest risk of damage is the myocardium, because RBCs are exposed to extreme hypothermia (4°C to 8°C) during the preparation of **blood cardioplegia** solution. Aggregates thus formed may be infused into the coronary vasculature, causing severe microcirculatory occlusion and preventing distribution of cardioplegia.

c. Symptoms usually are of vascular occlusion, manifesting as acrocyanosis on exposure to cold. Signs of hemolytic anemia may be present.

d. The idiopathic form of cold hemagglutinin disease is seen most frequently in older patients and probably represents a subclinical form of a lymphoproliferative or immunoproliferative disorder, either of which can induce cold agglutinins. The disease also occurs after mycoplasmal pneumonia, mononucleosis, and other infections.

2. **Diagnosis**

a. Routine **blood bank** cross-matching using the direct Coombs test may identify patients with critical temperatures at or above room temperature. However, autoantibodies responding to such warm temperatures are seen rarely (less than 1% of cardiac surgical patients). Direct Coombs tests run at varying temperatures will characterize a cold agglutinin.

   b. An RBC precipitate (hemagglutination) may form in the cold chamber when blood is mixed with a high K+ solution to form cold blood cardioplegia. A **rapid diagnostic test** has been proposed in which approximately 5 mL of the patient's blood is added to the chilled cardioplegia solution in the cold chamber during setup. Routine use of this test is advocated.

   c. Unexplained high aortic root pressure during cold blood cardioplegia infusion may indicate cold hemagglutinin disease.

   d. The sudden appearance of hemolysis with hemoglobinuria during hypothermic CPB or use of blood cardioplegia may be diagnostic.

3. Management

   a. If cold hemagglutinins are suspected preoperatively, careful assessment by a hematologist is warranted, including characterizing the type of antibody, its titer, and its critical temperature. The common immunoglobulin M (IgM) disease may be managed preoperatively with plasmapheresis and fresh frozen plasma replacement or (in extreme cases) exchange transfusion, whereas the rare IgG antibodies may respond to steroids, chlorambucil, or splenectomy.

   b. The thermal design of the operation should be reviewed and revised if possible. CPB should be avoided if alternative strategies (e.g., off-pump surgery) are feasible. If CPB is required, **systemic temperatures** (including arterial and venous blood values) should be maintained *above* the critical temperature. Systemic temperatures of 28°C or higher generally are safe in asymptomatic patients. Deep hypothermic circulatory arrest is feasible, provided the critical temperature is several degrees colder than the coldest blood temperature.

   c. **Cardioplegia** management includes avoidance of cold blood cardioplegia. Induction of cardiac arrest is achieved with **warm** crystalloid cardioplegia to wash all RBCs out of the myocardium. Subsequently, cold crystalloid cardioplegia is used to maintain arrest. Alternatives include warm blood–potassium cardioplegia or warm ischemic arrest with intermittent reperfusion.

   d. Intraoperative treatment with blood transfusion and use of a cellsaver with colloid and fresh frozen plasma infusions has been reported as an emergency substitute for plasmapheresis.

F. Cold urticaria. Patients with this disorder develop systemic histamine release and generalized urticaria in response to cold exposure. Marked histamine release occurs during CPB rewarming and can cause hemodynamic instability. The cardiovascular responses to histamine can be prevented by pretreatment with H_1- and H_2-receptor blockade; concomitant steroid administration may be useful [20].

G. Malignant hyperthermia [7,21]

1. During an acute malignant hyperthermia (MH) crisis, increased skeletal muscle metabolism may cause a mixed metabolic and respiratory acidosis, hyperthermia, rigidity, hyperkalemia, tachycardia, cardiac dysrhythmias, and rhabdomyolysis with myoglobinuria (and late renal failure). MH does not appear to affect cardiac muscle function directly.

2. Known MH **triggering factors** include succinylcholine and all modern volatile anesthetics. There is experimental evidence that rapid heating or therapy with α-adrenergic agonists or calcium may trigger MH, but this has not been shown clinically. Blood dantrolene concentration decreased during CPB in one patient, but it is not known whether additional dantrolene is necessary during CPB [22].

3. Management. For patients with known MH susceptibility, all known **triggering factors** should be meticulously avoided. An anesthesia machine that is free from all traces of volatile agent should be used. Recognition of MH crisis can be difficult, particularly during the active rewarming phase of CPB. A high index of suspicion is required for patients with known MH susceptibility. Monitoring the rate of CO_2 elimination (by monitoring oxygenator exhaust gas) or O_2 uptake (by arteriovenous O_2 measurements and pump flow rate) may permit early diagnosis of MH. It may be prudent to rewarm the patient gradually, avoid calcium administration unless Ca^{2+} concentration is low, and possibly avoid α-adrenergic agonists in favor of a pure β-adrenergic drug such as isoproterenol if this is appropriate for inotropic therapy [21]. If a patient is diagnosed with MH, it should be treated with dantrolene 1 to 2 mg/kg IV initially. Further doses may be required and should be titrated to effect. Active cooling and treatment of other MH complications may be necessary [21].

H. Hereditary angioedema [23]. A deficiency or abnormality in function of an endogenous inhibitor of the C1 complement protein leads to exaggerated complement pathway activation. Edema involving the airway, face, gastrointestinal tract, and extremities may follow even minor stresses. CPB can cause fatal complement activation in patients with hereditary angioedema; peak activation follows protamine administration. During acute attacks, management is mainly supportive, because epinephrine, steroids, and histamine antagonists are of little benefit, and fresh frozen plasma may exacerbate the reaction by providing additional complement substrates. A purified, vapor-heated C1 inhibitor concentrate is available commercially (Immuno AG, Vienna, Austria) but has not been approved for routine use in the United States [24]. Preoperative management to increase C1 inhibitor levels is critical. Subacute and chronic therapies include androgens (stanozolol) and antifibrinolytics.

I. Pregnancy [25]. Cardiac surgery with CPB during pregnancy involves a high risk of fetal demise or morbidity (10% to 50%), although maternal mortality appears to be no greater than in the nonpregnant patient. Longer duration of CPB appears to increase the risk to the fetus.

1. Physiology. Placental ischemia may be caused by microembolization, elevated IVC pressure due to obstructed drainage, or low pump flow rates (pregnant patients have a larger resting cardiac output and require higher than usual flows during CPB). In addition, uterine blood flow is not autoregulated, so hypotension of any origin is likely to cause placental hypoperfusion. Uterine contractions may be induced by CPB, possibly related to rewarming or to dilution of progesterone.

2. Management

a. Additional monitoring. Fetal heart rate monitoring is mandatory. Uterine contractile activity should be monitored using a tocodynamometer applied to the maternal abdomen.

b. Blood pressure and flow. Maintaining an adequate perfusion pressure (60 to 75 mm Hg) is advocated. Using increases in pump flow to elevate the blood pressure is preferable to using pressor drugs, due to the risk of uterine artery vasoconstriction with α-adrenergic stimulation. If required, ephedrine is the preferred vasopressor. Fetal bradycardia not related to hypothermia may indicate placental hypoperfusion and should be treated promptly by increasing the pump flow and perfusion pressure.

c. Metabolic state. Blood gas abnormalities (including hyperoxia), severe hemodilution, and profound hypothermia are best avoided if possible. An adequate blood glucose level must be maintained.

d. Tocolytic drugs such as magnesium sulfate, ritodrine, or terbutaline may be necessary.

e. Inotropic drugs ideally should not have unbalanced α-vasoconstrictor and uterine-contracting activity. Amrinone or milrinone, or low-to-moderate doses of epinephrine or dopamine, has theoretical advantage.

References

1. Wang JS, Lin CY, Hung WT, et al. Monitoring of heparin-induced anticoagulation with kaolin activated clotting time in cardiac surgical patients treated with aprotinin. *Anesthesiology* 1992;77:1080–1084.
2. Gravlee GR, Angert KC, Tucker WY, et al. Early anticoagulation peak and rapid distribution after intravenous heparin. *Anesthesiology* 1988;68:126–129.
3. Aldea GS, O'Gara P, Shapira OM, et al. Effect of anticoagulation protocol on outcome in patients undergoing CABG with heparin-bonded cardiopulmonary bypass circuits. *Ann Thorac Surg* 1998;65:425–433.

4. Nadolney EM, Svennson LG. Carbon dioxide field flooding techniques for open heart surgery: monitoring and minimising potential adverse effects. *Perfusion* 2000;15:151–153.

5. Oka Y, Inoue T, Hong Y, et al. Retained intracardiac air. Transesophageal echocardiography for definition of incidence and monitoring removal by improved techniques. *J Thorac Cardiovasc Surg* 1986;63:329–338.

6. Schwartz DS, Ribakove GH, Grossi EA, et al. Single and multivessel port access coronary artery bypass grafting with cardioplegic arrest: technique and reproducibility. *J Thorac Cardiovasc Surg* 1997;114:46–52.

7. **Kurusz M, Mills NL. Management of unusual problems encountered in initiating and maintaining cardiopulmonary bypass. In: Gravlee GR, Davis RF, Kurusz M, et al., eds. *Cardiopulmonary bypass: principles and practice*. Baltimore: Lippincott Williams & Wilkins, 2000:578–612.**

8. **Mills NL, Ochsner JL. Massive air embolism during cardiopulmonary bypass: causes, prevention, and management. *J Thorac Cardiovasc Surg* 1980;80:708–717.**

9. Moore RA, Geller EA, Gallagher JD, et al. Effect of hypothermic cardiopulmonary bypass on nitroprusside metabolism. *Clin Pharmacol Ther* 1985;37:680–683.

10. Hickey S, Gaylor JDS, Kenny GNC. In vitro uptake and elimination of isoflurane by different membrane oxygenators. *J Cardiothor Vasc Anesth* 1996;10:352–355.

11. Dawson PJ, Bjorksten AR, Blake DW, et al. The effects of cardiopulmonary bypass on total and unbound plasma concentrations of propofol and midazolam. *J Cardiothorac Vasc Anesth* 1997;11:556–561.

12. Murkin JM, Murphy DA, Finlayson DC, et al. Hemodialysis during cardiopulmonary bypass: report of twelve cases. *Anesth Analg* 1987;66:899–901.

13. Sebel PS. Central nervous system monitoring during open heart surgery: an update. *J Cardiothorac Vasc Anesth* 1998;12:3–8.

14. Wickey GS, Martin DE, Larach DR, et al. Combined carotid endarterectomy, coronary revascularization, and hypernephroma excision with hypothermic circulatory arrest. *Anesth Analg* 1988;67:473–476.

15. **Mangano CM, Hill L, Cartwright CR, et al. Cardiopulmonary bypass and the anesthesiologist. In: Kaplan JA, ed. *Cardiac anesthesia*, 4th ed. Philadelphia: WB Saunders, 1999:1061–1110.**

16. Heiner M, Teasdale SJ, David T, et al. Aorto-coronary bypass in a patient with sickle cell trait. *Can Anaesth Soc J* 1979;26:428–434.

17. Kingsley CP, Chronister T, Cohen DJ, et al. Anesthetic management of a patient with hemoglobin SS disease and mitral insufficiency for mitral valve repair. *J Cardiothorac Vasc Anesth* 1996;10:419–424.

18. Koshy M, Weiner SJ, Miller ST, et al. Surgery and anesthesia in sickle cell disease. Cooperative study of sickle cell diseases. *Blood* 1995;86:3676–3684.

19. Bracken CA, Gurkowski MA, Naples JJ, et al. Cardiopulmonary bypass in two patients with previously undetected cold agglutinins. *J Cardiothorac Vasc Anesth* 1993;7:743–749.

20. Johnston WE, Moss J, Philbin DM, et al. Management of cold urticaria during hypothermic cardiopulmonary bypass. *N Engl J Med* 1982;306:219–221.

21. Byrick RJ, Rose DK, Ranganathan N. Management of a malignant hyperthermia patient during cardiopulmonary bypass. *Can Anaesth Soc J* 1982;29:50–54.

22. Larach DR, High KM, Larach MG, et al. Cardiopulmonary bypass interference with dantrolene prophylaxis of malignant hyperthermia. *J Cardiothorac Anesth* 1987;1:448–453.

23. Jaering JM, Comunale ME. Cardiopulmonary bypass in hereditary angioedema. *Anesthesiology* 1993;79:1429–1433.

24. Waytes AT, Rosen FS, Frank MM. Treatment of hereditary angioedema with a vaporheated C1 inhibitor concentrate. *N Engl J Med* 1996;334:1630–1631.

25. Strickland RA, Oliver WC, Chamtigian RC. Anesthesia, cardiopulmonary bypass, and the pregnant patient. *Mayo Clin Proc* 1991;66:411–429.

8. WEANING FROM CARDIOPULMONARY BYPASS

Mark E. Romanoff and David R. Larach

Terminating cardiopulmonary bypass (CPB) requires the anesthesiologist to apply the basic tenets of cardiovascular physiology and pharmacology. The goal is a smooth transition from the mechanical pump back to the heart as the source of blood flow. Weaning from the pump involves optimizing cardiovascular variables including preload, afterload, heart rate (HR) and conduction, contractility, and the O_2 supply/demand ratio, as in the pre-CPB period. However, the time period for optimization is compressed to minutes or seconds, and decisions must be made quickly to avoid myocardial injury or damage to the other major organ systems.

   I. Preparation: CVP mnemonic. The major objectives in preparing for termination of CPB can be remembered with the aid of the mnemonic **CVP:**

C	V	P
Cold	Ventilation	Predictors
Conduction	Vaporizer	Protamine
Calcium	Volume expanders	Pressure
Cardiac output	Visualization	Pressors
Cells		Pacer
Coagulation		Potassium

   A. Cold. Core temperature (nasopharyngeal, tympanic membrane, bladder) should be greater than 36°C before terminating CPB. Shell, or rectal, temperature should be at least 33°C. Bladder temperature also may represent shell temperature. Ending CPB when cold causes prolonged hypothermia from equilibration of the cooler, vessel-poor group with the warmer and better perfused vessel-rich group when active rewarming is discontinued. Nasopharyngeal temperature correlates with brain temperature but may be artificially elevated during rapid rewarming (by a large volume of warm CPB blood) and should not be used for determining the temperature at which CPB is discontinued unless it has been stable for 20 to 30 minutes. Venous return temperature can be used in a similar manner to help confirm core temperature. The nasopharyngeal temperature should not exceed 38°C, as this may increase the risk of postoperative central nervous system dysfunction.
   B. Conduction. Cardiac rate and rhythm must be controlled as follows:
     1. Rate
        a. HR of 80 to 100 beats/min often is needed for adequate cardiac output (CO) post-CPB because of a potentially reduced ability to increase stroke volume. In coronary artery bypass graft (CABG) procedures, the O_2 supply/demand ratio is more favorable after grafting, so that a higher rate (80 to 100 beats/min) after CPB should carry less risk of ischemia than before CPB. Patients with severely limited stroke volume (aneurysmectomy or after ventricular remodeling) may require even higher rates.
        b. Sinus bradycardia may be treated with atropine or an inotropic drug, but epicardial pacing is more predictable.
        c. Sinus tachycardia of more than 120 beats/min should be treated before termination of CPB. Often the act of "filling the heart" and increasing preload will reflexly decrease the HR to an acceptable level. Other etiologies of increased HR must be addressed. **Common etiologies include:**
          (1) Hypoxia
          (2) Hypercapnia
          (3) Medications (inotropes, pancuronium, scopolamine)
          (4) Light anesthesia, awareness
            (a) "Fast track" anesthesia with its lower medication dosing schedule requires special attention to this complication. An additional dose of narcotic, benzodiazepine, or hypnotic (propofol infusion) should be given during the rewarming period or if tachycardia is present.
          (5) Anemia

(6) ST and T-wave changes indicative of ischemia should be treated and the surgeon should be notified. A nitroglycerin (NTG) infusion or an increase in the perfusion pressure often improves the situation. Refractory causes include residual air or graft occlusions.

2. Rhythm

   a. Normal sinus rhythm is preferable. In patients with poorly compliant, thick-walled ventricles (associated with aortic stenosis, hypertension, or ischemia), the atrial "kick" may contribute up to 40% of CO, so attaining synchronized atrial contraction [sinus rhythm, atrial or atrioventricular (AV) sequential pacing] is **very important** before attempting CPB termination. Atrial pacing is acceptable if there is no AV block, but often atrial and ventricular leads are needed.

   b. Supraventricular tachycardias (HR greater than 120 beats/min) such as regular narrow-QRS atrial flutters and atrial fibrillation, should be cardioverted with synchronized internal cardioversion before terminating CPB.

   c. Esmolol, calcium channel blockers, or adenosine may be used to chemically cardiovert or to control the ventricular response rate. A decrease in contractility is seen with some agents. Digoxin can be effective, but its onset is delayed.

   d. Third-degree AV block requires pacing, although atropine occasionally may be effective.

   e. Ventricular dysrhythmias are treated as indicated (see Chapter 2).

C. Calcium. Calcium salts should be immediately available to treat hypocalcemia and hyperkalemia, which commonly occur after CPB. However, the routine administration of calcium post-CPB is not recommended.

   1. Mechanism of action. Most studies suggest that calcium produces an elevation in systemic vascular resistance (SVR) primarily, when the ionized Ca^{2+} level is in the low–normal range or higher [1]. Despite this increase in afterload, contractility is maintained. At very low ionized calcium levels, contractility is increased by calcium administration. The usual dose is 5 to 15 mg/kg of CaCl. Calcium is clearly indicated when the ionized Ca^{2+} level is low and contractility is depressed after CPB. Also, elevating calcium levels will help counteract the dysrhythmogenic and negative inotropic actions of hyperkalemia.

   2. Measurement. Ionized Ca^{2+} levels should be evaluated after rewarming to help direct therapy. The usual range is 1.0 to 1.3 mmol/dL. Calcium levels are affected by pH: Low pH will increase Ca^{2+} levels, whereas elevated pH will decrease Ca^{2+} levels. Correction of pH should be attempted before treating abnormal values. Citrated blood cardioplegia reperfusion solutions can lower blood Ca^{2+} levels substantially.

   3. Risks of calcium administration [1]

   a. Inhibition of the hemodynamic action of inotropes (e.g., epinephrine, dobutamine) has been reported.

   b. Patients taking digoxin may experience life-threatening dysrhythmias.

   c. Coronary spasm might occur in rare susceptible patients.

   d. Augmentation of reperfusion injury is possible. Calcium administration should wait until 15 minutes after aortic cross-clamp release.

D. Cardiac output. Measuring CO helps to assess the function of the heart after CPB. This may be performed by using a pulmonary artery (PA) catheter or transesophageal echocardiography (TEE). If a PA catheter that permits continuous CO measurement is used, it may take up to 3 minutes to obtain the first CO after CPB. If the patient is stable, this is acceptable; if not, the equipment for a manual determination should be available.

E. Cells

   1. The hemoglobin concentration ordinarily should be greater than 7.0 g/dL before terminating CPB. If it is not, packed red blood cells or whole blood should be given during CPB to maintain O_2-carrying capacity after CPB. Patients with residual coronary stenoses, anticipated low CO, or end-organ damage may benefit from even higher hemoglobin concentrations.

   2. Packed red blood cells should be immediately available for use once the CPB pump volume is exhausted.
 F. Coagulation. Anticipate possible coagulation abnormalities requiring therapy. If needed, the following blood products should be administered only after CPB.
   1. Platelets should be available if indicated (thrombocytopenia, aspirin use, chronic renal failure, reoperation, long "pump run").
   2. Fresh frozen plasma or cryoprecipitate should be available if indicated for treatment of appropriate factor deficiencies.
   3. Desmopressin acetate (DDAVP) can be used to increase platelet aggregation in patients with chronic renal failure, von Willebrand disease, or other platelet abnormalities. In patients without preexisting platelet abnormalities, DDAVP has little effect on blood loss or replacement in CABG patients but may be effective in open-chamber surgery [2].
   4. These blood products and DDAVP should not be given until the heparin has been reversed and all surgical repairs are complete. Blood product therapy should be guided by the clinical situation and by laboratory findings (e.g., prothrombin time, partial thromboplastin time, thromboelastogram, platelet count).
 G. Ventilation
   1. Adequate oxygenation and ventilation while the patient is on CPB must be ensured by checking arterial and venous blood gas measurements at routine intervals. pH should be between 7.30 and 7.50 at normothermia before CPB separation.
   2. The lungs should be reexpanded with two to three sustained breaths (15 to 20 seconds each) to a peak pressure of 30 to 40 cm H_2O with visual confirmation of bilateral lung expansion and resolution of atelectasis. In patients with internal mammary artery grafts, care must be taken to prevent lung overdistention, which may cause graft avulsion. An estimate of lung compliance should be made (see Section 7 below). Rarely, tracheal suction may be indicated. Caution should be used in these anticoagulated patients. The surgeon may need to evacuate any hemothorax or pneumothorax.
   3. Inspired oxygen fraction (FIO_2) should be 1.0. If air was used during CPB to prevent atelectasis, it should be discontinued. Nitrous oxide should never be used during or after cannulation to avoid increasing the size of air emboli.
   4. The pulse oximeter should be turned on; if pulsatile flow exists, it should be functional.
   5. All airway monitors should be on line (apnea, FIO_2, end-tidal CO_2).
   6. Mechanical ventilation must be started before an attempt to terminate CPB. Terminating CPB without lung ventilation could have disastrous consequences. The timing for commencement of mechanical ventilation while the patient is still on CPB is controversial. Some practitioners believe that ventilation should begin when arterial or pulmonary pulsatile blood flow resumes in order to avoid hypoxemia. However, this may not be necessary in normothermic, nearly full-flow bypass [3] and may cause severe respiratory alkalosis of pulmonary venous blood. The pulse oximeter or the CPB circuit venous oxygen tension also can be used to assess the need for ventilation during partial CPB.
   7. Auscultation of breath sounds will confirm air movement and may reveal wheezing, rales, or rhonchi. Appropriate treatment should be instituted before terminating CPB.
 H. Vaporizer. Inhalation agents used during CPB for blood pressure (BP) control ordinarily should be turned off at least 10 minutes before terminating CPB. These agents will decrease contractility and may take as long as 15 to 20 minutes to clear from the circuit.
 I. Volume expanders. Albumin, hetastarch, or crystalloid solution should be available to increase preload if blood products are not indicated. Hetastarch may be contraindicated if excessive bleeding is anticipated or with impaired renal function.
 J. Visualization of the heart is important before terminating CPB. TEE is helpful in permitting a detailed examination. Primarily the right atrium and ventricle are visible in the chest to the naked eye. TEE can evaluate all four chambers. It is possible to evaluate the following parameters:

1. Contractility. The heart will beat vigorously and "snap" with each beat in a normal contractile pattern. Wall-motion abnormalities from ischemia or infarct can be compared to pre-CPB observations.
2. Distention of the chambers.
3. Residual air in left-sided structures [e.g., left atrium (LA), left ventricle (LV), pulmonary veins].
4. Conduction. Direct visual diagnosis of normal sinus rhythm or atrial dysrhythmias can be easier than using the electrocardiogram (ECG). Visualization of the LA appendage may prove especially helpful in this regard.
5. Valvular function or perivalvular leaks can be identified before attempting CPB termination.

K. Predictors

1. Assess the patient's risk for difficult weaning from CPB. Risk factors that can be identified **before** terminating CPB include [4]:
   a. Preoperative ejection fraction less than 0.45 or diastolic dysfunction
   b. Female patient undergoing CABG (tendency to incomplete revascularization because of smaller more diseased coronary arteries)
   c. Elderly patient
   d. Angiotensin-converting enzyme (ACE) use (excessive vasodilation)
   e. Ongoing ischemia or evolving infarct in the pre-CPB period
   f. Prolonged CPB duration (more than 2 to 3 hours)
   g. Inadequate surgical repair
      (1) Incomplete coronary revascularization
         (a) Small vessels (not graftable or poor "runoff")
         (b) Distal disease (especially in diabetic patients)
      (2) Valvular disease
         (a) Valve replacement with very small valve (high transvalvular pressure gradient post-CPB)
         (b) Suboptimal valve **repair** (residual regurgitation or stenosis)
   h. Incomplete myocardial preservation during cross-clamping
      (1) ECG not asystolic (incomplete diastolic arrest)
      (2) Prolonged ventricular fibrillation before cross-clamping
      (3) Warm myocardium
         (a) LV hypertrophy (incomplete cardioplegia)
         (b) High-grade coronary stenoses (no cardioplegia to that area of heart)
         (c) Choice of grafting order (grafts should be performed first in an area of the heart served by a high-grade lesion in the absence of retrograde cardioplegia, so cardioplegia may be infused early)
         (d) Noncoronary collateral flow washing out cardioplegia
         (e) Poor LV venting
2. **Additional preparations for high-risk patients**
   a. One common practice is to have a syringe of ephedrine (5 mg/mL) or dilute epinephrine prepared (4 to 10 µg/mL). Boluses can be used until a decision is made regarding the need for a continuous infusion.
   b. Discuss the need for additional **invasive monitoring** with the surgeon (i.e., LA or central aortic catheter).
   c. Check for immediate availability of other **inotropic or vasoactive** medications: epinephrine, dobutamine, milrinone, norepinephrine, prostaglandin E_1, and nitric oxide.
   d. As appropriate to the anticipated level of difficulty separating from CPB, check for immediate availability of an **intraaortic balloon pump** (IABP) and consider placement of a femoral arterial catheter to facilitate its rapid insertion and possibly for improved BP monitoring.
   e. Consider starting an inotropic infusion or the IABP before terminating CPB in patients with poor contractility. Note that the Frank–Starling law implies that an empty heart will not beat very forcefully. Often a sluggishly contracting heart will start to "snap" once it is filled

f. A good rule is "The first attempt off CPB is the best one." Optimizing all parameters before CPB termination is strongly advised. If in doubt, start an inotrope. Preemptive use of milrinone has been shown to improve cardiac function during and after cardiac surgery [5].

L. Protamine. The protamine dose should be calculated and drawn up in a syringe or be ready as an infusion. **Premature use of protamine is catastrophic.** Therefore, protamine should be prominently labeled and should not be placed where routine medications are stored, to avoid accidental use. The surgeon, anesthesiologist, and perfusionist must all coordinate the use of this medication.

M. Pressure. Check the calibration and zero level of all transducers before terminating CPB.

    1. Arterial pressure. Recognize that radial artery catheters may underestimate central aortic pressure following rewarming. Femoral artery catheters do not share this limitation. An aortic root vent, if present, may be connected to a transducer also. If the radial arterial catheter is not functioning, a needle placed in the aorta or aortic cannula can be transduced during and after termination of CPB until the cannula is removed.

    2. PA pressure. Ensure that the catheter has not migrated distally to a wedge position. Often the PA catheter must be withdrawn 3 to 5 cm even if this was done at CPB initiation.

N. Pressors and inotropes

    1. Medications that are likely to be used should be readily available, including a vasodilator (e.g., NTG, nitroprusside) and a potent inotropic agent (e.g., dopamine, dobutamine, epinephrine, milrinone).

    2. NTG and phenylephrine or norepinephrine should always be available to infuse after CPB even if their use is not expected. Some practitioners use prophylactic NTG infusion (approximately 50 μg/min) for all coronary revascularization procedures to prevent coronary vasoconstriction. It also can be used as a venodilator to allow additional volume to be infused in patients after CPB.

    3. Volumetric infusion pumps deliver vasoactive substances with the highest accuracy and reproducibility.

O. Pacer. An external pacemaker should be in the room, checked, and set to the initial settings by the anesthesiologist. A pacemaker often is needed for treatment of bradycardia or asystole. In patients with heart block, an AV sequential pacemaker is strongly advised to retain a synchronized atrial contraction. Use of a DDD pacer, when available, is recommended.

P. Potassium. Blood chemistries should be checked before terminating CPB.

    1. Hyperkalemia may induce conduction abnormalities and decreases in contractility. It is more common after long pump runs when large amounts of cardioplegic solution are used and absorbed, especially in patients with renal dysfunction.

    2. Hypokalemia can cause dysrhythmias and should be treated if less than 3.5 mEq/L and there is adequate urine output after CPB.

    3. Glucose levels in diabetic patients should be checked and treatment undertaken if indicated. High levels of glucose in any patient may contribute to central nervous system dysfunction and poor wound healing after CPB and should be treated.

    4. Ionized Ca^{2+} levels are discussed in Section **I.C** above.

    5. Other electrolytes should be evaluated as needed. In particular, low levels of magnesium are common after CPB and have been associated with dysrhythmias.

II. Sequence of events immediately before terminating CPB. Weaning from bypass describes the transition from total CPB (bypass pump supplies 100% of the required mechanical work) to a final condition in which the heart provides 100% of this work. The transition should be gradual, recognizing that cardiac function post-CPB is not usually normal. (At times, though, cardiac function may be **improved** after bypass if ischemia is relieved or valvular dysfunction repaired.)

A. Final checklist before terminating CPB

    1. Confirm

a. Ventilation
(1) Lungs are ventilated with 100% O_2, a visual confirmation.
(2) Ventilatory alarms are enabled.
(3) Breath sounds and heart tones are heard via the esophageal stethoscope.
(4) All vaporizers are off.
b. The patient is sufficiently rewarmed.
c. The heart, great vessels, and grafts have been properly de-aired.
d. The patient is in optimal metabolic condition.
e. All equipment and drugs are ready.
2. Do not proceed until these criteria have been met.
3. Weaning from CPB requires the utmost concentration and vigilance by the anesthesiologist, and all distractions should be eliminated.
B. **What to look at during weaning.** Key information is obtained from three sources: the invasive pressure display, the heart itself, and the ECG.
1. **Invasive pressure display**
   a. Pressure waveforms [arterial, central venous pressure (CVP), and PA or LA, if used] are best displayed using overlapping traces, and there are some benefits to the use of an identical scale as well. Advantages of this display format include the following:
      (1) Coronary perfusion pressure is graphically depicted as the vertical height between the arterial diastolic pressure and the filling pressure (PA diastolic or LA mean) during diastole.
      (2) The vertical separation between the PA mean and CVP waveforms estimates right ventricular (RV) work (see Section **II.B.1.d** below).
      (3) The slope of the rise in central aortic pressure during systole may give some indication of LV contractility and is most easily appreciated if the waveform is not compressed.
      (4) Valvular regurgitation can be diagnosed by examining CVP, pulmonary capillary wedge pressure (PCWP), or LA waveforms (e.g., mitral regurgitation may produce V waves in LA and PCWP tracings) as well as by TEE.
   b. **Arterial pressure.** The systolic and mean systemic arterial pressures should be checked continuously.
      (1) The **systolic** pressure describes the pressure generated by the heart's own contraction.
      (2) Before CPB separation, the **mean** pressure describes the work performed by the bypass pump and the vascular tone. After separation, it reflects the cardiac work and vascular tone.
      (3) The **diastolic pressure** reflects vascular tone and gives an indication of coronary perfusion pressure.
      (4) The **pulse pressure** reflects the mechanical work done by the heart. As the heart assumes more of the circulatory work, this pressure difference increases. LV failure is suggested by a decreased pulse pressure.
      (5) Difficulty in weaning (poor LV function) may be reflected by a low pulse pressure or systolic–mean pressure difference in the presence of high atrial filling pressures when the venous return line is partially occluded.
      (6) It is important to remember that a radial artery catheter may not be accurate following CPB. During the first 30 minutes after CPB, the radial artery tends to underestimate both the systolic and mean central aortic pressures [6]. Clinically significant radial artery hypotension should be confirmed by a noninvasive BP reading or with a central aortic or femoral artery pressure measurement before treatment or resumption of CPB.
   c. **Central venous pressure.** This provides an index of right heart filling before and during weaning.
   d. **CVP–PA mean pressure step-up.** The mechanical work performed by the RV is related to the difference between the CVP and the PA mean pressure.

2. **Inspection of the heart visually or echocardiographically** provides valuable information about contractility, wall-motion abnormalities, conduction, preload, and valvular function.
3. **ECG** changes, such as heart block, dysrhythmias, or ischemia, occur frequently, mandating frequent examination.
4. **Ventilation and oxygenation.** Routine airway management issues as well as problems in the other major organ systems must not be overlooked. The partial pressure of carbon dioxide (P_aCO_2) should be kept at or below 40 mm Hg in the post-CPB period. Minor elevations in P_aCO_2 can increase pulmonary vascular resistance (PVR) significantly [7].

III. **Sequence of events during weaning from CPB**
  A. **Step 1: Retarding venous return to the pump**
    1. **Consequences of partial venous occlusion.** Slowly the venous line is partially occluded (by the surgeon or perfusionist). This increase in venous line resistance causes right atrial pressure to rise and causes some blood to flow through the tricuspid valve into the RV instead of all draining to the pump. According to the Frank–Starling law, CO increases as preload rises; therefore, the heart begins to eject blood more forcefully as the heart fills and enlarges.
    2. **Preload.** The amount of venous line occlusion is adjusted carefully to attain and maintain a certain optimal preload or **LV end-diastolic volume** (LVEDV).
      a. **Estimating preload.** Unless TEE is in use, LV filling **volumes** cannot be measured directly. Instead, LVEDV is estimated from a filling **pressure** [PA diastolic, PCWP, or LA pressure (LAP)]. The relationship of LVEDV to LA pressure and PCWP can be quite variable after bypass secondary to changes in diastolic compliance. Decreased compliance is caused by myocardial edema and ischemia. Therefore, the PCWP is a relatively poor indicator of LVEDV in the post-CPB period [8], but this is usually the best available indicator.
      b. **Optimal preload** is the **lowest** value that provides an adequate CO. Preload greater than the optimal value may cause:
        (1) Ventricular distention and increased wall tension [increased myocardial oxygen consumption (Mvo_2)]
        (2) Decreased coronary perfusion pressure
        (3) Excessive or decreased CO
        (4) Pulmonary edema
      c. **Typical weaning filling pressures.** For patients with good LV function preoperatively, PCWP of 8 to 12 mm Hg or CVP of 6 to 12 mm Hg often suffices. Abnormal contractility or diastolic stiffness may necessitate much higher filling pressures to achieve adequate filling volumes (20 mm Hg or higher), but in such cases it is imperative to monitor **left** heart filling by a PA or LA line, or by TEE.
      d. **CVP/LAP ratio.** Normally, the CVP is lower than the LAP, which usually is estimated by the PCWP (CVP/LAP ratio less than 1). If the ratio is elevated (greater than 1), the intraventricular septum may be forced toward the left, limiting LV filling and CO. This "septal shift" often can be diagnosed by TEE as well. In this situation, termination of CPB may be impossible until the ratio is normalized by improving RV function [9].
  B. **Step 2: Lowering pump flow into the aorta**
    1. **Attaining partial bypass.** The rise in preload causes the heart to begin to contribute to the CO. This condition is termed *partial bypass* because the venous blood draining into the right atrium divides into two paths: Some goes to the pump, and some passes through the RV and lungs and is ejected into the aorta by the LV.
      a. Some institutions advocate keeping the patient on partial CPB for several minutes to wash vasoactive substances from the lungs before terminating CPB.
    2. **Reduced pump outflow requirement.** Because two sources of blood are now supplying the aorta, the amount of arterial blood returned from the pump to the patient can be reduced as native CO increases to maintain total aortic

blood flow. Therefore, the perfusionist lowers the pump flow rate in increments of 0.5 to 1.0 L/min. This step is repeated, allowing gradual reductions in pump flow rate while cardiac function and hemodynamics are carefully monitored.

   3. Readjusting venous line resistance. Some adjustment in the venous line resistance may be needed to maintain a constant filling pressure as the heart is given more work to perform. Also, as arterial pump outflow is reduced, less venous inflow is needed to keep the venous reservoir from being pumped dry. Therefore, the venous line clamp can be progressively tightened to achieve the desired increase in preload.

C. Step 3: Terminating bypass. If the heart is generating an adequate systolic pressure (typically 90 to 100 mm Hg for an adult) at an acceptable preload with pump flows of 1 L/min or less, the patient is ready for a trial without CPB, and bypass is terminated. The pump is stopped, and both pump cannulas are clamped shut. If these criteria are not met, CPB is reinstituted, and management of cardiovascular decompensation is begun (see Section **IV.D.** below).

There are **variant techniques.** At some institutions, weaning is accomplished by abruptly clamping the venous line shut, then lowering pump flow as the heart rapidly begins to eject blood in response to the precipitous filling. Although this technique may be satisfactory for patients with good heart function, it requires that pump flows be decreased quickly because the venous reservoir would otherwise be pumped dry in the absence of venous return. It is not recommended for patients with compromised cardiovascular function.

IV. Sequence of events immediately after terminating CPB

  A. Preload: infusing blood from the pump. If cardiac performance is inadequate, small increases in preload may be beneficial. For adult patients, volume is transferred in 50- to 100-mL increments from the venous pump reservoir to the patient through the aortic cannula. Before volume infusion, the aortic cannula should be inspected for air bubbles within its lumen. Increments of 10 to 50 mL are used in pediatric patients. During volume infusions from the pump, the BP, filling pressure, and heart should be watched closely. **Continuous** infusion is contraindicated because overdistention of the heart may occur and the oxygenator reservoir may be emptied, embolizing air to the patient.

    1. The almost instantaneous infusion of volume by the pump allows for evaluation of LV function. You can assume that during the infusion there is no change in SVR. According to the formula:

$$BP = CO \times SVR$$

If you make SVR a constant, then:

$$BP \cong CO,$$

so an increase in BP with a small volume infusion must indicate an increase in CO.

    2. If BP and CO do not change with increased preload, the patient probably is at the top (flat part) of the Frank–Starling curve, and further volume infusion is unlikely to be of benefit.

    3. If BP does rise, the rise probably is due to a rise in CO, and further volume administration may be beneficial. In this manner, the optimal preload can be titrated after CPB.

    4. Three factors often contribute to a need to give volume after CPB:

      a. Continued rewarming of peripheral vascular beds results in vasodilation.

      b. Changes in LV diastolic compliance alter optimal filling pressure.

      c. Continued bleeding.

  B. Measuring cardiac function

    1. Before taking the **relatively** irrevocable steps of removing the aortic cannula or administering protamine, cardiac function should be assessed. Particularly in adults, this is important because an adequate BP may be the result of a low CO and a high systemic vascular resistance. Cardiac function may be assessed by measuring CO or by echocardiography. The derived **cardiac index** (CO/body surface area) should be calculated. Generally, a cardiac index of more than 2.0 L/min/m^2 should be present to consider permanent termination of CPB, although an index of greater than 2.3 usually is considered "normal." If HR is high, a normal CO can exist despite a low stroke volume. Therefore, a calculation of the **stroke volume index** (cardiac index/HR) can be useful (normal is greater than 40 mL/beat/m^2).

2. **Measuring patient perfusion.** Signs of adequate **tissue** perfusion after CPB should be sought. Within the first 5 to 10 minutes after terminating CPB, arterial blood gases and pH should be measured, looking for lactic acidosis or gas exchange abnormalities. Mixed venous Po$_2$ indicates global body O$_2$ supply/demand balance. Urine output normally rises after CPB, and lack of such a rise should be evaluated and treated immediately. The ideal perfusion pressure for adequate tissue perfusion should be individualized. Patients with renal insufficiency, cerebrovascular disease, or hypertension may require higher perfusion pressures, although the increased BP may worsen bleeding.

3. **Afterload and aortic impedance.** In the presence of good LV function (and the absence of myocardial ischemia), the anesthesiologist should avoid elevated afterload (as reflected by systolic BP) to prevent excessive stress on the aortic suture lines and to reduce surgical bleeding. In adults, the usual desired range for systolic BP is 100 to 140 mm Hg.

   With impaired LV function or valvular regurgitation, SVR should be reduced to the lowest level possible while maintaining adequate BP for organ perfusion. Reducing the aortic impedance improves LV ejection and lowers systolic LV wall stress and myocardial O$_2$ demand. Impedance is related to BP and SVR, and lowering SVR can result in increased CO with no change in BP.

4. **HR and rhythm.** The optimal HR is usually 70 to 100 beats/min.
   a. **Bradycardia** (HR less than 60 beats/min). **Low HRs** can reduce CO substantially because the abnormal LV stiffness that often is present after CPB prevents the normal rise in stroke volume as HR falls. Pacing is the ideal means for increasing HR, especially atrial or AV sequential pacing, because of its controllability.
   b. **Tachycardia** (greater than **120 beats/min**) can be detrimental to LV filling by increasing Mvo$_2$ and should be treated promptly.
   c. **Dysrhythmias** require appropriate and timely treatment.

C. **Removing the cannulas.**
   1. **Venous cannula(s).** The presence of a large cannula(s) in the right atrium or in the vena cava will retard venous return to the heart and, if cardiac function is reasonable, the venous cannula should be removed as soon as practical. Removing the cannula will allow the perfusionist to "reprime" the pump and allow for further volume infusion through the aortic cannula.
   2. **Aortic cannula.** Removal of the aortic cannula should wait until at least half of the protamine dose has been infused.

D. **Cardiovascular decompensation**
   1. Refer to Chapter 2 for specific drug pharmacology and doses.
   2. Failure of the LV or RV, both of which are recovering from the insult of CPB, together with low SVR are the most common causes of cardiovascular insufficiency during the weaning process.
   a. **LV failure**
      (1) Differential diagnosis of LV failure after CPB is listed in Table 8.1.
      (2) Treatment of LV failure during weaning from CPB includes
         (a) Inotropic drug administration. Most commonly epinephrine or dobutamine is chosen as a first-line agent, although some institutions advocate the use of dopamine or milrinone initially. Regardless of choice, often ephedrine 10 to 20 mg or a 4- to 10-μg bolus of epinephrine is given to increase contractility and BP while commencing an inotrope infusion.
            (i) Epinephrine or dopamine may be appropriate if HR is normal and SVR is low or normal.

Table 8.1 Differential diagnosis of left ventricular failure after cardiopulmonary bypass

I. Ischemia
    A. Graft failure
        1. Clot in graft
        2. Distal suture causing constriction
        3. Kinking of graft
        4. Air in graft
        5. Graft sewn in backward (no flow through valves)
        6. Inadequate flow through internal mammary artery
    B. Inadequate coronary blood flow
        1. Incomplete revascularization (secondary to distal disease or inoperable vessels)
        2. Inadequate coronary perfusion pressure
        3. Emboli in native coronary arteries—air or particulate matter (clot, atherosclerotic plaque)
        4. Coronary spasm
        5. Tachycardia (decreased diastolic filling time)
        6. Increased myocardial O_2 demand
        7. Surgical injury to native coronary artery
    C. Myocardial ischemia leading to myocardial damage
        1. Incomplete myocardial preservation during cardiopulmonary bypass
        2. Evolving myocardial infarction
II. Valve failure
    A. Prosthetic valve
        1. Sewn in backward
        2. Paravalvular leak
        3. Mechanical obstruction (immobile disk)
    B. Native valve—acute mitral regurgitation (papillary muscle ischemia or rupture)
III. Gas exchange problems
    A. Hypoxemia
        1. Inadequate F_{IO_2}
        2. Mechanical ventilator failure
        3. Airway disconnected
        4. Severe bronchospasm
        5. Pulmonary edema ("pump lung" adult respiratory distress syndrome)
    B. Hypoventilation
IV. Inadequate preload
V. Excessive preload (can lead to distention of cardiac structures)
VI. Reperfusion injury
VII. Ventricular septal defect
VIII. Miscellaneous causes of decreased contractility
    A. Medications
        1. β-Blockade
        2. Calcium channel blockers
        3. Inhalational agents
    B. Acidemia
    C. Electrolyte abnormalities
        1. Hyperkalemia
        2. Hypocalcemia
    D. Preexisting left ventricular failure

         (ii) Dobutamine or milrinone may be more appropriate if SVR is increased.

         (iii) Epinephrine or milrinone may be appropriate if HR is elevated.

         (iv) Dobutamine or dopamine may be more appropriate if HR is low and pacing is not being used.

         (v) Norepinephrine or phenylephrine may be appropriate if SVR is low and CO is normal or elevated.

         (vi) Milrinone will significantly reduce SVR, so the use of an arterial vasoconstrictor (phenylephrine, norepinephrine) often is necessary.

    (b) Start NTG if ischemia is present (consider use of short acting β-blockers or calcium channel blockers).

b. RV failure

  (1) Diagnosis

    (a) The RV was once believed to be just a conduit to the pulmonary circulation. This is incorrect. Active pumping by the RV is mandatory for optimal cardiovascular function, particularly in the presence of elevated PA pressures.

    (b) Patients most at risk include those with

         (i) Pulmonary hypertension

             (a) Chronic mitral valve disease

             (b) Left-to-right shunts (atrial septal defect, ventricular septal defect)

             (c) Massive pulmonary embolism

             (d) Air embolism

             (e) Primary pulmonary hypertension

             (f) Acute or chronic mitral regurgitation

                (i) Valvular dysfunction

                (ii) Papillary muscle rupture

             (g) Diastolic LV dysfunction

         (ii) RV ischemia or infarct

         (iii) RV outflow obstruction

         (iv) Tricuspid regurgitation

    (c) Physiologic findings

         (i) Depressed cardiac index (CI)

         (ii) Inappropriate elevation in CVP compared to PCWP (unless biventricular failure exists)

         (iii) Increased PVR (more than 2.5 Wood units or greater than 200 dynes · sec/cm^5)

         (iv) Pulmonary hypertension

         (v) Reduced CVP to PA mean step-up pressure (less than 5 mm Hg) (see Section **II.B.1.d**).

  (2) Treatment

    (a) Treat signs of ischemia.

         (i) Start NTG infusion if systemic BP permits.

         (ii) Increase coronary perfusion pressure.

    (b) Increased preload usually is required.

    (c) Increase inotropic support. Milrinone, dobutamine, and isoproterenol often are effective because any of these will increase RV contractility and decrease PVR.

    (d) Use adjuncts to decrease PVR.

         (i) Hyperventilation will induce hypocapnia and decrease PVR. This should be accomplished by means of a high respiratory rate because an increase in tidal volume may increase PVR.

         (ii) Avoid hypoxemia, which will induce pulmonary vasoconstriction.

         (iii) Avoid acidemia.

(iv) Maintain normal core temperature.

(v) Use pulmonary vasodilators (nitroglycerin, nitroprusside).

(e) Prostaglandin E_1 (PGE_1) infusion through a right atrial line will induce pulmonary vasodilation. This often requires concomitant norepinephrine infusion into the systemic circulation through an LA catheter to avoid marked SVR reduction [10].

(f) Administer nitric oxide (NO) by inhalation (4 to 24 ppm). Some studies suggest that NO improves pulmonary hypertension and weaning parameters better than PGE_1 [11].

(g) Use an RV assist device.

E. **Inappropriate vasodilation** may prevent achievement of an adequate BP despite an acceptable or elevated CI.

   1. Causes include
      a. Preexisting medications (calcium channel blockers, ACE inhibitors)
      b. Electrolyte abnormalities
      c. Acid–base disturbances
      d. Sepsis
      e. Idiopathic condition (poorly characterized factors related to CPB)
      f. Hyperthermia
   2. Excessive hemodilution decreases viscosity and lowers the apparent SVR.
   3. Management includes vasoconstrictors (e.g., phenylephrine or norepinephrine) and red blood cell transfusion, when appropriate.

F. **Resumption of CPB**

   1. The decision to resume CPB after a trial of native circulation must not be made prematurely because there are dangers to resuming CPB (inadequate heparinization, hemolysis), but CPB must be restarted before permanent ischemic damage is sustained by the heart, brain, and kidneys. If diagnosis and treatment of cardiovascular derangements mentioned previously cannot be made within 3 to 5 minutes, reinstitution of CPB is indicated. While the patient is on CPB, diagnosis and treatment should continue but may proceed without markedly increasing the risk of organ failure.

   2. Heparin should be given as needed based on the last activated clotting time measurement made while the patient was on CPB. (If any protamine was given, a **full dose** of heparin, 300 units/kg, is needed before resuming CPB.)

   3. Any mechanical factors that could compromise cardiac performance must be sought and surgically corrected.
      a. Ongoing ischemia based on ECG changes or TEE wall-motion abnormalities may indicate graft occlusion and may require surgical reevaluation for graft patency. A Doppler probe can be used to assess flow.
      b. Valvular abnormalities may be inferred from the PA trace or more specifically by TEE. Evaluation for perivalvular leaks, prosthetic valve function, or residual stenosis/regurgitation should be undertaken at this time, if indicated.

   4. Unsuccessful weaning will necessitate the addition of more aggressive inotropic support. These are added to the first-line regimen.
      a. Second-line agents may include the following (any of which may also be first-line agents):
         (1) Epinephrine will cause increased contractility, a slight decrease in SVR at low-to-moderate dosages, and increased SVR at high dosages.
         (2) Norepinephrine will cause markedly increased SVR and an increase in contractility.
         (3) Milrinone will cause increased contractility and a moderate decrease in SVR.

   5. **Increase monitoring.** LA pressure is a better estimate of LV end-diastolic pressure than PA pressures. Aortic or femoral arterial pressures may be more accurate than radial pressures. Transesophageal or epicardial echocardiography, using a probe in a sterile sheath, can provide valuable data on function and filling and should be considered if reinstituting CPB.

    6. If the second attempt to wean is unsuccessful, continue to optimize preload and afterload with vasodilators or volume infusion as needed.

       a. IABP will augment diastolic BP, increase coronary perfusion, and decrease afterload and should be considered.

       b. If chest closure adversely affects hemodynamics in an edematous poorly functioning heart, then the chest can be left open and covered with a dressing. The patient can be brought to the intensive care unit in this condition and closed in the future.

       c. If available, ventricular assist devices can be life saving after multiple failed attempts to separate the patient from CPB. These usually are used either to rest the "stunned myocardium" or as a bridge to heart transplantation (see Chapter 21).

References

1. Royster RL, Butterworth JF IV, Prielipp RC, et al. A randomized, blinded, placebo-controlled evaluation of calcium chloride and epinephrine for inotropic support after emergence from cardiopulmonary bypass. *Anesth Analg.* 1992;74:3–13.
2. Marquez J, Koehler S, Strelec SR, et al. Repeated dose administration of desmopressin acetate in uncomplicated cardiac surgery: a prospective, blinded, randomized study. *J Cardiothorac Vasc Anesth* 1992;6:674–676.
3. Moore RA, Gallagher JD, Kingsley BP, et al. The effect of ventilation on systemic blood gases in the presence of left ventricular ejection during cardiopulmonary bypass. *J Thorac Cardiovasc Surg* 1985;90:287–290.
4. Bernard F, Denault A, Babin D, et al. Diastolic dysfunction is predictive of difficult weaning from cardiopulmonary bypass. *Anesth Analg* 2001;92:291–298.
5. **Kikura M, Sato S. The efficacy of preemptive milrinone or amrinone therapy in patients undergoing coronary artery bypass grafting. *Anesth Analg* 2002;94: 22–30.**
6. **Mohr R, Lavee J, Goor DA. Inaccuracy of radial artery pressure measurement after cardiac operations. *J Thorac Cardiovasc Surg* 1987;94:286–290.**
7. Salmenpera M, Heinonen J. Pulmonary vascular responses to moderate changes in $PaCO_2$ after cardiopulmonary bypass. *Anesthesiology* 1986;64:311–315.
8. **Hansen RM, Viquerat CE, Matthay MA, et al. Poor correlation between pulmonary arterial wedge pressure and left ventricular end-diastolic volume after coronary artery bypass graft surgery. *Anesthesiology* 1986;64:764–770.**
9. Kopman EA, Ferguson TB. Interaction of right and left ventricular filling pressures at the termination of cardiopulmonary bypass. *J Thorac Cardiovasc Surg* 1985;89:706–708.
10. D'Ambra MN, LaRaia PJ, Philbin DM. Prostaglandin E_1. A new therapy for refractory right heart failure and pulmonary hypertension after mitral valve replacement. *J Thorac Cardiovasc Surg* 1985;89:567–571.
11. **Rajek A, Pernerstorfer T, Kastner J, et al. Inhaled nitric oxide reduces pulmonary vascular resistance more than prostaglandin E1 during heart transplantation. *Anesth Analg* 2000;90:523–530.**

9. THE POSTCARDIOPULMONARY BYPASS PERIOD: A SYSTEMS APPROACH

Sibylle A. Ruesch and Jerrold H. Levy

The postcardiopulmonary bypass period represents a time in which the myocardium is recovering from the insult of surgery, cardiopulmonary bypass (CPB), and the potential inflammatory effects associated with extracorporeal circulation. During this period, major physiologic changes occur and they need to be understood in order to develop proper therapeutic approaches in patient management. The extent of these physiologic alterations and the time to recovery depend on numerous patient and surgical factors. This chapter identifies these physiologic changes and provides a systems approach to proper management of patients in the postbypass period.

   I. **Cardiovascular system.** The cardiovascular system is perhaps the system that undergoes the greatest physiologic stress during CPB and requires the most attention in the immediate postbypass period. Therefore, it is important to identify which factors may adversely affect cardiovascular outcome during this period.
   A. **Factors contributing to adverse cardiovascular outcome in the postbypass period**
      1. **Patient factors**
         a. **Age.** Patients older than 70 years suffer greater cardiac morbidity and mortality. Explanations for this observation include more extensive atherosclerosis, impairment of right ventricular (RV) or left ventricular (LV) function, and greater likelihood of coexistent medical illnesses, such as diabetes, chronic obstructive pulmonary disease, and peripheral vascular disease [1].
         b. **Female gender.** Women represent a high-risk group, particularly in those procedures involving myocardial revascularization. The reason for this is uncertain; however, it has been noted that women are older at the time of presentation for surgery, are less likely to be revascularized, have smaller coronary vessels, and more frequently are diabetic and hypertensive.
         c. **Congestive heart failure.** Preoperative ventricular dysfunction represents a significant risk factor and is associated with a higher mortality. Patients with the following conditions are likely to undergo a surgical procedure in congestive heart failure (CHF): (a) acute valvular dysfunction with hemodynamic deterioration, (b) recent myocardial infarction with ongoing ischemia despite optimal medical therapy, and (c) CHF secondary to significant impairment of LV/RV function.
         d. **Emergency operation.** Patients requiring emergent myocardial revascularization due to ongoing ischemia or hemodynamic deterioration after thrombolytic therapy, or unsuccessful angioplasty or stent placement also represent a high-risk group for multiple reasons. Some patients will be at greater risk for both prebypass and postbypass bleeding due to recent thrombolytic therapy, heparin administration, or recent use of platelet inhibitors including IIb/IIIa receptor antagonists and clopidogrel bisulfate (Plavix).
      2. **Surgical factors**
         a. **During CPB**
            (1) **Prolonged CPB.** Although every revascularization is associated with some kind of transient myocardial impairment in the early postbypass period, the extent of it is mainly dependent on prebypass RV and LV function and degree of dyssynergy. With adequate myocardial preservation, myocardial damage is unlikely to occur in most individuals with aortic cross-clamping of less than 2 hours' duration [2]. Cross-clamping times exceeding this interval may result in impairment of myocardial performance. Also, as the duration of CPB increases, functional platelet abnormalities and the potential for bleeding and coagulopathy also increase.
            (2) **Inadequate repair**
               (a) **Coronary artery.** Myocardial revascularization may be inadequate for several reasons. The most common etiology is diffuse vascular disease distal to the site of the coronary anastomoses, which is most likely to occur in patients with smaller distal vessels, such as the elderly individuals, diabetics, and women. Other

possible causes of impaired revascularization include technically difficult distal anastomoses as well as vein grafts or internal mammary arteries of poor quality, or, alternately, a diffusely atherosclerotic aorta where surgical technique was modified to avoid atheroembolic episodes.

(b) **Valves.** When a patient is hemodynamically unstable in the postbypass period after a valve replacement, first consideration must be given to a mechanical problem. Possibilities include (a) mechanical obstruction due to valve malfunction (stuck leaflet), (b) incorrect sewing of the valve (backward), (c) failure of a suture line resulting in a significant perivalvular leak, or (d) atrioventricular (AV) disruption after mitral valve replacement. Patients undergoing valve surgery also are placed at risk by the presence of intraventricular air, which may embolize to the coronary [preferably the right coronary artery (RCA) due to anatomic considerations] or carotid artery when the heart starts ejecting.

(3) **Inadequate myocardial protection**

(a) **Inadequate myocardial cooling and cardioplegia administration.** Optimal protection of the myocardium during CPB is essential for the prevention of prolonged postbypass cardiac dysfunction. The loss of cardiac contraction (asystole) has the greatest impact in reducing the cardiac metabolism, followed by hypothermia. Therefore, most surgeons use a combination of cold cardioplegia, moderate patient hypothermia, and topical application of ice slush to ensure adequate myocardial protection. Delivery of the cardioplegia is easier to the LV because several routes can be used (anterograde, retrograde, or combined). In contrast, the RV can only be correctly protected with anterograde cardioplegia because the retrograde delivery through the coronary sinuses is inhomogeneously distributed to the RV. Patients with significant RCA disease are therefore more at risk for postbypass RV dysfunction secondary to suboptimal myocardial protection and will rely on the topical cooling.

(b) **Improper venting of the heart.** Cardiac distention should be avoided because this leads to increased myocardial wall tension and increased O_2 consumption. Several factors that may promote distention include increase in coronary collateral blood flow, aortic insufficiency, ventricular fibrillation (VF), and repeated administration of cardioplegia. Decompression is most commonly achieved with the use of an LV vent, which usually is inserted at the junction of the left atrium and right superior pulmonary vein or through the pulmonary artery (PA). Alternately, the left atrial appendage may be cut to allow spontaneous decompression. When venting is utilized, it is important to ensure that air is removed before ventricular ejection.

(c) **Impaired myocardial perfusion.** Coronary perfusion pressure is defined as the mean pressure in the aortic root during diastole minus LV intracavitary pressure. Although extensive debate exists as to what is the ideal coronary perfusion pressure, it is believed that a pressure between 50 and 70 mm Hg is adequate in most circumstances during CPB. Higher pressures may be required in cases of severe coronary stenosis, marked LV hypertrophy, and in instances where there is temporary ventricular distention. Myocardial flow also may be impaired at the time of reperfusion when emboli in the form of air or atheromatous debris may be present.

(d) **Ventricular fibrillation** has a deleterious effect on the heart, resulting in increased O_2 consumption, elevated wall tension, and subsequent decrease in subendocardial flow. Appropriate management includes increasing coronary perfusion pressure, cooling the patient, and, if possible, immediately cross-clamping the aorta, with infusion of a cardioplegic agent to arrest the heart.

(4) Ventriculotomy. Ventriculotomy will lead to entrainment of air and debris into the heart and predispose to embolization of the coronary and cerebral circulations. It is a type of myocardial trauma that may contribute to impaired cardiac performance in the postbypass period.

(5) Reperfusion injury. Reperfusion injury describes a series of functional, structural, and metabolic alterations that result from reperfusion of myocardium after a period of temporary ischemia. The potential for this type of injury exists for all cardiac procedures where the aorta is clamped. The damage is characterized by (a) cytosolic accumulation of calcium; (b) marked cell swelling (myocardial edema), which decreases postischemic blood flow and ventricular compliance; and (c) generation of free radicals resulting from reintroduction of O_2 during reperfusion. These oxygen-free radicals can cause membrane damage by lipid peroxidation. Various strategies are used to minimize injury, including reoxygenation with warm blood to start aerobic metabolism as well as other evolving strategies.

b. Post-CPB

(1) Decannulation. When the patient is hemodynamically stable after separation from CPB, the venous cannula(s) is (are) removed. Blood loss and atrial dysrhythmias are the most common complications during repair of the atrial cannula site. After infusion of the appropriate volume of blood from the pump, the aortic cannula is clamped and removed. Although the timing and technique of removal vary among institutions, most centers remove the cannula before infusion of protamine. In addition, to minimize blood loss and prevent possible aortic disruption, the blood pressure frequently is lowered to reduce tension on the aortic wall. If, during aortic cannula removal, there is significant blood loss resulting in hemodynamic deterioration, a cannula may quickly be reinserted into the right atrium and the appropriate volume infused to achieve stability. However, some institutions will leave the aortic cannula in place during the initial infusion of protamine.

(2) Manipulation of the heart. The heart often is lifted after bypass, to allow examination of the distal anastomotic sites. The sequelae of this action include impaired venous return, atrial and ventricular dysrhythmias, and decreased ventricular ejection, all of which result in systemic hypotension. Manipulation such as this should be limited to brief periods in order to avoid ischemia and hemodynamic deterioration. Also, "overtreatment" of these hypotensive episodes with the administration of catecholamine boluses should be avoided, as it usually results in major hypertension when mechanical manipulation is stopped. Very high blood pressure at this stage can lead to graft disruption and increased bleeding.

(3) Myocardial ischemia

(a) Coronary artery spasm. Ischemia in the postbypass period may be secondary to spasm of the native coronary vessels or internal mammary artery. This typically manifests as ST-segment elevation, although dysrhythmias, severe hypotension, and cardiac arrest also may occur as sequelae. Mechanisms that have been proposed include intense coronary vasoconstriction from hypothermia, local trauma, respiratory alkalosis, excess sympathetic stimulation of the α-receptors on the coronary vessels, release of vasoconstricting agents from platelets (thromboxane), and injury to native vascular endothelium with the loss of endogenous vascular relaxing factors (i.e., endothelium-derived relaxing factor and prostacyclin). Therapeutic modalities that have been used successfully to treat coronary spasm include intra-coronary administration of drugs including nitroglycerin, pa-paverine, or systemic administration of nitroglycerin; calcium channel blockers (e.g., nicardipine); and other phosphodiesterase inhibitors (milrinone or inamrinone) [3].

   (b) Mechanical obstruction. Compression of vein or internal mammary artery grafts can produce myocardial ischemia and should be considered. Ventilation with large tidal volumes can intermittently impair internal mammary artery graft flow and the distended lung can lead to disruption of the graft at the anastomotic site.

   (c) Inadequate revascularization. See Section **(2)** above.

(4) Protamine administration. See Section **III.A.4.**

(5) Chest closure. During chest closure, hemodynamic deterioration may ensue. In general, patients with normal LV function and ade-quate intravascular volume tolerate closure without problems. Some patients experience mild hypotension and will respond promptly to volume administration. In individuals with poor ventricular function or patients currently receiving inotropic agents, additional volume or inotropic support may be required to maintain similar hemodynam-ics. If these interventions fail, the surgeon may be required to reopen the chest. Use of transesophageal echocardiography (TEE) can be es-pecially useful to sort out the causes of hemodynamic instability, in-cluding myocardial ischemia with new wall-motion abnormalities or hypovolemia.

   Chest closure may cause cardiovascular deterioration for the fol-lowing reasons. (a) In patients who have significant myocardial edema, closure will impair RV contractility and venous return. (b) Edematous, overdistended lungs can lead to a tamponade-like effect after closure in patient with severe chronic obstructive lung (pulmonary) disease (COPD). (c) A nonidentified source of bleeding before adaptation of the sternal borders can lead to cardiac tamponade with significant change in hemodynamics. (d) Finally, closure may result in a vein or internal mammary artery graft becoming kinked, with the develop-ment of ischemia in the area of the jeopardized myocardium. If these mechanical problems are eliminated and hemodynamics remain com-promised, the chest may need to be left opened temporarily.

B. Management of hemodynamics in the postbypass period. Proper manage-ment of patients in the postbypass period involves continuous assessment of five hemodynamic variables. These are preload, rate, rhythm, contractility, and after-load. Patients with new onset atrial fibrillation should be cardioverted and VF/ventricular tachycardia (VT) should be shocked as well. For the patient with re-current VT/VF despite defibrillation, intravenous amiodarone should be considered, based on the revised advanced cardiopulmonary life support (ACLS) guidelines, using a 150-mg load, 1 mg/min infusion, and additional 150-mg loads followed by defibrillation until an appropriate rhythm is established.

   1. Preload. Assessment of volume status is most commonly achieved by measur-ing the PA occlusion pressure (PAOP); however, the role of TEE in assessing ventricular volumes and preload is rapidly expanding in cardiac anesthesiology practice. What represents the ideal value will vary from one patient to another. Generally, however, a higher PAOP may be required postbypass to generate the same stroke volume because of a decrease in myocardial compliance. Other means of assessing preload include intermittent visualization of the heart until chest closure. Although administration of adequate volume is essential to opti-mize the patient's hemodynamics, it is of paramount importance to prevent ventricular distention.

   2. Rate. To achieve an adequate cardiac index, a faster heart rate may be re-quired. Although the lower limit of heart rate has not been determined, a rate greater than 70 bpm is generally acceptable and easy to achieve with atrial pacing. Slow heart rates or atrial/ventricular dyssynchronization are one of the most easily correctable parameters affecting cardiac output. Pacing should always be kept in mind to improve hemodynamics if the patient's cardiac index falls.

3. **Rhythm.** The ideal rhythm after bypass is sinus rhythm or atrial pacing in order to improve ventricular filling in the patient with a noncompliant LV after cardiac surgery, especially in the patient with preexisting ventricular dysfunction. Normally the "atrial kick" provides about 20% of ventricular filling, but this may be a significantly higher fraction after CPB, when ventricular dysfunction and reduced compliance are present. Other individuals will manifest variable degrees of AV block and require AV pacing after bypass. On occasion, rhythms such as supraventricular tachycardia or atrial fibrillation will occur and are best managed by cardioversion. Those patients with chronic atrial fibrillation usually are refractory to this therapy and require ventricular pacing. Even when pacing is not required postbypass, it is important to confirm that both the atrial and ventricular pacing wires are functional before chest closure and that pacing thresholds are not excessively high.

4. **Contractility.** Contractility may be best assessed with TEE, but it is a complex parameter that often is assessed indirectly with different measurements. However, TEE is the only examination that can make a distinction between regional or global impairment of myocardial function and quantify LV function. Direct visualization of the heart can be used to assess contractility and volume status; however, it is predominantly the RV that is viewed through a median sternotomy. Although determination of cardiac index should be made initially after separation from bypass, multiple factors affect it. Cardiac index then should be measured at any time when there is a significant change in patient hemodynamics as well as after chest closure. Although a cardiac index of 2.2 L/min/m^2 or greater is considered acceptable, the actual number is affected by rate, rhythm, and volume status. Before initiation of inotropic therapy, it is important to check heart rate and rhythm as well as the volume status of the patient. Optimization of these parameters may be all that is needed to augment cardiac index. If an inotrope is required, usually the choice of agent(s) will be based on preexisting ventricular dysfunction and down-regulation of β-adrenergic receptors as well as anticipated problems with systemic vascular resistance (SVR) and pulmonary vascular resistance (PVR) [4].

5. **Afterload.** Afterload is the force that opposes ventricular fiber shortening during systole. It is related directly to chamber dimension and inversely to wall thickness. In clinical practice, SVR is a parameter used to measure afterload. SVR; however, is only one component of ventricular afterload that is a derived hemodynamic parameter not routinely indexed to body surface area.

   Alterations in calculated SVR after bypass typically are manifested as changes in blood pressure and cardiac output. Increases in SVR may be related to an inadequate level of anesthesia, hypothermia, preexisting hypertension, intrinsic vascular disease, or use of drugs with vasoconstrictive properties. In patients with normal or elevated blood pressure and adequate cardiac index, reduction in vascular resistance can be achieved with a vasodilator (i.e., nitroglycerin, nicardipine, or nitroprusside) or an inhalational anesthetic agent. The intravenous calcium channel blockers (i.e., nicardipine) are arterial vasodilators, have no effects on the venous capacitance bed, and offer better choices when treating post-CPB hypertension in the patient with good ventricular function. If cardiac index is depressed, however, catecholamines alone or in combination with the cyclic adenosine monophosphate (cAMP)-specific (type III) phosphodiesterase inhibitors, such as milrinone, may be required.

   Etiologies of a low SVR postbypass include vasodilatory shock due to overwarming, use of angiotensin-converting enzyme (ACE) inhibitors, transfusion reactions, and anaphylactic/anaphylactoid reactions. Treatment will depend on the specific etiology. Management frequently includes use of an arteriolar vasoconstricting agent to maintain coronary perfusion pressure. Patients with an elevated cardiac index will benefit from either norepinephrine or phenylephrine. Patients with a depressed index will require an agent that has both β- and α-stimulating properties, such as norepinephrine. Norepinephrine is a safe and effective agent for treating hypotension in the postbypass period. For vasodilatory shock refractory to norepinephrine post-CPB, arginine vasopressin should be considered with a high cardiac index.

C. **Postbypass cardiovascular collapse.** Although profound cardiovascular collapse after bypass is uncommon, it is likely that a technical problem (ischemia, valvular dysfunction) or severe metabolic derangement exists, and TEE should be considered to help make the correct diagnosis. If cardiovascular deterioration is unresponsive to maximal inotropic therapy and no immediate reversible cause can be identified (Fig. 9.1), then reinstitution of CPB will be necessary. When this decision is made, protamine, if being administered, must be stopped and the patient must receive a standard bolus dose of heparin. During the period that it takes to reestablish CPB, it is important to maintain coronary and cerebral perfusion with inotropes and vasopressors. In extreme circumstances it may be necessary for the surgical assistant to initiate open chest massage, while the surgeon places the arterial and venous cannulas.

When CPB is initiated, all inotropes and vasopressors should initially be stopped, because patients in this situation frequently become hypertensive. If blood pressure elevation is marked, the perfusionist can lower pump flow briefly while appropriate vasodilator therapy is given. Resumption of extracorporeal circulation will significantly lower myocardial oxygen requirements. Maintenance of a reasonable perfusion pressure is critical to allow adequate O_2 delivery to potentially ischemic cells. This should be achieved with a pure α agent such as phenylephrine. Despite lower O_2 requirements and adequate supply, the ischemic cell may not be able to utilize O_2 efficiently. This has resulted in the use of secondary cardioplegia.

Additional recovery and reversal of damage can occur if the heart is rearrested with warm blood–enriched cardioplegia for a brief period. Consideration to separate from bypass should be made only after the surgeon is assured that technical difficulties did not account for impaired myocardial performance and that the heart is "adequately rested." In many cases, intraaortic balloon counterpulsation will be initiated to avoid the increased O_2 demands associated with maximal inotrope therapy.

II. **Respiratory system**
  A. **Pulmonary edema**
    1. **Post-CPB pulmonary dysfunction.** Pulmonary dysfunction after CPB is a common event; however, the extent and severity often vary. The alveolar-arterial (A-a) O_2 gradient increases after bypass and becomes maximal at approximately 18 to 48 hours postoperatively. The ethology of this ventilation–perfusion mismatch is presumed to be an increase in pulmonary interstitial fluid and results in hypoxemia and hypercapnia. In its most severe state, a form of adult respiratory distress syndrome develops and is referred to as *postperfusion lung syndrome* [5]. Numerous etiologic factors have been suggested, including loss of surfactant, hypoxic damage to lung tissue, and pulmonary vasculitis caused by hemolyzed blood, protein denaturation, and multiple pulmonary emboli. Another mechanism of damage is lung accumulation of activated neutrophils containing lysosomal enzymes that produce pulmonary capillary damage and subsequent leakage of plasma. Transfusion reactions and transfusion-related acute lung injury also might play a role in pulmonary dysfunction. Postperfusion lung syndrome has virtually been eliminated today with the use of membrane oxygenators, which has greatly diminished blood trauma.
    2. **LV dysfunction.** Poor ventricular function in the postbypass period will result in elevated pulmonary venous pressures. This, combined with reduced colloid osmotic pressure secondary to hemodilution, will result in increased pulmonary interstitial fluid.
    3. **Preexisting pulmonary edema.** Individuals presenting for surgery with pulmonary edema represent a significant risk. These patients may be extremely difficult to oxygenate or ventilate after CPB. Techniques that may improve oxygenation include ultrafiltration and aggressive diuresis while on bypass.

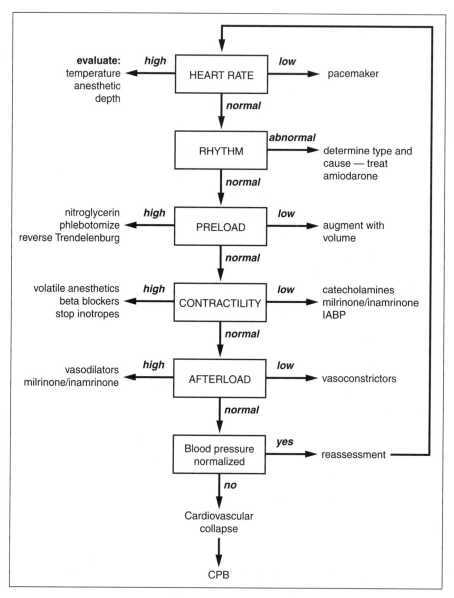

FIG. 9.1 Management scheme for cardiovascular dysfunction in the postbypass period. *CPB,* cardiopulmonary bypass; *IABP,* intraaortic balloon pump.

    4. Anaphylactic reactions. Certain drugs, such as protamine, and administration of blood products or colloid volume expanders may, on rare occasions, cause an increase in pulmonary capillary permeability.

B. Mechanical factors

    1. Pneumothorax occurs most commonly when the pleural cavity is entered during dissection of the internal mammary artery. Other etiologic factors include barotrauma from excess positive-pressure ventilation, particularly in patients with low lung or chest wall compliance, and entry into the pleural space as a complication of central venous access. A pneumothorax may manifest itself only after chest closure.

2. **Hemothorax.** Accumulation of blood in the pleural cavity can occur during bypass as blood from the mediastinum frequently overfills the pericardial sling. It also may occur with dissection of the internal mammary artery before administration of heparin, which results in the collection of clot in the pleural space. The pleural space should be examined, and adequate removal of blood and clot is imperative before termination of CPB and before chest closure.

3. **Movement of the endotracheal tube.** Draping the patient for cardiac procedures often will result in part of the head and endotracheal tube being obscured from direct vision. Even when the endotracheal tube is visualized, the surgeon frequently will push on this tube in an attempt to gain better surgical exposure, which may result in its displacement. Therefore, it is important intermittently to reconfirm proper positioning by checking all connections, observing bilateral chest movement, and visualizing one or both lung fields if the pleural cavities are exposed.

4. **Obstruction of the tracheobronchial tree**
    a. **Mucous plug.** Dry inspissated secretions may accumulate in the tracheobronchial tree or endotracheal tube and partially or completely obstruct the airway. In most cases, this can be diagnosed and managed by suctioning the airway with a small catheter.
    b. **Blood.** Injury to the upper airway or trachea due to laryngoscopy, placement of an endotracheal tube, or an unrecognized preexistent airway lesion followed by heparinization may result in aspiration of blood. If significant, this can result in varying degrees of airway obstruction. More likely, however, the blood will be aspirated into the distal airways and alveoli, causing marked ventilation–perfusion mismatch. Blood also may appear in the airway due to perforation of the PA secondary to inappropriate management of the PA catheter. Frequent manipulation of the heart and continuous changes in intravascular volume may result in movement of the catheter into the wedge position. Subsequent balloon inflation could perforate the PA. Risk factors for inadvertent pulmonary artery catheter (PAC) displacement include advanced patient age, anticoagulation, hypothermia, and pulmonary hypertension.

C. **Protamine administration.** See Section **III.A.4.**

D. **Intrapulmonary shunt**
    1. **Atelectasis.** Perhaps the most common cause of decreased arterial oxygenation postbypass is atelectasis. Although diffuse, chest radiographs postoperatively frequently reveal a pattern of left lower lobe infiltration and atelectasis. The likely explanation is that application of ice causes temporary phrenic nerve injury with subsequent paralysis of the left leaf of the diaphragm. Attempts to prevent or attenuate atelectasis by ventilation of the nonperfused lungs during bypass have been unsuccessful.
    2. **Inhibition of hypoxic pulmonary vasoconstriction.** Hypoxic pulmonary vasoconstriction is the mechanism believed to be responsible for the increase in PVR in regions of atelectasis. This selective increase in resistance diverts blood away from hypoxic areas toward normoxic ventilated lung segments, thereby minimizing shunt. This protective mechanism can be attenuated or inhibited by the use of vasodilators (nitroprusside, nitroglycerin) and inotropes.

E. **Intracardiac shunt.** When evaluating hypoxemia after CPB, the possibility of a right-to-left shunt must always be considered. Decreased RV contractility and compliance after CPB, in the presence of increased PVR associated with positive end-expiratory pressure (PEEP), frequently will elevate right atrial pressures above those on the left side. This equalization or reversal of pressure is the mechanism by which a patent foramen is opened. A helpful diagnostic tool in detecting a right-to-left shunt at the atrial level is TEE.

III. Hematologic system
A. Protamine

1. **Pharmacology.** Protamine is a highly alkaline polycationic protein derived from salmon sperm that is predominantly arginine. Protamine binds the polyanionic glycosaminoglycan heparin and therefore neutralizes its effect. The clinical applications of protamine include neutralizing the effects of heparin and delaying the absorption of subcutaneously administered insulin.

2. **Dose.** Various methods have been used to determine the appropriate dose of protamine needed to reverse the effects of heparin. Some of these are detailed here.

   In 1975, Bull et al. [6] recommended the quantitative neutralization of heparin. By using the *heparin dose–response curve based on activated clotting time* (ACT) just before separation from CPB, one could determine the amount of circulating heparin remaining. This relationship assumed that only heparin was responsible for ACT prolongation. Bull et al. recommended that 1.3 mg of protamine would adequately neutralize 100 units of circulating heparin in most individuals. However, this technique greatly overestimates the amount of protamine required at the end of CPB.

   The automated heparin protamine titration test represents a more precise method for determining the residual heparin concentration at the termination of bypass, by performing an in vitro neutralization of heparin based on different doses of protamine (Medtronic-HemoTec Heparin Monitoring System-HMS, Englewood, CO, U.S.A.). It automatically calculates the required dose of protamine. Using this technique, the total dose of protamine administered is less than that using a fixed protamine-heparin regimen.

   Most clinicians use *fixed dosing of protamine* for neutralizing heparin, which is based on a fixed protamine/heparin ratio determined by the total heparin administered during the initiation of CPB [7]. The ratio used is 0.5 to 1.0 mg of protamine for every 100 units of heparin given to the patient. Lower doses often are all that is required to reverse heparin, because heparin levels decrease with time.

3. **Route and rate.** Protamine may be administered safely by either a central or a peripheral route. The most important factor in keeping hemodynamic changes at their lowest possible level is the rate of administration. Although this rate varies considerably among institutions, a suggested interval for the initial dose of protamine is as an infusion over 10 to 15 minutes, but no faster than 25 to 50 mg/min. Infusing protamine over 30 minutes may reduce the incidence of heparin rebound compared with administration over 5 minutes.

4. **Classification of protamine reactions.** Multiple reactions to protamine have been described. The most life-threatening types of reactions are called *anaphylaxis* [8]. Anaphylactic reactions are mediated by immunoglobulin E antibodies, which bind to the surface of mast cells and basophils. Prior exposure to protamine or similar antigen is required to produce this sensitization. On reexposure, these cells will release histamine, prostaglandins, and chemotactic factors, thereby initiating an anaphylactic response characterized by vascular collapse. *Anaphylactoid reactions* are nonimmunologic and therefore do not require previous exposure to the antigen. Both immunoglobulin G (IgG) antibodies to protamine and heparin–protamine complexes can activate the complement system with the generation of fragments called *anaphylatoxins*. Complement-mediated reactions can range from mild changes to acute cardiovascular collapse, pulmonary vasoconstriction, and RV failure. The hemodynamic consequences of catastrophic pulmonary vasoconstriction include a several-fold increase in PA pressure followed by RV distention and hypokinesis. This obstruction to RV outflow results in severe systemic hypotension requiring inotropic support to restore circulatory stability. The presumed mechanism is the activation of complement, which results in the generation of thromboxane causing acute pulmonary vasoconstriction. This reaction may represent an anaphylactic reaction mediated by complement-fixing IgG antibodies. Therapy for these protamine reactions is listed in Table 9.1.

Table 9.1 Therapy for idiosyncratic protamine reactions

Initial therapy
1. Stop administration of protamine
2. Maintain airway with 100% O_2
3. Discontinue all anesthetic agents
4. Start intravascular volume expansion (2–4 L of crystalloid with hypotension)
5. Give epinephrine (5–10 µg IV bolus with hypotension, titrate as needed; 0.1–1.0 mg IV with cardiovascular collapse)
6. Reinstitute cardiopulmonary bypass for severe reactions to allow time for drug therapy to take effect

Secondary treatment
1. Antihistamines (0.5–1 mg/kg diphenhydramine)
2. Catecholamine infusions (starting doses: epinephrine, 5–10 µg/min, norepinephrine, 5–10 µg/min as an infusion, titrated to desired effects), arginine vasopressin (0.1 units/min)
3. Aminophylline (5–6 mg/kg over 20 min with persistent bronchospasm) followed by infusion
4. Corticosteroids (0.25–1.00 g hydrocortisone; alternatively, 1–2 g methylprednisolone)[a]
5. Sodium bicarbonate (0.5–1.0 mEq/kg with persistent hypotension or acidosis)

Specific treatment for catastrophic pulmonary vasoconstriction
Therapy as above; once diagnosed, treatment of pulmonary hypertension, right ventricular failure, and bronchoconstriction should include immediate hyperventilation and one or more of the following treatments: milrinone or inamrinone; prostaglandin E_1 and left atrial norepinephrine; inhaled nitric oxide.

[a] Methylprednisolone may be the drug of choice if the reaction is suspected to be mediated by complement.
IV, intravenous.
Modified from Levy JH. *Anaphylactic reactions in anesthesia and intensive care,* 2nd ed. Boston: Butterworth-Heinemann, 1992: 162.

5. **Alternatives to protamine.** Unfortunately, there are no current protamine alternatives available; however, several alternatives have been used for potential protamine allergic patients. *Platelet factor 4 or heparinase* has been used in clinical studies to reverse heparin in cardiac surgery [9]. Hexadimethrine (polybrene) is no longer available for clinical use.

One alternative is removal of a major element in the coagulation cascade. *Defibrinogenemia* has been achieved with ancrod, an enzyme found in the Malayan pit viper. This form of anticoagulation for bypass has been used in a small group of individuals only. To assure its effectiveness as an anticoagulant, it is necessary to monitor fibrinogen levels.

Protamine may be avoided by allowing the *spontaneous termination of heparin's action.* Although this has been used in individuals who are at risk for a protamine reaction, it represents a technique that results in increased blood product administration.

B. **Blood conservation**
   1. **Autologous transfusions**
      a. **Preoperative donation.** Although preoperative autologous blood donations in patients undergoing cardiac surgery have been used, this is not practical for the majority of cardiac surgical patients, and it may not be cost effective.
      b. **Prebypass phlebotomy/autologous normovolemic hemodilution.** Intraoperative hemodilution by means of phlebotomy may reduce the requirement for homologous red blood cell transfusion [10]. Patients should have a hematocrit greater than 0.35 before blood is removed. The amount of removed blood varies from 1 to 3 units (500 to 1,500 mL) and depends on the baseline hematocrit as well as the age of the patient, the patient's body surface area, and the presence of any coexisting diseases [11]. Prebypass

phlebotomy may be accomplished before heparinization and the blood placed in citrate phosphate dextrose (CPD) blood bags, or it may be done just before initiation of bypass, when blood is collected from the venous line of the CPB circuit.

   c. **Intraoperative blood salvage.** Blood that is lost before systemic heparinization or after protamine administration can be retrieved by a system that adds heparin or other anticoagulants. This salvaged blood is washed and filtered such that the remaining product is packed red blood cells. Several systems are commercially available for this purpose.

   d. **Shed blood.** Blood collected from both the mediastinum and pleural cavities in the postoperative period can be reinfused to the patient; however, this product collected from these sites does not clot due to defibrination, has an increased free hemoglobin content, and contains a spectrum of other hemostatic activation products that may not be ideal for reinfusion unless urgently needed or washed and spun.

2. **Acceptance of a lower hematocrit.** What constitutes an acceptable postbypass hematocrit in patients undergoing cardiac surgery still remains controversial and varies among institutions. Patients who are healthy and demonstrate good ventricular function after bypass generally tolerate hematocrits in the range from 23% to 25%. Those individuals who have a reduced capacity to increase cardiac output, who continue to have limited coronary blood flow, or who have increased metabolic demands will require the increased O_2-carrying capacity afforded by a higher hematocrit. Therefore, in patients with ventricular dysfunction and incomplete revascularization, as well as in older patients, packed red blood cells should be considered for the treatment of hypovolemia.

3. **Pharmacologic therapy**

   a. **Erythropoietin.** Recombinant human erythropoietin stimulates the bone marrow to produce red blood cells. Current use of this product requires considerable amounts of time that often is not afforded in cardiac surgery and requires concomitant iron administration.

   b. **Aprotinin.** When administered before and during CPB, aprotinin significantly decreases postoperative bleeding and reduces the need for allogenic transfusions in cardiac surgical patients requiring CPB [12]. Aprotinin has been shown to be safe and effective in reducing transfusions in high-risk patients, and it is the only agent approved by the US Food and Drug Administration for this purpose. Multiple mechanisms of action are likely responsible, including antiinflammatory effects, inhibition of multiple proteases, and antifibrinolytic effects [13]. Aprotinin therapy should be instituted before incision and sternotomy.

   c. **E-Aminocaproic acid or tranexamic acid.** Both E-aminocaproic acid (EACA) and tranexamic acid are synthetic fibrinolytic inhibitors that act by occupying the lysine binding sites on plasminogen and plasmin. This, in turn, displaces these proteins from the lysine residues on fibrinogen and fibrin and interferes with the ability of plasmin to split fibrinogen. Although the routine use of fibrinolytic inhibitors in open heart surgery is controversial, it has been shown to result in modest reductions of bleeding after primary coronary bypass procedures.

   d. **Desmopressin acetate.** Desmopressin acetate (DDAVP) is believed to exert its effects by increasing the release of factor VIII(C) and von Willebrand factor. Von Willebrand factor multimers play a role in enhancing platelet adhesiveness. The prophylactic use of DDAVP (0.3 µg/kg administered after bypass) in patients undergoing elective coronary artery bypass grafting was shown not to decrease blood loss or blood product administration. DDAVP may have a beneficial effect in certain subsets of patients including those with preexisting uremia.

IV. **Renal system**

   A. **Effects of CPB on the kidneys.** Many of the variables introduced with initiation of CPB have an effect on the renal system. Hemodilution, for example, reduces renal vascular resistance, resulting in increased flow to the outer renal cortex and subsequent enhanced urine flow. If systemic hypothermia is used as a form of myocardial protection, renal vascular resistance increases and renal blood flow, glomerular filtration rate, and free water clearance all decrease. Other variables that have the potential to impair renal function significantly in the postoperative period include microemboli and hemolysis of red blood cells.

B. Postbypass renal dysfunction. Certain factors have been identified that place patients at risk for renal dysfunction in the postbypass period. These include elevated preoperative serum creatinine, combined valve and bypass procedures, and advanced age. Prolonged bypass times also may place patients at risk. Although a topic of some debate, the mode of perfusion (pulsatile vs. nonpulsatile) does not appear to influence perioperative renal function.

C. Management. Pharmacologic therapy may have some benefit in patients with severe renal dysfunction or failure. A frequent observation is that urine flow is diminished during bypass compared with individuals who have normal renal function. This may result in significant hyperkalemia and accumulation of extracellular fluid. Administration of furosemide (initial dose 5 mg) or mannitol (0.5 to 1.0 mg/kg) has been shown to increase urine output in these patients. Fenoldopam in low dose (0.05 to 0.1 µg/kg/min) will increased renal blood flow and may provide an important therapeutic option. Despite these interventions, some patients will require ultrafiltration during bypass or potentially dialysis in the early postoperative period.

V. Central nervous system

A. Anesthetic depth. The modern assessment of anesthetic depth with the bispectral index monitor adds important information for the proper management of the patient. In the postbypass period there are varying levels of surgical stimulation, with the highest being the placement of sternal wires and chest closure. If an increase in the depth of anesthesia is needed, the choice of agent(s) will depend primarily on the hemodynamic status of the patient.

Small doses of opioids or benzodiazepines can be titrated incrementally in patients with stable hemodynamics. Additionally, judicious use of a volatile agent may be considered, particularly in patients who are hypertensive.

Use of *nitrous oxide should be avoided* after bypass for several reasons. Nitrous oxide has the capability of enlarging air emboli that may have been generated during bypass. Many patients require high inspired concentrations of O_2 during this period for reasons already mentioned. Finally, nitrous oxide can elevate PA pressures in those with preexisting pulmonary hypertension and can depress RV function.

It must be remembered that all patients have some degree of postbypass ventricular dysfunction. Even small doses of narcotics have the potential to cause adverse hemodynamic consequences.

B. Neuromuscular blockade. Patients frequently require additional neuromuscular relaxation in the postbypass period. The main objective is to prevent shivering, which in some circumstances can increase O_2 consumption by 500%. To ensure adequate O_2 delivery to tissues in this circumstance, an increase in cardiac output would be required that may not be possible without inotropic support. The muscle relaxant can be selected for its specific hemodynamic characteristics and duration of action.

VI. Metabolic considerations

A. Electrolyte disturbances

1. Hypokalemia is a relatively common electrolyte abnormality in the postbypass period. Although the etiologic factors of hypokalemia are numerous, only those unique to bypass will be mentioned. The kidney represents a major source of potassium loss. Both the preoperative and intraoperative use of diuretics, including mannitol administration on bypass, promotes significant potassium wasting. Glucose may be administered as a myocardial substrate during bypass. If significant hyperglycemia occurs, an osmotic diuresis with potassium loss will ensue. Hypokalemia also may result from the shift of potassium to the intracellular space. Such a shift may occur with alkalemia, from either hyperventilation or excess bicarbonate administration and with concomitant administration of insulin in a diabetic patient. In addition, use of inotropes capable of stimulating β_2-receptors will promote the intracellular shift of potassium. Treatment will vary depending on the severity of hypokalemia. In most instances, intravenous administration up to 10 mEq/hour (in adults) will be effective. In life-threatening situations, potassium may be administered at a rate of 20 mEq/hour with continuous cardiac monitoring.

2. **Hyperkalemia** occurs uncommonly after bypass. In most cases, hyperkalemia occurs when large doses of cardioplegic agents are administered, particularly in patients with impaired renal function. Hyperkalemia may persist in the postbypass period but generally resolves spontaneously without intervention. Depending on the cardiac rhythm, moderate hyperkalemia (potassium levels between 6.0 and 7.0 mEq/L) may require therapy with one of the treatment modalities listed in Table 9.2. With severe hyperkalemia (potassium levels greater than 7.0 mEq/L), all therapeutic interventions may be needed.

3. **Hypocalcemia** can occur after bypass, although the incidence is unknown. Common etiologic factors include hemodilution from the pump prime, particularly in children; acute alkalemia; and calcium sequestration. Alkalemia that occurs with hyperventilation or rapid administration of parenteral bicarbonate results in enhanced binding of calcium to protein. Sequestration of calcium occurs with administration of a large volume of blood that contains the chelating agent citrate. Severe hypocalcemia results in myocardial depression and vasodilation.

   Calcium administration after CPB is indicated in the presence of severe hyperkalemia or in cases of hypotension associated with a low serum ionized calcium. Calcium may be administered as 10% calcium chloride (272 mg of elemental calcium) in a dose of 5 to 10 mg/kg.

   Routine administration of calcium after CPB is controversial because of its potential adverse effects. During the period of ischemia, there is a decrease in the production of high-energy phosphates, which results in the accumulation of cytosolic calcium. This increase in calcium during reperfusion reduces diastolic compliance and impairs relaxation. This fact must be considered when administering calcium in the postbypass period; however, the exact relationship between exogenously administered calcium and its intracellular accumulation has yet to be delineated.

4. **Hypomagnesemia** commonly occurs in patients undergoing cardiac surgery. England and colleagues [14] suggested that large quantities of magnesium-free fluids with subsequent hemodilution most likely contribute to this observation. Other etiologic factors include loss of the cation in the extracorporeal circuit and redistribution of magnesium to other body stores. These authors conducted a randomized, controlled trial with patients in the treatment group receiving 2 g of magnesium chloride after termination of CPB. Magnesium-treated patients had a lower incidence of postoperative ventricular dysrhythmias and an increased cardiac index in the early postoperative period.

B. **Hyperglycemia.** Certain groups of patients are at risk for developing hyperglycemia during cardiac surgery. Diabetics, particularly those who are insulin dependent, usually require an intraoperative insulin infusion to maintain glucose hemostasis. Glucose-containing solutions are used at some centers as the sole priming solution for the CPB circuit. Marked hyperglycemia may occur in patients on bypass and may persist into the postoperative period. Reported benefits from

Table 9.2 Treatment of hyperkalemia

1. Diuresis
2. Sodium bicarbonate, 1–2 mEq/kg in children and one ampule (44.6 mEq) in adults
3. Infusion of dextrose and insulin, 1–2 g glucose per kilogram with 0.3 units regular insulin per gram of glucose in children; 25 g (1 ampule of D50) of glucose and 10 units of regular insulin in adults
4. Calcium, 20 mg/kg of calcium gluconate over a 5-min period for children and 500–1,000 mg of calcium chloride for adults

the use of such solutions include a reduction in perioperative fluid requirements and decreased fluid retention postoperatively. Use of inotropes, particularly epinephrine, after bypass may contribute to hyperglycemia by stimulating hepatic glycogenolysis and gluconeogenesis. The deleterious effects associated with hyperglycemia include an osmotic diuresis and the resulting electrolyte abnormalities, a potential to enhance both focal and global ischemic neurologic injury, and, if severe, coma. The use of glucose-containing solutions is no longer recommended.

VII. **Postbypass temperature regulation**
   A. **Effects of hypothermia.** All patients who undergo hypothermic CPB experience variable degrees of hypothermia in the postbypass period. This can have a profound effect on the cardiovascular system, particularly in individuals with borderline cardiac reserve. As the temperature decreases, arteriolar tone will increase, resulting in elevated SVR. The hemodynamic consequences of this include hypertension, a decrease in cardiac output, and increased myocardial O_2 consumption. Total body O_2 consumption may be increased because of the presence of shivering.
   B. **Etiology of postbypass hypothermia.** Hypothermic CPB results in a vasoconstricted state. During rewarming, many of these peripheral vascular beds (i.e., muscle and subcutaneous fat) do not adequately dilate and therefore act as a reserve of cold blood, which eventually will equilibrate with the central circulation. Opening and warming these vascular beds with pharmacologic vasodilation will diminish the "after-drop" in core temperature. The drop in temperature usually reaches its nadir 80 to 90 minutes after bypass.
   C. **Prevention and treatment of hypothermia.** The most effective way to attenuate postbypass hypothermia is to be assured that effective rewarming occurs during CPB. In many instances, the nasopharynx is the site of temperature measurement used to determine adequacy of rewarming. However, the nasopharynx reflects temperature of the central core, which receives a large percentage of the cardiac output and is not an indicator of the temperature in the peripheral tissues. A more appropriate site for monitoring the peripheral or shell temperature, therefore, is the rectum or the bladder. After-drop may be reduced by terminating CPB at a rectal temperature greater than 36°C.

   Other techniques that have been suggested to attenuate hypothermia include heating inspired gases, increasing ambient temperature, and using warm irrigation fluids in the chest cavity and warming blankets. The contribution of these techniques to preventing postbypass hypothermia is likely to be minor for the rewarming process but is of importance in maintaining the patient's temperature until he or she leaves the operating room.

Useful Internet Sites

AmiodaroneIV.com
DocMD.com
BleedingWeb.com
CTSnet.org
Milrinone.com

References

1. Bailey JM, Levy JH, Hug CC. Cardiac surgical pharmacology. In: Edmunds H, ed. *Adult cardiac surgery.* New York: McGraw-Hill, 1997:225–254.
2. Verrier ED. Cardiac surgery. *J Am Coll Surg* 1999;188:104–110.
3. Huraux C, Makita T, Montes F, et al. A comparative evaluation of the effects of multiple vasodilators on human internal mammary artery. *Anesthesiology* 1998;88:1654–1659.
4. **Levy JH, Bailey JM, Deeb M. Intravenous milrinone in cardiac surgery. *Ann Thorac Surg* 2002;73:325–330.**
5. Byrick RJ, Kolton M, Hart JT, et al. Hypoxemia following cardiopulmonary bypass. *Anesthesiology* 1980;53:172–174.
6. Bull BS, Huse WM, Brauer FS, et al. Heparin therapy during extracorporeal circulation. *J Thorac Cardiovasc Surg* 1975;69:685–689.

7. **Despotis GJ, Filos K, Gravlee G, et al. Anticoagulation monitoring during cardiac surgery: a survey of current practice and review of current and emerging techniques.** *Anesthesiology* **1999;91:1122–1151.**
8. Levy JH. *Anaphylactic reactions in anesthesia and intensive care,* 2nd ed. Boston: Butterworth-Heinemann, 1992.
9. Mochizuki T, Olson PJ, Ramsay JG, et al. Protamine reversal of heparin affects platelet aggregation and activated clotting time after cardiopulmonary bypass. *Anesth Analg* 1998;87:781–785.
10. Owings DV, Kruskall MS, Thurer RL, et al. Autologous blood donations prior to elective cardiac surgery. *JAMA* 1989;262:1963–1968.
11. **Levy JH. Blood conservation strategies. In: Cameron DE, Yang P, eds.** *Current therapy in thoracic and cardiovascular surgery.* **St. Louis: Mosby** *(in press).*
12. Levy JH, Pifarre R, Schaff H, et al. A multicenter, placebo-controlled, double-blind trial of aprotinin to reduce blood loss and the requirement of donor blood transfusion in patients undergoing repeat coronary artery bypass grafting. *Circulation* 1995;92:2236–2244.
13. **Mojcik C, Levy JH. Systemic inflammatory response syndrome and anti-inflammatory strategies.** *Ann Thorac Surg* **2001;71:745–754.**
14. England MR, Gordon G, Salem M, et al. Magnesium administration and dysrhythmias after cardiac surgery. *JAMA* 1992;268:2395–2402.

10. POSTOPERATIVE CARE OF THE CARDIAC SURGICAL PATIENT

Russell P. Woda and Robert E. Michler

Planning for postoperative management of a cardiac surgery patient begins preoperatively. This has become increasingly important in an era of fast tracking and cost-saving initiatives. Developing strategies to maximize postoperative resources poses an ever-increasing challenge. The purpose of this chapter is to describe many of the postoperative issues that must be considered when caring for the cardiac surgical patient.

I. Transition from operating room to intensive care unit

A. General principles

1. The termination of the surgical procedure begins the process of preparing for the transition from the operating room to the postoperative recovery area. This may be represented by a move to an intensive care unit (ICU) or to an intermediate high acuity recovery area depending upon the local style of practice. The transition period from the operating room is a time where the anesthesia provider must exercise marked attention to details. Many factors must be addressed simultaneously.

2. Hemodynamic monitoring must be carried out continuously. Careful attention must be given to systemic arterial blood pressure and intravascular volume status.

3. Airway management must be a top priority, as careful attention to endotracheal tube patency and security must be maintained if the patient remains intubated. If a patient is extubated at the end of the surgery, close attention to the patient's anatomic airway must be maintained.

4. Adequacy of ventilation must also be assessed. This may be done by providing adequate positive-pressure ventilation or by ensuring the patient's ability to spontaneously maintain an adequate tidal volume and respiratory rate. Attention must also be given to the status of any chest tubes to assure proper functioning in order to avoid a pneumothorax and be aware of any ongoing bleeding.

B. The transport process

1. The **transport process** begins with having a planned system for providing safe, efficient transport while maintaining a constant state of monitoring and vigilance. Transportation should not occur in a random, haphazard manner but rather a routine efficient system should be developed. Petre et al. [1] described an effective, well-organized transport method. Their system required modification of the operating room and ICU to create a transport technique that allowed for uninterrupted hemodynamic monitoring and continuous intravenous infusions. They pointed out that transport periods could vary from just a few minutes to substantially longer, depending upon the proximity of the operating suites to the recovery area.

2. **Transport to ICU**

   a. **Patient transport** begins with patient movement from the operating room table to the transport bed. Movement can cause hemodynamic instability, as fluid shifts may occur or arrhythmias develop. Having ready access to a large-bore intravenous infusion port and to any ongoing or continuous infusions of medications is critical to managing this period safely and being able to respond promptly.

   b. The anesthesia provider must ensure adequate **supplemental oxygen** and adequate ventilation during transport. Smith and Crul [2] demonstrated that postoperative patients transported without supplemental oxygen had a high incidence of early postoperative hypoxia during transport. They attributed the hypoxic events to ventilation–perfusion mismatch that may result from dependent atelectasis. In the event of pretransport extubation, one also must consider the possibility of hypoventilation from the residual effects of anesthetics or neuromuscular blocking agents.

   c. **Ventilation** can be assured during transport in an intubated patient by using a bag-valve mask device or a transport ventilator. Several companies have developed compact ventilators that can be used during transport to ensure adequate positive-pressure ventilation and appropriate amounts of positive end-expiratory pressure (PEEP) if necessary. Other ventilators designed for use in the postoperative period have battery backup systems that can be used for transportation. Portable ventilators can be very effective but may be cumbersome in view of all of the components that go into the transport process. If a bag-valve mask is used for transport, it must be assured that it is attached to an oxygen source to provide an increased fractional inspired concentration of oxygen (FIO_2) to prevent the possibility of an hypoxic event. Many bag-valve systems also can be modified to provide PEEP during transport, but careful attention must be given to the fact that PEEP impairs cardiac preload and can depress cardiac function. Extubated cardiac patients must receive supplemental oxygen via mask or nasal cannula during transport. Adequacy of ventilation can be monitored by using a precordial or esophageal stethoscope and by direct observation of an adequate chest rise and a patent airway. Adequacy of oxygenation should be monitored with a transportable pulse oximeter, ideally one that is relatively resistant to motion artifact.

    d. Hemodynamic monitoring must be continuous and visible to the transport team and anesthesia provider. Systems have been designed that can transfer cables and transducers to the transport bed to allow uninterrupted monitoring. Some commercial systems allow transfer of the cables and transducers to the monitors in the recovery area, thereby providing the advantage of continuous monitoring throughout the transport process.

    e. Continuous infusions of medications and fluids must be maintained during transport. Due to the often variable time periods of transport between locations, discontinuation of drug infusions seems imprudent. Identifying and purchasing infusion devices that are compact and have adequate battery life is essential, as the amount of equipment that may be necessary for transporting a cardiac patient can be excessive. If the patient is stable, it may be reasonable to discontinue one or more intravenous infusions after flushing them in order to reduce "transport clutter" while assuring uninterrupted access to at least one large-bore intravenous cannula or port.

    Other variables that must be considered during transport depend on the operative interventions. Patients may be connected to pacemakers, intraaortic balloon pumps (IABPs), ventricular assist devices, nitric oxide, and multiple chest tubes, requiring diligence toward each device to ensure function and accessibility. Proper planning requires an assignment of duties to the transport team to determine who is responsible for which device so none is overlooked or to ensure no one person has more to manage than is feasible. Cooperation among the surgeons, perfusionist, respiratory therapists, and nurses directed by the anesthesia provider facilitates this process and results in a smooth transport process.

C. Transfer of care to ICU personnel. Transferring the care of a cardiac patient to the ICU staff must be done in an orderly and methodical fashion. Upon arrival to the recovery area, it is important that the anesthesia provider identify the nurse who will assume responsibility for the patient and direct the transfer of equipment and information. When an uninterrupted system is developed, the transfer can be smooth and without incident. If all monitors and infusions must be disconnected and then reconnected, this period can be somewhat destabilizing. Careful attention must be given to prioritizing tasks, such as ventilator connection and continuous electrocardiogram (ECG) and arterial pressure monitoring while deferring extemporaneous personnel and clinical issues (e.g., drawing blood for laboratory tests) to a more appropriate time. The surgical team should provide transition information about the patient.

II. The early intensive care unit period

    A. Initial review of the patient

        1. The **initial review** of the patient upon his or her arrival to the recovery area includes the patient's history, with information such as age, height, weight, preexisting medical conditions, a list of preoperative medications, and review of the most current laboratory findings (with special emphasis on potassium and hematocrit). The report should include a detailed review of the patient's cardiac status, including ventricular dysfunction, valvular disease, coronary anatomy, and details of the surgical procedure.

2. An **anesthetic review** should be presented, which would include types and location of intravenous catheters and invasive monitors, along with any complications that occurred during their placement. A brief description of the anesthetic technique used should be discussed to help plan for a smooth emergence. A postcardiopulmonary synopsis should be reported, including the use of vasoactive, inotropic, and antiarrhythmic drugs, as well as any untoward events such as arrhythmias and presumed drug reactions.

3. Early upon arrival to the ICU, the patient's **heart rate and rhythm** should be determined. If the patient is being paced, the settings should be reviewed and all electrodes identified and secured, as the patient may be dependent on the device.

B. **Transition to ICU monitors.** The patient should remain hemodynamically monitored throughout the reporting period. If it is required that the patient be disconnected from hemodynamic monitoring and reconnected to the ICU system, careful detail should be used to assure a smooth transition, as early postoperative hemodynamics can fluctuate. An invasive arterial blood pressure and central filling pressures should promptly be achieved to help direct therapy for hemodynamic changes. If a pulmonary artery catheter is present, it should be connected and a baseline cardiac output established. Circulatory support devices, such as IABPs and ventricular assist devices, should be checked for adequate functioning.

C. **Laboratory tests. Few laboratory tests are needed in the early postoperative period.** An initial arterial blood gas (ABG) should be drawn to ensure the adequacy of oxygenation and ventilation, whether the patient is on a mechanical ventilator or breathing spontaneously. A baseline potassium and hematocrit should be obtained. Acid–base status should be reviewed from ABGs and corrected as appropriate. Baseline coagulation parameters, including prothrombin time (PT), activated partial thromboplastin time (aPTT), and platelet count, should be acquired if the patient is bleeding excessively.

D. **Initial ventilator settings.** Intubated patients must have their endotracheal tube evaluated for patency, security, and position. Patients who have no respiratory effort need to be placed in a full-support mode of ventilation, such as assist-control or synchronized intermittent mandatory ventilation (SIMV) with an adequate rate, tidal volume, and a small amount of PEEP (e.g., 5 cm H_2O) to prevent postoperative atelectasis. Patients who have regained spontaneous ventilatory effort can be placed on a weaning mode of ventilation, such as SIMV at a lower rate with addition of some **pressure support ventilation (PSV).** PSV is used for two physiologic purposes:

1. to overcome the resistance of the ventilatory system, which includes the ventilator, tubing, and endotracheal tube;
2. to reduce the patient's work of breathing during weaning.

An advantage of PSV is its titratable ability to match a patient's work of breathing, whereas SIMV is an all-or-none mode with any given breath. PSV by itself constitutes a true weaning mode in that the patient must "trigger" the ventilator with respiratory effort that is unaccompanied by a backup mode for apnea periods. PSV and SIMV modes can be combined. PEEP may be used with any of the aforementioned modes to prevent atelectasis, but caution must be exercised because excessive use of PEEP impedes venous return and may impair cardiac performance. Some suggestions have been made that the application of PEEP may decrease mediastinal bleeding [3]. The literature on this topic is inconsistent and this technique must be used with caution, as PEEP's adverse effects on hemodynamics are well established [4].

III. **Mechanical ventilation after cardiac surgery**

A. **Hemodynamic response to positive-pressure ventilation.** The normal physiology associated with spontaneous ventilation derives from negative-pressure development inside the chest cage and resultant airflow into the lungs. Placing a patient on a positive-pressure ventilator induces variable degrees of physiologic and hemodynamic change. Woda et al. [5] demonstrated that certain patterns of positive-pressure breathing in patients with preexisting lung disease can induce intrinsic PEEP. This intrinsic PEEP, also known as auto PEEP or occult PEEP, results from preexisting poorly compliant lungs as found in chronic obstructive lung (pulmonary) disease (COPD). This tendency toward the development of intrinsic PEEP increases in the presence of increased airways resistance from conditions such as bronchospasm, a small-caliber artificial airway, or marked amounts of secretions or debris in the airway. Many patients presenting for cardiac surgery have COPD in varying degrees of severity. Rapid respiratory rates and lower inspiratory to expiratory (I/E) ratios promote the development of intrinsic PEEP. Intrinsic PEEP has the same physiologic effects as applied PEEP. Lambermont et al. [6] demonstrated that application of PEEP decreased right and left ventricular enddiastolic volumes because of a reduction in venous compliance and an increase in peripheral blood pooling (increased venous capacitance). This venous pooling reduces cardiac output because of decreased cardiac preload.

Transesophageal echocardiography (TEE) has demonstrated that PEEP can cause leftward displacement of the interventricular septum and an attendant restriction of left ventricular filling. Jardin et al. [7] demonstrated that **increasing amounts of PEEP were associated with a progressive decline in cardiac output, mean arterial pressure, and left ventricular dimensions and with equalization of right and left ventricular filling pressures.** These findings suggest the need for careful application of PEEP in postoperative cardiac surgical patients.

B. **Pulmonary changes after sternotomy and thoracotomy.** Performing cardiac surgery requires either a midline sternotomy or a thoracotomy to gain access to the heart and its surrounding anatomic structures. Both of these approaches temporarily compromise the function of the thoracic cage, which acts as a respiratory pump. Van Belle et al. [8] demonstrated significant reduction in total lung capacity, inspiratory vital capacity, forced expiratory volumes, and functional residual capacity 1 week postoperatively compared to preoperative values. Even at 6 weeks postoperatively, total lung capacity, inspiratory vital capacity, and forced expiratory volume remained significantly below preoperative values. These findings suggest a marked tendency toward postoperative atelectasis and the resultant possibility of hypoxemia from increased physiologic shunting. These changes in chest wall function can increase physiologic shunt to as much as 13% (compared to a baseline normal value of 5%).

Impaired pulmonary function after cardiac surgery can result from increases in total lung water and dysfunctional diaphragmatic movement. Cold cardioplegia solutions may injure the left phrenic nerve, which impairs left diaphragmatic movement. This occurrence most often is temporary (days to weeks), but the decreased diaphragmatic movement creates a propensity for atelectasis.

C. **Choosing modes of ventilation**
   1. **Extubated patient.** The patient's condition upon arrival to the ICU or recovery area strongly influences the selection of a ventilatory mode. If the patient was **extubated in the operating room,** supplemental oxygen may be all that is necessary postoperatively. Nevertheless, aggressive pulmonary toilet and frequent incentive spirometry must be performed to prevent the atelectasis and hypoxemia that may develop from the changes in chest wall function. If hypoxemia develops, continuous positive airway pressure (CPAP) using a face mask can be applied to improve the physiologic shunt that occurs from progressive atelectasis. If ventilation should become impaired, as evidenced by a rising P_aCO_2, facemask positive-pressure ventilation can be used if available to temporize and potentially avoid reintubation of the trachea. This technique utilizes an apparatus similar to what is used for face-mask CPAP, and a rate of ventilation can be selected to deliver positive-pressure tidal volumes. Using face-mask ventilation requires an awake patient with a patent airway, confidence that the stomach is empty to ensure against aspiration, and the presence of a functioning nasogastric tube to remove any air that enters the gastrointestinal tract.
   2. **Intubated patient**
      a. If a patient returns from the operating room with an **endotracheal tube in place,** the choice of mechanical ventilation mode is based on the patient's inherent respiratory effort. If a patient is demonstrating an inspiratory

effort, a weaning mode can be selected. The most common weaning method used is SIMV or PSV. SIMV allows selection of a guaranteed basal respiratory rate with intermittent spontaneous breaths taken by the patient. The delivered breaths are synchronized to avoid initiation of a breath during spontaneous exhalation. This avoids breath stacking and reduces the possibility of barotrauma. The number of mandatory breaths per minute can be weaned as the patient recovers and more frequent or deeper spontaneous breathing occurs. The spontaneous breaths can be supported by adding PSV and CPAP to assist in the work of breathing and in avoiding atelectasis. **The weaning process progresses until the patient is spontaneously triggering all of the breaths in the breathing cycle and receiving minimal amounts of CPAP and PSV.**

If a patient returns from the operating room with an endotracheal tube in place and is not demonstrating any spontaneous respiratory effort, a full-support mode, such as assist control (AC) or SIMV, should be selected. AC is a full-support mode of ventilation where a set respiratory rate is delivered regardless of the patient's respiratory effort. If a spontaneous breath is initiated, the ventilator detects the trigger and delivers a set tidal volume breath. Weaning cannot be performed during this mode unless the ventilator is disconnected intermittently and the patient is connected to a T-piece apparatus.

b. Patients who have marked difficulty with oxygenation after cardiac surgery may be given a full-support mode of ventilation with advancing amounts of PEEP. Often these patients require continuation of sedation and muscle paralysis to tolerate this type of ventilation scheme. If advancing amounts of PEEP are required, it may be helpful to place a pulmonary artery catheter (if one is not already present) to evaluate the hemodynamic effects of the positive pressure.

c. Weaning from mechanical ventilation is a multifactorial event requiring diligence directed toward many issues. In many postoperative environments, this can best be accomplished by using an algorithm so that weaning can proceed methodically and without interruption. Figure 10.1 shows an algorithm that could facilitate efficient weaning.

(1) One must be sure that cardiac surgical patients are warm after surgery, as a cool environment is used in the operating room. **Postoperative hypothermia** can occur, which results in shivering, high oxygen consumption, and increased cardiac stress. Acid–base disorders must be identified and corrected according to their underlying cause. Residual anesthetics need to be cleared and a plan for sedation and analgesia during weaning established. Many centers have adopted routine use of propofol for sedation during weaning from mechanical ventilation due to its short, predictable duration of action. Laboratory abnormalities of electrolytes and hematocrit must be corrected to achieve successful weaning from mechanical ventilation. An appropriate heart rate and rhythm must be identified and any dysrhythmias managed. Bleeding from the chest tubes must be assessed and documented in order to avoid prematurely weaning the unstable patient who may require surgical reexploration.

(2) Weaning typically starts out in a volume ventilation mode such as SIMV by decreasing the number of guaranteed breaths by the ventilator. The ventilator does less as the patient is able to do more. During SIMV weaning, some CPAP can be added to the spontaneous breaths to prevent atelectasis. PSV can be added to the spontaneous breaths to overcome the resistance created by the breathing circuit and the endotracheal tube. Once the patient is breathing spontaneously with minimal CPAP and PSV, an evaluation for extubation can be done. Weaning can be performed without drawing ABGs after each ventilation change if noninvasive monitoring systems, such as pulse oximetry and end-tidal carbon dioxide measurement, are uti-

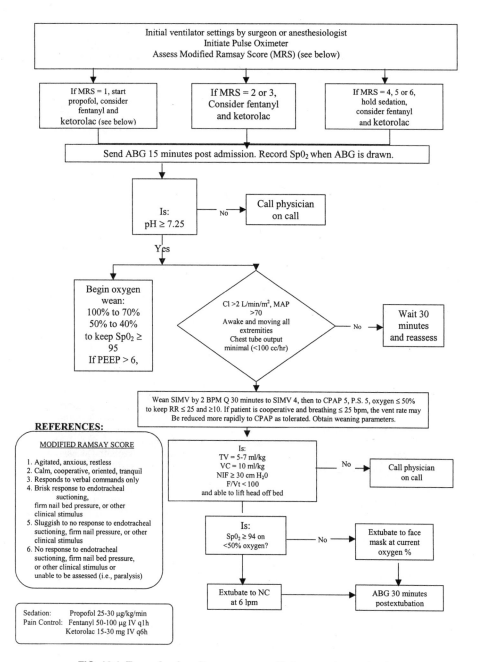

FIG. 10.1 Example of cardiac surgery ventilator weaning protocol.

lized. ABGs typically should be checked before extubation with minimal ventilator settings and a low F_{IO_2} in order to evaluate the adequacy of oxygenation and ventilation under those conditions.

(3) **Extubation can be carried out once evaluation of airway protective mechanisms, oxygenation, ventilation, and muscle strength are established.** Some traditional weaning criteria, such as a negative inspiratory force (NIF) of 30 mm H_2O or more or a vital capacity of 15 mL/kg or more require an alert, cooperative patient. It also is useful to establish a patient baseline respiratory rate and tidal volume, but these parameters may be altered by discontinuation of sedation immediately before extubation. One method for predicting the ability to be extubated is to evaluate the frequency of respiratory rate (f) as a ratio to tidal volume (TV) or the "rapid shallow breathing test" (f/V_T). This weaning parameter was carefully evaluated by Yang and Tobin [9], who determined that if f/V_T was 100 or less, there was an 80% chance of successful extubation. This is an attractive test to use because it is simple, does not require patient effort, and has a high predictive value.

(4) Patients must be encouraged to use **incentive spirometry** and to do **deep breathing** and coughing maneuvers after extubation to reduce atelectasis. One must be mindful of a variety of other physiologic causes of hypoxemia while managing the postextubation patient. Diffusion abnormality, low F_{IO_2}, hypoventilation, and V/Q mismatch along with shunt comprise the list of possibilities, with atelectasis being the most common. If hypoxemia persists and atelectasis is the presumed cause, mask CPAP can be used to improve oxygenation and decrease shunt.

(5) If **hypercarbia** is present in the postextubation period in an awake patient who can maintain a patent airway, noninvasive positive-pressure ventilation (NPPV) with a mask can be used for a short period of time. NPPV may be associated with a decreased incidence of nosocomial pneumonia as compared to endotracheal intubation. This mode of ventilation may be useful for certain cases of mild respiratory failure. Table 10.1 lists conditions in which NPPV would be contraindicated.

IV. **Principles of fast tracking**

A. **Goals of fast tracking.** It has long been suggested that patients may do better after cardiac surgery if they are weaned from the ventilator and extubated as early as possible so they may be discharged earlier from the ICU and begin their postoperative cardiac rehabilitation programs, a technique that has been termed fast tracking. Other goals of fast tracking include early ambulation, early resumption of a regular diet, and prevention of potential complications of prolonged intubation (e.g., nosocomial pneumonia). This concept initially was conceived for the healthiest of cardiac surgery patients but has since become the goal for many patient groups representing varying severities of illness [10–12]. A combination of improving patient care via early

Table 10.1 Contraindications to noninvasive positive-pressure ventilation

Cardiac or respiratory arrest
Nonrespiratory organ failure
Severe encephalopathy (e.g., Glasgow Coma Score <10)
Severe upper gastrointestinal bleeding
Hemodynamic instability or unstable cardiac dysrhythmia
Facial surgery, trauma, or deformity
Upper airway obstruction
Inability to cooperate
Inability to clear respiratory secretions
High risk for aspiration

extubation along with cost containment has driven the development of fast-track cardiac surgery techniques. Cost containment can be separated into various components. Respiratory therapists and nurses may find less time is spent managing patients who are extubated earlier, which could reduce staffing requirements. Reducing hospital and ICU lengths of stay reduces cost in cardiac surgery patients. Early postoperative extubation has long been thought to potentially benefit patients by restoring their cough reflexes earlier, thereby reducing atelectasis. Early extubation also may improve hemodynamics by restoring the normal physiology of negative intrathoracic pressures. Patient comfort may improve and less pain medication may be required with earlier extubation. Elderly patients, emergency cases, patients on an IABP, and those receiving inotropic support may not be good candidates for early extubation, however [13]. Also, those patients who have postoperative instability and complications such as stroke, bleeding, or dysrhythmias may fail early extubation protocols.

Some investigators dispute the value of early extubation, finding that early extubation does not reduce ICU length of stay and may result in more complications. Montes et al. [14] showed that an early extubation population had more reintubations than did a group extubated in the ICU, with no difference in the length of stay in the ICU or total hospital time.

B. **Methods of fast tracking.** A variety of anesthetic techniques can be used to facilitate fast tracking. Shorter-acting narcotics, such as alfentanil and remifentanil, provide opportunities for faster weaning from the ventilator. These shorter-acting intravenous narcotics can be combined with intrathecal opioids to enhance postoperative analgesia [15,16]. Propofol infusions have been added to the cardiac anesthetic repertoire because of a predictable and rapid recovery profile that is almost independent of the duration of infusion. This property makes this technique desirable not only as a component of general anesthesia, but also as a sedative agent in the early postoperative management of fast-track cardiac surgery patients. Caution is needed when short-acting agents are used to set the stage for early extubation, as the incidence of intraoperative awareness may be as high as 0.3% [17].

C. **Fast tracking in the postanesthesia care unit.** Many institutions prepare for the postoperative management of cardiac surgery patients by developing enhanced step-down or postanesthesia care units (PACUs), where postoperative management can occur safely and efficiently. These units require nurses who understand fast-tracking techniques, so that patients who have undergone cardiac surgery can move smoothly through early extubation in preparation for early transfer to a regular nursing unit. These specialized postanesthesia care units can be very effective in providing fast-track techniques because of their focused effort in caring for fast-track cardiac surgery patients.

D. **Utilizing protocols.** Developing and utilizing institution-specific fast-track protocols revolves around systematic plans for weaning patients from ventilators and managing routine postoperative issues to facilitate the progression toward early ICU and hospital discharge. Protocols ideally address most issues before they occur. Protocol development should be carried out jointly by all members of the perioperative care team before a fast-tracking program is initiated.

V. **Hemodynamic management in the postoperative period**

A. **Monitoring for ischemia.** Monitoring the postoperative cardiac surgical patient for myocardial ischemia is essential, and it is important to treat clinically significant changes in blood pressure, heart rhythm, and cardiac output as if they either result from or may cause myocardial ischemia. Ischemia can be detected by utilizing a continuous ECG with ST-segment analysis, although there is a slight delay in diagnosis of ischemia using this method. Many bedside ECG monitoring systems have ST-segment analysis built into their software algorithms, which is a cost-effective method of monitoring for ischemic events. Other indicators of myocardial ischemia include pulmonary artery pressures and cardiac output, which tend to be less reliable and often late markers of myocardial ischemia. TEE segmental wall-motion abnormalities represent the most sensitive early detector of myocardial ischemia, but continuous monitoring usually is unfeasible because the TEE probe (if used) typically is removed at the end of surgery [18].

Intraoperative and ongoing postoperative ischemia can be detected as soon as 6 hours after the event begins by examining some specific cardiac markers. The earliest and most useful marker is cardiac troponin I (cTnI) [19]. The ability to measure cTnI is particularly useful in cases where ECG monitoring is difficult to interpret, such as with left bundle branch block or left ventricular hypertrophy. This biologic marker gives clear evidence for an ischemic event.

B. Ventricular dysfunction after cardiac surgery. Ventricular dysfunction after cardiac surgery may be multifactorial. **Inadequate myocardial protection, myocardial hyperthermia, small blood vessels, incomplete revascularization, and reperfusion injury all can contribute to postoperative ventricular dysfunction.** Preoperative predictors of postoperative ventricular dysfunction include cardiac enlargement, advanced age, diabetes mellitus, female gender, high left ventricular end-diastolic pressures at cardiac catheterization, small coronary arteries, and ejection fraction less than 0.40. Intraoperative predictors include longer cardiopulmonary bypass (CPB) and aortic cross-clamp times. These factors increase the likelihood of needing inotropic support in the postoperative period. When patients present to the operating room with impaired ejection fractions and have long CPB periods, there is a high incidence of requiring inotropic support postoperatively. Patients who have normal cardiac performance and short periods of CPB have a much lower likelihood of requiring postoperative inotropic support.

Most practitioners utilize β-adrenergic agonists (β-agonists) when there is a need to improve ventricular function after CPB. Depletion of endogenous catecholamines and the resulting β-receptor down-regulation can blunt the response to β-agonists. Increased G-inhibitory proteins, reperfusion injury, tachycardia, incomplete revascularization, and nonviable myocardium also may attenuate the inotropic response to β-agonists.

Agents chosen to treat ventricular dysfunction after cardiac surgery typically utilize $β_1$-agonism as their primary method of improving cardiac function. Other mechanisms available include phosphodiesterase inhibitors such as amrinone and milrinone, which work to augment β-adrenergic stimulation by inhibiting the breakdown of cyclic adenosine monophosphate (cAMP). The agents most frequently used to cause $β_1$-agonism are dobutamine, dopamine and epinephrine, each of which has its own inherent hemodynamic profile and side effects.

C. Fluid management. Managing postoperative fluids after cardiac surgery can be challenging. Cardiac surgical procedures, especially those involving CPB, typically result in fluid sequestration by "third spacing." Therefore, most cardiac surgery patients reach the recovery area with excess fluids present that must be mobilized. Healthy patients who have adequate cardiac and renal function typically diurese these fluids over the first 2 postoperative days without assistance. Other cardiac surgery patients, such as the elderly or those with renal or cardiac dysfunction, may require diuretic drugs to remove excess body water.

Cardiac surgical patients frequently require allogenic blood products. CPB priming solutions cause hemodilution, which causes patients to arrive in the ICU with relatively low hemoglobin and hematocrit measurements. Many times the mobilization of free water through diuresis returns the red cell mass to an acceptable level. Some patients require administration of packed red blood cells to arrive at adequate hematocrit values due to excessive intraoperative or postoperative bleeding or to preexisting anemia. Controversy exists over what is the lowest postoperative acceptable hematocrit for cardiac surgery patients. Although no absolute number has been proven, maintaining adequate oxygen-carrying capacity in the face of a potentially limited ability to increase cardiac output or coronary blood flow must be considered. **In patients with limited reserve, it may be necessary to maintain a higher hemoglobin concentration, e.g., 9 to 10 g/dL, than in patients who can compensate normally for anemia.** For most cardiac surgical patients, a hemoglobin concentration of 8 to 9 g/dL is adequate for postoperative recovery.

Administration of coagulation factors must be addressed. Patients who leave the operating room and arrive in the recovery area with coagulopathy may require administration of fresh frozen plasma or platelet concentrates to improve clot formation. Many patients may have a postoperative bleeding propensity because of residual effects from the preoperative administration of various platelet inhibitors (e.g., aspirin, clopidogrel). Platelet concentrates or possibly desmopressin may be necessary to reverse this state. One must consider the possibility that residual heparin effect or heparin rebound may be present, which may require neutralization with protamine.

D. Managing hypotension. Postoperative cardiac surgery patients frequently can have hypotension, the etiology of which must be evaluated in order to optimize therapy. If adequate preload and a normal cardiac rhythm are present, hypotension represents either inadequacy in cardiac function or vasodilation. Inadequate cardiac function sometimes can be managed by administering fluids to increase cardiac preload. However, it is critical to recognize that ventricular function or myocardial ischemia may be worsened by excessive fluid administration. Vasodilation demands scrutiny for contributory drugs such as vancomycin, nitroglycerin, or diltiazem.

E. Dysrhythmia management. Continuous monitoring of the ECG may identify dysrhythmias in postoperative cardiac surgery patients. A variety of dysrhythmias can occur that are either atrial or ventricular in origin. Patients with ongoing myocardial ischemia, possibly from incomplete revascularization or myocardial stunning, probably are predisposed to dysrhythmias. Managing postoperative dysrhythmias constitutes an important part of ICU care in cardiac surgery patients. Atrial fibrillation is the most common clinically significant dysrhythmia to occur after cardiac surgery, and it may occur in as many as one third of patients who undergo myocardial revascularization using CPB. Useful drugs for treating atrial fibrillation include procainamide, digoxin, diltiazem, esmolol, and amiodarone. **It has been shown that various preoperative or postoperative pharmacologic prophylactic strategies may reduce the incidence of postoperative atrial fibrillation or other atrial dysrhythmias** [20]. Using prophylaxis against atrial fibrillation may benefit the patient by decreasing both the number of days spent in the ICU and the total length of stay in the hospital.

F. Perioperative hypertension. Perioperative hypertension can result from a number of causes.

1. One of the most important and earliest mechanisms is emergence from anesthesia. This may present a challenge in hypertensive management as the anesthetics are cleared.

2. Another cause of postoperative hypertension is withdrawal from preoperative antihypertensive medications. β-Blockers and centrally acting α_2-agonists are known to elicit rebound hypertension upon withdrawal.

3. **Some causes of acute postoperative hypertension include hypercarbia, hypoxemia, deficient analgesia, intravascular volume excess, and hypothermia.** One must consider iatrogenic causes, such as administration of the wrong medication or use of a vasoconstrictor when it was not necessary.

4. Unusual causes include intracranial hypertension (from cerebral edema or massive stroke) and bladder distention. Rare causes to consider include endocrine or metabolic disorders such as hyperthyroidism, pheochromocytoma, renin–angiotensin disorders, and malignant hyperthermia.

G. Pulmonary hypertension. Pulmonary hypertension may occur after cardiac surgery, the causes of which can be divided into new-onset acute pulmonary hypertension and continuation of a more chronic pulmonary hypertensive state.

1. Chronic pulmonary hypertension is less responsive to traditional therapeutic interventions. Chronic elevation in the pulmonary vascular resistance (PVR) creates a challenging scenario with respect to the ability of the right ventricle to function adequately against increased resistance. Chronic pulmonary hypertension is managed by continuing any ongoing medications that the patient has been taking, such as calcium channel blockers, along with utilizing therapeutic agents mentioned below (see Section **V.G.2**) for management of acute pulmonary hypertension.

2. Acute postoperative pulmonary hypertension must be managed aggressively to avoid right ventricular failure. First and foremost, hypoxemia and hypercarbia must be ruled out and managed as treatable causes of acute pulmonary hypertension. Ongoing acidosis (metabolic or respiratory) that has been untreated

also contributes to the development of pulmonary hypertension. Left ventricular failure, mitral stenosis or regurgitation, and pulmonary venous thrombosis should be considered. Therapeutic interventions that can be useful to treat pulmonary hypertension include inhaled nitric oxide, nitroglycerin, sodium nitroprusside, prostacyclin, and phosphodiesterase III inhibitors. With the exception of nitric oxide, these agents also can reduce systemic vascular resistance (SVR) to cause systemic arterial hypotension. The balance of managing pulmonary hypertension and systemic hypotension can be very challenging, often requiring a combination of agents. It may become necessary to infuse a vasoconstrictive agent to increase SVR while administering an agent to lower PVR. This maneuver can be very complex and contradictory in that most agents that increase SVR also increase PVR. Vasopressin should be considered as an agent that may increase SVR without proportionately increasing PVR.

VI. Postoperative pain and sedation management techniques. Managing postoperative pain and agitation are paramount in caring for the postoperative cardiac surgery patient. Pain represents a response to nociceptor stimulation from the surgical intervention. Patients may be agitated after cardiac surgery for a variety of reasons. Table 10.2 lists some possible causes of agitation that must not be overlooked because of the potential that they might be inappropriately "masked" by administration of a sedative drug.

   A. Systemic opioids. A variety of techniques can be used to manage postoperative pain. It is very useful to initially discern the type, quality, and location of pain before administering an analgesic agent. Commonly used opioids include fentanyl, morphine, hydromorphone, and meperidine. All of these agents are narcotic agonists that work through the μ-receptor mechanism to provide analgesia. Butorphanol and nalbuphine are narcotic agonist–antagonists that can be used to provide analgesia while minimizing the chance of respiratory depression. Table 10.3 lists commonly used analgesic agents for postoperative pain along with loading and maintenance dosing.

   B. Intrathecal opioids. In the era of fast-tracking patients through the postoperative period, several regional analgesic techniques have been pursued to improve patient comfort. Systemic (intravenous, intramuscular, transcutaneous, or oral) opioids can cause respiratory depression and somnolence, making them potentially undesirable for fast tracking. Intrathecal narcotics constitute an alternative to systemic opioids. This route has been explored in an attempt to improve patient comfort with less respiratory depression and other side effects. Intrathecal opioids can facilitate early extubation and discharge from an ICU without compromising pain control or increasing the likelihood of myocardial ischemia [21]. Intrathecal morphine may be useful in attenuating the postsurgical stress response in coronary artery bypass graft (CABG) patients as measured by plasma cortisol and epinephrine concentrations [22]. **This evidence suggests that intrathecal opioids may be an excellent pain management choice in preparing the cardiac surgical patient for early extubation and fast tracking in the ICU.**

Table 10.2 Causes of postoperative agitation

Hypoxemia
Hypercapnea
Residual anesthetics/emergence from anesthesia
Gastric or urinary retention
Electrolyte abnormalities (hyponatremia)
Residual premedication (scopolamine, phenothiazines)
Aggravation of preoperative psychologic conditions (anxiety)
Other medications (atropine, cimetidine, propranolol)
Ischemia or hemorrhage of the central nervous system
Delirium tremens
Wernicke encephalopathy

Table 10.3. Analgesics

	Intravenous loading dose	Maintenance dose	Special considerations
Fentanyl	0.5–3.0 µg/kg	1–4 µg/kg/hr	May cause bradycardia, tachyphylaxis to infusion
Morphine	0.08–0.12 mg/kg	0.03 mg/kg every 10 min	Histamine release Metabolites accumulate in renal failure
Ketorolac	15–30 mg	15 mg IV every 6 hr	Caution in renal failure, coagulopathy
Hydromorphone	0.02 mg/kg	25–50 µg/kg every 10 min	No metabolites in renal failure
Meperidine	1.0–1.5 mg/kg	0.30 mg/kg every 10 min	May cause tachycardia Avoid with monoamine oxidase inhibitors Metabolites may accumulate in renal failure and may reduce seizure threshold
Butorphanol	0.02–0.04 mg/k	0.01 mg/kg every 10 min	Mixed agonist/antagonist
Nalbuphine	0.08–0.15 mg/kg	0.03 mg/kg every 10 min	Mixed agonist/antagonist
Codeine	0.5–1.0 mg/kg	⅙ total bolus every 15 min	Nausea

C. **Nonsteroidal antiinflammatory drugs.** Nonsteroidal antiinflammatory drugs (NSAIDs) can be helpful when managing postoperative pain in cardiac surgery. A small amount of drug can provide analgesia without excessive sedation and other complications associated with narcotic use. A concern with NSAIDs is their inhibition of platelet function and the potential for increased bleeding. NSAIDs also have been considered a poor choice after cardiac surgery because of their tendency to induce gastric ulcer formation and impair renal function. Renal insufficiency, active peptic ulcer disease, history of gastrointestinal bleeding, and bleeding diathesis should exclude the use of NSAIDs in the postoperative cardiac surgery patient [23].

D. **Nerve blocks.** A variety of systemic and intrathecal analgesic techniques have been reviewed. Although these techniques are useful, each has inherent risks and complications. Nerve blocks constitute a potential alternative to these methods. Intercostal nerve blocks can be performed with ease during thoracic surgery procedures, as the intercostal nerves are easily accessible through the surgical field. These blocks also can be performed percutaneously by the anesthesia provider preoperatively or postoperatively. Intercostal blocks do not provide satisfactory analgesia for a median sternotomy. Thoracic epidural analgesia for cardiac surgical procedures requiring CPB is considered acceptable by some practitioners. Others consider the risk of epidural hematoma, however small, to be a deterrent in the face of the hypocoagulable state present during and after CPB.

VII. **Metabolic abnormalities.** Many metabolic abnormalities can occur in the perioperative period. These irregularities result from large fluid and electrolyte shifts that can result from intravenous infusions or from CPB priming or myocardial protectant solutions.

A. **Electrolyte abnormalities**

1. **Hyperkalemia** can present from cardioplegia, overaggressive replacement, or from secondary extracellular shifts associated with respiratory or metabolic

acidosis. Hypokalemia is more common than hyperkalemia, and it is commonly associated with dilution or ion shifts associated with hyperventilation and urinary losses. Potassium supplementation can be infused carefully at a maximum rate of 20 mEq/hour via a central venous catheter, as rapid potassium infusion can induce lethal arrhythmias.

2. **Hypocalcemia** may be present and may be related to rapid transfusion of large amounts of citrate-preserved bank blood. Hypocalcemia can be treated with 250- to 1,000 mg intravenous doses of calcium chloride or calcium gluconate, while paying careful attention to the development of dysrhythmias. When following the calcium status, it is important to measure ionized calcium and not total calcium, because low albumin levels may decrease total calcium levels, while ionized calcium remains normal.

3. **Hypomagnesemia** is a common perioperative electrolyte abnormality. Hypomagnesemia may result from dilution by large CPB primes and by urinary excretion. If magnesium supplementation is required, it can be given in amounts of 2 to 4 g intravenously over 30 to 45 minutes. An infusion of 1 g/hour of magnesium sulfate can be used as well to assure a slow, steady infusion of this substance. If given too fast, it may cause hypotension. In refractory dysrhythmias, particularly of the ventricular type, a normal serum magnesium concentration may not exclude the possibility of decreased total body stores of magnesium.

B. **Shivering.** Many patients arrive in the ICU with a tendency toward shivering. The exact mechanism of shivering is difficult to discern, but it is thought to be associated with inadequate rewarming and temperature fluctuation. Many patients are hypothermic when they arrive in the ICU and develop shivering as they emerge from anesthesia. Shivering can result in a 300% to 600% increase in oxygen demand, which potentially places unachievable oxygen delivery demand upon a compromised myocardium. The associated increase in CO_2 production may cause respiratory acidosis. Effective first-line treatments include active rewarming and prevention of further temperature loss or meperidine and sedation. Sustained shivering frequently will require mechanical ventilation.

C. **Acid–base disorders.** Acid–base disorders can occur as a result of inadequate blood flow during a period of increased metabolic demand. Respiratory acidosis most often results from hypoventilation or increased CO_2 production. Residual anesthetics or an awakening patient with inadequate analgesia combined with impaired respiratory mechanics may lead to hypoventilation. Metabolic acidosis, when present, is associated frequently with inadequate systemic perfusion because of compromised cardiac function. In the presence of acid–base disorders, repeated ABG measurement will be required in the early postoperative period. Metabolic acidosis in a cardiac surgery patient may require administration of sodium bicarbonate to correct the underlying acidosis. This should be done with caution, as the etiology of the metabolic acidosis should be determined and managed as well. Lactic acidosis, a frequent finding in cardiac surgery patients, needs to be managed by assuring adequate cardiac output, intravascular volume, and appropriate management of shivering.

D. **Glucose management.** Many patients presenting for cardiac surgery have a history of either adult-onset or juvenile diabetes. Many of these patients withhold their therapy, either insulin or oral hypoglycemic agents, on the day of surgery. This can result in wide swings in serum blood glucose, which must be assessed and addressed early in the patient's postoperative care. Careful control of blood glucose levels, preferably by maintaining blood glucose at less than 200 mg/dL with frequent monitoring, is important in these patients. **Unrecognized hyperglycemia can result in excessive diuresis and the potential for a hyperosmolar or ketoacidotic state.** Elevated serum glucose can be managed by using a continuous infusion of regular insulin and a dextrose-containing solution, often starting at a dose of 0.1 units/kg/hour or less with titration to the desired serum blood glucose level.

Perioperative hyperglycemia may be especially prevalent in programs where fast-track clinical pathways are used [24]. One institution examined this potential and discovered that preoperative diabetes, pre-CPB administration of glucocorticoids, volume of glucose-containing cardioplegia solutions administered, and use of epinephrine infusions were associated with the development of perioperative hyperglycemia. These conditions frequently occur and can precipitate the need for aggressive management of postoperative hyperglycemia using insulin.

VIII. Complications in the first 24 hours postoperatively. A number of life-threatening complications can occur in the first 24 hours after cardiac or thoracic surgery. Due to the relative instability of these patients in their early postoperative care, it is essential that the postoperative care provider identify and respond promptly to the development of the most common postoperative complications.

  A. Respiratory failure. Respiratory failure may be the most common postoperative complication of cardiac or thoracic surgery. Pulmonary dysfunction develops from the surgical incision and its attendant disruption of the thoracic cage. Uncontrolled postoperative pain exacerbates this effect. Respiratory failure can present as hypoxemia, hypercarbia, or both. Prompt identification and appropriate treatment of respiratory failure are essential to managing postoperative cardiac and thoracic surgery patients. Respiratory failure causes must be scrutinized to avoid overlooking such serious complications as pneumothorax, acute congestive heart failure, and prosthetic valve failure.

  B. Bleeding. Some patients experience persistent bleeding after cardiac or thoracic surgery. Bleeding typically is monitored by the amount of blood that drains into the chest tubes after surgery. Persistent postoperative bleeding must be managed by providing the appropriate therapy based on the etiology of the blood loss. It is critical to differentiate a bleeding diathesis from a surgical bleeding situation requiring reoperation; therefore, it is essential to determine the status of the coagulation system, which traditionally is done by acquiring (at a minimum) PT, activated partial thromboplastin time (aPTT), and platelet count. This panel of tests does not give any indication about the functional status of the platelets. This is particularly important in managing cardiac patients who have received preoperative therapy with aspirin or other platelet inhibitors to prevent thrombosis during the period leading up to corrective surgery. Transfusion of platelet concentrates may be appropriate when one suspects that the bleeding results from platelet dysfunction, which may be caused by either preoperative platelet inhibitors or CPB.

  During this process, one must consider surgical bleeding as a cause of high blood losses. Surgical bleeding often is considered once coagulopathy has been ruled out, and it may require a return to the operating room for mediastinal or thoracic exploration to identify and cauterize or ligate a bleeding site. Transport of these patients may be difficult because of hemodynamic instability.

  Sudden hemorrhage from a suture line or cannulation site can cause profound hypotension due to hypovolemia or tamponade. Rapid volume infusion of blood products, colloids, or crystalloids is necessary to maintain intravascular volume. Patients who are quickly stabilized are transferred to the operating room for sternotomy or thoracotomy to repair the bleeding site. In some instances, emergency sternotomy must be performed in the ICU to stop a bleeding site that has created relative instability. In general, chest tube drainage greater than 500 mL/hour or sustained drainage exceeding 200 mL/hour justifies surgical reexploration.

  C. Cardiac tamponade. Excessive mediastinal bleeding with inadequate drainage or sudden massive bleeding can result in cardiac tamponade. Cardiac tamponade after cardiac surgery may be confusing if the pericardium has been opened, suggesting to the inexperienced observer that tamponade cannot occur. However, this is not true because tamponade may occur in loculated areas. The differential diagnosis typically includes biventricular failure, and transthoracic echocardiography or TEE may be required to make a definitive diagnosis.

  D. Pneumothorax. Pneumothorax can occur in patients who have undergone sternotomy or thoracotomy. Most often this patient population arrives in the recovery or ICU area with one or more chest tubes in place. It is essential for patients to have a baseline postoperative chest x-ray film to confirm the adequacy of the placement of the chest tubes and the absence of a pneumothorax. Pneumothorax can convert to tension pneumothorax when a one-way valve is present, causing elevated intrapleural pressure. The result can be a shift of mediastinal structures causing mechanical obstruction of the vena cava or the heart itself to cause a low cardiac output state and hypotension.

E. Hemothorax. Hemothorax can occur after coronary artery bypass surgery and must be considered in all patients who have undergone internal mammary artery dissection, which most often involves opening the left intrapleural space. These patients may need to be returned to the operating room for surgical management.

F. Acute graft closure. Acute coronary graft closure is uncommon and can result in myocardial ischemia or infarction. If cardiac decompensation does occur and graft closure is the suspected cause, reexploration should be performed to evaluate graft patency. However, it usually is difficult to know whether a graft has closed, and reexploration for this reason is uncommon. These patients may need to be taken to the cardiac catheterization laboratory, where emergent cardiac catheterization can be performed to discern the presence of an occluded graft.

G. Prosthetic valve failure. Acute prosthetic valve failure should be suspected when sudden hemodynamic changes occur following open heart surgery, particularly if the rhythm is unchanged and intermittent loss of the arterial waveform is noted on the monitor screen. Immediate surgical correction is necessary. Valve dehiscence with a perivalvular leak usually does not present in the early postoperative period.

H. Postoperative neurologic dysfunction. Neurologic complications can occur in the postoperative period. These complications can be divided into three groups: focal ischemic injury (stroke), diffuse encephalopathy (global hypoperfusion syndrome), and peripheral nervous system injury. Normothermic CPB and continuous blood cardioplegia have become popular. This technique, while sparing the myocardium, may be associated with an increased risk of neurologic complications. Few laboratory tests exist that help predict and monitor neurologic complications after bypass. The serum S100β protein has been shown to correlate with long CPB perfusion times and with postoperative central nervous system dysfunction.

IX. Discharge from the intensive care unit. Discharge from the ICU historically has occurred 1 to 3 days after cardiothoracic surgery. Reducing the amount of time spent in the ICU after cardiac surgery recently has become a priority. Many patients now are discharged from the ICU on the morning after routine CABG operations, with no compromise in patient care or safety. Complications such as those noted earlier often delay ICU discharge. Some centers place routine CABG patients in an ICU-level recovery area for several hours before discharging them to a "step-down" or intermediate care area, or even to a "monitored bed" postoperative nursing unit.

The criteria for ICU discharge vary depending upon the type of surgery. Predicting which patients can leave the ICU in an early fast-track style can be accomplished by reviewing a variety of preoperative risk factors. Ejection fraction can be a valid predictor of mortality, morbidity, and resource utilization when statistically applied to a cardiac surgery population [25]. Other preoperative predictors of prolonged ICU stays include cardiogenic shock, age greater than 80 years, dialysis-dependent renal failure, and surgery performed emergently [26]. These factors and others can be used to predict a patient's length of stay and plan for resource utilization.

X. Economics of postoperative planning and strategies. With the ever-increasing interest in fast-tracking patients through an ICU or recovery room, opportunities to reduce the costs of cardiac and thoracic surgery have arisen. Postoperative cost reduction can be divided into a variety of categories. By adopting a fast-track program, one might realize cost reduction via decreased length of stay in the ICU, decreased laboratory testing, decreased time on a ventilator, and decreased overall length of time in the hospital. Fast-tracking strategies can reduce length of stay in the ICU, yet this reduction has not consistently resulted in a decreased overall length stay in the hospital. Finding techniques and methods to shorten overall length of stay and reduce costs continues to generate strong interest and investigation.

Off-pump coronary artery bypass surgery (OPCAB) constitutes a further attempt to decrease postoperative complications and resource utilization. The economic aspects of this type of surgery, where patients are not placed on CPB, have been evaluated in some studies. Studies have suggested that OPCAB reduces costs by decreasing ICU length of stay, but these savings may be offset by increased intraoperative costs (depending upon techniques and equipment utilized) or by an increased incidence of required cardiac interventions after hospital discharge. At this time, it is not possible to state with certainty that OPCAB reduces long-term costs or improves long-term clinical outcomes. The OPCAB technique has proven safe in many different types of patients, including the elderly [27]. Continuing improvements in pain relief and early extubation should enhance economic savings.

XI. The transplant patient. Cardiac transplant patients historically have spent long periods postoperatively on mechanical ventilation, with attendant prolonged ICU stays. Recent application of fast-track strategies has shortened times to extubation and provided earlier postoperative mobilization for these patients.

XII. Patients with mechanical assist devices. Recent technologic advances have facilitated development of mechanical assist devices for cardiac surgery patients with severely impaired right or left ventricular functions. The number of assist devices available continues to grow, resulting in options for left ventricular, right ventricular, or biventricular mechanical assistance. Postoperative management of patients with mechanical assist devices requires a thorough understanding of the technology underlying any device that may be chosen. Often perfusionists participate continuously in the ICU to manage the ventricular assist devices.

The list of clinical considerations for a patient on a mechanical assist device is lengthy. Device-specific considerations include maintenance of an appropriate heart rate and filling status, as many of these devices are preload dependent. Coagulation abnormalities are a frequent concern when patients are brought to the ICU with implanted mechanical devices. These patients have clear tendencies toward coagulopathy and need to be treated carefully with appropriate blood products to achieve the targeted coagulation status.

Other considerations that must be met during the ICU period include adequate oxygenation and ventilation using a mechanical ventilator, along with maintenance of temperature, nutrition, acid–base balance, and electrolyte balance. Patients with mechanical assist devices can be weaned from the ventilator using standard weaning protocols depending upon their hemodynamic, blood gas exchange, and neurologic stability. Often a mechanical device can be implanted as a short-term technique for managing a patient's unstable hemodynamic state with an anticipated plan to return to the operating room at a later date to remove the device. This influences one's decision about weaning a patient from mechanical ventilation by possibly carrying out the weaning process without actually removing the endotracheal tube because of an impending trip back to the operating room. In other circumstances, mechanical assist devices are used as bridges to cardiac or cardiopulmonary transplantation when patients' hemodynamic stability cannot be maintained without this intervention. In these situations, each individual patient's cardiopulmonary stability dictates the plan for weaning from mechanical ventilation.

XIII. Family issues in the postoperative period. Interaction with families is important in communicating any patient's status and in giving appropriate expectations concerning recovery. Cardiac surgeons consider communication with family members to be a vital part of surgical planning, and information is made readily available at a variety of venues.

   A. The preoperative discussion. The preoperative discussion is important because the surgeon and anesthesiologist can give a detailed description of what can be anticipated in the postoperative period. This information can be relayed to patients either through preoperative visitations or through video or web site access describing typical postoperative events. Preoperative visitation allows patients the opportunity to ask questions and to understand the plan of movement through the postoperative course. Many times anesthesiology preoperative visitation may be complicated or precluded by admission day surgery patterns whereby cardiac surgery patients arrive at the hospital on the day of surgery. In these circumstances, opportunities for discussions with anesthesia care providers can be limited and must be anticipated at the preoperative visit with the surgeon, when information can be disseminated and questions can be answered.

   B. Family visitation. Family visitation occurs in the ICU or recovery room for many postoperative cardiac and thoracic surgery patients. The ability for patients to be visited by a family member provides reassurance about their course progression and encouragement toward postoperative care. Family members can be very important in encouraging adequate pulmonary toilet, coughing, deep breathing, and early ambulation to improve postoperative outcomes. Most cardiac surgery programs have designated personnel for the liaison between the professional staff caring for postoperative cardiac surgery patients and family members who need education, encouragement, and the opportunity to assist in postoperative care.

C. The role of family support. Family support is a vital link toward the early success of a fast-tracking program. Family members need adequate education by surgical and anesthesia staff, who can outline the expected events in the early postoperative course. The role of family support is heightened when patients spend very short periods in postoperative areas such as the recovery room or ICU. Family members who are educated about the expected postoperative course can facilitate postoperative care and smooth the transition from the ICU to a regular nursing floor and finally to the patient's home.

References

1. Petre JH, Bazaral MG, Estafanous FG. Patient transport: an organized method with direct clinical benefits. Biomedical instrumentation and technology. *Biomed Instrument Technol* 1989;23:100–107.
2. **Smith DC, Crul JF. Early postoperative hypoxia during transport.** *Br J Anaesth* **1988;61:625–627.**
3. Ilabaca PA, Ochsner JL, Mills NL. Positive end-expiratory pressure in the management of the patient with a postoperative bleeding heart. *Ann Thorac Surg* 1980;30:281–284.
4. Zurick AM, Urzua J, Ghattas M, et al. Failure of positive end-expiratory pressure to decrease postoperative bleeding after cardiac surgery. *Ann Thorac Surg* 1982;34:608–611.
5. **Woda RP, Dzwonczyk R, Bernacki BL, et al. The ventilatory effects of auto-positive and end-expiratory pressure development during cardiopulmonary resuscitation.** *Crit Care Med* **1999;27:2212–2217.**
6. Lambermont B, Detry O, D'Orio V, et al. Effects of PEEP on systemic venous capacitance. *Arch Physiol Biochem* 1997;105:373–378.
7. Jardin F, Farcot JC, Boisante L, et al. Influence of positive end-expiratory pressure on left ventricular performance. *N Engl J Med* 1981;304:387–392.
8. **van Belle AF, Wesseling GJ, Penn OC, et al. Postoperative pulmonary function abnormalities after coronary artery bypass surgery.** *Respir Med* **1992;86:195–199.**
9. Yang KL, Tobin MJ. A prospective study of indexes predicting the outcome of trials of weaning from mechanical ventilation. *N Engl J Med* 1991;324:1445–1450.
10. Royse CF, Royse AG, Soeding PF. Routine immediate extubation after cardiac operation: a review of our first 100 patients. *Ann Thorac Surg* 1999;68:1326–1329.
11. Marianeschi SM, Seddio F, McElhinney DB, et al. Fast-track congenital heart operations: a less invasive technique and early extubation. *Ann Thorac Surg* 2000;69:872–876.
12. Walji S, Peterson RJ, Neis P, et al. Ultra-fast track hospital discharge using conventional cardiac surgical techniques. *Ann Thorac Surg* 1999;67:363–370.
13. **Wong DT, Cheng DCH, Kustra R, et al. Risk factors of delayed extubation, prolonged length of stay in the intensive care unit, and mortality in patients undergoing coronary artery bypass graft with fast-track cardiac anesthesia.** *Anesthesiology* **1999;91:936–944.**
14. Montes FR, Sanchez SI, Girlado JC, et al. The lack of benefit of tracheal extubation in the operating room after coronary artery bypass surgery. *Anesth Analg* 2000;91:776–780.
15. Zarate E, Latham P, White PF, et al. Fast-track cardiac anesthesia: use of remifentanil combined with intrathecal morphine as an alternative to sufentanil during desflurane anesthesia. *Anesth Analg* 2000;91:283–287.
16. Latham P, Zarate E, White PF, et al. Fast-track cardiac anesthesia: a comparison of remifentanil plus intrathecal morphine with sufentanil in a desflurane-based anesthetic. *J Cardiothorac Vasc Anesth* 2000;14:645–651.
17. Dowd NP, Cheng DCH, Karski JM, et al. Intraoperative awareness in fast-track cardiac anesthesia. *Anesthesiology* 1998;89:1068–1073.
18. Owall A, Ehrenberg J, Brodin LA. Myocardial ischaemia as judged from transesophageal echocardiography and ECG in the early phase after coronary artery bypass surgery. *Acta Anaesthesiol Scand* 1993;37:92–96.
19. Jacquet L, Noirhomme P, Khoury GE, et al. Cardiac troponin I as an early marker of myocardial damage after coronary bypass surgery. *Eur J Cardiothorac Surg* 1998;13:378–384.
20. Daoud EG, Strickberger A, Man C, et al. Preoperative amiodarone as prophylaxis against atrial fibrillation after heart surgery. *N Engl J Med* 1997;337:1785–1791.

21. **Shroff A, Rooke GA, Bishop MJ. Effects of intrathecal opioid on extubation time, analgesia, and intensive care unit stay following coronary artery bypass grafting.** *J Clin Anesth* **1997;9:415–419.**
22. Hall R, MacLaren C, Barker R, et al. Does intrathecal morphine alter the stress response following coronary artery bypass grafting surgery? *Can J Anesth* 2000;47:463–466.
23. Hynninen MS, Cheng DCH, Hossain I, et al. Nonsteroidal anti-inflammatory drugs in treatment of postoperative pain after cardiac surgery. *Can J Anesth* 2000;47:1182–1187.
24. London MJ, Grunwald GK, Shroyer LW, et al. Association of fast-track cardiac management and low-dose to moderate-dose glucocorticoids administration with perioperative hyperglycemia. *J Cardiothorac Vasc Anesth* 2000;14:627–630.
25. Kay GL, Sun GW, Aoki A, et al. Influence of ejection fraction on hospital mortality, morbidity, and costs for CABG patients. *Ann Thorac Surg* 1995;60:1640–1651.
26. **Doering LV, Esmailian F, Laks H. Perioperative predictors of ICU and hospital costs in coronary artery bypass graft surgery.** *Chest* **2000;118:736–743.**
27. Boyd WD, Desai AND, Del Rizzo DF, et al. Off-pump surgery decreases postoperative complications and resource utilization in the elderly. *Ann Thorac Surg* 1999;68:1490–1493.

II. ANESTHETIC MANAGEMENT OF SPECIFIC CARDIAC DISORDERS

11. ANESTHETIC MANAGEMENT FOR MYOCARDIAL REVASCULARIZATION

Alann Solina, Steven H. Ginsberg, Jay C. Horrow, and Frederick A. Hensley, Jr.

I. Introduction

A. Prevalence and economic impact of coronary artery disease. Although the death rate for coronary heart disease has declined over the last several decades, it is still the leading cause of death in the United States. In the United States, more than 12 million people have a history of angina pectoris, myocardial infarction, or both [1]. More than 500,000 coronary artery bypass graft (CABG) revascularization procedures are performed annually [1].

The economic consequence of coronary heart disease is enormous. It is estimated that the total annual cost of cardiovascular disease in the United States is close to $300 billion, which represents almost 17% of the total health care costs due to major illnesses [2]. Additionally, coronary heart disease accounts for almost a fifth of all disability disbursements by the Social Security Administration [1].

B. Symptoms and progression of coronary artery disease. A complete description of angina pectoris and other symptoms related to coronary artery disease is given in Chapter 1. Unlike the usually predictable time course and progression of symptoms in patients with valvular heart disease, patients with coronary artery disease may have variable onset of symptoms as well as progression of disease characterized by discrete events such as angina or myocardial infarction. Many patients suffer ischemia without symptoms; these "silent" ischemic events require diligence for detection and prompt treatment before and after operation. Only 20% of myocardial infarctions are preceded by long-standing angina [1]. All aspects of preoperative evaluation of these patients (i.e., exercise stress testing and cardiac catheterization) are discussed in Chapter 1.

C. Historical perspective of CABG. Early unsuccessful attempts at myocardial revascularization by inducing pericardial adhesions took place before the 1950s. In 1951, Vineburg implanted the internal mammary artery (IMA) directly into the myocardium. Subsequent research showed that although myocardial blood flow was improved by this procedure, the additional blood flow was not enough to lead to symptomatic improvement of angina pectoris. In 1967, Favalaro and Effler at the Cleveland Clinic began performing reversed saphenous vein bypass grafting procedures, as we know them today. In 1968, Green performed an anastomosis of the IMA directly to a coronary artery. There was a resurgence of interest in the IMA grafting procedure in the late 1970s and early 1980s after a number of studies showed far greater graft patency rates for IMA grafts compared with saphenous vein grafts. In addition, better long-term survival was evident in patients receiving IMA grafts, regardless of ventricular function.

An interest in enhanced recovery ("fast track") cardiac surgery in the 1990s perhaps was initially engendered by economic concerns over efficient resource utilization, especially in view of the increased penetration of managed care, but subsequently was fueled by recognized improvements in clinical outcome. The 1990s also gave rise to minimally invasive revascularization techniques, which allow for revascularization through smaller incisions or through the use of port-access devices. Additionally, in select cases, the advent of new myocardial stabilization devices obviated the need for exposure to cardiopulmonary bypass for myocardial revascularization. Transmyocardial laser revascularization, introduced in the late 1990s, attempts to promote angiogenesis and physically create new channels for blood flow. This procedure more typically is performed in patients with poor targets for coronary revascularization. These techniques and the anesthetic concerns that they engender are discussed thoroughly elsewhere (see Chapter 13). The use of intraoperative transesophageal echocardiography (TEE) was one of the more important clinical developments affecting the quality of care during coronary revascularization surgery in the 1990s (see Chapter 4).

The clinical acuity of cardiac surgery patients has continued to increase over the last decade. High-risk, multivessel angioplasty and the use of intracoronary stents both are associated with a risk of vessel patency failure. An aging patient population and an increase in the number of redo revascularization operations also has increased the risk faced by CABG patients. An increased patient risk profile, the development of new surgical techniques, and the increasing use of intraoperative echocardiography has increased the complexity and sophistication of perioperative anesthetic management and has helped to drive the development of the subspecialty of cardiac anesthesia.

D. **Evaluating risk of morbidity and mortality for CABG surgery**
   1. **Introduction.** Assessment of perioperative risk for morbid events and mortality is important because it (a) is crucial in the analysis of outcome and performance improvement data, (b) serves as a basis of comparison for different therapeutic approaches within and across care-giver systems, (c) is a requisite part of the informed consent process, and (d) may help to determine optimal resource utilization. A comprehensive review of the myriad risk stratification schema is beyond the scope of this text; however, a brief discussion of some of the more popular risk stratification tools follows.
   2. **Risk factor models.** Although risk stratification tools may differ in the specific weights assigned to certain risk factors, there is agreement that certain factors are associated with increased risk of morbidity and mortality. These factors include poor left ventricular (LV) function (history of congestive heart failure or LV ejection fraction less than 30%), advanced age, obesity, emergency surgery, concomitant valve surgery, prior cardiac surgery, history of diabetes, and history of renal failure [3,4].

      The composite score of the individually weighted risk factors is associated with a certain predicted risk of short- and long-term morbidity and mortality, length of stay, and hospital costs. Some of the more recognized risk stratification tools include the Society of Thoracic Surgeons (STS) Model, the Parsonnet Model, the Cleveland Clinic Preoperative Cardiac Surgical Severity Score, the New York State Model, and the Northern New England Model (Table 11.1).
   3. **Model evaluation.** Individual risk stratification models are crudely assessed for accuracy by determining the relationship of predicted to observed morbidity and mortality. Physicians and hospital administrators frequently are concerned that the various models do not completely capture risk in sicker patients. Some models do not allow for adequate flexibility with regard to the dynamic nature of the patient's physiology during the preoperative period. For example, a patient's LV ejection fraction at the time of cardiac catheterization will be used in the evaluation process, instead of that derived from TEE at the time of surgery.

II. **Myocardial oxygen supply**
   A. **Introduction.** The viability and function of the heart are predicated upon a relatively delicate balance of oxygen supply and demand. It is of paramount importance

Table 11.1 Risk factor inclusion in various risk stratification models for coronary artery bypass grafting

	Montreal	Cleveland	Newark	New York	Northern New England	Society of Thoracic Surgery
Emergency	+	+	+	+	+	+
Poor left ventricular function/ congestive heart failure	+	+	+	+	+	+
Redo operation	+	+	+	+	+	+
Gender/ small size	–	+	+	+	+	+
Valve disease	–	+	+	+	–	–
Advanced age	+	+	+	+	+	+
Renal disease	–	+	+	+	+	–
Obesity	+	–	+	–	–	–

for the cardiac anesthesiologist to understand the intricacies of this relationship. The following two sections delineate the components and regulation of the myocardial oxygen supply/demand equality. The myocardium maximally extracts O_2 from arterial blood at rest. With exertion or hemodynamic stress, the only way the O_2 supply can increase acutely to meet the myocardial energy demand is by increasing coronary blood flow (CBF). Ischemia occurs when CBF does not increase to a level sufficient to meet myocardial demand, and aerobic metabolism is impaired. The following approach achieves the clinical goal of ensuring that O_2 supply at least matches demand:

- Optimize the determinants of myocardial O_2 supply and demand
- Select anesthetics and adjuvant agents and techniques according to their effects on O_2 supply and demand
- Monitor for ischemia to detect its occurrence early and intervene rapidly

B. Coronary anatomy
　　1. Introduction. One must have a thorough understanding of the coronary artery anatomy and distribution of blood flow to the myocardium to understand the surgical procedure as well as the extent and degree of myocardium at risk for ischemia and infarction during anesthesia and surgery. The blood supply to the myocardium derives from the aorta through two main coronary arteries (see Fig. 1.2), the left and right coronary arteries. The left main coronary artery extends for a short distance (0 to 40 mm) before dividing into the left anterior descending artery and the circumflex coronary artery.
　　2. Left anterior descending coronary artery. The left anterior descending artery begins as a continuation of the left main coronary artery and courses down the interventricular groove, giving rise to the diagonal and septal branches. The septal branches vary in number and size, arise in an almost perpendicular fashion from the left anterior descending artery, and provide the predominant blood supply to the interventricular septum. The septal branches also supply the bundle branches and the Purkinje system. One to three diagonal branches of variable size exist, and these branches distribute blood to the anterolateral aspect of the heart. The left anterior descending artery continues down the interventricular groove and usually passes all the way around to the apex of the LV.
　　3. Circumflex coronary artery. The circumflex artery arises from the left main coronary artery at almost a 90-degree angle and passes down the left atrioventricular groove. Its main vessels are the obtuse marginal branches, which range from one to three in number. They supply the lateral free wall of the LV. In 15% of patients, the circumflex artery gives rise to the posterior descending coronary artery (see Section II.B.4). In 45% of patients, the sinus node artery arises from the circumflex distribution.
　　4. Right coronary artery. The right coronary artery passes down the right atrioventricular groove. It gives rise to acute marginal branches that supply the right anterior wall of the right ventricle. In approximately 85% of individuals, the right coronary artery gives rise to the posterior descending artery to supply the posterior inferior aspect of the LV. This blood supply pattern is classified as a right dominant system. In the majority of the population, the right coronary artery supplies a significant portion of blood flow to the LV. In the other 15% of the population, the posterior-inferior aspect of the LV is supplied by the circumflex coronary artery (left dominant system) or both right coronary and circumflex arteries (codominant system). The sinus node artery arises from the right coronary artery in 55% of patients. The atrioventricular node artery derives from the dominant coronary artery and is responsible for blood supply to the node, the bundle of His, and the proximal part of the bundle branches.

C. Determinants of myocardial oxygen supply. In broad terms, the supply of oxygen to the myocardium is determined by the arterial oxygen content of the blood and the blood flow in the coronary arteries.
　　1. O_2 content = (hemoglobin) (1.34) (% saturation) + (0.003) (Po_2)

Ensuring maximal O_2 content therefore involves having a high hemoglobin level, highly saturated blood, and a high P_{O_2}. Warm temperature, normal pH, and high levels of 2,3-diphosphoglyceric acid all favor release of O_2 at the tissues.

2. **Determinants of blood flow in normal coronary arteries.** CBF varies directly with the **pressure differential** across the coronary bed [coronary perfusion pressure (CPP)] and inversely with coronary vascular resistance (CVR): **CBF = CPP/CVR.** However, coronary artery blood flow is autoregulated (i.e., resistance varying directly with perfusion pressure) so that flow is relatively independent of CPP between 50 and 150 mm Hg but is pressure dependent outside of this range. Metabolic, autonomic nervous system, hormonal, and anatomic parameters alter CVR, and hydraulic factors influence CPP. Coronary stenoses also increase CVR.

   a. **Control of CVR.** Factors affecting CVR are outlined in Table 11.2.

      (1) **Metabolic factors.** When increased coronary flow is required secondary to increased myocardial workload, metabolic control factors are primarily responsible. Hydrogen ion, CO_2, and lactate all may play a role in metabolic regulation of CBF by inducing changes in CVR. Adenosine probably is an important metabolic regulator of blood flow [5]. When the O_2 supply of the myocardium is exceeded, adenosine from adenosine triphosphate breakdown causes coronary vasodilation and increases blood flow.

      (2) **Autonomic nervous system.** The coronary arteries and arterioles are endowed with α- and β-receptors. In general, α_1-receptors are responsible for coronary vasoconstriction, whereas β-receptors mediate a vasodilatory effect. α_2-Receptors on endothelial cells appear to be involved in a nitric oxide-mediated decrease in coronary vascular tone [6]. Muscarinic signaling also may be involved in nitric oxide-mediated control of coronary vascular tone. An increased population of α-receptors may cause episodes of coronary spasm in individuals with nonobstructed coronaries. α_1-Mediated constriction of the coronary circulation may counter some of the metabolic vasodilation, especially in the resting basal state. However, under most circumstances such as increasing demand or ischemia, metabolic control factors will override α-mediated vasoconstriction.

      (3) **Hormonal factors.** Two stress hormones, vasopressin (antidiuretic hormone) and angiotensin, are known to be potent coronary vasoconstrictors. It still is unclear whether the blood levels of these hormones

Table 11.2 Control of coronary vascular resistance

	Increase CVR	Decrease CVR
Metabolic	$\uparrow O_2$, $\downarrow CO_2$ $\downarrow H^+$	$\downarrow O_2$, $\uparrow CO_2$ $\uparrow H^+$ Lactate Adenosine
Autonomic nervous system	$\uparrow$ α-Adrenergic tone $\uparrow$ Cholinergic tone	$\uparrow$ β-Adrenergic tone
Hormonal	$\uparrow$ Vasopressin (antidiuretic hormone) $\uparrow$ Angiotensin $\uparrow$ Thromboxane	$\uparrow$ Prostacyclin
Endothelial modulation		$\uparrow$ Nitric oxide $\uparrow$ Endothelium-derived hyperpolarizing factor $\uparrow$ Prostaglandin I_2

$\uparrow$, increased; $\downarrow$, decreased; CVR, coronary vascular resistance.

during major stress are high enough to produce clinical coronary vaso-constriction.

Thromboxane may cause thrombosis and coronary vasospasm during myocardial infarction. Prostaglandin I_2 (PGI_2) decreases coronary vascular tone.

(4) **Endothelial modulation.** Nitric oxide, which is released from the endothelium in response to chemical stimuli and mechanical vessel stress, is responsible for a cyclic guanosine monophosphate (c-GMP)–mediated vasodilatory effect on vascular smooth muscle. Nitric oxide also may contribute to vessel patency and blood flow by inhibiting platelet adhesion. PGI_2 and endothelium-derived hyperpolarizing factor, which are released by the vascular endothelium, also cause relaxation of vascular smooth muscle. Endothelin, an extremely potent vasoconstrictor that is released by vascular endothelium, does not appear to be significantly involved in the regulation of myocardial blood flow under normal physiologic conditions [6].

(5) **Anatomic factors**

   (a) **Capillary/myocyte ratio.** There is an almost 1:1 ratio of capillaries to myocytes in the human myocardium. However, only three to four fifths of these capillaries function during normal conditions. During exercise, episodes of hypoxia, or extreme myocardial O_2 demand, the additional unopened capillaries are recruited and increase blood flow, causing a decrease in CVR. This decreases the intercapillary distance and thus the diffusion distance of O_2 to a given myocyte. This adaptation, along with coronary vasodilation, contributes to coronary vascular reserve.

   (b) **Coronary collaterals.** Coronary collateral channels exist in the human myocardium. Under most circumstances, they are nonfunctional. However, in the presence of impeded CBF, these coronary channels may enlarge over time and become functional.

(6) **Other factors affecting CVR.** CVR may be partly regulated by myogenic control of vessel diameter, which dynamically responds to the distending pressure inside the vessel. CVR varies linearly with blood viscosity. High hematocrit and hypothermia both increase viscosity dramatically, thus adversely increasing CVR. For these reasons, hemodilution is necessary when inducing hypothermia. It should be noted that there is a transmural gradient of vascular tone, with vascular resistance being lower in the subendocardium than in the subepicardium [5].

b. **Hydraulic factors and subendocardial blood flow**

(1) **LV subendocardial blood flow.** Unlike CBF in the low-pressure right ventricular system, LV subendocardial blood flow is intermittent and occurs only during the diastolic portion of the cardiac cycle. Because of the increased intracavitary pressure and excessive subendocardial myocyte shortening, subendocardial arterioles are essentially closed during systole. Of the total LV coronary flow, 85% occurs during diastole and 15% occurs in systole (primarily in the epicardial region). Thus, the majority of blood flow to the epicardial and middle layers of the LV and **all** the blood flow to the endocardium occur during diastole.

(2) **Coronary perfusion pressure.** CPP equals the arterial driving pressure less the back-pressure to flow across the coronary bed. For the LV, the driving pressure is the aortic blood pressure during diastole. The back-pressure to flow depends on the area of myocardium under consideration. Most blood returns via the coronary sinus, and the corresponding back-pressure is that of the right atrium. However, for the endocardium, drainage occurs through thebesian veins directly into the ventricular cavities. Because the endocardium is the area most at risk, attention focuses on its flow. Thus, the calculation

for subendocardial CPP uses LV end-diastolic pressure (LVEDP) as the back-pressure:

CPP = Aortic diastolic blood pressure – LVEDP

Because diastole shortens relative to systole as heart rate increases, subendocardial blood flow is decreased at extremely rapid heart rates. Figure 11.1 demonstrates the total time per minute spent in diastole as a function of heart rate. Elevations in LVEDP (e.g., heart failure, ischemia) also will impede subendocardial blood flow. **Thus, to optimize CPP, one should aim for normal-to-high diastolic blood pressure, low LVEDP, and low heart rate.**

3. **Determinants of myocardial blood flow in stenotic coronaries.** In addition to the physiologic determinants of myocardial blood flow in normal coronary arteries, stenotic vessels add pathologic determinants of myocardial blood flow. Stenoses increase CVR and decrease CBF.
    a. **Types of coronary stenoses**
        (1) **Fixed or dynamic.** A fixed stenosis is composed of an atherosclerotic plaque. A dynamic stenosis can occur in a region of a normal coronary artery, such as occurs in Prinzmetal variant angina or vasospastic angina. A combination of dynamic stenosis superimposed on an obstructive lesion may occur, particularly in patients with unstable angina pectoris.
        (2) **Focal or segmental.** The length of a coronary artery lesion can be short (focal) or long (segmental). Given the same decrease in cross-sectional area, a longer segmental stenosis of a coronary artery increases CVR more, thus reducing coronary flow more than would a short focal coronary stenosis (Poiseuille's law).
    b. **Degree of stenosis.** CBF is reduced in proportion to the fourth power of the vessel diameter. Angiographically, a 50% diameter decrease in lumen size corresponds to a 75% reduction in cross-sectional area, which is

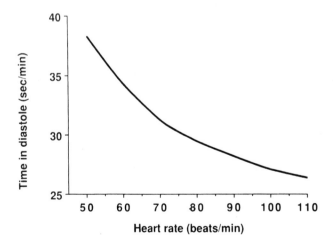

FIG. 11.1 Total time spent in diastole each minute is plotted as a function of heart rate in beats per minute (beats/min). The reduction in diastolic interval leads to diminished left ventricular blood flow as heart rate increases.

hemodynamically consistent with symptoms of angina on exertion. A 75% reduction in diameter at angiography corresponds to a 94% reduction in cross-sectional area, which corresponds clinically to symptoms of angina at rest. Two discrete lesions in the same coronary artery will result in two tandem pressure drops, creating an impact on coronary flow in an additive fashion.

  c. **Collateral channels.** If the stenotic coronary lesion develops slowly, then collateral channels will enlarge to provide additional blood supply to a jeopardized region of the myocardium. These channels directly connect one coronary artery to another or different segments of the same coronary artery without an intervening capillary bed. Often in the presence of a low-grade obstructive lesion, these channels supply enough blood flow to prevent ischemia. However, as the degree of **coronary stenosis increases, the collateral channels may not be adequate.**

  d. **Patterns of stenoses.** Certain patterns of stenoses have important clinical implications related to the amount of myocardium supplied and placed in jeopardy by the stenotic lesion(s). A left main coronary stenosis limits blood flow to a large amount of the LV muscle mass. High-grade, very proximal stenotic lesions of both the circumflex and left anterior descending systems have the same **physiologic** implications as does a left main stenosis. **Prognostically,** however, a left main stenosis is more severe because only one vessel needs to become completely occluded to compromise a large amount of myocardial muscle. In addition, similar "left main equivalent" situations may exist when a severely stenosed coronary provides collateral blood flow to a region with a totally occluded vessel (Fig. 11.2).

  e. **Diffuse distal coronary disease.** In addition to discrete focal and segmental coronary lesions in graftable vessels, diffuse distal disease may be present in the small branches of the coronary vessels distal to where a graft could be placed. This diffuse disease further reduces blood flow to the myocardium and lessens the effectiveness of bypassing proximal coronary obstructions.

  f. **Associated disease states**
     (1) **Diabetic patients.** Diabetic patients have been shown to have abnormal coronary microvasculature consisting of thickened capillary basement membranes that limit the diffusion of O_2 to the myocytes.

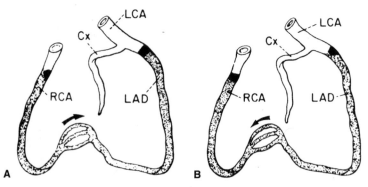

FIG. 11.2 Two examples of possible left main "equivalency." Two-vessel coronary disease with an occluded left anterior descending coronary artery (*LAD*) and myocardium jeopardized by a right coronary artery (*RCA*) stenosis (**A**) or an occluded RCA and myocardium jeopardized by a stenotic LAD (**B**). Cx, circumflex coronary artery; *LCA*, left coronary artery. (From Hutter AM Jr. Is there a left main equivalent? *Circulation* 1980;62:209, with permission.)

(2) **Hypertensive patients.** Hypertensive patients are at increased risk for subendocardial ischemia. Hypertension is associated with LV hypertrophy. Because of increased wall thickness, the compressive forces on the coronary arteriole and O_2 demand in hypertensive patients are even greater in the subendocardium compared to those in normal individuals. A combination of LV hypertrophy with severe coronary stenosis places a patient at increased risk for development of subendocardial ischemia.

III. Myocardial oxygen demand. Direct measurement of myocardial oxygen demand is not feasible in the clinical setting. The product of heart rate and systolic pressure (rate–pressure product) sometimes is used as an easily obtainable clinical indicator of myocardial oxygen demand. The three major determinants of myocardial O_2 demand are heart rate, contractility, and wall stress.

   A. Heart rate. If a relatively fixed amount of O_2 were consumed per heartbeat, one would expect the O_2 demand per minute to increase linearly with heart rate. Thus, a doubling of heart rate would yield a doubling of O_2 demand. In fact, demand more than doubles with a two-fold increase in heart rate. The source of this additional O_2 demand is the staircase phenomenon, in which increased heart rate causes a small increase in contractility and increases in contractility mean more O_2 consumed (see Section **B** below).

   B. Contractility. More O_2 is used by a highly contractile heart compared with a more relaxed heart.

      1. Quantitative assessment. Strictly defined, the contractile state of the heart is a dynamic intrinsic characteristic that is not influenced by preload or afterload. The rate of rise of LV pressure, dP/dt, has been used as a quantitative measure of contractility. Clinically it is possible to quantify dP/dt echocardiographically by measuring the rate of rise in the velocity of the mitral regurgitant jet using Doppler technology. Unfortunately, loading conditions and chamber compliance significantly affect the acceleration of the mitral regurgitant jet. Additionally, although mitral regurgitation frequently is observed echocardiographically, it is not universally present. Contractility can be approximated in a load-independent fashion using the slope of the end-systolic pressure–volume relationships of a family of LV pressure–volume loops. This method usually is not available in clinical settings.

      2. Qualitative measures. One can easily observe the contractile state of the heart when the pericardium is open. Remember, though, that the right ventricle is more easily and most often viewed this way, whereas the left is more obscured. TEE provides a means for qualitative estimation of LV contractility. Clinically, we infer that contractility is good when there is a brisk rise in the arterial pressure tracing. However, the shape of the radial arterial tracing is heavily influenced by confounding factors (e.g., system resonant frequency, damping by air bubbles, compliance of the arterial tree, and reflections of pressure waves from arteriolar sites).

      3. Increased subendocardial myocyte shortening. In addition to the intermittent decrease in subendocardial blood flow, the subendocardial region has higher rates of oxidative metabolism secondary to the increased myocyte shortening in this region. Little reserve for increased coronary vasodilation occurs in the subendocardium because most of these vessels already are maximally dilated. Because of the increased demand and intermittent limitations of blood flow in the subendocardial region, myocardial O_2 tension falls first here (Fig. 11.3). Thus, this region is more susceptible to an ischemic insult.

   C. Wall stress. The stress in the ventricular wall depends on the pressure in the ventricle during contraction (afterload), the chamber size (preload), and the wall thickness. The calculation for a sphere (which we shall assume for the shape of the ventricle, for the sake of simplicity) is as follows:

$$\text{Wall stress} = \text{Pressure} \times \frac{\text{radius}}{2\ (\text{wall thickness})}$$

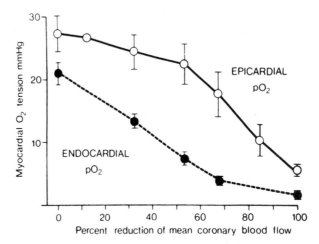

FIG. 11.3 Relationship of subendocardial O_2 supply (represented by myocardial O_2 tension) to reductions in coronary blood flow. Demonstrated is the increased vulnerability of the subendocardial zone compared to the epicardial zone. (Modified from Winbury MM, Howe BB. Stenosis: regional myocardial ischemia and reserve. In: Winbury MM, Abiko Y, eds. *Ischemic myocardium and antianginal drugs.* New York: Raven, 1979:59.)

1. **Chamber pressure.** Oxygen demand increases with chamber pressure. Doubling the pressure doubles the O_2 demand. Systemic blood pressure usually reflects the chamber pressure; thus, we equate systemic blood pressure with LV afterload. The heart's true afterload is more complex because there are elastic and inertial components that affect ejection. Mean systemic pressure, not peak systolic pressure, correlates with O_2 demand. In aortic stenosis, however, the LV experiences very high chamber pressures despite more modest systemic pressures. The clinical goal is to keep afterload (and thus wall stress) low.

2. **Chamber size.** Doubling the ventricular volume increases the radius by only 26% (volume varies with the radius cubed). Thus, increased chamber size is associated with more modest increases in O_2 demand. Nevertheless, because preload determines ventricular size, we desire a low preload to keep wall stress (and thus O_2 demand) low. For example, much of the beneficial effect of nitroglycerin stems from venodilation and its attendant decrease in preload.

3. **Wall thickness.** A thicker wall means less stress over any part of the wall. Ventricular hypertrophy serves to decrease wall stress, although the additional tissue requires more O_2 overall. Hypertrophy occurs in response to the elevated afterload that occurs in chronic systemic hypertension or aortic stenosis. Although wall thickness is essentially uncontrollable clinically, its effects should be considered. LV aneurysms, seen after transmural infarction, increase wall stress because of their affect on LV volume (radius) and reduced wall thickness.

D. **Summary. The factors that increase O_2 demand are increases in heart rate, chamber size, chamber pressure, and contractility.** Table 11.3 and Figure 11.4 summarize the myocardial supply and demand relationship. **Note that tachycardia and increases in LVEDP both lead to increased demand and decreased supply of oxygen.**

IV. **Monitoring for myocardial ischemia**

A. **Introduction.** Monitoring for cardiac surgery is discussed in Chapter 3. Typical monitoring for CABG surgery includes the standard American Society of

Table 11.3 Regulation of O_2 supply and demand

Parameter	Demand	Supply	O_2 balance
Low heart rate	↓	↑	Positive
Low RAP or PCWP	↓	↑[a]	Positive
High heart rate	↑	↓	Negative
High RAP or PCWP	↑	↓	Negative
High temperature	↑	0	Negative
Low temperature	↑↓	↓	Variable
Low MAP	↓	↓	Variable
High MAP	↑	↑	Variable
Low hemoglobin	↓	↓↑	Variable
High hemoglobin	↑	↑↓	Variable

[a] However, a drastic decrease in filling pressure will decrease cardiac output.
↑, increased; ↓, decreased; ↑↓, may increase or decrease; 0, unchanged; MAP, mean arterial pressure; PCWP, pulmonary capillary wedge pressure; RAP, right atrial pressure.

Anesthesiology (ASA) monitors and invasive arterial blood pressure monitoring. Although TEE is used more frequently in current practice, it is not considered the standard of care for routine procedures. The use of PA catheters for routine CABG also is highly variable. Detection and treatment of intraoperative ischemia is critically important because intraoperative ischemia is an independent predictor of postoperative myocardial infarction [7]. Only half of intraoperative ischemic events can be related to a hemodynamic alteration (tachycardia, hypotension, or hypertension). Because patients who develop intraoperative ischemia are more likely to suffer a perioperative transmural myocardial infarction, we must monitor patients closely to detect and treat every ischemic episode. Angina is a symptom, not a sign; therefore, an awake, communicative patient with an intact warning system is necessary. Ischemia is diagnosed with certainty by decreased lactate extraction of a regional myocardial circulatory bed. This technique is not feasible on a routine clinical basis, so we turn to picking up the clues that ischemia leaves in its wake: changes on the electrocardiogram (ECG), pulmonary arterial (PA) pressure changes, and myocardial wall-motion abnormalities.

B. ECG monitoring

1. Introduction. Despite the increasing use of intraoperative TEE to detect new ischemic wall-motion abnormalities, continuous multilead ECG monitoring still is a standard monitor of intraoperative ischemia. ECG monitoring is relatively inexpensive, easy to use and read, and can be automated. A particular advantage of ECG monitoring for myocardial ischemia is that it may be accomplished before and during the induction of anesthesia, when it is impossible to use TEE. ECG monitoring is, of course, easily accomplished in the intensive care unit (ICU) setting postoperatively, when it is more difficult and logistically impossible to use continuous TEE as a monitor of ischemia. ECG changes tend to occur later in the temporal cascade of events that follow myocardial ischemia. This is especially true with less dramatic coronary supply/demand inequality.

2. ST-segment analysis. The ST segment of the ECG changes with ischemia. Depression denotes endocardial ischemia, and elevation denotes transmural ischemia. ST-segment changes occur at least 60 to 120 seconds after the start of ischemia. The reference for the ST segment usually is taken as 80 ms after the J-point, which is the end of the QRS wave (Fig. 11.5). Significant changes usually are defined as 0.1 mV or 1 mm of ST-segment elevation or depression at normal gain. ECG monitoring systems include automated real-time ST-segment analysis. Although this feature constitutes a definite advance in the "human engineering" aspects of ischemia monitoring, the machine is only as smart as the person interpreting its data. Beware of intraventricular conduction delays,

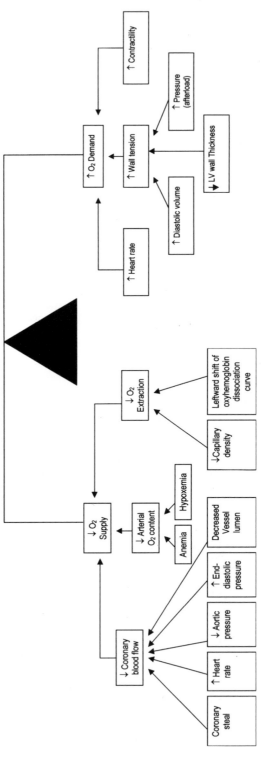

FIG. 11.4 Summary of factors that affect myocardial oxygen supply and demand. (Adapted from Crystal GJ. Cardiovascular physiology. In: Miller RD, ed. *Atlas of anesthesia: vol. VIII. Cardiothoracic anesthesia.* Philadelphia: Churchill Livingstone, 1999;1:1, with permission.)

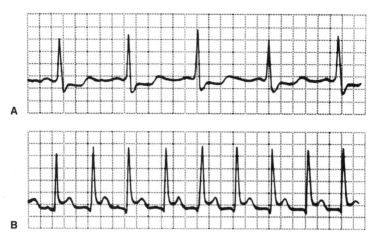

FIG. 11.5 A: ST-segment depression, an indicator of subendocardial ischemia. **B:** Transmural ischemia, one cause of ST-segment elevation, produces the pattern appearing in the **lower tracing.**

bundle branch blocks, and ventricular pacing, all of which can render ST-segment analysis invalid. Check the machine's determination of where the ST segment occurs: 80 ms after the J-point is not always appropriate.
  a. **Differential diagnosis of ST-segment changes.** The differential diagnosis of ST-segment elevation includes the several causes of transmural ischemia (atherosclerotic disease, coronary vasospasm, intracoronary air), pericarditis, and ventricular aneurysm (Fig. 11.5). One also must consider improper lead placement, particularly reversal of limb and leg leads, and improper selection of electronic filtering. **The diagnostic mode should always be chosen on machines equipped with a diagnostic–monitor mode selection switch.**
3. **T-wave changes.** New T-wave alterations (flipped or flattened) may indicate ischemia. These may not be detected by viewing the ST segment alone. Likewise, pseudonormalization of the ST segment or T wave (an ischemic-looking tracing in a patient without ischemia reverting to a more normal-looking one) may indicate a new onset of ischemia and should be treated appropriately.
4. **Multilead ECG monitoring.** Simultaneous observation of an inferior lead (II, III, or aVF) and an anterior lead (V_5) provides detection superior to single-lead monitoring. Five-lead monitoring is thought to detect approximately 90% of ischemic events. Ischemia limited to the posterior of the heart is difficult to detect with standard ECG monitoring. Modified chest leads may be necessary when the surgical incision precludes usual placement.
C. **PA pressure monitoring**
  1. **General indications for a PA catheter for revascularization procedures.** A PA catheter should be placed when the risks are outweighed by the benefits. The clinical utility of PA catheters is broad based. Some of its many functions include provision of a conduit for infusions and as a monitor of blood temperature, ventricular preload, myocardial ischemia, cardiac output, vascular resistance, and right ventricular ejection fraction (with special catheters equipped with particularly fast thermistors). Additionally, the oximetric capabilities of special PA catheters can be used to determine mixed venous oxygen saturation. Claims that PA catheterization does not affect outcome [8,9]

should be doubted until randomized studies provide validation. At many institutions, PA catheters are not considered necessary for the intraoperative management of routine coronary bypass surgery. However, at times, PA catheters are placed by the anesthesiologist for use in the postoperative setting, when it often is more difficult to utilize TEE.

   2. **Detection of ischemia: PA pressures.** The absolute PA pressure is not diagnostic of ischemia. Pulmonary hypertension, whether primary or secondary to valvular heart disease, is not uncommon. Elevations of PA pressure or pulmonary capillary wedge pressure may occur secondary to rapid volume infusion, alterations in table positioning, use of vasoactive agents, or light anesthesia in the absence of ischemia. The morphology of the waveform, however, is more predictive. Appearance of a new V wave on the pulmonary capillary wedge pressure waveform indicates functional mitral regurgitation, which is due to valvular pathology or papillary muscle dysfunction from ischemia (see Fig. 3.13). A new V wave suggestive of ischemia may occur before or in the absence of ECG changes. However, detection of changes on the pulmonary capillary wedge waveform requires frequent wedging of the PA catheter, a questionable practice in heparinized patients because of the possibility of PA rupture. Often the morphology of the PA pressure tracing will change when a new V wave appears on the wedge tracing. When the PA pressure wave changes shape, check the wedge for a new V wave.

D. **Transesophageal echocardiography**
   1. **General indications for TEE during revascularization procedures.** TEE is used to assess ventricular preload and contractility, detect myocardial ischemia-induced regional wall-motion abnormalities (RWMAs), evaluate the aortic cannulation site, detect concomitant valve pathology, detect the presence and pathophysiologic effect of pericardial effusion, aid the placement of intraaortic balloon catheters and coronary sinus catheters, and detect the presence of ventricular aneurysms and ventricular septal defects. TEE has become an invaluable clinical tool and is used routinely at many institutions for most CABG surgery. New RWMAs in the postbypass period have been found to be prognostically related to adverse outcomes. See Chapter 4 for a detailed discussion of intraoperative TEE.
   2. **Detection of myocardial ischemia with TEE**
      a. **Regional wall-motion abnormalities**
         (1) **Introduction.** The heart quickly and reliably develops RWMAs as a consequence of myocardial ischemia. RWMAs resulting from myocardial ischemia temporally precede both ECG and PAP changes. Normal wall motion consists of symmetrical systolic circumferential radial shortening and thickening. Abnormalities of wall motion include hypokinesis (impaired shortening and thickening), akinesis (no shortening or thickening), and dyskinesis (systolic lengthening and thinning). One advantage of using RWMA for detection of ischemia is that it is possible to simultaneously interrogate regions of the heart that are representative of all three major coronary arteries (including the posterior wall, which is not easily monitored with ECG). This is, perhaps, most easily accomplished in the short-axis, midpapillary muscle view. However, it must be appreciated that ischemia confined to regions that are not being interrogated will not be detected. Proper interrogation of the heart involves performing a comprehensive examination in multiple tomographic planes.
         (2) **Limitations of monitoring RWMA**
            (a) **Tethering.** Nonischemic tissue that is adjacent to ischemic tissue may move abnormally simply because it is attached to tissue exhibiting an RWMA. This tends to exaggerate the RWMA.
            (b) **Pacing/bundle branch blocks.** In the presence of a bundle branch block or myocardial pacing, a temporal heterogeneity of the onset of ventricular contraction exists that may mimic an RWMA.

        (c) Interventricular septum. Septal motion is dependent upon ventricular loading conditions, the presence or absence of the pericardium, and conduction abnormalities.

        (d) Stunned myocardium. Myocardium, which presently is well perfused, may exhibit an RWMA predicated upon antecedent ischemia. This eventuality may prompt therapeutic intervention, which is no longer necessary or appropriate.

        (e) Induction/ICU. Use of TEE for detection of ischemia is not possible during induction of anesthesia and is not logistically pragmatic in the ICU.

  b. Diastolic LV filling patterns. Doppler echocardiography may be used to evaluate the pattern of LV filling. Normally the transmitral velocity filling pattern is biphasic. The initial component, called the E wave, is due to passive emptying of the left atrium (LA), and the second component, the A wave, is due to atrial contraction. Because the LA–LV pressure gradient is higher at the beginning of ventricular diastole, the E wave normally is larger than the A wave. With ischemia-induced reductions in LV compliance, there is an increase in LA pressure that results in a larger LA–LV pressure gradient at the beginning of diastole. This causes an increase in the E-wave velocity (i.e., an increase in the E/A ratio). Additionally, with decreased ventricular compliance, the LA–LV pressure gradient decreases more rapidly, so there is a more rapid deceleration of the E wave. Unfortunately, it is difficult to use ventricular filling patterns as an indicator of ischemia because they are affected by ventricular loading conditions and are critically affected by the site of Doppler interrogation within the ventricular inflow tract.

  c. Intraoperative stress TEE. Low-dose dobutamine (2.5 μg/kg/min), when administered for 3 to 5 minutes, will improve coronary flow without significantly affecting demand. This will lead to improved myocardial energetics and may improve existing wall-motion abnormalities. A demonstration of contractile reserve of this sort is an indication of tissue viability and may help to determine whether it is worthwhile to attempt revascularization of a particular region.

  d. Contrast echocardiography. When introduced into the coronary circulation, sonicated albumin will distribute in the myocardium according to tissue perfusion. The ability to identify qualitative perfusion of the myocardium eventually may prove to be of significant clinical utility. For example, it eventually may be possible to demonstrate flow in an area of stunned myocardium that presently is demonstrating an RWMA, thus obviating the need for therapeutic intervention. At present, contrast agents are not approved by the U.S. Food and Drug Administration for this indication. Additionally, there are some technical imaging issues that must be resolved before this technique can become a real clinical tool.

  e. Detection of infarction complications. TEE can be used to detect complications of ischemia/infarction such as acute mitral insufficiency, ventricular septal defect, and pericardial effusion.

V. Anesthetic effects on myocardial oxygen supply and demand. Several well-designed studies have failed to reveal a relationship between anesthetic agent selection and clinical outcome in the setting of cardiac surgery [10,11]. This finding probably is predicated, at least in part, upon the fact that cardiac anesthesiologists are keenly aware of the effects that anesthetic agents have on myocardial oxygen supply/demand dynamics and have the ability to effectively monitor for and treat myocardial ischemia.

  A. Intravenous nonopioid agents

    1. Thiopental and thiamylal. Induction doses of the ultra-short-acting barbiturates **decrease systemic vascular resistance (SVR) and cardiac contractility and increase heart rate.** Oxygen demand is decreased by the first two effects and increased by the third effect. Oxygen supply is decreased by all three hemodynamic perturbations. The net effect on myocardial O_2 balance is not easily predicted. It depends on the initial conditions. For example, the hyperdynamic, hypertensive patient may benefit from restoration of more appropriate conditions of blood pressure and contractility, whereas a patient whose O_2 balance depends on a normal heart rate may respond to the resultant tachycardia with ischemia.

2. **Ketamine.** The hallmark of ketamine administration is an increase in sympathetic tone leading to **increases in SVR, filling pressures, contractility, and heart rate.** Myocardial O_2 demand is strongly increased, whereas O_2 supply may be only slightly augmented, thus producing ischemia. The patient who already is maximally sympathetically stimulated may respond with decreased contractility and vasodilation. Ketamine is not recommended for routine use in patients with ischemic heart disease. It is, however, sometimes used in the setting of tamponade physiology because of its ability to preserve heart rate, contractility, and SVR.

3. **Etomidate.** Induction doses of etomidate (0.2 to 0.3 mg/kg) **do not alter heart rate or cardiac output,** although mild peripheral vasodilation may lower blood pressure slightly. As such, it is an ideal drug for rapid induction of anesthesia in patients with ischemic heart disease. Etomidate offers little protection from the increases in heart rate and blood pressure that accompany intubation. It usually is necessary to supplement etomidate with other agents (e.g., opioids, benzodiazepines, volatile agents, β-blockers, and nitroglycerin) in order to control the hemodynamic profile and prevent myocardial oxygen supply/demand inequality. An induction dose will block adrenal steroidogenesis for 6 to 8 hours.

4. **Benzodiazepines.** Midazolam (0.2 mg/kg) or diazepam (0.5 mg/kg) may be used to induce anesthesia. Although both agents are compatible with the goal of maintaining hemodynamic stability, blood pressure may decrease more with midazolam owing to more potent peripheral vasodilation. Negative inotropic effects are inconsequential. Blood pressure and filling pressures decrease with induction, whereas heart rate remains essentially unchanged. Addition of induction doses of a benzodiazepine to a moderate-dose opioid technique, however, may result in profound peripheral vasodilation and hypotension.

5. **Propofol.** The cardiovascular effects of induction doses of propofol are similar to those of the thiobarbiturates: **systemic blood pressure, SVR, and cardiac contractility decrease.** Heart rate may increase less with propofol compared to thiopental.

6. **α₂-Adrenergic agonists.** Centrally acting α₂-adrenergic agonists result in a reduction in stress-mediated neurohumoral response and therefore are associated with decreases in heart rate and blood pressure. These agents typically are used during maintenance of anesthesia or postoperatively. There is some evidence suggesting that use of oral clonidine may be associated with a reduced incidence of perioperative myocardial ischemia in patients undergoing CABG surgery. Dexmedetomidine is associated with a greater relative α₂ selectivity than clonidine. Both agents have sedative and antinociceptive characteristics. Use of α₂-adrenergic agonists is associated with a reduced opioid requirement. Additionally, α₂-adrenergic agonists do not result in respiratory depression.

B. **Volatile agents.** In general, **volatile anesthetics decrease both O_2 supply and demand. The net effect on the myocardial supply/demand equality depends upon the hemodynamic profile that prevails at the time of administration.** Halothane and enflurane, although seldom used in contemporary practice, have been included in this section for the sake of completeness.

1. **Heart rate.** If heart rate is high, halothane decreases it; if heart rate is low, halothane has little effect. Sevoflurane is associated with a negligible effect on heart rate. Enflurane, desflurane, and isoflurane often cause an increase in heart rate. Isoflurane also may decrease heart rate if the decrease in SVR is not profound, if the carotid baroreceptor function is impaired, or if the patient is fully β-blocked. Junctional rhythms, most often associated with enflurane, may occur with any volatile agent. Junctional rhythms deprive the heart of an atrial kick and lead to decreased stroke volume, cardiac output, and CBF, which may offset the salubrious effects of low heart rate.

2. **Contractility.** All volatile anesthetics decrease contractility, which lowers O_2 demand. However, isoflurane and probably desflurane and sevoflurane are less depressant than halothane or enflurane. In decompensated hearts, however, all volatile anesthetics may decrease ventricular function.
3. **Afterload.** Decreases in cardiac output and SVR result in decreased systemic blood pressure with volatile anesthesia. Venodilation and blunted contractility account for the decrease in cardiac output. SVR decreases with isoflurane and desflurane, and perhaps with enflurane and sevoflurane, but is essentially unchanged during halothane administration. The decrease in diastolic blood pressure reduces myocardial O_2 supply, whereas the decreased afterload reduces O_2 demand. In the steady state, the cardiovascular actions of desflurane are similar to those of isoflurane. However, during induction without opioids, heart rate and systemic and PA blood pressures may increase and require therapeutic intervention.
4. **Preload.** Volatile agent anesthesia is characterized by maintenance of filling pressures. Therefore, CPP (diastolic aortic pressure minus LVEDP) may decrease during volatile anesthesia.
5. **Coronary steal.** A coronary "steal" phenomenon has been described in which dilation of normal vascular beds diverts blood away from other beds that are ischemic and thus maximally dilated (Fig. 11.6). Steal prone anatomy is thought to exist in 23% of patients undergoing CABG [12]. Coronary steal has been observed in canine models of steal-prone coronary anatomy with isoflurane administration under circumstances that caused collateral flow to be pressure dependent. It is doubtful that isoflurane-induced coronary steal is of significant clinical importance to patients undergoing coronary revascularization surgery so long as hypotension and consequent pressure-dependent coronary artery perfusion are avoided. Coronary steal has not been observed with halothane, enflurane, or desflurane.
6. **Preconditioning.** Volatile anesthetics may confer a degree of preconditioning-like protective effect against ischemia-reperfusion injury in human myocardial tissue [13] (see Section **VII.D.6**).

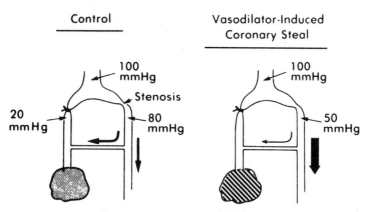

FIG. 11.6 Theoretical basis of coronary steal. The shaded, marginally ischemic area normally receives barely enough flow **(left)**. A potent vasodilator improves flow to the normal myocardium but does not affect the already maximally dilated area in jeopardy. This process decreases flow through the collateral from the nonischemic bed. This further impoverishment of the marginally ischemic area produces frank ischemia **(right)**. (Modified from Becker LC. Conditions for vasodilator-induced coronary steal in experimental myocardial ischemia. *Circulation* 1978;57:1108.)

C. **Nitrous oxide.** The mild negative inotropic effects of nitrous oxide yield a decrease in contractility, producing a reduction in both O_2 supply and demand. Adding nitrous oxide to an opioid-oxygen anesthetic will decrease SVR due, in part, to the removal of the vasoconstrictive effects of 100% O_2. The sympathomimetic effects of nitrous oxide counterbalance any direct depression of contractility except in patients with poor LV function in whom the myocardium already is highly stimulated intrinsically.

If nitrous oxide is used in a technique that provides a "light" anesthetic that is inadequate to cover attendant stimulation, increases in SVR and afterload are likely. Nitrous oxide does not appear to cause myocardial ischemia in patients with coronary artery disease.

D. **Opioids**
1. **Heart rate.** All opioids except meperidine decrease heart rate by a centrally mediated vagotonic effect (meperidine has an atropine-like effect). The dose of drug and speed of injection affect the degree of bradycardia. The result is decreased O_2 demand. By releasing histamine, morphine or meperidine may elicit a reflex tachycardia that decreases O_2 supply and increases O_2 demand.
2. **Contractility.** Aside from meperidine, which decreases contractility, the opioids have little effect on contractility in clinical doses.
3. **Afterload.** In compromised patients, who often depend on elevated sympathetic tone to maintain cardiac output and systemic resistance, the loss of sympathetic tone associated with opioid induction of anesthesia may result in a sudden drop in blood pressure and consequent decreases in both O_2 supply and demand.
4. **Preload.** Despite a lack of histamine-releasing properties, fentanyl and sufentanil will reduce preload when administered in either moderate doses (25 µg/kg for fentanyl) or larger doses by decreasing intrinsic sympathetic tone. Oxygen demand is decreased.
5. **Hyperdynamic state.** Elevations of heart rate, blood pressure, and cardiac output with or without decreased filling pressures are common during pure opioid-oxygen anesthetic techniques in patients with good ventricular function. This high-supply/high-demand state may be less preferable than the low-demand state achieved with volatile anesthesia. Additional opioid, which often fails to treat the hypertension associated with a hyperdynamic cardiac state, frequently decreases systemic blood pressure excessively when hypertension originates from increased SVR alone.

E. **Muscle relaxants**
1. **Succinylcholine.** This drug may cause a variety of **dysrhythmias** (bradycardia, tachycardia, extrasystoles), which may negatively affect myocardial O_2 balance.
2. **Tubocurarine, metocurine iodide, and atracurium besylate.** These drugs **release histamine** at one, two, and three times the dose for 95% twitch depression ED_{95}, respectively. None is the drug of choice for patients with ischemic heart disease.
3. **Pancuronium.** Heart rate increases 20% when pancuronium is combined with a volatile anesthetic. With high-dose opioid anesthesia, heart rate usually remains stable. Occasionally a patient will develop tachycardia and ischemia during induction or intubation. Pancuronium also is known to increase systemic blood pressure, although the effects on O_2 balance in the heart are not predictable.
4. **Vecuronium.** Vecuronium has a **flat cardiovascular profile** that is ideal with a low- or moderate-dose opioid anesthetic supplemented by volatile agent. Bradycardia may occur when it is given in conjunction with **rapid** injection of high doses of the highly lipid-soluble opioids.
5. **Doxacurium.** Although devoid of cardiovascular perturbation when injected slowly by a peripheral vein, this long-acting agent may release sufficient histamine when given rapidly by a central vein to induce a reflex tachycardia.
6. **Mivacurium.** Histamine release at doses greater than twice the ED_{95} and a short duration of action render this drug inappropriate for routine myocardial revascularization procedures.

7. **Rocuronium.** Although the drug is a more potent vagal blocker than vecuronium, it is less potent than pancuronium. Consequently, tachycardia is possible but less likely than with pancuronium. Rocuronium administration does not result in significant perturbations in other hemodynamic parameters.

F. **Summary.** Volatile anesthesia provides a **low-supply/low-demand** environment. The opioid-oxygen technique provides a **high-supply/high-demand** environment. Success with either technique depends on maintaining proper balance, with O_2 supply exceeding demand.

VI. **Anesthetic approach for myocardial revascularization procedures**
   A. **Fast-track cardiac anesthesia**
      1. **Historical perspective**
         a. **High-dose narcotic technique.** Until the 1990s, anesthesia for cardiac surgery was based on a high-dose narcotic technique that was considered to be compatible with minimal impairment of cardiac function and, therefore, was conducive to the maintenance of perioperative hemodynamic stability. Additionally, it was believed that the delayed awakening associated with high-dose narcotic technique allowed time for the heart to recover from the obligatory ischemia suffered during cardiopulmonary bypass, decreased stress hormone release and attendant myocardial ischemia in the immediate postoperative period, and allowed time requisite for temperature and hemostatic homeostasis [14].
            (1) **Anesthetic management for high-dose narcotic technique.** Typical premedication consists of morphine [0.1 mg/kg administered intramuscularly (IM)] and scopolamine (0.3 to 0.4 mg, IM). Induction of anesthesia is accomplished with fentanyl (25 to 100 μg/kg). Anesthesia is maintained with fentanyl (total cumulative dose of approximately 100 μg/kg), volatile agent, benzodiazepine, and long-acting muscle relaxants.
            (2) **Indications for high-dose narcotic technique.** In the present economic climate, high-dose narcotic technique is less frequently considered to be necessary or appropriate. However, high-dose narcotic technique may be used when early extubation is not considered a realistic goal. Additionally, high-dose narcotic technique may be used when it is absolutely necessary to avoid precipitous changes in hemodynamic conditions, such as when there are surgical concerns about anastomotic or aortic cannulation site integrity.
         b. **Impetus for change.** In the late 1980s and early 1990s, with the increased economic pressure engendered by greater penetration of managed care in the United States and mushrooming health care costs, an interest in alternate clinical management strategies that focused on shorter hospital stays and reduced costs developed. It became apparent that with the judicious use of narcotics supplemented by volatile agents or short-acting intravenous (IV) agents, it was possible to simultaneously integrate economic and clinical priorities [15]. In contradistinction to earlier work, more recent studies have suggested that heavy postoperative sedation is not requisite to avoid myocardial ischemia [16]. In the last decade, the emergence of new surgical techniques, improved myocardial protection, warmer bypass temperatures (32° to 34°C), improvements in anesthetic technique, management of perioperative coagulopathy, and temperature homeostasis (e.g., warmer operating room temperatures and use of active warming devices) have allowed the further development of fast-track cardiac anesthesia.
      2. **Definition and goals.** Fast-track cardiac anesthesia is a method of anesthetic management that promotes rapid recovery. It may be associated with reduced health care costs and improved clinical outcome.
      3. **Inclusion guidelines.** Early fast-track initiative exclusion criteria included obesity, moderate-to-severe pulmonary disease, emergency operations, poor ventricular function, combined procedures, redo operations, and advanced age. Early reports indicated that in view of these exclusion criteria, it was

possible to safely fast track 40% to 60% of surgical revascularization patients. Subsequently, inclusion criteria have been significantly liberalized. Presently, an attempt to deliver anesthesia that is compatible with enhanced recovery is made in most patients unless they are hemodynamically compromised or difficult airways. Poor LV function is not necessarily considered to be an absolute contraindication to fast tracking so long as hemodynamic stability is maintained. It is imperative to continuously evaluate the patient for the appropriateness of enhanced recovery as the operation progresses.

4. **Anesthetic management (Table 11.4)**
   a. **Premedication.** Long-acting agents such as scopolamine are preferentially avoided. Same-day admission patients may not have adequate time to be properly sedated with slow-onset agents. In this scenario, it may be useful to allay anxiety with a rapid-acting agent such as midazolam (0.03 to 0.07 mg/kg IV).
   b. **Intraoperative anesthetic agent management**
      (1) **Induction of anesthesia.** In order to limit the total opioid dose (e.g., 10 to 15 µg/kg fentanyl), it is necessary to supplement opioid with IV and/or volatile anesthetic agents. Typically etomidate, propofol, or thiopental is used to accomplish the induction of anesthesia. If etomidate is used (0.3 mg/kg), it often is necessary to use an additional agent, such as a low-dose narcotic, to avoid tachycardia and hypertension. Additionally, judicious use of short-acting β-blocking agents (e.g., esmolol) and/or nitroglycerin may be required to maintain hemodynamic stability during induction with a low-dose narcotic technique.
      (2) **Maintenance of anesthesia.** Anesthesia is maintained with a variable combination of volatile agents, low-dose narcotics, and IV hypnotic agents. The ultra-short-acting opioid remifentanil is associated with good hemodynamic stability, adequate attenuation of the neurohumoral stress response, and early awakening. However, due to its short half-life, it requires supplemental analgesia in the postoperative period. When volatile agents are used, it is important to reduce the reliance upon the volatile agent in advance of patient transport to the ICU. Otherwise, the patient may become acutely hyperdynamic upon arrival to the ICU, prompting the use of long-duration sedatives by the ICU staff.

      α_2-Agonists (e.g., dexmedetomidine and clonidine) are used adjunctively because of their ability to reduce the neurohumoral stress response in addition to their sedative and antinociceptive properties. These agents may reduce the anesthetic requirement and therefore

Table 11.4 Typical fast track cardiac anesthetic at Robert Wood Johnson Medical School

Induction	Etomidate[a]	0.3 mg/kg
	Fentanyl	0–10 µg/kg
	Midazolam	0–0.05 mg/kg
	Pentothal[a]	5.0 mg/kg
	Propofol[a]	2.0–3.0 mg/kg
	Succinylcholine	1.5–2.0 mg/kg
Maintenance	Fentanyl	5–10 µg/kg
	Midazolam	0.05 mg/kg
	Rocuronium	As needed by train-of-four monitoring
	Propofol	0–30 µg/kg/min
	Volatile agent	0.5–1.0 minimum alveolar concentration
Intensive care unit	Propofol	0–30 µg/kg/min

[a] It is typical to use one of these three induction agents, depending on hemodynamic status and ventricular function.

may facilitate a more rapid emergence from anesthesia. Dexmedetomidine is approved for use as a postoperative sedative and is administered as an infusion (0.2 to 0.7 µg/kg/hour).

Intrathecal and epidural analgesia may facilitate recovery by decreasing the perioperative opioid requirements [17]. Concern about neuroaxial hematoma formation in the presence of systemic anticoagulation limits the clinical application of regional anesthesia.

c. **Intraoperative awareness.** When avoiding high-dose narcotic technique, it is imperative to match the level of anesthesia to the operative stress at different times during the procedure to avoid harmful hemodynamic response to stimulation. It also is important to be aware of the possibility of intraoperative recall, although recent literature indicates that significant intraoperative awareness may occur in only 0.3% of fast-track patients, which is similar to the rate observed in general surgery [18]. Frequently, volatile agents are administered while the patient is on bypass with a vaporizer attached to the cardiopulmonary bypass circuit. Recently, the bispectral index (BIS) monitor (Aspect Medical Systems, Napick, MA, USA) has been used during cardiac surgery in an effort to avoid intraoperative awareness. Although intraoperative recall has been anecdotally reported at relatively low BIS scores, there may be a role for BIS monitoring, particularly when using an anesthesia technique that is consistent with early awakening.

d. **Temperature homeostasis.** Attention to heat preservation is critically important when early extubation is anticipated because hypothermia will delay respiratory weaning and may be associated with postoperative arrhythmias and coagulopathy [19]. Additionally, hypothermia may precipitate shivering, which significantly raises myocardial oxygen consumption. Fluid-filled warming blankets and heated-humidified breathing circuits are relatively ineffective mechanisms of intraoperative heat preservation because their nominal ability to conserve heat is far outweighed by the large deficits in body heat experienced by these patients. IV fluid warmers may be of greater clinical utility, especially when there are large transfusion requirements [20]. The cardiopulmonary bypass circuit heat exchanger provides the best means of restoring body temperature. Target a PA blood temperature greater than 37°C and a bladder temperature greater than 34°C. Forced hot-air convective warming is the best means of preserving body temperature during off-bypass revascularization.

e. **Hemostatic homeostasis.** Scrupulous surgical attention to hemostasis may be supplemented by the use of pharmacologic hemostatic agents such as aminocaproic acid and aprotinin (see Chapter 18). Use of these agents generally is restricted to revascularization that involves the use of bypass. Both agents are associated with reduced bleeding and subsequent need for transfusion of blood products in the postoperative period.

f. **Intraoperative extubation.** In the absence of ventricular impairment, hemodynamic instability, hypothermia, or significant coagulopathy, intraoperative tracheal extubation may be considered. However, extubation in the operating room may not confer any significant clinical or economic benefit to the patient [21].

5. **ICU management.** It is of paramount importance that the ICU staff appreciates the goal of fast tracking and the mechanism by which it is achieved so that they can help to deliver care that is consistent with enhanced recovery. The goal is to maintain a degree of sedation with a relatively short-acting agent that is devoid of significant hemodynamic effect, until such time as the patient is deemed ready for weaning from mechanical ventilation. For an uncomplicated patient, it is reasonable to tailor the level of sedation to accomplish extubation 4 to 8 hours postoperatively. This amount of time allows the patient to recover from inadequate myocardial protection during cardiopulmonary bypass, to achieve temperature homeostasis, and to be treated for perioperative coagulopathy (Fig. 11.7).

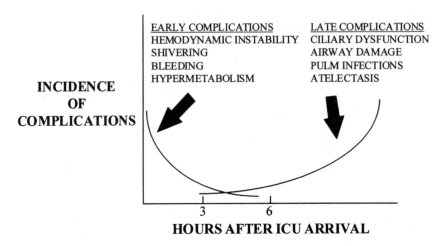

EARLY COMPLICATIONS   LATE COMPLICATIONS
HEMODYNAMIC INSTABILITY   CILIARY DYSFUNCTION
SHIVERING   AIRWAY DAMAGE
BLEEDING   PULM INFECTIONS
HYPERMETABOLISM   ATELECTASIS

INCIDENCE
OF
COMPLICATIONS

3   6

HOURS AFTER ICU ARRIVAL

FIG. 11.7 Early and late complications seen in patients undergoing coronary revascularization in the immediate postoperative period. (Adapted from Higgins T. Pro: early endotracheal extubation is preferable to late extubation in patients following coronary artery surgery. *J Cardiothorac Vasc Anesth* 1992;6:488–493.)

Propofol frequently is used to provide a smooth transition from intraoperative anesthesia to postoperative sedation. Propofol is easy to titrate, has a short onset, has a predictable duration of action, and has manageable effects upon the hemodynamic profile. It may be advisable to have nitroglycerin immediately available as an IV drip for rapid titration to desired blood pressure.

Sedation and weaning protocols are especially designed and implemented for fast-track patients (see Chapter 10). Point-of-care arterial blood gas monitoring may facilitate weaning from mechanical ventilation. Many institutions track the effect of the fast-track anesthesia program on resource utilization, hospital costs, and clinical outcome as a continuing performance improvement project.

6. **Clinical and economic benefits**
   a. **Clinical benefits of enhanced recovery.** Early extubation may be associated with reduced postoperative lung atelectasis and improved pulmonary shunt fraction [22,23]. Positive-pressure ventilation has deleterious effects on cardiac output and organ perfusion that may be minimized by early extubation. Early chest tube removal facilitates patient mobilization. Early extubation yields greater patient satisfaction as long as appropriate analgesia is maintained.
   b. **Economic benefits.** Early extubation protocol reduces ICU stay and hospital stay, and it may reduce the total cost of surgery by as much as 25% [24,25].

B. **Special circumstances**
   1. **Off-bypass revascularization** is associated with unique risks and benefits, which are detailed in Chapter 13.
   2. **Urgent CABG**
      a. **Introduction.** Patients present for urgent coronary artery bypass surgery for treatment of angina refractory to maximal nonsurgical management or in the setting of a clinical misadventure in the catheterization/angioplasty suite. These patients frequently are actively ischemic or may be in the process of an acute myocardial infarction. Often these patients are hemodynamically unstable and should be transported by physicians who are

knowledgeable about the patient's present medical condition, with full monitoring, oxygen, and emergency medications.

b. **Monitoring and IV access.** Upon arrival in the operating room, it is essential to establish monitoring and proper IV access in an expeditious and safe fashion. Frequently it is possible to use preexisting femoral arterial and venous catheters to start the operation. Although it is difficult to determine intraoperative thermodilution cardiac output and pulmonary capillary occlusion pressure with a PA catheter inserted through the femoral vein, it is customary to begin the operation without the delay that would be engendered by establishing alternate central venous access.

c. **Anesthetic management.** Induction of anesthesia usually is accomplished with short-acting agents (e.g., etomidate) that do not compromise hemodynamic conditions. Short-acting agents are preferable in the event that induction of anesthesia and consequent attenuation of sympathetic tone result in hemodynamic collapse. Every effort should be made to place the patient on cardiopulmonary bypass without delay. In the event that the patient is unable to tolerate adequate anesthesia, an effort should be made to provide protection from intraoperative awareness with an amnestic agent (e.g., scopolamine). Depending upon the extent of preoperative myocardial damage and the success of revascularization, inotropic support and/or mechanical assistance may be necessary to successfully separate the patient from bypass.

3. **Poor LV function.** Patients with poor ventricular function (ejection fraction less than 35%) should receive a reduced dose of premedication. It is customary to administer 0% to 50% of the usual premedication to these patients and then supplement the premedication when necessary with more rapidly acting agents (e.g., midazolam) under monitored conditions in the preoperative holding area. With severe ventricular compromise, it may be necessary to initiate therapy with inotropic agents before the induction of anesthesia. Induction of anesthesia is accomplished with short-acting agents that are devoid of significant hemodynamic effect (e.g., etomidate). It usually is possible to slowly titrate IV opioids to achieve adequate anesthetic depth. If ventricular function is not expected to improve significantly as a result of revascularization, appropriate inotropic agents should be used to separate the patient from cardiopulmonary bypass.

4. **Patients with critical coronary artery disease.** In patients with severe coronary artery disease (left main or left main equivalent disease), even brief episodes of myocardial oxygen supply/demand imbalance may not be tolerated. It is necessary to assiduously avoid increases in heart rate, contractility, or wall tension. It also is imperative to maintain CPP. If nitroglycerin is being used, it should be continued until the cross-clamp is applied (i.e., abolishment of coronary flow). These patients generally fare better with a high-supply/high-demand anesthetic technique rather than a low-supply/low-demand technique (see Section **V.F**).

5. **CABG for patients previously treated with antiplatelet medications.** Patients treated with antiplatelet agents are at risk for significant coagulopathy and consequent bleeding. It often is necessary to treat these patients empirically with platelet infusions to avoid catastrophic blood loss and high transfusion requirements.

6. **CABG for patients with heparin-induced thrombocytopenia.** Management of cardiopulmonary bypass for patients with heparin-induced thrombocytopenia is discussed in Chapter 18.

7. **Redo CABG procedures.** An increased incidence of bleeding, perioperative ischemia, infarction, and pump failure are the main concerns that lead to increased morbidity and mortality in this subgroup of patients undergoing myocardial revascularization. Table 11.5 summarizes these special concerns as well as their causes and appropriate perioperative anesthetic management.

8. **Patients with acute ischemic mitral regurgitation.** Patients with acute mitral regurgitation on the basis of ischemic papillary muscle dysfunction or

Table 11.5 Perioperative management of the myocardial revascularization reoperation patient

Perioperative problem	Cause	Management
Bleeding	Pericardial adhesions Preoperative antiplatelet or anticoagulant medication	Large-bore IV access Blood readily available and checked in the OR Careful dissection on reopening chest Femoral area exposed and ready for emergency cannulation Anticipated need for clotting factors and platelets in the postbypass period Availability of blood salvage equipment (cell saver) Prophylactic antifibrinolytic therapy
Ischemia or infarction	Increased incidence of unstable angina Long period before bypass instituted Thrombus in vein grafts embolize to native vessels Interruption of vein graft flow (associated with 50%–60% mortality) Longer bypass and cross-clamp times Increased amount of noncoronary collateral flow	Close monitoring of ischemia (ECG, PA catheter, two-dimensional TEE) Expeditious treatment of ischemia once detected Careful manipulation of vein grafts; retrograde cardioplegia Careful dissection around vein grafts Minimal cross-clamp time Mean perfusion pressure <60 mm Hg when cross-clamp is applied to limit noncoronary flow
Pump failure after bypass	Perioperative ischemia and infarction	Same as above Treat ischemia aggressively after bypass to improve myocardial function Anticipate need for intravenous inotropic and mechanical support

ECG, electrocardiogram; IV, intravenous; OR, operating room; PA, pulmonary artery; TEE, transesophageal echocardiography.

ruptured chordae tendineae often are hemodynamically unstable and may present for surgical repair and revascularization without the benefit of maximal preoperative preparation. The pathophysiology of acute mitral regurgitation is discussed elsewhere (see Chapter 12). In brief, acute mitral insufficiency is associated with tachycardia, high LVEDP, and increased contractility, which all may serve to worsen the already compromised myocardial oxygen supply/demand dynamic. Because the intraaortic balloon pump frequently stabilizes these patients sufficiently to permit survival until operation, its continued use until establishment of bypass is essential.

VII. Causes and treatment of perioperative myocardial ischemia. Multiple factors may lead to development of ischemia in the perioperative period. Often several causes occur simultaneously. For purposes of discussion, causes of ischemia will be divided into those that are most common in the prebypass, bypass, and postbypass periods (Table 11.6). Factors leading to ischemia during one time period may enhance or worsen ischemia in subsequent time periods.

Any of the hemodynamic alterations (tachycardia, hypertension, hypotension, ventricular distention) outlined in the initial chapters on anesthetic management for cardiac surgery may be responsible for ischemia during any phase of the perioperative period. In addition, factors that decrease O_2 content and delivery, such as poor oxygenation or anemia, may be additive to any ischemic event throughout the operative procedure.

A. **Causes of ischemia in the prebypass period**
   1. **Ischemia associated with specific high-risk anesthetic-surgical events.** Events precipitating ischemia in the prebypass period include endotracheal intubation, surgical stress (skin incision, sternal split), cannulation, and initiation of bypass [7]. Episodes of ischemia may occur during these high-risk events even in the absence of hemodynamic changes [7].
   2. **Ischemia associated with hemodynamic abnormalities.** Some episodes of ischemia during high-risk periods are associated with hemodynamic abnormalities, especially tachycardia (greater than 100 beats/min). Every attempt should be made to minimize hemodynamic alterations to prevent myocardial ischemia. Ischemia triples the likelihood of perioperative infarction.
   3. **Coronary spasm.** Coronary spasm in a normal coronary vessel or around an atherosclerotic lesion may cause myocardial ischemia in the prebypass period. Intense sympathetic stimulation or light levels of anesthesia theoretically could trigger coronary vasospasm. In addition, manipulation of the heart and coronary vessels by the surgeon may induce coronary spasm.
   4. **Spontaneous thrombus formation.** Spontaneous thrombus formation at an atherosclerotic plaque leading to occlusion of a coronary vessel may be responsible for myocardial infarction. Although uncommon, nothing precludes this scenario from occurring in the operating room in the prebypass period.

B. **Causes of ischemia during bypass**
   1. **Periods without aortic cross-clamp.** Hemodynamic alterations, mechanical factors during bypass, and ventricular fibrillation can influence the occurrence of ischemia before application or after removal of the aortic cross-clamp. In addition, particulate microemboli (thrombus, plastic, and other foreign material)

Table 11.6 Causes of perioperative ischemia in the myocardial revascularization patient

Prebypass	Bypass	Postbypass
Hemodynamic alterations[a]	Hemodynamic alterations[a]	Hemodynamic alterations[a]
Coronary spasm	Coronary spasm	Coronary spasm
	Cardioplegic arrest	
Thrombus formation	Emboli (air, thrombus particulate matter)	Thrombus (native vessel, graft)
High-risk anesthetic-surgical events[b]	Ventricular fibrillation	
	Ventricular distention	
	Surgical complications[b]	Surgical complications[b]
		Incomplete revascularization
		Excessive use of inotropes
		Distention of the lungs leading to occlusion of internal mammary artery graft flow

[a] Includes tachycardia, hypotension, hypertension, ventricular distention.
[b] See text for details.

are present in all bypass circuits and may lead to ischemia when the coronaries are perfused on bypass. Coronary air emboli can occur with imperfect de-airing of the vein grafts. Whenever the heart or aorta is opened, air embolism to the native coronary circulation is a potential problem.

2. **During aortic cross-clamp.** Once the aortic cross-clamp is applied, ischemia is inevitable regardless of the myocardial preservation technique used. As cross-clamp time increases, so does the potential for ischemic injury and subsequent infarction. Washout of cold cardioplegic solution owing to excessive noncoronary collateral flow may be responsible for ischemia during this period. Unfortunately, once the aorta is cross-clamped and the cardioplegic solution is administered, the electrical and mechanical quiescence precludes monitoring for ischemia.

3. **After removal of aortic cross-clamp**
   a. **Surgical and technical complications.** Surgical complications include the following:
      (1) Inadvertent incision of the coronary back wall, leading to coronary dissection
      (2) Improper handling of the vein graft with endothelial cell loss, leading to graft thrombus formation
      (3) Twisting of vein grafts
      (4) Anastomosis of the vein graft to the coronary vein
      (5) Suturing the artery closed while grafting or poor-quality anastomoses
      (6) Inadequate vein graft length, leading to stretching of the vein when the heart is filled
      (7) Excess length of vein graft, leading to vein kinking
   b. **Etiology of ST-segment elevation after cross-clamp removal.** After removal of the aortic cross-clamp, ST-segment elevation may occur. The length of cardioplegic arrest, residual electrophysiologic effects of cardioplegia, coronary air or atheromatous debris embolus, or coronary artery spasm all may contribute to the etiology of this ECG abnormality. Often the ST-segment elevation is located in the inferior leads (i.e., right coronary distribution), implicating air embolus as the etiology (air seeks the high location of the right coronary ostium). Persistence of ST-segment changes after aortic cross-clamp removal may indicate ongoing ischemia secondary to coronary artery spasm or coronary air embolus, and appropriate therapy is required. Recall that ventricular aneurysm and pericarditis also cause ST-segment elevations.

C. **Causes of ischemia in the postbypass period**
   1. **Incomplete revascularization.** It is important for the anesthesiologist to know whether the patient has been completely revascularized before terminating cardiopulmonary bypass.
      a. **Ungraftable vessels.** Sometimes vessels are deemed ungraftable once the surgeon palpates and examines the caliber of the vessel. That region of the myocardium supplied by the unrevascularized stenotic vessel may have a greater chance of developing ischemia in the postbypass period than in the prebypass period because of the added insult of cardioplegic arrest.
      b. **Diffuse distal disease and diabetes.** Diffuse distal disease, often present in diabetic patients, increases the risk for ischemia in the postbypass period. Severe distal disease also is a risk factor for early vein graft closure because the small distal vessels provide poor runoff for vein graft flow.
      c. **Stress.** Historically it was thought that patients who received intensive analgesia had a lower incidence of ischemia after operation [14]. More recent literature suggests that the incidence of ischemia in patients who are more lightly sedated is similar to that of patients managed with deeper planes of sedation so long as the coronary supply/demand dynamic is properly maintained [16].
   2. **Coronary spasm.** Coronary spasm can occur in the postbypass period, most commonly in right coronary arteries that are not diseased. Surgical manipulation and exogenous as well as endogenous catecholamines may contribute to this problem.

3. **Mechanical factors.** Mechanical factors such as vein graft kinking or stretching or occlusion of IMA flow secondary to overinflation of the lungs may cause ischemia in the postbypass period.

4. **Surgical and technical complications** (see Section **B**).

5. **Thrombus formation.** Thrombus formation in the native vessel or the bypass graft may occur after bypass, leading to severe ischemia and infarction. Coronary vasospasm or hypercoagulability arising from coagulation system manipulations or from patient disease may contribute to clot formation in vessels.

6. **Inotropes.** Improper use of inotropes, including calcium, during weaning from bypass or in the postbypass period may increase the risk of ischemia or potentiate ischemia during this period.

D. **Treatment of myocardial ischemia.** Table 11.7 lists conventional treatments of ischemia in the patient undergoing myocardial revascularization.

1. **Treatment of ischemia secondary to hemodynamic abnormalities**
   a. Increase or decrease anesthetic depth.
   b. Administer vasodilators or vasopressors when SVR is either high or low, respectively.
   c. Administer a β-blocker, specifically esmolol, to treat tachycardia.
   d. Use atrioventricular sequential pacing. (Specifically in the postbypass period, this can be extremely beneficial to improve rate, rhythm, and hemodynamic stability.)
   e. Use inotropes when failing ventricular function is diagnosed by decreased cardiac output and increased ventricular filling pressures. (Pump failure leads to severe decreases in CPP because diastolic blood pressure is decreased and LVEDP is increased.) *Note:* Indiscriminate use of inotropes may aggravate ischemia. Therefore, preload, heart rate rhythm, and afterload all should be maximized before inotropes are used.

2. **Correction of surgical complications and mechanical problems**
   a. Any surgical correctable factors leading to ischemia should be attended to in the postbypass period.
   b. Overinflation of the lungs when an IMA graft is present should be avoided.
   c. If residual air in the coronary arteries is suspected, pharmacologic elevation of systemic blood pressure or manual myocardial contraction may help dislodge air from the coronary circulation.

3. **Treatment of coronary spasm.** IV and/or sublingual nifedipine and IV nitroglycerin, diltiazem, and nicardipine are therapeutic options for treating coronary spasm. For specific doses of each drug for this indication, refer to Chapter 2.

4. **Specific pharmacologic treatment of ischemia.** This treatment includes (a) nitroglycerin, (b) β-blockers, and (c) calcium channel blockers. Refer to Chapter 2 for mechanisms of action and doses of these drugs. IV nitroglycerin probably is the most frequently used pharmacologic treatment of ischemia in

Table 11.7 Treatment of ischemia

Adequate oxygenation
Hemodynamic stability (e.g., adequate anesthetic depth)
Surgical correction
Specific pharmacologic treatment
Nitroglycerin
Calcium channel blockers
β-Blockers (esmolol)
Heparin
Inotropic support (ischemia secondary to a failing ventricle)
Mechanical support
Intraaortic balloon pump
Left ventricular assist device
Right ventricular assist device

the operating room throughout the perioperative period. Specific prophylactic use includes postbypass administration of nitroglycerin in incompletely revascularized patients, patients with severe distal coronary disease, and diabetic patients.

Because ischemia frequently occurs from thrombus formation on atheroma, many nonsurgical patients receive heparin as acute therapy and antiplatelet agents (most commonly aspirin) for long-term prophylaxis. These agents should be withheld after bypass until the threat of surgical hemorrhage ceases.

5. **Mechanical support.** Refer to Chapter 21 for a complete discussion of circulatory assist devices.

   a. **Intraaortic balloon pumps.** Intraaortic balloon pumps have been used for many years as a treatment of ischemia by increasing CPP and decreasing afterload for LV ejection. In patients with angina, insertion of a balloon pump often relieves symptoms in the presence of normal ventricular function. In patients with impaired ventricular function, elevation of CPP and improved ventricular ejection may relieve ischemia and improve pump performance.

   b. **Right and LV assist devices.** These devices may be useful for treating severe ischemia caused by myocardial failure or ischemia that led to myocardial failure. Data on their use as treatment of ischemia is still in question.

6. **Ischemic preconditioning.** Tissue injury resulting from ischemia and subsequent tissue reperfusion may involve a reduction in adenosine triphosphate (ATP) levels, free oxygen radicals, and calcium-mediated injury. A brief period of tissue ischemia ("ischemic preconditioning") may protect against the damage caused by subsequent prolonged ischemia and tissue reperfusion. Endogenously produced adenosine may mediate ischemic preconditioning via enhanced preservation of ATP, inhibition of platelet and neutrophil-mediated inflammatory tissue injury, vasodilation, and decreased basal cellular energy requirements related to intracellular hyperpolarization [13]. Adenosine and some volatile anesthetics may confer a degree of a preconditioning-like protective effect.

References

1. American Heart Association. *National Vital Statistics Reports, Volume 48, No. 11. Heart and Stroke Statistical Update, American Heart Association.*
2. National Institutes of Health. *Disease Statistics, Fact Book, Fiscal Year 2000, National Heart, Lung, and Blood Institute.*
3. **Higgins T. Quantifying risk and assessing outcome in cardiac surgery. *J Cardiothorac Vasc Anesth* 1998;12:330–340.**
4. Dupuis J, Feng W, Nathan H, et al. The cardiac anesthesia risk evaluation score. *Anesthesiology* 2001;94:194–204.
5. Dole W. Autoregulation of the coronary circulation. *Prog Cardiovasc Dis* 1987;XXIX: 293–323.
6. Berkowitz DE. Vascular function: from human physiology to molecular biology. In: Schwinn DA, ed. *New advances in vascular biology and molecular cardiovascular medicine.* Baltimore: Williams & Wilkins, 1998:25–47.
7. **Slogoff S, Keats A. Does perioperative ischemia lead to postoperative myocardial infarction? *Anesthesiology* 1985;62:107–114.**
8. Tuman KJ, McCarthy RJ, Spiess BD, et al. Effect of pulmonary artery catheterization on outcome in patients undergoing coronary artery surgery. *Anesthesiology* 1989;70: 199–206.
9. Connors A, Speroff T, Dawson NV, et al. The effectiveness of right heart catheterization in the initial care of critically ill patients. *JAMA* 1996;276:889–896.
10. **Slogoff S, Keats A. Randomized trial of primary anesthetic agents on outcome of coronary artery bypass operations. *Anesthesiology* 1989;70:179–188.**
11. **Tuman K, McCarthy R, Spiess B, et al. Does choice of anesthetic agent significantly affect outcome after coronary artery surgery? *Anesthesiology* 1989;70: 189–198.**

12. Buffington CW, Davis KB, Gillispie S, et al. The prevalence of steal-prone anatomy in patients with coronary artery disease: an analysis of the Coronary Artery Surgery Study Registry. *Anesthesiology* 1988;69:721–727.
13. Lee T. Mechanisms of ischemic preconditioning and clinical implications for multiorgan-reperfusion injury. *J Cardiothorac Vasc Anesth* 1999;13:78–91.
14. **Mangano DT, Siliciano D, Hollenberg M, et al. Postoperative myocardial ischemia: therapeutic trials using intensive analgesia following surgery. *Anesthesiology* 1992;76:342–353.**
15. Prakash O, Johson B, Meij S, et al. Criteria for early extubation after intracardiac surgery in adults. *Anesth Analg* 1977;56:703–708.
16. **Hall R, MacLaren C, Smith M, et al. Light versus heavy sedation after cardiac surgery: myocardial ischemia and the stress response. *Anesth Analg* 1997;85: 971–978.**
17. **Scott NB, Turfrey DJ, Ray D, et al. A prospective randomized study of the potential benefits of thoracic epidural anesthesia and analgesia in patients undergoing coronary artery bypass grafting. *Anesth Analg* 2001;93:528–535.**
18. Dowd N, Cheng D, Karski J, et al. Intraoperative awareness in fast track cardiac anesthesia. *Anesthesiology* 1998;89:1068–1073.
19. **Leslie K, Sessler D. The implications of hypothermia for early extubation following cardiac surgery. *J Cardiothorac Vasc Anesth* 1998;12[6 Suppl 2]:30–34.**
20. Ginsberg S, Solina A, Papp D, et al. A prospective comparison of three heat preservation methods for patients undergoing hypothermic cardiopulmonary bypass. *J Cardiothorac Vasc Anesth* 2000;14:501–505.
21. Montes F, Sanchez S, Giraldo J, et al. The lack of benefit of tracheal extubation in the operating room after coronary artery bypass surgery. *Anesth Analg* 2000;91:776–780.
22. **Cheng D, Karski J, Peniston C, et al. Morbidity outcome in early versus conventional tracheal extubation after coronary artery bypass grafting: a prospective randomized trial. *J Thorac Cardiovasc Surg* 1996;112:755–764.**
23. Johnson D, Thomson D, Mycyk T, et al. Respiratory outcomes with early extubation after coronary artery bypass surgery. *J Cardiothorac Vasc Anesth* 1997;11:474–480.
24. **Cheng D, Karski J, Peniston C, et al. Early tracheal extubation after coronary artery bypass graft surgery reduces costs and improves resource use. *Anesthesiology* 1996;85:1300–1310.**
25. **Cheng D. Fast-track cardiac surgery: economic implications in postoperative care. *J Cardiothorac Vasc Anesth* 1998;12:72–79.**

12. ANESTHETIC MANAGEMENT FOR THE TREATMENT OF VALVULAR HEART DISEASE

Roger A. Moore and Donald E. Martin

I. Cardiac response to valvular heart disease. The anesthetic management of patients undergoing valvular heart surgery requires a thorough understanding of the following:

- Abnormal pressure and volume loads imposed by abnormal valves
- Structural and functional mechanisms by which the heart attempts to compensate
- Events that may signal the limits of compensation, such as arrhythmias, ischemia, and cardiac failure
- Secondary complications, such as endocarditis or emboli

   A. Ventricular function. To anticipate the effect of valvular lesions on ventricular function, it is helpful to separate ventricular function into its two distinct components [1].

      1. Systolic function represents the ventricle's ability to contract and eject blood against an afterload. Systolic function allows the ventricle to respond to a pressure load and is best described by the ratio of end-systolic pressure to end-systolic volume. As end-systolic pressure (afterload) increases, the ventricle cannot empty completely, and end-systolic volume increases. However, the ratio of end-systolic pressure to volume remains almost constant under most circumstances and is directly related to ventricular **contractility.**

      2. Diastolic function represents the ventricle's ability to relax and accept inflowing blood, or preload. Diastolic function is necessary for the ventricle to respond to a volume load and is best described by the relationship between end-diastolic pressure and end-diastolic volume, or ventricular **compliance.**

         Both systolic and diastolic function require energy and can be compromised by ventricular ischemia.

   B. Ventricular hypertrophy. Chronic volume and pressure loads each evokes a characteristic ventricular response. Pressure loads usually result in **concentric** ventricular hypertrophy, with an increase in ventricular wall thickness that allows the heart to maintain its normal, or concentric, position within the chest cavity. Volume loading, on the other hand, leads to **eccentric** hypertrophy. The word *eccentric* in this context means that the heart dilates and, because of increased chamber size, assumes an eccentric position in the chest.

   C. Pressure–volume relationship. Both systolic and diastolic components of ventricular function, along with the corresponding pressure and volume loads, can be represented graphically by a pressure–volume loop, which shows the pressure–volume relationship at each instant during a single cardiac cycle [2]. Figure 12.1 shows a representative pressure–volume loop under normal conditions. Diastolic function is represented by a dashed line and includes phase 1, isovolumetric relaxation, and phase 2, ventricular filling. Systolic function is represented by a solid line and includes phase 3, isovolumetric contraction, and phase 4, ventricular ejection. The area inside the loop provides a rough index of the energy used to eject blood, or the stroke work. The shape of this loop changes with variations in ventricular load, ventricular compliance, and ventricular contractility. Each valvular lesion imposes its own unique set of stresses on the left ventricle (LV) and the right ventricle (RV). These variations lead to specific hemodynamic profiles for each lesion that suggest the anesthetic and therapeutic priorities for patients with each type of valvular heart disease.

II. Aortic stenosis

   A. Natural history

      1. Etiology. Aortic stenosis is classified as valvular, subvalvular, or supravalvular based on the anatomic location of the stenotic lesion. Pure valvular aortic stenosis is the most common, accounting for more than 75% of patients. In the past, the primary cause of valvular aortic stenosis was **rheumatic** valvular degeneration. Because of improved recognition and treatment of streptococcal infections, rheumatic carditis has now become less common. Calcific degeneration of a **congenitally bicuspid aortic valve** currently is the most common etiology. A congenitally bicuspid aortic valve occurs in approximately 1% to 2% of the general population, making it one of the most common congenital malformations. **Senile degeneration** of normal aortic valves also can occur. Thirty percent of patients older than 85 years are found to have significant degenerative

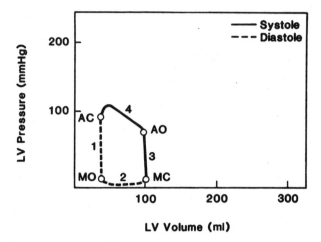

FIG. 12.1 Pressure–volume loop for the normal ventricle. *AC*, aortic valve closure; *AO*, aortic valve opening; *MC*, mitral valve closure; *MO*, mitral valve opening; phase *1*, isovolumetric relaxation; phase *2*, ventricular filling; phase *3*, isovolumetric contraction; phase *4*, ventricular ejection. (Modified from Jackson JM, Thomas SJ, Lowenstein E. Anesthetic management of patients with valvular heart disease. *Semin Anesth* 1982;1:240.)

changes of the aortic valve on autopsy. A characteristic finding of senile valvular degeneration is progression of calcification from the base of the valve toward the edge, as opposed to rheumatic degeneration, in which calcification spreads from the edge toward the base.

2. **Symptomatology.** Patients with rheumatic aortic stenosis may be asymptomatic for 40 years or more. Patients with congenitally bicuspid aortic valves may develop symptomatic aortic stenosis any time between the ages of 15 and 65 years, but calcification of the valve more often occurs after age 30 and usually in the seventh or eighth decade of life. The onset of any one of a triad of symptoms is an ominous sign and indicates a life expectancy of less than 5 years:

    a. **Angina pectoris.** Angina is the initial symptom in 50% to 70% of patients with severe aortic stenosis. Angina secondary to aortic stenosis alone most commonly occurs with exertion. In contrast, angina at rest commonly indicates associated coronary artery disease.

    b. **Syncope.** Syncope is the first symptom in 15% to 30% of patients. Once syncope appears, the average life expectancy is 3 to 4 years.

    c. **Congestive heart failure.** Once signs of LV failure occur, the average life expectancy is only 1 to 2 years. All patients with aortic stenosis are at increased risk for sudden death. Only 18% of patients are alive 5 years after stenosis has progressed to the point of peak systolic pressure gradient greater than 50 mm Hg or effective aortic valve orifice size less than 0.7 cm^2 (aortic valve index less than 0.5 cm^2/m^2).

B. **Pathophysiology**

    1. **Natural progression**

        a. **Stage 1: mild aortic stenosis—asymptomatic with physiologic compensation.** The normal adult aortic valve area is 2.6 to 3.5 cm^2, representing a normal aortic valve index of 2 cm^2/m^2. As stenosis progresses, the maintenance of normal stroke volume is associated with an increasing systolic pressure gradient between the LV and the aorta. LV systolic pressure increases to as much as 300 mm Hg, whereas the aortic systolic pressure and stroke volume remain relatively normal. This higher gradient results in a compensatory **concentric LV hypertrophy** (increased muscle mass in the LV wall without dilation of the ventricular chamber). The resultant increase in LV end-diastolic pressure (LVEDP) is not a sign of systolic dysfunction or failure but rather an indication of the decreased LV diastolic function or reduced compliance.

b. **Stage 2: moderate aortic stenosis—symptomatic impairment.** As stenosis progresses toward the critical orifice size of 0.7 to 0.9 cm² (aortic valve index 0.5 cm²/m²), **dilation** as well as hypertrophy of the LV may occur, leading to increases in both LV end-diastolic volume (LVEDV) and LVEDP. A decrease in ejection fraction may be noted, indicating compromise of LV contractility. Ventricular contractility decreases more rapidly in some patients than in others but eventually is reduced in all untreated patients.

The increased LVEDV and LVEDP leads to increased myocardial work and O₂ demand. In this situation, two of the primary determinants of myocardial O₂ demand (tension developed by the myocardium and duration of systole) are increased. At the same time, myocardial O₂ supply is impeded because of the elevated LVEDP, causing a decrease in coronary perfusion pressure. Finally, the Venturi effect of the jet of blood flowing through the aortic valve and past the coronary arteries may lower pressure in the coronary ostia enough to reverse systolic coronary blood flow. These factors produce a heart particularly at risk for ischemia and sudden death, even in the absence of concurrent atherosclerotic coronary disease.

The initial appearance of symptoms in patients with aortic stenosis often is associated with the development of atrial fibrillation. Normal patients depend on atrial contraction for approximately 20% of the stroke volume. However, with the reduced ventricular compliance and increased LVEDP that is present in patients with aortic stenosis, passive ventricular filling is reduced, and atrial contraction can supply as much as 40% of ventricular filling during diastole. Therefore, loss of sinus rhythm and atrial contribution to cardiac output can lead to rapid clinical deterioration.

c. **Stage 3: critical aortic stenosis—terminal failure.** Continuation of the disease process with reduction of the aortic valve index to less than 0.5 cm²/m² leads to further decreases in ejection fraction and increases in LVEDP. Pressure builds up in the pulmonary venous circuit, leading to pulmonary edema when the left atrial pressure increases to more than 25 to 30 mm Hg. Normally, sudden death will intervene, but if the patient is able to survive, the increasing pulmonary arterial hypertension eventually will produce RV failure.

2. **Pressure–volume relationship** (Fig. 12.2). As the pressure gradient across the aortic valve develops, stroke volume is preserved by an increase in LV systolic pressure. During the early stages of LV compensation, LV hypertrophy leads to reduced LV compliance, with elevation of LVEDP, whereas the LV end-systolic volume stays relatively normal. In the later stages of the disease, myocardial ischemia and compromise of LV function can lead first to marked elevations of LVEDP and LVEDV and, finally, to elevation of LV end-systolic volume and depression of stroke volume. Each of these changes, but especially elevated ventricular pressures, increases O₂ cost to an already compromised myocardium.

3. **Calculation of stenosis.** Determination of the aortic valve area is performed using the Gorlin modification of standard hydraulic formulas [3]. The formula for calculating aortic valve area is summarized as follows:

$$\text{Aortic valve area (cm}^2) = \frac{\dfrac{\text{Cardiac output}}{(\text{systolic ejection period} \times \text{HR})}}{1 \times 44.5 \times \sqrt{\text{mean aortic pressure gradient}}}$$

where 1 is the aortic orifice constant and HR is heart rate.

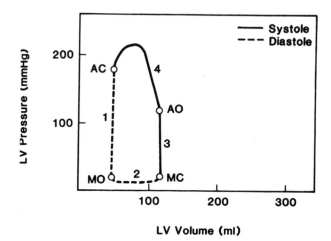

FIG. 12.2 Pressure–volume loop of a patient with moderate aortic stenosis and left ventricular compensation showing markedly elevated left ventricular systolic pressure, elevated end-systolic and end-diastolic volumes, and increased diastolic pressure. *AC*, aortic valve closure; *AO*, aortic valve opening; *MC*, mitral valve closure; *MO*, mitral valve opening; phase *1*, isovolumetric relaxation; phase *2*, ventricular filling; phase *3*, isovolumetric contraction; phase *4*, ventricular ejection. (Modified from Jackson JM, Thomas SJ, Lowenstein E. Anesthetic management of patients with valvular heart disease. *Semin Anesth* 1982;1:241.)

A simplified version of the Gorlin formula that is accurate enough to be clinically useful at normal heart rates is as follows:

$$\text{Aortic valve area (cm}^2) = \frac{\text{Cardiac output (L/min)}}{\sqrt{\text{Mean pressure gradient}}}$$

This simplified version of the formula is valid only because the product of the heart rate, systolic ejection period, and the constant approximates unity.

There is a direct relationship between the aortic valve area and the flow across the aortic valve. A series of relationships can be established between the rate of aortic valve blood flow and the mean systolic pressure gradient for any aortic valve area (Fig. 12.3). Blood flow is not significantly impeded until the aortic valve area falls below a critical level of 0.5 to 0.7 cm².

    4. Pressure wave disturbances
        a. Arterial pressure. Arterial pulse pressure usually is reduced to less than 50 mm Hg in severe aortic stenosis. The systolic pressure rise is delayed with a late peak and a prominent anacrotic notch. As stenosis increases in severity, the anacrotic notch occurs lower in the ascending arterial pressure trace. The dicrotic notch is relatively small or absent.
        b. Pulmonary arterial wedge pressure. Because of the elevated LVEDP, which stretches the mitral valve annulus, a prominent V wave can be observed but, with progression of the disease and the development of left atrial hypertrophy, a prominent A wave becomes the dominant feature.
   C. Goals of perioperative management
      1. Hemodynamic profile

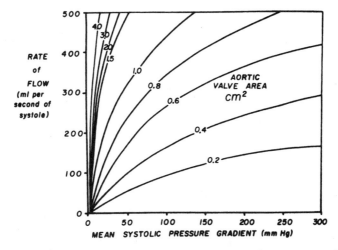

FIG. 12.3 Comparison between rate of blood flow and mean systolic pressure gradient across the aortic valve in individuals with different aortic valve areas, as determined by the Gorlin formula. (From Schlant RC. Altered cardiovascular function of rheumatic heart disease and other acquired valvular disease. In: Hurst JW, Logue RB, Schlant RC, et al., eds. *The heart,* 4th ed. New York: McGraw-Hill, 1978:968, with permission.)

	LV preload	Heart rate	Contractile state	Systemic vascular resistance	Pulmonary vascular resistance
Aortic stenosis	↑	↓ (sinus)	Maintain constant	↑	Maintain constant

a. **LV preload.** Because of the decreased LV compliance as well as the increased LVEDP and LVEDV, **preload augmentation** is necessary to maintain a normal stroke volume. Use of nitroglycerin may dangerously reduce cardiac output.

b. **Heart rate.** Extremes of heart rate are not tolerated well. A high heart rate can lead to decreased coronary perfusion. A low heart rate can limit cardiac output in patients with a fixed stroke volume. If a choice must be made, however, **low heart rates (50 to 70 beats/min) are preferred to rapid heart rates (greater than 90 beats/min)** to allow time for systolic ejection across a stenotic aortic valve. Because of the importance of atrial contraction for LV filling, it is **essential to maintain a sinus rhythm.**

c. **Contractility.** Stroke volume is maintained through preservation of a heightened contractile state. **β-Blockade is not well tolerated** and can lead to an increase in LVEDV and a decrease in cardiac output significant enough to induce clinical deterioration.

d. **Systemic vascular resistance.** Most of the afterload to LV ejection is caused by the stenotic aortic valve itself and thus is fixed. Systemic blood pressure reduction does little to decrease LV afterload. However, the hypertrophied myocardium of the patient with aortic stenosis is at great risk for development of subendocardial ischemia. Coronary perfusion depends on maintenance of an adequate systemic diastolic perfusion pressure.

Therefore, **early use of α-adrenergic agonists is indicated to prevent drops in blood pressure** that can lead quickly to sudden death [4]. Because the primary impedance to ventricular ejection occurs at the aortic valve, blood pressure augmentation using α-adrenergic agonists does little to reduce total forward flow.

e. **Pulmonary vascular resistance.** Except for end-stage aortic stenosis, **pulmonary artery pressures remain relatively normal.** Special intervention for stabilizing pulmonary vascular resistance is not necessary.

2. **Anesthetic techniques**

a. **Light premedication** is necessary to provide a calm patient without tachycardia. However, the use of a heavy premedicant with agents that markedly reduce either preload or afterload should be avoided. A combination of morphine, 0.05 to 0.10 mg/kg intramuscularly (IM), and scopolamine, 0.2 to 0.3 mg IM; lorazepam, 1 to 2 mg by mouth (PO), alone; or midazolam, 1 to 3 mg PO or IM, can be used with little adverse hemodynamic effect. Dosage of premedication should be adjusted for each patient based on individual considerations, including the patient's age and physical status.

b. **Thermodilution cardiac output pulmonary artery catheters** are helpful for evaluating the cardiac output of patients before repair of the aortic valve. Pulmonary capillary wedge pressure, however, may underestimate the true end-diastolic pressure of a noncompliant LV. There is also a small dysrhythmogenic risk during transventricular passage of a pulmonary artery catheter. If a patient shows dysrhythmias during advancement of a pulmonary artery catheter, the catheter tip should be left in a central venous position until repair of the aortic valve is completed. Mixed venous oxygen saturation monitoring via an oximetric pulmonary artery catheter may be used to provide a continuous index of cardiac output. However, because postbypass management is not likely to be marked by myocardial failure or low-output states, this technique may be best reserved for patients with other valve lesions.

c. Any **anesthetic agent** that causes myocardial depression, blood pressure reduction, tachycardia, or other dysrhythmias should be used with caution. Each of these physiologic changes can lead to rapid deterioration. A narcotic-based anesthetic usually is chosen for this reason.

d. During the induction and maintenance of anesthesia, a potent **α-adrenergic agent** such as phenylephrine should be readily available for early and aggressive treatment of reductions in systemic systolic or diastolic pressure.

e. If the patient develops signs or symptoms of ischemia, **nitroglycerin** should be used with caution because its effect on preload or arterial pressure may worsen the patient's condition.

f. **Supraventricular dysrhythmias should be treated aggressively** with **synchronized** direct-current shock because both tachycardia and the loss of effective atrial contraction can lead to rapid reduction of cardiac output and hemodynamic deterioration. Ventricular ectopy also should be treated aggressively because patients whose rhythm deteriorates into ventricular fibrillation often cannot be successfully resuscitated.

g. **An experienced cardiac surgeon should be present, and the perfusionist should be prepared before induction of anesthesia, in the event that rapid cardiovascular deterioration necessitates emergency use of cardiopulmonary bypass.**

h. In the presence of myocardial hypertrophy, adequate myocardial preservation with **cardioplegic solution** during bypass is essential to avoid myocardial "contracture" or "stone heart." The traditional cold potassium cardioplegia, which must be administered via coronary ostial catheters during valve replacement, may be inadequate. Retrograde administration of warm blood cardioplegia via the coronary sinus may have an important role in preserving myocardial integrity.

      i. In the absence of preoperative ventricular dysfunction and associated coronary disease, inotropic support often is not required after cardiopulmonary bypass because valve replacement decreases ventricular afterload.

      j. **Omniplanar transesophageal echocardiography (TEE)** is suggested for intraoperative monitoring of LV function and detection of intracavitary thrombi. If commissurotomy is performed rather than valve replacement, TEE is a highly effective method for quantitating residual aortic regurgitation. With total valve replacement, TEE will readily identify perivalvular leaks.

  3. Surgical intervention. Because of the high risk of sudden death, all symptomatic patients should undergo surgery. Asymptomatic patients with a transvalvular gradient greater than 50 mm Hg or valve index less than 0.5 cm^2/m^2 should undergo surgery. The initial surgical procedure often is a valvular commissurotomy performed under direct vision, which frequently results in some residual aortic stenosis and aortic regurgitation. Eventually, most patients require prosthetic valve replacement. Surgical intervention should not be denied to patients no matter how severe the symptomatology because irreparable LV failure occurs only very late in the disease process. After isolated aortic valve replacement, hospital mortality is 3% to 5%. Of the patients leaving the hospital, 85% can expect to survive for at least 5 years.

  4. Postoperative care. After aortic commissurotomy or valve replacement, pulmonary capillary wedge pressure and LVEDP immediately decrease and stroke volume rises. **Myocardial function improves rapidly, although the hypertrophied ventricle still may require an elevated preload to function normally. Over a period of several months, LV hypertrophy regresses.** It must be remembered that if a prosthetic valve has been used, a residual gradient of 7 to 19 mm Hg may be present and, if a commissurotomy has been performed, concurrent aortic regurgitation may be present. Most patients do very well after surgery for aortic stenosis, provided intraoperative myocardial preservation is adequate.

D. Idiopathic hypertrophic subaortic stenosis (hypertrophic cardiomyopathy). This disease process represents a **dynamic stenosis** of the aortic outflow tract, unlike valvular aortic stenosis, which is fixed. The response of the myocardium to this disease process is similar to that seen in valvular aortic stenosis; however, the increased muscle mass in the subaortic region eventually leads to severe obstruction of LV outflow. In this special situation, β-blockade may be beneficial. These patients also **benefit from preload augmentation for maintaining LV volume, from afterload augmentation for increasing diastolic perfusion through the hypertrophied muscle mass and from slow heart rates.** Patients with hypertrophic cardiomyopathy are at increased risk from arrhythmias, particularly tachyarrhythmias, during surgery.

III. Aortic regurgitation

  A. Natural history

    1. Etiology. Rheumatic fever and syphilitic aortitis were the primary causes of aortic regurgitation in the past. However, with early identification and successful treatment of these diseases, they now are seen infrequently as causes of aortic regurgitation. Increasingly, **bacterial endocarditis, trauma, aortic dissection,** and a variety of congenital diseases leading to abnormal collagen formation, such as **Marfan syndrome** or **cystic medionecrosis,** are becoming the primary etiologies.

    2. Symptomatology. Patients with **chronic aortic regurgitation** may be asymptomatic for up to 20 years. The 10-year mortality for asymptomatic aortic regurgitation varies between 5% and 15%. However, once symptoms develop, patients progressively deteriorate and have an expected survival rate of 5 to 10 years. Early symptoms include dyspnea, fatigue, and palpitations. Angina pectoris normally is a late symptom and is an ominous sign. Patients with **acute aortic regurgitation,** on the other hand, may deteriorate rapidly, and the prognosis is guarded.

B. Pathophysiology

1. **Natural progression**

   a. **Acute aortic regurgitation.** The sudden occurrence of acute aortic regurgitation places a major volume load on the LV. An immediate compensatory mechanism for maintenance of adequate forward flow is increased sympathetic tone, producing tachycardia and an increased contractile state. Fluid retention increases preload. However, the combination of increased LVEDV and increased total stroke volume and heart rate may not be sufficient to maintain normal cardiac output. Rapid deterioration of LV function can occur, necessitating emergency surgical intervention.

   b. **Chronic aortic regurgitation**

      (1) **Stage 1: mild aortic regurgitation—asymptomatic with physiologic compensation.** The onset of aortic regurgitation leads to LV systolic and diastolic volume overload. The increased volume load leads to eccentric hypertrophy of the LV, with increases in both the thickness of the LV wall and the size of the ventricular cavity. Because the LVEDV increases slowly, the LVEDP remains relatively normal. Because volume work is less expensive metabolically than pressure work, no major increase in myocardial O_2 demand occurs, despite an increased ejection fraction. Forward flow is aided by the presence of chronic peripheral vasodilation, which occurs along with a large stroke volume in patients with mild aortic regurgitation. There is minimal symptomatology as long as the regurgitant fraction remains less than 40% of the stroke volume.

      (2) **Stage 2: moderate aortic regurgitation—symptomatic impairment.** As the amount of aortic regurgitation progresses to more than 60% of stroke volume, continued LV dilation and hypertrophy occur, finally leading to irreversible LV myocardial tissue damage. An early sign of these changes is an increase in LVEDP to greater than 20 mm Hg, indicating LV dysfunction. The onset of LV dysfunction is followed by an increase in pulmonary arterial pressure with symptoms of dyspnea and congestive heart failure.

      (3) **Stage 3: severe aortic regurgitation—terminal failure.** After the onset of symptomatology, LV dysfunction continues to progress and eventually becomes irreversible. Symptomatology is rapidly progressive, and surgical intervention at this point is not always successful. Angina pectoris may occur because of the reduction in diastolic aortic pressure with decreased diastolic coronary perfusion, ventricular dilation with increased wall tension, and the presence of a hypertrophied LV. As a compensatory mechanism for poor cardiac output and poor coronary perfusion, sympathetic constriction of the periphery occurs, leading to further decreases in cardiac output.

2. **Pressure–volume relationship** (Fig. 12.4). In acute aortic regurgitation, a sudden volume load is placed on a normally compliant LV. This leads to increases in both LV end-diastolic and end-systolic volumes. Because the LV does not have time to compensate through eccentric hypertrophy, the result is a sudden increase in LVEDP. The compensatory mechanism of sympathetic stimulation may not be sufficient to maintain adequate stroke volume.

   In chronic aortic regurgitation, eccentric hypertrophy occurs, leading to massive increases in LV end-diastolic and end-systolic volumes. An increase in LV compliance over time allows the LVEDP to remain only mildly elevated. With this compensatory mechanism, stroke volume can be maintained for some time. Ejection fraction is an unreliable index of LV function in patients with aortic regurgitation.

3. **Determination of severity**

   a. **Qualitative estimate.** The amount of aortic regurgitation usually is estimated based on angiocardiographic clearance of injected dye into the aortic root [5].

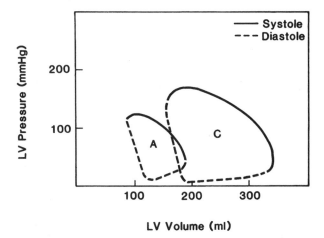

FIG. 12.4 Pressure–volume loops, aortic insufficiency. Loop *A,* from a patient with acute aortic insufficiency, shows moderately elevated left ventricular systolic and diastolic volumes as well as an increase in ventricular volume during ventricular relaxation. Loop *C,* from a patient with chronic aortic insufficiency, shows markedly increased systolic and diastolic volumes but lower end-diastolic pressure. (Modified from Jackson JM, Thomas SJ, Lowenstein E. Anesthetic management of patients with valvular heart disease. *Semin Anesth* 1982;1:247.)

+1   Slight reflux of dye into the LV during LV diastole with opacification limited to the LV outflow tract; dye is completely cleared with next systole

+2   Moderate reflux of dye into the LV during diastole; dye is not completely cleared with the next systole

+3   Complete opacification of the LV for several systoles

+4   Complete opacification of the LV by the end of the first diastole, with maintenance of opacification for several systoles; density of the dye in the LV is greater than that in the aorta

  b. **Calculation of regurgitant fraction.** A more quantitative estimate of the severity of aortic regurgitation can be obtained by comparing forward flow (thermodilution cardiac output) with total volume of blood ejected by the LV (angiographic cardiac output). The regurgitant fraction, or fraction of each stroke volume flowing back into the LV, can be calculated using the following equation:

$$\text{Regurgitant fraction} = \frac{[(\text{EDV} - \text{ESV}) \times \text{HR}] - \text{CO}}{(\text{EDV} - \text{ESV}) \times \text{HR}}$$

  where EDV is end-diastolic volume, ESV is end-systolic volume, HR is heart rate, and CO is thermodilution cardiac output (forward flow).

4. **Pressure wave disturbances**
  a. **Arterial pressure.** Patients with aortic regurgitation show a wide pulse pressure with a rapid rate of rise, a high systolic peak, and the presence of a low diastolic pressure. The pulse pressure may be as high as 80 to 100 mm Hg. The rapid upstroke is due to the large stroke volume, and the rapid downstroke is due to the rapid flow of blood from the aorta back into the ventricle and into the dilated peripheral vessels. The occurrence

of a double peaked or bisferiens pulse trace is not unusual owing to the occurrence of a "tidal" or back wave.
   b. **Pulmonary capillary wedge trace.** Normally, stretching of the mitral valve annulus leads to functional mitral regurgitation, a prominent V wave, and a rapid Y descent. The V wave is more prominent in acute regurgitation and with the onset of LV failure.
C. **Goals of perioperative management**
   1. **Hemodynamic management**

	LV preload	Heart rate	Contractile state	Systemic vascular resistance	Pulmonary vascular resistance
Aortic regurgitation	↑	↑	Maintain	↓	Maintain

   a. **LV preload.** Because of the increased LV volumes, **maintenance of forward flow depends on preload augmentation. Pharmacologic intervention that produces venous dilation may significantly impair cardiac output in these patients by reducing preload.**
   b. **Heart rate.** Patients with aortic regurgitation show a significant increase in forward cardiac output with an increase in heart rate. The decreased time spent in diastole during tachycardia leads to a decreased regurgitant fraction. Actual improvement in subendocardial blood flow is observed with tachycardia due to a higher systemic diastolic pressure and a lower LVEDP. This explains why a patient who is symptomatic at rest may show improvement in symptomatology with exercise. **A heart rate of 90 beats/min seems to be optimal, improving cardiac output while not inducing ischemia.** Maintenance of sinus rhythm is not as important as it is in patients with stenotic lesions, and the presence of atrial fibrillation is common.
   c. **Contractility.** LV contractility must be maintained. In patients with impaired LV function, use of pure β-agents can increase stroke volume through a combination of peripheral dilation and increased contractility.
   d. **Systemic vascular resistance.** Normally, patients with chronic aortic insufficiency initially compensate for the limitation in cardiac output by dilation of the peripheral arterioles. The forward flow can be improved further with afterload reduction. Increases in afterload result in increased stroke work and can significantly increase the LVEDP. The patient in end-stage aortic regurgitation with LV impairment benefits most from therapy with afterload-reducing agents.
   e. **Pulmonary vascular resistance.** Pulmonary vascular pressure remains relatively normal except in patients with end-stage aortic regurgitation associated with severe LV dysfunction.
   2. **Anesthetic technique**
      a. **Premedication** that dilates the capacitance vessels should be avoided. **Light premedication** is recommended to maintain myocardial contractility and heart rate because tachycardia actually can be helpful for these patients. Increases in systemic vascular resistance that may arise from anxiety, however, may be detrimental.
      b. A pulmonary artery catheter is essential for maintaining cardiac output and LV filling pressures, particularly when vasodilators are required to maintain forward flow.
      c. The agent of choice for **induction** and maintenance of anesthesia should be directed at preserving the patient's preload, maintaining the peripheral arterial dilation, improving contractility, and keeping the heart rate near 90 beats/min. Use of isoflurane and pancuronium in combination with fluid augmentation is acceptable, except in patients with end-stage disease with reduced ventricular function in whom a synthetic narcotic in combination with pancuronium is better tolerated.

    d. In patients with acute aortic regurgitation associated with poor ventricular compliance, LV pressure may increase fast enough to close the mitral valve before end diastole. In this situation, the continued regurgitation of blood raises LVEDP above left atrial pressure, and **pulmonary capillary wedge pressure** can significantly underestimate the true LVEDP.

    e. Use of an intraaortic balloon pump is contraindicated in the presence of aortic regurgitation because augmentation of diastolic pressure will increase the amount of regurgitant flow.

    f. Omniplanar TEE is beneficial for monitoring LV function and quantitating regurgitation before valve repair. If annuloplasty or plication is performed, TEE is valuable for providing immediate feedback concerning the integrity of valvular function. In total valve replacement, TEE allows assessment of perivalvular leaks.

  3. Surgical intervention. Surgical repair can be performed with an annuloplasty or valvular plication but most frequently is provided through the use of valvular replacement with a prosthetic valve. Surgery is indicated if the patient is symptomatic or preferably as soon as echocardiographic evidence of LV dysfunction exists in the asymptomatic patient. It is important to intervene surgically before LV dysfunction progresses.

  4. Postoperative care. Immediately after aortic valve replacement, LVEDP and LVEDV decrease. However, LV hypertrophy and dilation persist. In the immediate postbypass period, **preload augmentation** must be continued to maintain filling of the dilated LV. In the early postoperative period, a decline in LV function may necessitate **inotropic or intraaortic balloon pump support.** If surgical intervention is delayed until major LV dysfunction has occurred, the prognosis for long-term survival is not good. The 5-year survival rate for patients whose hearts do not return to a relatively normal size within 6 months after surgical repair is only 43%. If surgery is performed early enough, the heart will return to relatively normal dimensions, and a long-term survival rate of 85% to 90% after 6 years can be expected.

IV. Mitral stenosis

  A. Natural history

    1. Etiology. In adults, mitral stenosis almost always is secondary to rheumatic heart disease, which leads to scarring and fibrosis of the free edges of the mitral valve leaflets. Fusion of the valvular commissures, progressive scarring of the leaflets, and contraction of the chordae tendineae lead to the development of a funnel-shaped mitral apparatus that can become secondarily calcified. Women are affected twice as frequently as men. Mitral stenosis, of rheumatic origin, often occurs along with mitral regurgitation or aortic regurgitation.

    2. Symptomatology. Patients are normally asymptomatic for 20 years or more after an acute episode of rheumatic fever. However, as stenosis develops, symptoms appear, associated at first with exercise or high cardiac output states. Twenty percent of patients in whom the diagnosis of symptomatic mitral stenosis is made die within 1 year, and 50% die within 10 years after diagnosis, without surgical intervention. The natural history is a slow progressive downhill course with repeated episodes of **pulmonary edema, dyspnea, paroxysmal nocturnal dyspnea, fatigue, chest pains, palpitations,** and **hemoptysis,** as well as hoarseness due to compression of the left recurrent laryngeal nerve by a distended left atrium and enlarged pulmonary artery. Symptoms often become apparent with the onset of atrial fibrillation, and patients in atrial fibrillation are at increased risk for formation of left atrial thrombi and subsequent cerebral or systemic emboli. Medical management can be successful if it is initiated early. Chest pain may occur in 10% to 20% of patients with mitral stenosis, but it is a poor predictor of the coexistence of coronary disease, which may be present in approximately 25% of patients.

  B. Pathophysiology

    1. Natural progression

      a. Stage 1: mild mitral stenosis—asymptomatic with physiologic compensation. The normal mitral valve area is 4 to 6 cm^2 (mitral valve index,

4.0 to 4.5 cm²/m²). The patient can remain essentially symptom-free during the 20- to 30-year period of slow progression of stenosis until a valve area of 1.5 to 2.5 cm² (or valve index of 1.0–2.0 cm²/m²) is reached. At this point, moderate exercise may induce dyspnea. Exercise testing in the cardiac catheterization laboratory, by detecting increased filling pressures with exercise, can identify this stage of the disease. Further progression of mitral stenosis leads to increases in left atrial pressure and volume that are reflected back into the pulmonary circuit.

   b. **Stage 2: moderate mitral stenosis—symptomatic impairment.** Between a valve area of 1.0 and 1.5 cm², increasing symptomatology appears with only mild-to-moderate exertion. Severe congestive failure can be induced either by the onset of atrial fibrillation or by a variety of disease processes leading to high cardiac output states, such as thyrotoxicosis, pregnancy, anemia, or fever. In all these conditions, the left atrial and pulmonary artery pressures suddenly rise as a result of the increased cardiac demand. The increase in pulmonary vascular resistance in response to high left atrial pressure eventually can lead to RV failure. Pulmonary arterial constriction, pulmonary intimal hyperplasia, and pulmonary medial hypertrophy eventually result in a picture of chronic pulmonary arterial hypertension associated with restrictive lung disease. Because atrial contraction contributes 30% of LV filling in mitral stenosis, the onset of atrial fibrillation can lead to significant impairment in cardiac output.

   c. **Stage 3: critical mitral stenosis—terminal failure.** With a valve area less than 1.0 cm², a patient is considered to have critical mitral stenosis, and symptoms are present even at rest. Not only are left atrial pressures on the border of producing congestive failure, but cardiac output also may be reduced. Chronic pulmonary hypertension eventually leads to RV dilation. The dilated RV can cause a leftward shift of the intraventricular septum, thereby limiting the already reduced LV size and further impairing LV ejection. With further RV dilation, tricuspid regurgitation results, leading to signs of peripheral congestion. A mitral valve area of 0.3 to 0.4 cm² is the smallest area compatible with life.

2. **Pressure–volume relationship** (Fig. 12.5). Due to the restriction of flow from the left atrium to the ventricle, patients with significant mitral stenosis have reduced LVEDV and LVEDP. Stroke volume also is reduced. The actual LV performance is relatively normal. The limitation of stroke volume in these patients is entirely due to inadequate filling of the LV.

3. **Calculation of mitral valve area.** Quantitative evaluation of mitral stenosis based only on the diastolic pressure gradient across the mitral valve is inaccurate, as with the aortic valve, because it does not take into consideration the important factor, **flow.** The Gorlin formula for determination of the mitral valve area is as follows:

$$\text{Mitral valve area (cm}^2) = \frac{\text{Mitral valve flow (mL/s)}}{0.85 \times 44.5 \times \sqrt{\text{mean mitral gradient}}}$$

   where 0.85 is the mitral orifice constant and mitral valve flow (mL/s) is cardiac output (mL/min)/diastolic filling period (s/beat) × HR (beats/min).

   Because tachycardia shortens the diastolic filling period, it compromises LV filling and leads to clinical deterioration. Comparisons of the rate of blood flow and the mean diastolic pressure can be graphically represented (Fig. 12.6). It is apparent that when the mitral valve area is 1.0 cm² or less, little additional flow can be obtained by increasing the pressure gradient across the valve.

4. **Pressure wave disturbances**

   a. **Pulmonary capillary wedge pressure.** Mitral stenosis produces a large A wave and, if it is associated with an element of mitral regurgitation, a prominent V wave. With increased impairment of left atrial contractility secondary to severe mitral obstruction, the A wave may become small. In the presence of atrial fibrillation, the A wave is obviously absent.

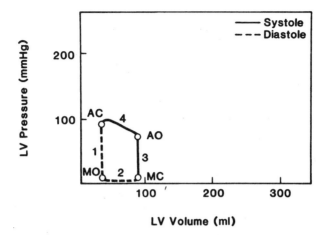

FIG. 12.5 Pressure–volume loop, mitral stenosis, showing decreased left ventricular systolic and diastolic volumes, reduced stroke volume, and decreased systolic and end-diastolic pressures. *AC,* aortic valve closure; *AO,* aortic valve opening; *MC,* mitral valve closure; *MO,* mitral valve opening; phase *1,* isovolumetric relaxation; phase *2,* ventricular filling; phase *3,* isovolumetric contraction; phase *4,* ventricular ejection. (Modified from Jackson JM, Thomas SJ, Lowenstein E. Anesthetic management of patients with valvular heart disease. *Semin Anesth* 1982;1:244.)

C. Goals of perioperative management
1. Hemodynamic management

	LV preload	Heart rate	Contractile state	Systemic vascular resistance	Pulmonary vascular resistance
Mitral stenosis	↑	↓	Maintain	Maintain	↓

a. **LV preload. Forward flow across the stenotic mitral valve is dependent on adequate preload.** On the other hand, patients with mitral stenosis already have elevated left atrial pressures so that overly aggressive use of fluids can easily send a patient who is in borderline congestive failure into florid pulmonary edema.

b. **Heart rate.** Blood flow across the mitral valve occurs during ventricular diastole. Tachycardia shortens the diastolic period so that at increased heart rates, the flow across the stenotic mitral valve must be increased to maintain the same level of cardiac output. Based on Poiseuille's law, the atrial–ventricular pressure gradient is proportional to the fourth power of the instantaneous flow across the mitral valve; hence, any increase in instantaneous flow requires a large increase in left atrial pressure. At the same time, excessive bradycardia can be dangerous because stroke volume is relatively fixed.

Atrial contraction in patients with mitral stenosis contributes approximately 30% of the LV stroke volume. If atrioventricular pacing is initiated in these patients, a **long PR interval of 0.15 to 0.20 ms is optimal** to allow blood adequate time, after atrial contraction, to cross the stenotic mitral valve. Decreases in the PR interval will drop diastolic

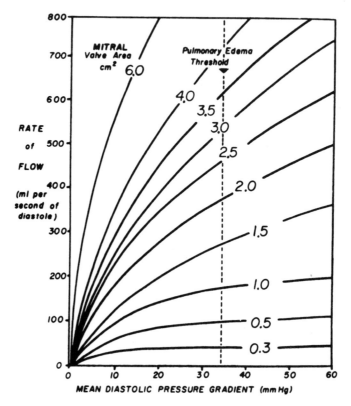

FIG. 12.6 Comparison between rate of blood flow across the mitral valve and mean diastolic pressure gradient across the mitral valve in individuals with different mitral valve areas, as determined by the Gorlin formula. Below a critical mitral valve area of 1.0 cm², a large increase in mean diastolic pressure gradient across the mitral valve produces a minimal increase in blood flow. The point at which pulmonary capillary pressure exceeds normal plasma oncotic pressure leading to the transudation of fluid and the development of pulmonary edema is indicated on the graph. (From Schlant RC. Altered cardiovascular function of rheumatic heart disease and other acquired valvular disease. In: Hurst JW, Logue RB, Schlant RC, et al., eds. *The heart,* 4th ed. New York: McGraw-Hill, 1978:972, with permission.)

flow and result in a reduced cardiac output. In patients with atrial fibrillation, the contribution of atrial contraction is lost.

c. **Contractility.** Adequate forward flow depends on adequate RV and LV contractility. Chronic underfilling of the LV, however, leads to cardiomyopathy with depressed ventricular contractility even in the face of restored filling. In end-stage mitral stenosis, depression of LV contractility may lead to severe congestive heart failure. Depression of RV contractility limits left atrial filling and, eventually, cardiac output. Many patients will require inotropic support before and especially after cardiopulmonary bypass.

d. **Systemic vascular resistance.** To maintain blood pressure in the presence of limited cardiac output, patients with mitral stenosis normally develop increased systemic vascular resistance. **Afterload reduction is not helpful in improving forward flow** because the limiting factor for cardiac output is the stenotic mitral valve. It is recommended that the afterload be kept in the normal range for these patients.

    e. Pulmonary vascular resistance. These patients frequently have **elevated pulmonary vascular resistances** and are prone to exaggerated pulmonary vasoconstriction in the presence of hypoxia. **Particular attention should be paid to avoiding any increases in pulmonary artery pressure due to injudicious use of anesthetic agents, particularly nitrous oxide, or to inadvertent acidosis, hypercapnia, or hypoxemia.**

2. **Anesthetic technique**

    a. Premedication should be light to avoid an acute decrease in preload or the possibility of sedation with resultant hypoxemia and hypercapnia. Avoidance of an anticholinergic should be considered to minimize tachycardia.

    b. Continue digitalis for heart rate control right up to the morning of surgery.

    c. Avoid pharmacologic agents or conditions that produce tachycardia, increased pulmonary vascular resistance, decreased preload, or decreased contractility. In particular **tachycardia,** whether it is due to a sinus mechanism or atrial fibrillation, must be treated aggressively. An attempt should be made to maintain sinus rhythm at all times with **immediate use of cardioversion** if new atrial fibrillation should occur. A narcotic anesthetic technique with high inspired O_2 concentration usually is chosen for these patients [6].

    d. Pulmonary artery catheters almost always are indicated for perioperative management. However, the catheters often must be inserted further than usual because of the dilated pulmonary arteries. Special care should be taken when placing the catheters because of the increased risk of pulmonary artery rupture. Further, the pressure data obtained from the catheters must be interpreted carefully. Pulmonary artery diastolic pressure often is not an accurate estimate of left atrial pressure because of significant pulmonary hypertension. Even pulmonary capillary wedge pressure that does reflect left atrial pressure overestimates LV filling pressure because of the stenotic mitral valve.

    Because of the risk of pulmonary artery rupture and the questionable information obtained from a wedge pressure, final placement of the pulmonary artery catheter in a wedge position usually is not necessary.

    e. TEE evaluation is particularly helpful for monitoring the adequacy of mitral valve repair. Mitral commissurotomy may result in significant mitral regurgitation, which can be identified in the immediate postbypass period so that further surgical intervention can be provided promptly. In addition, complications associated with mitral valve replacement, such as paravalvular leak, which otherwise would require a repeat procedure, can be identified rapidly and repaired while still in the operating room.

3. **Surgical intervention.** Surgical intervention should occur before the development of severe symptomatology because irreversible ventricular dysfunction may result if surgery is delayed too long. Surgery is not recommended for the asymptomatic patient unless there is evidence of systemic embolization or progressive pulmonary hypertension. Mitral commissurotomy is the operation of choice if the valve is not significantly calcified or severely fibrotic. Commissurotomy does not totally relieve the stenosis but rather makes it less severe. Restenosis of the mitral valve will occur in as many as 30% of patients within 5 years after commissurotomy and in 60% after 9 years. Nevertheless, during this time the patient does not require anticoagulation and is at risk for less morbidity than with an indwelling prosthetic valve. If the valve is not amenable to commissurotomy, mitral valve replacement should be performed. After isolated mitral valve replacement, 95% of patients survive to leave the hospital and, of these hospital survivors, 80% survive 5 years. A balloon-dilating technique at catheterization can be used to delay the necessity for open heart surgery by effectively relieving the mitral obstruction but with the risk of significant postdilation mitral regurgitation.

4. **Postoperative care.** Successful surgical intervention leads to a drop in pulmonary vascular resistance, pulmonary arterial pressure, and left atrial

pressure while increasing cardiac output in the first postoperative day. However, immediately after bypass, even patients with seemingly normal preoperative LV function may have major depression of myocardial contractility owing to their underlying cardiomyopathy exacerbated by ischemic arrest during cardiopulmonary bypass. These patients frequently require inotropic and intraaortic balloon pump support.

Pulmonary vascular resistance in most patients will continue to decrease with time after surgery. Failure of the pulmonary artery pressure to decrease usually is indicative of irreversible pulmonary hypertension and probably irreversible LV dysfunction. This places the patient in a prognostically poor group. **Preload augmentation as well as afterload reduction should be undertaken in the immediate postbypass period** to improve forward blood flow. Patients previously in chronic atrial fibrillation occasionally can be converted to sinus rhythm by prophylactic treatment with a bolus of procainamide (500 mg to 1 g) or amiodarone (150 mg) during bypass. If the patient does convert to a sinus rhythm, this rhythm can be maintained, at least for short periods of time, with continuous infusion of procainamide (2 mg/min) or amiodarone (33 mg/min) and overdrive atrial pacing at a rate of approximately 110 beats/min. It must be remembered that after prosthetic valve placement, a residual 4 to 7 mm Hg gradient across the mitral valve will still be present.

One catastrophic complication that can occur within the first few days after valve replacement is atrioventricular disruption. One method suggested to help avoid this complication is to **reduce LVEDP to as low a level as possible** while maintaining adequate cardiac output. Atrioventricular disruption is a particular risk for the elderly patient with a relatively noncompliant LV who experiences increased diastolic tension on the LV wall after surgery. Thus, inotropes in the postbypass period can serve two functions by (a) increasing contractility and (b) reducing LV size and wall tension.

V. Mitral regurgitation
  A. Natural history. The spectrum of mitral regurgitation varies from acute forms, in which rapid deterioration of myocardial function can occur, to chronic forms, which have slow indolent courses. Mitral regurgitation can be either primary or secondary to LV dilation or ischemia.
  1. **Etiology—chronic mitral regurgitation.** In the United States, the most common cause of mitral regurgitation probably is mitral valve prolapse, a common disorder that leads to significant regurgitation in 10% to 15% of cases. **Rheumatic** disease is an uncommon cause of mitral regurgitation. When it does occur, it is rarely pure. Usually it exists in combination with mitral stenosis. Rheumatic mitral regurgitation is a slow indolent process with an asymptomatic period that lasts 20 to 40 years. There is a gradual onset of fatigue and increasing dyspnea. Although mitral regurgitation can be tolerated for many years without ill effect, the onset of significant symptomatology (fatigue, dyspnea, or orthopnea) usually heralds a relatively rapid downhill course, with death occurring within 5 years. A sequela such as bacterial endocarditis, atrial fibrillation, reactive pulmonary hypertension, or systemic embolization leads to rapid clinical deterioration. **Atrial fibrillation** occurs in nearly 75% of cases. Survival rates are better in patients when surgery is performed before the development of irreversible LV dysfunction.
  2. **Etiology—acute mitral regurgitation.** Acute mitral regurgitation is being seen more frequently, especially mitral regurgitation on the basis of **papillary muscle dysfunction** due to myocardial ischemia. Papillary muscle dysfunction occurs in approximately 40% of patients who sustain a posterior septal myocardial infarction and in 20% of patients with an anterior septal infarction. **Bacterial endocarditis** is another frequent cause of nonrheumatic mitral regurgitation.
  B. Pathophysiology
  1. **Natural progression**
    a. **Acute.** Sudden development of mitral regurgitation leads to marked left atrial volume overload. Because of the normal compliance of the left atrium,

the sudden volume overload leads to significant increases in left atrial pressure that are passed on to the pulmonary circuit. As immediate compensation for decreased cardiac output, sympathetic stimulation increases contractility and produces tachycardia. In addition, the LV functions on a higher portion of the Frank–Starling curve because of increased LV volumes. The acute increases in left atrial and pulmonary artery pressures can lead to pulmonary congestion and edema. Of concern, the compensatory sympathetic stimulation can lead to increased myocardial O_2 consumption in myocardium already rendered ischemic by increased LVEDP and decreased subendocardial blood flow, and to peripheral constriction, further compromising systemic blood flow. Because LV ischemia is a common cause, acute mitral regurgitation often presents as biventricular failure.

b. Chronic

(1) Stage 1: mild mitral regurgitation—asymptomatic with physiologic compensation. During the slow development of chronic mitral regurgitation, eccentric hypertrophy of the LV occurs, with the heart shifting eccentrically to the left side of the chest. Both LV dilation and hypertrophy occur. The dilation of the LV allows preservation of a relatively normal LVEDP despite a markedly increased LVEDV. The forward cardiac output is preserved by an overall increase in total LV stroke volume (combined forward stroke volume and regurgitant stroke volume). In addition, the left atrium enlarges and becomes distensible. A large distensible left atrium can maintain near-normal left atrial pressures despite large regurgitant volumes, which helps to protect the pulmonary vascular bed. Most of these patients eventually develop atrial fibrillation.

(2) Stage 2: moderate mitral regurgitation—symptomatic impairment. LV dilation and hypertrophy continue to compensate for increasing regurgitation until eventually the forward stroke volume is compromised. Continued left atrial dilation may lead to further increases in regurgitation owing to stretching of the mitral annulus. At this point, the symptoms of forward heart failure, including increased fatigability and generalized weakness, may intervene. Once the regurgitant fraction is greater than 60%, congestive heart failure occurs. LV ejection fraction usually is elevated in patients with mitral regurgitation because of the ease of ejecting blood backward into the low-pressure pulmonary circuit. An ejection fraction of 50% or less indicates the presence of significant ventricular dysfunction in these patients.

(3) Stage 3: severe mitral regurgitation—terminal failure. Continued severe compromise of forward cardiac output leads to increases in pulmonary artery pressure and eventually RV failure. In addition, LV function continues to deteriorate, and the depression of ventricular function becomes irreversible even after cardiac valve replacement.

2. Pressure–volume relationship (Fig. 12.7). In chronic mitral regurgitation, LVEDP may remain relatively normal until the disease is far advanced despite major increases in LV end-diastolic and end-systolic volumes. The eccentric hypertrophy of the ventricle allows preservation of forward stroke volume by increasing total stroke volume. Blunting of the LV pressure increase during LV contraction occurs secondary to rapid early runoff of LV volume into the low-pressure left atrium. In contrast, in acute mitral regurgitation the compensatory increases in LV end-diastolic and end-systolic volumes are attenuated by acute increases in LVEDP until compensatory dilation can intervene.

3. Calculation of severity. The regurgitant fraction, which indicates the severity of mitral regurgitation, can be calculated quantitatively in the same way as in patients with aortic regurgitation (see Section **III.B.3.b**).

Mitral regurgitation consisting of less than 30% of total LV stroke volume is considered mild, 30% to 60% is considered moderate, and greater than 60% is considered severe.

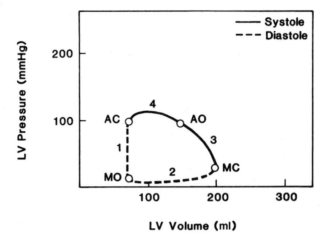

FIG. 12.7 Pressure–volume loop, moderate mitral insufficiency, showing markedly increased left ventricular end-systolic and end-diastolic volumes, along with some increase in left ventricular end-diastolic pressure. *AC,* aortic valve closure; *AO,* aortic valve opening; *MC,* mitral valve closure; *MO,* mitral valve opening; phase *1,* isovolumetric relaxation; phase *2,* ventricular filling; phase *3,* isovolumetric contraction; phase *4,* ventricular ejection. (Modified from Jackson JM, Thomas SJ, Lowenstein E. Anesthetic management of patients with valvular heart disease. *Semin Anesth* 1982;1:248.)

Normally, determination of regurgitant volume is made only qualitatively through the use of angiographic dye injection into the LV:

1+   Minimal opacification of the left atrium is rapidly cleared
2+   Moderate opacification of left atrium is rapidly cleared
3+   Left atrial opacification is as intense as LV and aortic opacification
4+   Left atrial opacification is more intense than LV and aortic opacification

Severe mitral regurgitation can be detected perioperatively on Doppler TEE by noting sustained reversal in the direction of pulmonary venous blood flow during systole and quantitated by the area of the regurgitant plume.

4. **Pressure wave disturbances**
    a. **Pulmonary capillary wedge tracing.** The size of the regurgitant wave is not directly related to the severity of mitral regurgitation. The size of the regurgitant wave or **"giant V wave"** depends on the compliance of the left atrium, the compliance of the pulmonary vasculature, the amount of pulmonary venous return, and the regurgitant volume. In patients with sudden onset of mitral regurgitation, a relatively noncompliant left atrium leads to large V waves. Patients with chronic mitral regurgitation have a large compliant left atrium that can accept the regurgitant volume without passing the pressure wave on to the pulmonary circuit [7].
    In patients with giant V waves or regurgitant waves, differentiation between the pulmonary arterial pressure trace and the pulmonary capillary wedge pressure trace can be difficult (Fig. 12.8). One easy way to make this differentiation, however, is by **superimposition of the pulmonary arterial trace and the arterial pressure trace.** Normally, the pulmonary arterial upstroke occurs slightly before the systemic arterial upstroke but, when a wedge position is achieved, an immediate rightward shift is ob-

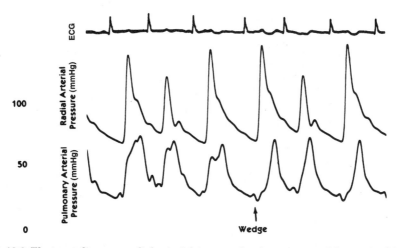

FIG. 12.8 Electrocardiogram, radial arterial trace, and pulmonary arterial trace in the unwedged and wedged positions for a patient with severe mitral regurgitation. The amplitude of the "giant V wave" or regurgitant wave is greater than the peak pulmonary artery pressure. (From Moore RA, Neary MJ, Gallagher JD, et al. Determination of the pulmonary capillary wedge position in patients with giant left atrial V waves. *J Cardiothorac Anesth* 1987;1:110, with permission.)

served in the position of the upstroke and peak to the position of the giant V wave, which occurs later than the arterial pressure upstroke. Therefore, when placing pulmonary artery catheters in patients with mitral regurgitation or patients at risk for having giant V waves, it is imperative to perform simultaneous observation of pulmonary arterial and systemic arterial traces [8].

C. **Goals of perioperative management**
   1. **Hemodynamic management**

	LV preload	Heart rate	Contractile state	Systemic vascular resistance	Pulmonary vascular resistance
Mitral regurgitation	↑,↓	↑ Maintain	Maintain	↓	↓

   a. **LV preload.** Augmentation and **maintenance of preload** frequently are helpful for ensuring adequate forward stroke volume. Unfortunately, a universal recommendation for preload augmentation cannot be made because in some patients dilation of the left atrial and LV compartments dilates the mitral valve annulus and increases the regurgitant fraction. A decision about **the best level of preload augmentation for an individual patient must be based on that patient's clinical response to a fluid load.**
   b. **Heart rate.** Bradycardia is harmful in patients with mitral regurgitation because it leads to an increase in LV volume, reduction in forward cardiac output, and increase in regurgitant fraction. **The heart rate should be kept in the normal to elevated range** in these patients. Atrial contribution to preload is not as important in patients with mitral regurgitation

as in those with stenotic lesions, and many of these patients, particularly those with chronic mitral regurgitation, come to the operating room in atrial fibrillation.

    c. **Contractility.** Maintenance of forward stroke volume is dependent on maximal function of the eccentrically hypertrophied LV. Depression of myocardial contractility can lead to major LV dysfunction and clinical deterioration. **Inotropic agents that increase contractility have a tendency to provide increased forward flow and actually can decrease regurgitation due to constriction of the mitral annulus.**

    d. **Systemic vascular resistance.** An increase in afterload leads to an increase in regurgitant fraction and reduction in systemic cardiac output. For this reason, **afterload reduction normally is desired, and α-adrenergic agents should be avoided.** Typically, sodium nitroprusside will decrease LV filling pressure and cause a significant increase in forward cardiac index. However, in patients with acute mitral regurgitation secondary to ischemic papillary muscle dysfunction, nitroglycerin might be a more logical choice for use as a dilating agent.

    e. **Pulmonary vascular resistance.** Most patients with extensive mitral regurgitation will develop increased pulmonary vascular pressure and even can present in right-sided heart failure. **Extreme caution must be taken to avoid hypercapnia, hypoxia, nitrous oxide, and pharmacologic or other interventions that might lead to pulmonary constrictive responses.**

2. **Anesthetic management**

    a. **Premedication** should be used **judiciously** because oversedation can lead to hypercapnia and marked increases in pulmonary vascular resistance.

    b. **Pulmonary artery catheters** are extremely helpful in guiding fluid management. They also help in evaluating the changing clinical state and significance of regurgitation for any particular patient as judged by changes in the height of the giant V wave.

    c. **Anesthetic agents** that lead to decreased contractility should be avoided. **High-dose narcotic relaxant anesthetics** are used most commonly.

    d. Patients with papillary muscle dysfunction secondary to ischemia frequently are helped by preoperative insertion of an **intraaortic balloon pump.** Inotropic support frequently is required in the postbypass period [9].

    e. Evaluation of the patient's regurgitant fraction is aided by the use of TEE. In addition, TEE can be invaluable for assessing the adequacy of valvular repair should annuloplasty or plication be chosen. When the valve is completely replaced, TEE is important for detecting the presence of a perivalvular leak in the immediate postbypass period so that repairs can be undertaken immediately.

    f. Nitric oxide, as a specific pulmonary artery dilator, may have an important role in the management of patients with reversible pulmonary hypertension. Hyperventilation is a second therapeutic modality available for selectively dilating the pulmonary vasculature without affecting the patient's systemic blood pressure. Prostaglandin E_1 also has been used but is accompanied by a decrease in systemic pressure.

3. **Surgical intervention** is not recommended if the patient can be treated medically with adequate relief of symptoms. However, once significant LV dysfunction occurs, surgery should be performed as soon as possible before the LV failure becomes irreversible. The surgical procedure usually performed is valve replacement using a mechanical or biologic valve, although occasionally annuloplasty can be performed with good results.

4. **Postoperative care.** A primary concern after valve replacement is the need to maintain LV performance. Once the valve is in place, the LV has to eject a full-stroke volume into the aorta without the protection of a low-pressure popoff into the left atrium. The result is an increase in LV wall tension that can compromise ejection fraction. Therefore, **in the postbypass period, LV performance frequently must be augmented using intraaortic balloon**

counterpulsation or inotropic support until the LV can adjust to the new hemodynamic state. After valve replacement, left atrial and pulmonary arterial pressures should decrease. Patients with long-standing mitral regurgitation will continue to need elevated left atrial pressure for maintenance of adequate forward flow. Immediately after weaning from cardiopulmonary bypass, patients who have been in chronic atrial fibrillation occasionally may revert to a sinus rhythm for a short period. An attempt should be made to keep the patient in sinus rhythm by using overdrive atrial pacing and treatment with procainamide or amiodarone.

VI. Tricuspid stenosis

A. Natural history

1. **Etiology.** The primary cause of acquired tricuspid stenosis is **rheumatic valvulitis.** Other causes of tricuspid stenosis include **systemic lupus erythematosus, endomyocardial fibroelastosis,** and **carcinoid syndrome.**

2. **Symptomatology.** Isolated tricuspid stenosis is manifest by the signs and symptoms of right-sided heart failure, including hepatomegaly, hepatic dysfunction, ascites, edema, and jugular venous distention with giant A waves visible on the central venous pressure recording. As stenosis progresses, cardiac output may be limited, at least during exercise. However, patients with tricuspid stenosis frequently have associated mitral stenosis, which is the primary cause of symptomatology and clinical deterioration.

B. Pathophysiology

1. **Natural progression.** The tricuspid valve area normally is 7 to 9 cm^2 in the typical adult. Significant impairment to forward blood flow does not occur until the valve orifice decreases to less than 1.5 cm^2. Therefore, there is a long asymptomatic period as stenosis develops. With progression of the stenosis, right atrial pressure increases and forward blood flow decreases. Preservation of sinus rhythm is important for maintaining flow across the tricuspid valve, and rapid clinical deterioration can occur if the sinus rhythm is lost.

2. **Calculation of severity.** Normally the gradient across the tricuspid valve is only 1 mm Hg. A mean gradient of 3 mm Hg across the tricuspid valve indicates significant tricuspid stenosis and usually corresponds to a valve area of 1.5 cm^2. A gradient of 5 mm Hg across the tricuspid valve indicates severe stenosis and corresponds to a valve area of 1.0 cm^2.

C. Goals of perioperative management

1. **Hemodynamic management**

	RV preload	Heart rate	Contractile state	Systemic vascular resistance	Pulmonary vascular resistance
Tricuspid stenosis	↑	↓ Maintain	Maintain	↑	Maintain

a. **RV preload.** Adequate forward flow of blood across the stenotic tricuspid valve depends on maintenance of adequate preload.

b. **Heart rate.** Patients with tricuspid stenosis depend on maintenance of sinus rhythm. **Supraventricular tachyarrhythmias can cause rapid clinical deterioration and should be controlled with either immediate cardioversion or pharmacologic intervention.** At the same time, bradycardia can be harmful because it reduces total forward flow.

c. **Contractility.** RV filling is impeded by tricuspid stenosis. Adequate cardiac output is maintained by an increase in RV contractility. A sudden depression in ventricular contractility can severely limit cardiac output and elevate right atrial pressure.

d. **Systemic vascular resistance. Changes in systemic afterload have little effect** on the hemodynamic state of patients with tricuspid stenosis unless there is associated mitral valve involvement, particularly mitral regurgitation. However, systemic vasodilatation may lead to hypotension in patients with limited blood flow across the tricuspid valve.

   e. Pulmonary vascular resistance. Because the limitation to forward flow is at the tricuspid valve, reducing pulmonary vascular resistance has little positive effect on improving forward flow. Keeping pulmonary vascular resistance in the normal range is adequate.

2. Anesthetic technique

   a. Extensive preoperative preparation—including salt restriction, digitalization, and diuretics—may reduce hepatic congestion, improve hepatic function, and reduce surgical risks.

   b. In patients with coexisting mitral valve disease, anesthetic technique is determined by the mitral valve lesion, as previously described. In patients with isolated tricuspid stenosis, the need to maintain high preload, high afterload, and adequate contractility favors the use of a narcotic-based anesthetic technique.

   c. Passage of a pulmonary artery catheter through the stenotic tricuspid valve may be impossible, and the catheter will have to be removed during bypass even if it can be placed. Therefore, use of a central venous pressure catheter, with surgical placement of a left atrial catheter and possibly a surgically placed pulmonary artery thermistor for cardiac output determination, may represent the best possible monitoring in this setting. Alternatively, a Swan–Ganz catheter placed into the superior vena cava until after bypass and then floated into the pulmonary artery is another approach.

3. Surgical intervention. Commissurotomy of the tricuspid valve is commonly the procedure of choice. However, in cases of extensive calcification, valve replacement with a low-profile prosthetic valve may be necessary. In the postcardiopulmonary bypass period, preload augmentation must be continued.

VII. Tricuspid regurgitation

A. Natural history. Isolated tricuspid regurgitation most frequently is seen in association with drug abuse, endocarditis, or chest trauma. More commonly, tricuspid regurgitation is associated with other cardiac abnormalities, such as end-stage aortic or mitral valve disease, most often mitral stenosis. With severe aortic or mitral valve disease, elevated pulmonary artery pressure leads to RV strain and, eventually, RV failure with tricuspid regurgitation. Carcinoid syndrome may produce isolated tricuspid regurgitation. The primary congenital cause of tricuspid regurgitation is Ebstein anomaly.

B. Pathophysiology

   1. Natural progression. Isolated tricuspid regurgitation is well tolerated because the RV can compensate for volume overload. On the other hand, a pressure load is not well tolerated by the RV. Most symptoms associated with tricuspid regurgitation are directly related to an increased RV afterload. Therefore, when tricuspid regurgitation is associated with pulmonary vascular hypertension, the impedance to RV ejection produces significant clinical deterioration from decreased cardiac output. Most patients with tricuspid regurgitation have associated atrial fibrillation due to distention of the right atrium.

   2. Pressure wave abnormalities. Central venous pressure tracings may show the presence of **giant V waves.** However, as with mitral regurgitation, the compliance of the right atrium, filling of the right atrium, and regurgitant volume each helps to determine the size of the regurgitant wave.

C. Goals of perioperative management

   1. Hemodynamic management

	RV preload	Heart rate	Contractile state	Systemic vascular resistance	Pulmonary vascular resistance
Tricuspid Regurgitation	↑	↑ Maintain	Maintain	Maintain	↓

      a. RV preload. To provide adequate forward flow, **preload augmentation** is desirable. A drop in central venous pressure can severely limit RV stroke volume.

      b. Heart rate. Normal to high heart rates are beneficial in these patients to sustain forward flow and prevent peripheral congestion. Most of these patients are in **chronic atrial fibrillation,** so maintenance of a sinus mechanism is rarely possible.

      c. Contractility. RV failure is the primary cause of clinical deterioration in patients with tricuspid regurgitation. Because the RV is designed geometrically to accommodate volume but not pressure loads, it may require perioperative inotropic support, especially in the setting of positive-pressure ventilation or elevated pulmonary vascular resistance. Any suppression of contractility with myocardial depressants may induce severe RV failure.

      d. Systemic vascular resistance. Variations in systemic afterload have **little effect** on tricuspid regurgitation unless there is concurrent aortic or mitral valve dysfunction.

      e. Pulmonary vascular resistance. Because the RV does not tolerate pressure loads, RV function and forward blood flow are improved with decreases in pulmonary vascular resistance. **Hyperventilation is helpful** in reducing pulmonary vascular resistance by producing hypocapnia. However, **high airway pressures during pulmonary ventilation and agents such as nitrous oxide that can increase pulmonary arterial pressure should be avoided. If inotropic support is necessary, dobutamine, isoproterenol, or milrinone, which dilate the pulmonary vasculature, should be used.** Inhalation of nitric oxide may have an important role in selectively reducing pulmonary vascular resistance in these patients.

   2. Surgical intervention. Many patients can be treated successfully with tricuspid valvular plication or annuloplasty. If the valve has deteriorated, valve replacement may be necessary. If a prosthetic valve is placed, residual tricuspid stenosis will occur because the valve prosthesis is smaller than the native valve, and postbypass preload augmentation will be necessary. In addition, in the immediate postbypass period, the RV will be under increased strain because the entire stroke volume will have to be ejected against the higher pulmonary vascular resistance, with no popoff pressure lowering back into the right atrium. Therefore, RV failure requiring inotropic support may occur.

VIII. Pulmonic stenosis
A. Natural history
   1. Etiology. Pulmonic stenosis may be valvular, infundibular, or located in a pulmonary arterial branch (distal pulmonary artery). Nearly all cases of pulmonic stenosis are congenital, although rarely rheumatic heart disease can lead to pulmonic stenosis.

   2. Symptomatology. Patients with pulmonic stenosis may live for extended periods completely without symptoms and frequently survive past the age of 70 years without surgical intervention. Symptoms, when they do occur, include tachypnea, syncope, angina, or hepatomegaly and peripheral edema. Intervening bacterial endocarditis or RV failure due to severe stenosis may lead to death.

B. Pathophysiology
   1. Natural progression. The normal pressure gradient across the pulmonic valve orifice usually is between 5 and 10 mm Hg. The diagnosis of pulmonic stenosis can be made when the gradient across the pulmonic valve reaches 15 mm Hg and RV systolic pressure reaches 30 mm Hg in the absence of an intracardiac shunt. Stenosis of the valve of more than 60% can occur before any significant obstruction to flow is generated. A peak systolic gradient of 50 mm Hg or less is considered mild pulmonic stenosis, between 50 and 100 mm Hg is considered moderate stenosis, and more than 100 mm Hg is considered severe pulmonic stenosis. As the pulmonic stenosis progresses from mild to moderate, concentric hypertrophy of the RV occurs. The increased hypertrophy

and pressure within the RV lead to a situation in which RV subendocardial blood flow no longer occurs throughout the cardiac cycle but only during diastole, similar to the LV. **Coronary perfusion pressure must be maintained to provide an adequate RV subendocardial coronary blood supply.**

  2. **Pressure wave abnormalities**
      a. **Pulmonary arterial pressure trace.** The pulmonary artery pressure upstroke is delayed, and there is a late systolic peak owing to impedance of blood flow through the stenotic pulmonary valve.
      b. **Central venous pressure trace.** A prominent A wave frequently is found in the central venous pressure trace.

C. **Goals of perioperative management**
  1. **Hemodynamic management**

	RV preload	Heart rate	Contractile state	Systemic vascular resistance	Pulmonary vascular resistance
Pulmonic stenosis	↑	↑	Maintain	Maintain	↓ Maintain

  a. **RV preload. RV performance depends on adequate preload** for the RV. Decreases in central venous pressure will lead to inadequate filling of the RV and decreased RV stroke volume.
  b. **Heart rate.** As pulmonic stenosis progresses, the patient becomes increasingly dependent on **atrial contraction** to provide adequate RV filling. Unfortunately, in severe pulmonic stenosis, tricuspid regurgitation can develop, leading to right atrial distention and atrial fibrillation. Because blood flow across the stenotic pulmonary valve occurs primarily during ventricular systole, **increases in heart rate usually provide increased flow.** Rarely, RV hypertrophy in combination with angina symptoms dictates the need for a slower heart rate to allow adequate time in diastole for subendocardial coronary blood flow.
  c. **Contractility.** With severe pulmonic stenosis, the RV **hypertrophies** in response to the pressure load. Depression of the contractile state can lead to RV failure and clinical deterioration. Pharmacologic intervention that depresses RV function should be avoided.
  d. **Systemic vascular resistance. Afterload should be maintained to provide adequate coronary perfusion to the hypertrophied RV.**
  e. **Pulmonary vascular resistance.** Because the primary impedance to forward flow is the pulmonic valve, reducing pulmonary vascular resistance will do little to enhance forward blood flow. However, especially in patients with mild or moderate pulmonary stenosis, major increases in pulmonary vascular resistance potentially can harm forward blood flow and lead to RV dysfunction. Therefore, **pulmonary vascular resistance should be kept in the low-to-normal range.**
  2. **Surgical intervention.** Any patient who develops significant symptomatology, a peak systolic gradient across the pulmonic valve of more than 80 mm Hg, or a peak systolic RV pressure of 100 mm Hg should have surgical intervention. Normally, valvulotomy is all that is necessary. Rarely, the pulmonic valve must be replaced. An attractive alternative to open heart surgery is the use of transluminal balloon angioplasty, which frequently is used for congenital pulmonic valvular stenosis.

IX. **Mixed valvular lesions.** For all mixed valvular lesions, management decisions emphasize the most severe or the most hemodynamically significant lesion.
  A. **Aortic stenosis and mitral stenosis.** Pathophysiologically, the progression of the disease follows a course similar to that seen in patients with pure mitral stenosis with development of pulmonary hypertension and, eventually, RV failure. Symptomatology is primarily referable to the pulmonary circuit, including dyspnea,

hemoptysis, and atrial fibrillation. This combination of valvular heart disease may lead to underestimation of the severity of the aortic stenosis because the aortic valve gradient may be relatively low because of low aortic valvular flow. Such a combination of lesions can be extremely serious because of the **limitations of blood flow at two points.**

    1. Hemodynamic management

	LV preload	Heart rate	Contractile state	Systemic vascular resistance	Pulmonary vascular resistance
Mitral stenosis alone	↑	↓	Maintain	↑	↓
Aortic stenosis alone	↑	↓	Maintain	↑	Maintain
Typical management for combined lesion	↑	↓	Maintain	↑	↓

        a. The best hemodynamic management for a patient with both aortic and mitral stenosis includes **preload augmentation, normal-to-low heart rates, and preservation of contractility.** Due to the high risk of decreased coronary perfusion, systemic vascular resistance must be increased whenever the diastolic perfusion pressure falls. All agents or conditions that might augment pulmonary vascular resistance must be aggressively avoided. Pco_2 should be maintained in the low-to-normal range, and a high inspired O_2 concentration should be supplied to minimize pulmonary vasoconstriction.

    B. Aortic stenosis and mitral regurgitation. This combination is relatively rare but should be suspected in patients with aortic stenosis who also have left atrial enlargement with atrial fibrillation. Mitral regurgitation can be exacerbated by LV dysfunction due to severe aortic stenosis. In this situation, the mitral valve does not require replacement, and the mitral regurgitation regresses after the aortic valve is replaced.

        1. Hemodynamic management

	LV preload	Heart rate	Contractile state	Systemic vascular resistance	Pulmonary vascular resistance
Aortic stenosis alone	↑	↓	Maintain	↑	Maintain
Mitral regurgitation alone	↑,↓	↑	Maintain	↓	↓
Typical management for combined lesion	↑	Maintain	Maintain	Maintain	↓

    In managing these patients, the hemodynamic requirements for aortic stenosis and mitral regurgitation are contradictory. **Because aortic stenosis most frequently will lead these patients into deadly intraoperative situations, it should be given priority when managing the hemodynamic variables.**

    Preload augmentation normally is beneficial and, for coronary perfusion, maintenance of at least normal afterload is desirable. Obviously, increased systemic vascular resistance may hurt forward flow, but the stenotic aortic valve provides the primary impedance to forward flow no matter what the systemic vascular resistance is. Heart rate should be kept at least in the normal range, and tachycardia should be avoided at all costs. Contractility should not be depressed, and conditions or pharmacologic agents that increase pulmonary vascular resistance should be avoided.

C. Aortic stenosis and aortic regurgitation. The combination of aortic regurgitation and aortic stenosis is not well tolerated because it provides the LV with both severe pressure and volume overloading. These stresses lead to major increases in myocardial O_2 consumption (Mvo_2) and, as might be expected, angina pectoris is an early symptom with this combination. Once symptomatology develops, the prognosis is similar to that of pure aortic stenosis.

   1. Hemodynamic management

	LV preload	Heart rate	Contractile state	Systemic vascular resistance	Pulmonary vascular resistance
Aortic stenosis alone	↑	↓	Maintain	↑	Maintain
Aortic regurgitation alone	↑	↑	Maintain	↓	Maintain
Typical management for combined lesion	↑	Maintain	Maintain	Maintain	Maintain

     Normally, augmentation of preload is beneficial for both aortic stenosis and aortic regurgitation. However, the hemodynamic requirements for afterload and heart rate for these two lesions are contradictory. Generally, **maintaining a hemodynamic profile consistent with aortic stenosis** is logical because compromise of this lesion intraoperatively is potentially more deadly than increasing the aortic regurgitation. Despite the risk of decreasing cardiac output, systemic vascular resistance should be augmented whenever systemic pressures begin falling to preserve coronary blood flow. Maintaining a normal heart rate, contractility, and pulmonary vascular resistance will help stabilize the patient.

D. Aortic regurgitation and mitral regurgitation. The combination of aortic and mitral regurgitation occurs frequently, and this combination can cause rapid clinical deterioration.

   1. Hemodynamic management

	LV preload	Heart rate	Contractile state	Systemic vascular resistance	Pulmonary vascular resistance
Mitral regurgitation alone	↑,↓	↑	Maintain	↓	↓
Aortic regurgitation alone	↑	↑	Maintain	↓	Maintain
Typical management for combined lesion	↑	↑	Maintain	↓	Maintain

     The hemodynamic requirements of aortic regurgitation and mitral regurgitation are similar. The primary problem is providing adequate forward flow and peripheral circulation. The development of acidosis leading to peripheral vasoconstriction and an increased impedance to LV outflow can lead to rapid clinical deterioration. Therefore, keeping the systemic vascular resistance relatively low while maintaining adequate perfusion pressure is the fine clinical balance needed until cardiopulmonary bypass can be initiated.

E. Mitral stenosis and mitral regurgitation. Rheumatic mitral stenosis rarely is pure and commonly exists in conjunction with mitral regurgitation. When dealing with patients with combined mitral stenosis and mitral regurgitation, decisions concerning hemodynamic management must consider which lesion is predominant. As a rule of thumb, **normalization of afterload, heart rate, and contractility,** while avoiding agents or conditions that lead to reactive pulmonary constriction and providing adequate preload, leads to optimal hemodynamic stabilization.

1. Hemodynamic management

	LV preload	Heart rate	Contractile state	Systemic vascular resistance	Pulmonary vascular resistance
Mitral stenosis alone	↑	↓	Maintain	Maintain	↓
Mitral regurgitation alone	↑,↓	↑	Maintain	↓	↓
Typical management for combined lesion	↑	Maintain	Maintain	↓ Maintain	↓

X. Prosthetic cardiac valves. The first successful prosthetic cardiac valve was placed in the descending thoracic aorta in 1952 by Charles Hufnagel in a patient with severe aortic regurgitation. Over the past 50 years, the available prosthetic valves have expanded to include stentless porcine bioprostheses, stented porcine and pericardial bioprostheses, allografts, and a wide range of mechanical prostheses. The decision regarding which prosthetic valve should be used for a particular patient is based upon a variety of factors, including the life expectancy of the patient (mechanical prostheses last longer), the ability of the patient to comply with anticoagulation therapy (mechanical prostheses require ongoing anticoagulation), the anatomy and pathology of the existing valvular disease, and the experience of the operating surgeon [10,11].

A. Essential characteristics of prosthetic heart valves

An ideal prosthetic heart valve is nonthrombogenic, chemically inert, preserves blood elements, and allows physiologic blood flow. The large number of different prosthetic valves that have been developed indicates that no ideal valve has yet been found.

B. Types of prosthetic valves

1. Mechanical. Current mechanical prosthetic valves are durable but thrombogenic. At present, all patients with mechanical prosthetic valves require anticoagulation therapy for the remainder of their lives. Normally, anticoagulation is provided with warfarin sodium, administered at a dose that will elevate the prothrombin time to 1.5 to 2.0 times control. There are four basic types of mechanical prosthetic valves.

a. Caged-ball valve prosthesis (Fig. 12.9). The initial Starr–Edwards caged-ball valve prosthesis had a high rate of thromboembolic phenomena. However, improvements were made to this valve, including covering all metal parts with cloth, to stimulate the growth of surrounding tissue and allow the valve to develop a neointima that decreases thrombus formation.

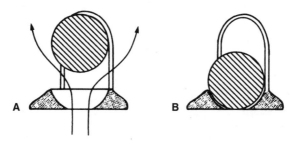

FIG. 12.9 Caged-ball valve prosthesis showing the movement of the ball in the open (**A**) and closed (**B**) positions.

The Starr–Edwards valve has been used in the aortic, mitral, and tricuspid positions. Other valves of this type include the Smeloff–Cutter, Braunwald–Cutter, Magovern–Cromie, and DeBakey–Surgitool. Because these valves are bulky and the most thrombogenic of all current valves, and because the ball tends to interfere with central laminar blood flow, they currently are used very rarely.

b. **Caged-disk valve prostheses** (Fig. 12.10). In an attempt to overcome the obstruction to blood flow presented by a bulky caged-ball valve, especially during cardiac tachyarrhythmias, a caged-disk valve was developed. Because of rapid disk breakdown, which included notching of the disk and even embolization, caged-disk valve prostheses are no longer used clinically. However, the widespread use of these valves in the 1970s has produced a reservoir of patients with these valves in place who still may be encountered. Other caged-disk valve prostheses once used include the Starr–Edwards 6500 series, Kay–Shiley, Cross–Jones, Harken, and Cooley–Bloodwell–Cutter valves.

c. **Monocuspid tilting-disk valve prosthesis** (Fig. 12.11). In an attempt to decrease the postoperative pressure gradient across valves in which a ball or disk occludes the center of the path of blood flow (i.e., caged-ball, caged-disk), the monocuspid, central flow, tilting-disk valve was developed. Although flow characteristics were better than those associated with central occluding valves, thromboembolic complications still occurred even with adequate anticoagulation. Monocuspid tilting-disk valves that may be seen in clinical use at this time are the Sorin Allcarbon (pyrolytic carbon-coated chromium alloy housing with a pyrolytic carbon monoleaflet), Medtronic Hall (titanium housing with pyrolytic carbon leaflet), Omnicarbon (titanium housing with pyrolytic carbon monoleaflet), and Bjork–Shiley Monostrut (cobalt-chromium alloy housing with Pyrolyte carbon monoleaflet).

d. **Bileaflet tilting-disk valve prosthesis** (Fig. 12.12). In 1977, a bileaflet St. Jude cardiac valve was introduced as a low-profile device to allow central blood flow through two semicircular disks that pivot on supporting struts. The St. Jude valve can be placed in the aortic, mitral, or tricuspid positions. These valves produce low resistance to blood flow and have a lower incidence of thromboembolic complications, although anticoagulation still is necessary. Studies indicate little difference in the hemodynamic profiles or outcome after implantation of either the monocuspid Medtronic–Hall or bicuspid St. Jude prosthesis. Bileaflet mechanical valve prostheses that may be seen in clinical use include the St. Jude Medical (pyrolytic carbon-coated graphite housing and Pyrolyte leaflets with tungsten for radiopacity), CarboMedics (solid Pyrolyte housing with pyrolytic carbon-coated graphite and tungsten substrate leaflets), Edwards Tekna (solid pyrolyte housing with pyrolytic carbon-coated graphite and tungsten leaflets), Bicarbon (Pyrolyte-coated titanium alloy housing with pyrolytic carbon-coated graphite and tungsten substrate leaflets), and Advancing the Standard (Pyrolyte housing with pyrolytic carbon-coated graphite substrate leaflets).

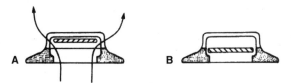

FIG. 12.10 Caged-disk valve prosthesis showing the disk in the open (**A**) and closed (**B**) positions.

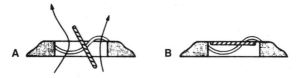

FIG. 12.11 Monocuspid tilting-disk valve prosthesis showing the disk in the open (**A**) and closed (**B**) positions.

2. **Bioprosthetic valves.** Bioprosthetic valves fall into two classifications: stented and nonstented. The Hancock porcine aortic bioprosthesis was introduced in 1970, followed by the Ionescu–Shiley bovine pericardial prosthesis in 1974 and the Carpentier–Edwards porcine aortic valve bioprosthesis in 1975. In contrast to modern mechanical prostheses, current bioprostheses are less durable but much less thrombogenic. Long-term anticoagulation for a bioprosthesis placed in the aortic position usually is unnecessary, although aspirin, dipyridamole, or other antiplatelet drugs often are used. Unfortunately, bioprostheses placed in the mitral position still place patients at risk for thromboembolism and require warfarin anticoagulation.

The overall 11-year outcomes for patients receiving mechanical prostheses and bioprostheses were found to be similar, leading to the recommendation that bioprostheses be used in patients older than 60 years who are undergoing aortic valve replacement because of the higher risk of bleeding and lower risk of mechanical valve failure during the remaining life span of these patients. In contrast, mechanical prostheses should be used in patients from ages 35 to 60 years and in those undergoing mitral valve replacement because of the greater risk of structural failure of the bioprosthesis in the mitral position and the higher likelihood that younger patients will outlive their bioprostheses. Because of the teratogenic effects of warfarin, young women who desire to become pregnant should receive a bioprosthesis.

a. **Stented bioprostheses.** Bioprostheses constructed from porcine aortic valves or bovine pericardium are placed on a polypropylene stent attached to a silicone sewing ring covered with Dacron. These valves allow for improved central annular flow and less turbulence, but the stent does cause some obstruction to forward flow, thereby leading to a residual pressure gradient across the valve.

Calcification of the bioprosthesis is a major long-term problem with porcine valves, which appear to calcify at the commissures, whereas bovine pericardial valves calcify at the regions of flexion.

Stented valves that can be found in clinical use today include the Carpentier–Edwards Supra-annular Porcine, the Hancock II Porcine,

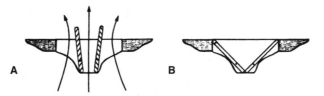

FIG. 12.12 Bileaflet tilting-disk valve prosthesis showing disks in the open (**A**) and closed (**B**) positions.

Medtronic Intact Porcine, Medtronic Mosaic Porcine, Hancock Modified Orifice Porcine, Biocor Porcine, St. Jude Medical Bioimplant Porcine, St. Jude Medical X-Cell Porcine, Carpentier–Edwards Pericardial, Mitroflow Pericardial, Sorin Pericarbon Pericardial, and Pericarbon Pericardial.

   b. **Stentless bioprostheses.** Porcine valves fixed in a pressure-free glutaraldehyde solution but without the use of a stent make up the category of stentless bioprostheses. The primary types of valves clinically encountered in this category include the St. Jude Medical–Toronto SPV Stentless Porcine, Medtronic Freestyle Stentless Porcine, Cryolife Bravo Stentless Porcine, Baxter Prima Stentless Porcine, and Biocor Stentless Porcine.

3. **Human valves.** The first use of a bioprosthesis taken from a cadaver occurred in 1962. However, techniques such as irradiation or chemical treatment used to sterilize and preserve the early homografts for implantation led to a shortened life span. More recently, antibiotic solutions have been used to sterilize human valves, which then are frozen in liquid nitrogen until implantation. Using these techniques, weakness of the prosthesis leading to cusp rupture occurs infrequently, with more than 75% of prostheses lasting for more than 10 years regardless of patient age. The incidence of prosthetic valve endocarditis and hemolysis resulting from blood flow through the homograft is very low. When homografts are used in the aortic position, anticoagulation is not required. However, in the mitral position a somewhat higher incidence of thromboembolism makes the use of anticoagulation somewhat more controversial.

Homografts may be most useful for aortic valve replacement in patients younger than 35 years and in patients with native valve endocarditis. Homografts are contraindicated in diseases associated with progressive dilation of the aortic root, which would stretch the valve prosthesis and lead to early regurgitation, and in patients with poorly controlled hypertension, which would place increased stress on valve leaflets.

XI. Prophylaxis of subacute bacterial endocarditis. Prosthetic heart valves, as well as abnormal native valves, provide a nidus for infection. They are not as well protected by the body's immune defenses as are normal heart valves. When any invasive procedure puts the patient with valvular heart disease at risk for bacteremia, precautions should be taken to prevent seeding of an abnormal or artificial valve with bacteria that, once present, are very hard to eradicate. Practically, this concern translates into

1. Strict aseptic technique for all procedures performed in patients with valvular heart disease
2. Elimination of existing sources of infection before implantation of a prosthetic valve
3. Antibiotic prophylaxis before, during, and after invasive procedures

Guidelines for antibiotic prophylaxis of patients with valvular heart disease are listed in Table 12.1.

XII. Anticoagulation management

   A. **Chronic management**

Because prosthetic heart valves are constructed of foreign materials, they pose the risk of thrombosis and systemic embolization. The extent of this risk depends on the type of prosthetic valve, its location within the heart, and any other coexisting risk factors for thrombosis. In general, mechanical valves are much more thrombogenic than bioprostheses, and valves in the mitral position are at more risk than those in the aortic position.

Warfarin sodium (Coumadin) is the agent most commonly used to prevent thrombus formation on prosthetic valves on a chronic basis. However, unfractionated heparin, low-molecular-weight heparin, and/or platelet inhibitors such as aspirin are used in special situations.

Controversy still exists regarding the optimal coumadin dose, and the subsequent target international normalized ratio (INR), to use in many situations and the place that antiplatelet agents should have in therapy. The most recent guidelines proposed by the American College of Chest Physicians are listed in Table 12.2.

Table 12.1 Suggested regimens for prevention of bacterial endocarditis in patients with prosthetic cardiac valves (defined as high-risk patients for subacute bacterial endocarditis)

	Agent	Adult dose	Pediatric dose[a]
Dental and upper respiratory tract procedures			
Standard general prophylaxis	Amoxicillin	2 g PO within 1 hr of procedure	50 mg/kg PO
Patients unable to take oral medications	Ampicillin	2.0 g IM or IV within 30 min of procedure	50 mg/kg IM or IV
Penicillin- and amoxicillin-allergic patients	Cephalexin or Cefadroxil[b]	2 g PO within 1 hr of procedure	50 mg/kg PO
	or		
	Clindamycin	600 mg PO within 1 hr of procedure	20 mg/kg PO
	or		
	Azithromycin	500 mg PO within 1 hr of procedure	15 mg/kg PO
	or		
	Clarithromycin		
Penicillin- and amoxicillin-allergic patients unable to take oral medications	Clindamycin	300 mg IV within 30 min of procedure	10 mg/kg
	or		
	Cefazolin[b]	1.0 gm IM or IV within 30 min of procedure	25 mg/kg IM or IV
Genitourinary and gastrointestinal procedures			
Standard general prophylaxis	Ampicillin	2.0 g IM or IV within 30 min of procedure	50 mg/kg
	plus		
	Gentamicin[c]	1.5 mg/kg (not to exceed 120 mg) within 30 min of procedure	1.5 mg/kg
	followed by		
	Amoxicillin	1.0 g PO 6 hr after initial dose	25 mg/kg PO
	or		
Penicillin-allergic patients	Ampicillin	1.0 g IM or IV 6 hr after initial dose	25 mg/kg IM or IV
	Vancomycin[c]	1.0 g IV over 1–2 hr within 30 min of procedure	20 mg/kg
	plus		
	Gentamicin[c]	1.5 mg/kg IM or IV (not to exceed 120 mg) within 30 min of procedure	1.5 mg/kg

[a] Total pediatric dose should not exceed the adult dose.
[b] Cephalosporins should not be used in patients with immediate-type hypersensitivity reaction (urticaria, angioedema, or anaphylaxis) to penicillins.
[c] No second dose of vancomycin or gentamicin is recommended.
IM, intramuscular; IV, intravenous; PO, by mouth.
Adapted from Dajani AS, Taubert KA, Wilson W, et al. Prevention of bacterial endocarditis. *JAMA* 1997;277:1794–1800, with permission.

Table 12.2 Recommendations for chronic anticoagulation management of patients with prosthetic cardiac valves—American College of Chest Physicians

Mechanical heart valves	Bioprosthetic heart valves
1. All patients should receive oral anticoagulants 2. Unfractionated or low-molecular-weight heparin to be used until INR is therapeutic for 2 d 3. Target INR of 2.5 (range 2.0–3.0) for St. Jude Medical bileaflet valve, Carbomedics bileaflet valve, Medtronic-Hall tilting disk valve in aortic position, with normal size atrium and sinus rhythm 4. Target INR of 3.0 (range 2.5–3.5) for tilting disk and bileaflet mechanical mitral valves 5. Target INR of 3.0 (range 2.5–3.5) for bileaflet aortic valves with atrial fibrillation 6. Alternative target INR of 2.5 (range 2.0–3.0) along with aspirin 80–100 mg/d for patients with tilting disk or bileaflet mitral valves or bileaflet aortic valves with atrial fibrillation 7. Target INR of 3.0 (range 2.5–3.5) along with aspirin 80–100 mg/d for patients with caged ball or caged disk valves 8. Target INR of 3.0 (range 2.5–3.5) along with aspirin 80–100 mg/d for patients with mechanical valves and additional risk factors 9. Target INR of 3.0 (range 2.5–3.5) along with aspirin 80–100 mg/d for patients with systemic embolism despite adequate anticoagulant therapy	1. All patients receive oral anticoagulants for the first 3 mo after valve insertion, with a target INR of 2.5 (range 2.0–3.0) 2. Unfractionated or low-molecular-weight heparin to be used until INR is therapeutic for 2 d 3. Aspirin 80 mg/d chronically for patients in sinus rhythm 4. Oral anticoagulants with target INR of 2.5 (range 2.0–3.0) for patients with atrial fibrillation or left atrial thrombus at the time of surgery 5. Oral anticoagulants are optional for patients who also have a permanent pacer (target INR 2.5, range 2.0–3.0) 6. Oral anticoagulants with target INR of 2.5 (range 2.0–3.0) for 3–12 mo for patients with systemic embolism

INR, international normalized ratio.
Adapted from Stein PD, Alpert JS, Bussey HI, et al. Antithrombotic therapy in patients with mechanical and biological prosthetic heart valves. *Chest* 2001;119:220S–227S.

B. Perioperative management

Although there is universal agreement that the presence of a mechanical heart valve requires systemic anticoagulation chronically, there is less agreement about anticoagulation management immediately before and after surgery [12,13]. Kearon and Hirsh [14] reported that the rate of thromboembolism associated with mechanical heart valve, even without therapy, is only an average of eight events per year, or 0.02 events per day. Based on these statistics, and the expense and complications associated with intravenous heparin use, these authors recommend that warfarin be stopped several days before elective surgery in order to allow the INR to drop to 1.5 or lower and then resumed as soon as possible postoperatively, but with no intervening heparin therapy. Other authors suggest the use of heparin therapy when the INR is less then 2.0, at least for patients with prosthetic mitral valves or other risk factors. Recommendations for perioperative management of anticoagulants for patients with mechanical heart valves who are undergoing non-cardiac surgery are listed in Table 12.3.

Table 12.3 Preoperative and postoperative anticoagulation management for noncardiac surgery

For patients with mechanical aortic valves and with no other risk factors:
- Discontinue warfarin 4 d preoperatively
- Perform surgery when INR <1.5
- Resume warfarin as soon as possible postoperatively
- Administer heparin only if INR <2.0 for ≥5 d

For patients with mechanical mitral valves, or aortic valves and other thromboembolic risk factors:
- Discontinue warfarin 4 d preoperatively
- Administer heparin IV, or low-molecular-weight heparin SQ, when INR <2.0
- Discontinue IV heparin 12 hours before surgery, or low-molecular-weight heparin 24 hours before surgery
- Perform surgery when INR <1.5
- Resume warfarin and heparin as soon as possible postoperatively
- Discontinue heparin when INR ≥2.0

INR, international normalized ratio; IV, intravenous; SQ, subcutaneous.
Adapted from Teide DJ, Nishimura RA, Gastineau DA, et al. Modern management of prosthetic valve anticoagulation. *Mayo Clin Proc* 1998;73:665–680.

References

1. **Jackson JM, Thomas SJ. Valvular heart disease. In: Kaplan JA, Reich DL, Konstadt SN, eds. *Cardiac anesthesia*, 4th ed. Philadelphia: WB Saunders, 1999:727–785.**
2. **Jackson JM, Thomas SJ, Lowenstein E. Anesthetic management of patients with valvular heart disease. *Semin Anesth* 1982;1:239–252.**
3. Gorlin R, McMillan IKR, Medd WE, et al. Dynamics of the circulation in aortic valvular disease. *Am J Med* 1955;18:855–870.
4. Goertz AW, Lindner KH, Schutz W, et al. Influence of phenylephrine bolus administration on left ventricular filling dynamics in patients with coronary artery disease and patients with valvular aortic stenosis. *Anesthesiology* 1994;81:49–58.
5. Yang SS, Bentivoglia LG, Maranhao V, et al. Assessment of valvular regurgitation. In: Yang SS, Bentivoglia LG, Maranhao V, et al., eds. *From cardiac catheterization data to hemodynamic parameters,* 2nd ed. Philadelphia: FA Davis, 1988:152–165.
6. Howie MB, Black HA, Romanelli VA, et al. A comparison of isoflurane versus fentanyl as primary anesthetics for mitral valve surgery. *Anesth Analg* 1996;83:941–948.
7. Fuchs RM, Heuser RR, Yin FCP, et al. Limitations of pulmonary wedge V waves in diagnosing mitral regurgitation. *Am J Cardiol* 1982;49:849–854.
8. Moore RA, Neary M, Gallagher J, et al. Determination of pulmonary capillary wedge position in patients with giant v-waves. *J Cardiothorac Anesth* 1987;1:108–113.
9. Butterworth JF, Legault C, Royster RL, et al. Factors that predict the use of positive inotropic drug support after cardiac valve surgery. *Anesth Analg* 1998;86:461–467.
10. **Edmunds L. Evolution of prosthetic heart valves. *Am Heart J* 2001;141:849–855.**
11. Birkmeyer NJ, Birkmeyer JD, Tosteson AN, et al. Prosthetic valve type for patients undergoing aortic valve replacement: a decision analysis. *Ann Thorac Surg* 2000;70:1946–1952.
12. Tiede DJ, Nishimura RA, Gastineau DA, et al. Modern management of prosthetic valve anticoagulation. *Mayo Clin Proc* 1998;73:665–680.
13. **Stein PD, Alpert JS, Bussey HI, et al. Antithrombotic therapy in patients with mechanical and biological prosthetic heart valves. *Chest* 2001;119:220S–227S.**
14. **Kearon C, Hirsh J. Management of anticoagulation before and after elective surgery. *N Engl J Med* 1997;336:1506–1511.**

13. ALTERNATIVE APPROACHES TO CARDIAC SURGERY WITH AND WITHOUT CARDIOPULMONARY BYPASS

James G. Ramsay, Michael G. Licina, Hamdy Awad, Charles J. Hearn, Lee K. Wallace, and Randall K. Wolf

The last 10 years have witnessed a major evolution in cardiac surgery in parallel with "minimally invasive" and laparoscopic developments in other surgical fields [1]. Two major objectives have been a reduction in the use of cardiopulmonary bypass (CPB) for revascularization and a reduction in the invasiveness of the surgical approach. The overall goals are to preserve and enhance the quality of the procedure(s) while providing faster recovery, reduced procedural costs, and reduced morbidity and mortality. The anesthesia care team facilitates cost-effective early recovery while providing safe, excellent operating conditions both for the patient and the surgeon. Anesthetic techniques and monitoring modalities have evolved with changes in surgical practice. Anesthesiologists have learned more about how to support the circulation during cardiac manipulation and periods of coronary occlusion. We have been charged with providing monitoring and support while the surgeon operates with minimal exposure while at the same time facilitating early recovery and discharge. Surgical techniques and their anesthetic considerations discussed in this chapter include coronary artery bypass grafting (CABG) without the use of CPB [off-pump CABG (OPCAB) and minimally invasive direct coronary artery bypass (MIDCAB)]; minimally invasive valve surgery (MIVS); computer-enhanced, endoscopic robotic-controlled CABG; and transmyocardial laser revascularization (TMLR), as an alternative revascularization technique.

I. **Off-pump coronary artery bypass and minimally invasive direct coronary artery bypass**
   A. **Historical perspective**
      1. **Early revascularization surgery**
         a. Early attempts at coronary artery surgery without the use of CPB included the Vineberg procedure in Canada [tunneling the internal mammary artery (IMA) into the ischemic myocardium] in the 1950s and internal mammary to coronary anastomosis in the 1960s by Kolessov in Russia.
         b. Sabiston in the United States and Favolaro from South America reported use of the saphenous vein for aorta-to-coronary artery bypass grafts (CABG), performed without CPB, in the same period.
         c. Introduction of CABG in the late 1960s expanded the indications for CPB, which had enabled congenital heart repairs and heart valve surgery since the 1950s. CPB with use of cardioplegia became the standard of care in the 1970s, providing a motionless field and myocardial "protection" with asystole and hypothermia.
      2. **Reports in the early 1990s**
         a. South American surgeons with limited resources continued to develop techniques for surgery without CPB, publishing in North American journals in the 1980s and early 1990s. In 1991, Benetti et al. [2] reported on 700 CABG procedures without CPB performed over a 12-year period with very low morbidity and mortality.
         b. North American and European interest grew in the 1990s, fueled by a desire to make surgery more appealing (vs. angioplasty) as well as the need to reduce cost and length of stay. Alternative incisions were explored, and techniques and devices to facilitate surgery on the beating heart were developed. The terms "OPCAB" and "MIDCAB" were coined.
      3. **Port-access cardiac surgery**
         a. Simultaneous with attempts to perform CABG without CPB, a group from Stanford University introduced a technique permitting surgery to be done with endoscopic instrumentation through small (1 to 2 cm) ports and a small thoracotomy incision. This is termed port-access surgery or the trade name of Heartport (Johnson and Johnson, Inc., New Brunswick, NJ, U.S.A.). A motionless surgical field was required, necessitating CPB. Extensive use of transesophageal echocardiography (TEE) is required to assist in placement and to monitor the position of the various cannulas.
         b. Heartport contributed new knowledge in two major areas: percutaneous endovascular instrumentation for CPB and instrumentation for performing surgery through the small thoracotomy incision. The latter techniques continue to develop to permit "minimally invasive" valve surgery through partial sternotomy or thoracotomy incisions.

    4. MIDCAB. A number of **alternative incisions** to midline sternotomy have facilitated access to specific coronary artery distributions to allow CABG without CPB. **The most popular and sustaining approach is a left anterior thoracotomy to allow left IMA harvest and grafting to the left anterior descending (LAD) artery territory. This is the procedure usually referred to as MIDCAB.**

    5. North American/European experience after 1998

        a. Initially viewed by most as experimental, off-pump techniques now are established as an acceptable alternative to CABG with CPB. Approximately 10% to 20% of all CABG surgeries are performed using these techniques; however, the range in practice is wide. Some surgeons perform virtually all revascularizations as OPCAB. Most large cardiac surgery practices have at least one surgeon who performs a significant number of off-pump procedures.

        b. MIDCAB procedures are more technically demanding because they require specialized instrumentation and operating through a small incision. These procedures are performed in a smaller number of institutions than are OPCAB procedures.

B. Rationale for avoiding sternotomy and CPB for coronary artery surgery

    1. Reduction in complications

        a. A change in surgical practice should provide better or equivalent results at a reduced cost. When OPCAB and MIDCAB procedures are performed by experienced surgeons using modern epicardial stabilizer techniques, short-term vessel patency appears to be equivalent for OPCAB and on-pump CABG, both for arterial and venous grafts. Limited data currently suggest inferior long-term patency, but these data do not reflect recent improvements in coronary artery stabilizers.

        b. Avoidance of aortic manipulation and cannulation might reduce embolic complications such as stroke. With multivessel OPCAB, a partial or side-biting aortic clamp may be necessary to perform proximal venous anastomoses. This can be avoided by using the IMA as the only proximal vessel with its origin intact.

        c. MIDCAB and OPCAB reduce the whole-body "inflammatory response" induced by surgery and especially by extracorporeal circulation. This might be expected to reduce fluid requirements and coagulopathy.

        d. Most published reports indicate a reduced need for transfusion. This probably is multifactorial, owing to the lack of hemodilution (avoidance of pump prime), and hypothermia, as well as the lack of blood exposure to extracorporeal surfaces and to high doses of heparin and protamine.

    2. Competition with angioplasty. Refinements in interventional cardiology and reductions in postprocedure restenosis have allowed an ever-increasing population of patients to have coronary lesions treated in the catheterization laboratory. Patients are unlikely to choose surgery if nonsurgical results are nearly equivalent. Evolution of surgical techniques to provide the same (or better) excellent results with less physiologic trespass will be necessary if coronary artery surgery is to survive.

    3. Progress toward truly "minimally invasive" surgery

        a. Avoidance of CPB is of more physiologic importance than avoidance of sternotomy, but it is the postoperative recovery from sternotomy that is foremost in patients' minds. From a patient's perspective, the smaller the surgical scar, the better. MIDCAB addresses this issue, but this can only access LAD coronary artery distribution.

        b. Endoscopic techniques have been slow to be adopted in cardiac surgery, partly because until recently existing technology did not provide the range of motion/control required for vascular anastomoses.

        c. Heartport represented the first published use of endoscopic techniques. Surgeons now are working with computer-assisted instruments to perform surgery on the beating heart (see following). Techniques developed for off-pump surgery are likely to contribute to the ability to perform such procedures endoscopically.

C. Refinement of the surgical approach
   1. Development of modern epicardial stabilizers
      a. In early reports, compressive devices (e.g., metal extensions rigidly attached to the sternal retractor) were used to reduce the motion of the coronary vessel during the cardiac and respiratory cycles. These devices often interfered with cardiac function and were impossible to use for circumflex-distribution lesions.
      b. Modern devices typically apply gentle pressure or epicardial suction, reducing the effect on myocardial function yet providing greater fixation in space. These devices also allow greater flexibility in accessing vessels on the inferior and posterior surfaces of the heart (Fig. 13.1).
   2. Techniques to position the heart (through midline sternotomy)
      a. Surgery on the anterior wall of the heart (LAD and diagonal branches) usually requires only mild repositioning, such as a laparotomy pad under the cardiac apex. This has minimal impact on cardiac function.
      b. Surgery on the right coronary artery or left circumflex coronary artery marginal branches requires turning or twisting of the heart. If done manually (i.e., by an assistant), this is cumbersome and often induces hemodynamic compromise. Use of posterior pericardial stitches and a gentle retracting "sock" (web roll wrapped around the apex in a "sling" to pull the heart to either side) greatly facilitates hemodynamic tolerance of these abnormal positions.
      c. For circumflex vessel distribution surgery, dissection of the right pericardium to prevent the right ventricle from being compressed as it is being turned allows preservation of function.

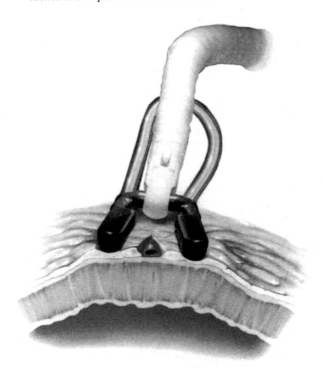

FIG. 13.1 The Octopus 2 tissue stabilizer (Medtronic Inc., Minneapolis, MN, U.S.A.). Through gentle suction the device elevates and pulls the tissue taut, thereby immobilizing the target area. (Courtesy of Medtronic Inc.)

3. Surgical adjuncts to reduce ischemia

   a. Performing CABG surgery on the beating heart requires a mandatory period of coronary occlusion for each distal anastomosis.

   b. Intracoronary shunts can maintain coronary flow at the possible cost of trauma to the endothelium.

   c. "Ischemic preconditioning" involves a brief (e.g., one to four 5-minute periods) occlusion followed by a generally equivalent period of reperfusion before performing the anastomosis. In animal models of myocardial infarction, this technique reduces the area of necrosis. An equivalent physiologic effect can be provided by 1 MAC end-tidal isoflurane [3]. A single 5-minute period of preconditioning preceding OPCAB or MIDCAB probably does not provide the same benefit as that seen in animal models using more periods of occlusion, but this technique is used by some surgeons.

   d. Perfusion-assisted direct coronary artery bypass (PADCAB) allows immediate perfusion of a vein graft once the distal anastomosis is performed. This preserves the usual practice of performing distal coronary artery anastomoses first, then performing proximal aortic vein graft anastomoses with the heart in its physiologic position. To accomplish this technique, a small arterial cannula is placed in the aorta or femoral artery and blood is withdrawn passively, then pumped at the desired flow and pressure into the vein graft [4].

   e. The proximal anastomosis of a vein graft can be performed first in order to allow immediate perfusion once the distal anastomosis is completed.

   f. Regional hypothermia techniques have been described for use during coronary artery occlusion.

   g. Preoperative insertion of an intraaortic balloon pump (IABP) has been used for patients with reduced ventricular function who require multivessel OPCAB.

D. Patient selection

   1. High risk versus low risk

   a. Early reports of OPCAB often described single-vessel or double-vessel bypass performed on low-risk patients. This was promoted as permitting early recovery and discharge. MIDCAB is performed by some surgeons for disease that is limited to the LAD distribution and can be accessed through a small thoracotomy.

   b. OPCAB now is promoted for multivessel bypass in patients at high risk for adverse outcomes. Elderly patients at risk for stroke, patients with severe lung disease, or patients with severe vascular disease and/or renal dysfunction often are selected. Prospective randomized studies have not yet demonstrated reduced adverse outcomes with OPCAB in these populations.

   c. Zenati et al. [5] have described combining MIDCAB (i.e., IMA to LAD) with angioplasty/stent to other vessels in high-risk patients.

   d. As mentioned earlier, a small number of surgeons attempt to perform virtually all CABG procedures as OPCAB regardless of preoperative risk status.

E. Anesthetic management

   1. Preoperative assessment

   a. The cardiac catheterization report should be reviewed and then discussed with the surgeon. This allows the anesthesiologist to predict the effect of each coronary occlusion and to discuss the planned sequence of grafting with the surgeon as well as the potential for use of specific adjuncts (e.g., shunts, PADCAB). This requires knowledge of the coronary anatomy and its usual nomenclature (Fig. 13.2).

   b. The vessel, location, and degree of stenosis determine the functional response to intraoperative coronary occlusion. Even with a proximal stenosis, an important vessel (e.g., LAD) may supply adequate resting flow to a large area of myocardium. Acute loss of flow to this large area (with surgical occlusion) may cause ventricular failure. A stenosis further down the vessel may be less important to overall ventricular performance.

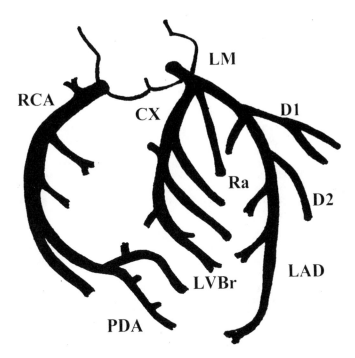

FIG. 13.2 Coronary anatomy. The main branches from the circumflex artery (*CX*) are named "marginal" or "obtuse marginal" vessels. *D1,* first diagonal; *D2,* second diagonal; *LAD,* left anterior descending artery; *LM,* left main; *PDA,* posterior descending artery; *RCA,* right coronary artery; *LVBr,* left ventricular branch; *Ra,* Ramus intermedius (<40% of individuals).

    c. High-grade stenosis (e.g., 90%) is likely to be associated with some collateral blood flow from adjacent regions, as flow through the stenosis may be inadequate even at rest. A 10-minute occlusion of such a vessel may have surprisingly little effect on regional function and hemodynamics because of the collateral flow. A lesser degree of stenosis (e.g., 75% to 80%) may not affect resting flow; hence, there may be little or no collateral blood flow. Occlusion of such a vessel may cause severe myocardial dysfunction in the distribution of that vessel.

    d. If incisions other than sternotomy are to be used to access specific coronary regions, positioning of the arms and the body, the potential need for one-lung anesthesia, and the sites for vascular access need to be discussed.

2. Measures to avoid hypothermia

    a. Unlike on-pump CABG, it is difficult to restore heat to a hypothermic OPCAB patient. In order to maintain hemostasis and facilitate early recovery, **prevention of heat loss needs to be planned before the patient enters the room.**

    b. While in the preoperative area, the patient should be kept warm with blankets.

    c. The operating room should be warmed to the greatest degree tolerated by the operating team. The temperature can be reduced once warming devices have been placed and the patient is fully draped.

    d. The period and degree to which the patient is uncovered for preoperative procedures and surgical skin preparation and draping should be minimized.

This requires vigilance on the part of the anesthesiology team and frequent reminders to the surgical team.

   e. Various adjuncts to preserve heat include heated mattress cover or insert; forced-air warming blankets, including sterile "lower body" blankets placed after vein harvesting; and circumferential heating tubes.

   f. Fluid warmers should be used for all high-volume intravenous infusions.

   g. Low fresh-gas flows with circle/CO_2 reabsorption circuits will help prevent heat loss.

3. Monitoring (Table 13.1)

   a. Preoperative assessment of ventricular function

      (1) One of the determinants of the need for extensive monitoring is preoperative ventricular function. **Patients with normal or near-normal left ventricular function are less likely to need diagnosis and therapy guided by invasive monitoring.**

      (2) A patient with an elevated left ventricular end-diastolic pressure (at cardiac catheterization) may have a "stiff" ventricle, or diastolic dys-

Table 13.1 Monitoring approaches for OPCAB and MIDCAB

Monitor	Advantages	Disadvantages	Comment
ECG	Universal Simple Inexpensive Recognized criteria	Insensitive Position dependent (lead and heart) Incision dependent Loss of V4-5 (MIDCAB)	Best if multilead Should be calibrated ST-segment trending helpful
Central venous pressure	Simple Inexpensive	Insensitive for LV dysfunction No cardiac output	Important for drug infusions Affected by position of heart and patient Use of "introducer" allows rapid insertion of PAC
Pulmonary artery catheter	LV filling pressure Cardiac output Options may be helpful (Svo₂, CCO, pacing)	Expensive Insensitive for acute regional dysfunction Postoperative nuisance	Controversial monitor May prolong ICU stay due to "abnormal numbers"
Transesophageal echocardiography	Gold standard for acute ischemia Verify restoration of function Guide surgical cannula placement	Expensive User dependent Distracting May not have good view of heart	Requires expertise May give false sense of security
Cardiac output (bioimpedance, aortic flow, CO₂ rebreathing)	Less invasive than PAC Can give beat-to-beat flow	Expensive No measure of LV filling May be user dependent	Bioimpedance questionable with open chest Cannot get readings on all patients

CCO, continuous cardiac output; ICU, intensive care unit; LV, left ventricular; MIDCAB, minimally invasive direct coronary artery bypass grafting; OPCAB, off-pump coronary artery bypass grafting; PAC, pulmonary artery catheter; Svo₂, mixed venous oxygen saturation.

function. This commonly is caused by hypertrophy or ischemia. Left ventricular filling pressures obtained intraoperatively must be interpreted in this context. Volumetric assessment of preload (by TEE) may be more valuable in this type of patient.

(3) Patients with poor ventricular function may tolerate coronary occlusions poorly. Appropriate responses may be best guided by monitors of cardiac output and filling pressures or by TEE [6,7].

(4) Repeated occlusions in multiple regions of the myocardium (i.e., for multivessel OPCAB) are likely to result in a cumulative effect. There may be a period of myocardial dysfunction requiring inotropic support, even in patients with good underlying function. The combination of reduced ventricular function and the need for multiple bypass grafts is likely to result in a need for inotropic and/or vasopressor infusions. Such patients are likely to benefit from monitoring with a pulmonary artery catheter (PAC) and/or TEE.

(5) Preoperative placement of a large-bore central venous introducer, but with an obturator of some kind rather than a PAC, may be a reasonable first approach in most patients. This avoids use of the PAC in uncomplicated patients while allowing for rapid PAC placement should this be necessary at any time in the perioperative period.

b. **Specific monitors**

(1) Lead V_5 of the electrocardiogram (ECG) detects 75% of the ischemia found on all 12 leads. This lead should be monitored in all patients undergoing OPCAB or MIDCAB, as permitted by the surgical incision. Lead II gives clear p waves but increases ischemia detection by only 5% to 10%.

(2) The PAC is variably useful during OPCAB. For single- or double-vessel bypass in patients with preserved left ventricular function, there is little need for this monitor. **The worse the ventricular function and the greater the number of planned bypass grafts, the more likely it is that information from the PAC will be useful.**

(3) Continuous cardiac output from the PAC or other devices and continuous mixed venous oximetry may provide incremental benefit in assessing the adequacy of cardiac function, especially in high-risk patients. Use patterns for these devices may be institution specific or even surgeon or anesthesiologist specific.

(4) **Monitoring with TEE can provide detailed information about the effects of coronary occlusion and recovery, and it provides the earliest, most specific information about acute deterioration during interventions.** Development of acute ventricular dilation and mitral regurgitation that may occur when a large region of the myocardium becomes ischemic are detected immediately with this monitor. Obtaining adequate images may be distracting to clinical care. With the heart in an unusual position (e.g., apex up for circumflex marginal artery grafting), images may be difficult or impossible to obtain. A reversible wall-motion abnormality that resolves with restoration of flow is reassuring; however, this does not guarantee a good-quality graft or anastomosis.

(5) Carbon dioxide elimination is dependent on cardiac output. If ventilation is constant, an acute decline in cardiac output will cause an acute decrease in end-tidal carbon dioxide concentration.

c. **Monitoring for specific procedures**

(1) For MIDCAB or other reduced-access procedures, provision must be made for transcutaneous defibrillation and pacing.

(2) For port-access surgery (Heartport or related procedures), TEE is required to guide and monitor cannula placement and function.

4. **Anesthetic technique**

a. **Early recovery usually is desired. Extubation immediately or shortly after surgery should be the goal.**

   b. A vapor-based anesthetic technique facilitates early recovery. Keys to prevention of delayed awakening are avoiding the use of scopolamine, minimizing the dose of benzodiazepines; using modest doses of opioids (or short-acting opioids); and avoiding residual paralysis at the end of surgery. Use of bispectral index (BIS) monitoring can help guide administration of hypnotic agents.

   c. Transfer of the intubated yet awakening patient to the intensive care unit (ICU) and early ICU care are facilitated by use of short-acting sedative drugs such as propofol or dexmedetomidine.

   d. Thoracic epidural or lumbar spinal anesthetic and analgesic techniques have been promoted by some as suitable adjuncts to off-pump approaches. There are reports of OPCAB procedures done without general anesthesia. Most centers are reluctant to risk major neuraxial techniques shortly before full heparinization for CPB, which is a possible occurrence with OPCAB or MIDCAB. Use of such techniques seems unlikely to shorten postoperative length of stay and has not yet been subjected to the rigors of a prospective clinical trial.

   e. For MIDCAB (thoracotomy), postoperative epidural analgesia [8], paravertebral blocks or, intercostal blockade may be useful for pain control.

5. Anticipation and management of ischemia

   a. Knowledge of the coronary anatomy and surgical plan is essential. This allows appropriate timing of pharmacologic and other interventions before ischemia is induced. **Use of isoflurane anesthesia may provide pharmacologic "preconditioning,"** as mentioned earlier. Avoidance of hemodynamic alterations associated with ischemia, such as tachycardia (especially in the presence of hypotension), must be avoided. Intravenous β-adrenergic blockade may be beneficial; however, this must be balanced with the possibility of impaired myocardial performance during coronary occlusion.

   b. Maintenance of adequate coronary perfusion pressure is of great importance in allowing collateral blood flow to ischemic regions. Intravascular volume loading, Trendelenburg position (see below), reduction in the depth of anesthesia, and/or use of α-adrenergic agonists all may be indicated.

   c. Early experience without modern stabilizers suggested bradycardia (to reduce motion) was helpful to the surgeon. This is no longer an issue. Grafting to the right coronary territory (supplying the sinus and atrioventricular nodes) can be associated with bradycardia. Thus, although β-blockade may be useful to treat tachycardia, epicardial pacing may be required for ischemia-induced bradycardia.

6. Intravascular volume loading

   a. Positioning of the heart may kink or partially obstruct venous return and/or compress the right ventricle. Intravascular volume loading and head-down (Trendelenburg) position can help reduce this effect (Fig. 13.3) [9]. Close observation of the heart, filling pressure, and blood pressure to provide feedback to the surgeon is essential.

   b. Intravenous vasodilators (e.g., nitrates) can exacerbate reductions in cardiac filling. More commonly, intravenous vasoconstrictors (phenylephrine or norepinephrine) will be required during abnormal cardiac positions.

7. Surgery–anesthesiology interaction. With all of the above considerations, it should be clear that there must be excellent communication between the surgeon and anesthesiologist for OPCAB or MIDCAB. Anticipation of and planning for problems allow the anesthesiologist to intervene in a timely manner. The surgeon must say in advance what he or she is planning to do. Similarly, changes in cardiac performance and the need for intervention must be communicated continuously to the surgeon. The anesthesiologist must observe the surgical field, watching the procedure as well as the position, size, and function of the heart. An observant, communicative team with basic monitoring (ECG, blood pressure, and central venous pressure) is likely to produce better results than a team that communicates poorly and uses extensive monitoring.

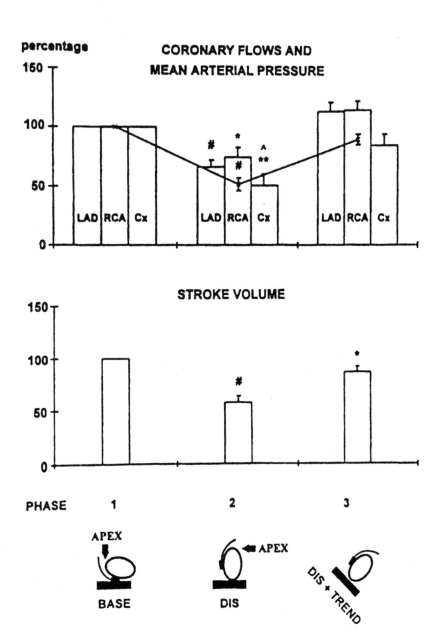

FIG. 13.3 Relative changes in hemodynamic parameters during vertical displacement of the beating porcine heart by the Medtronic Octopus tissue stabilizer and the effect of head-down tilt. *BASE*, pericardial control position; *Cx*, circumflex coronary artery; *DIS*, displacement of the heart by the Octopus; *DIS + TREND*, Trendelenburg maneuver (20-degree head-down tilt while the heart remains retracted 90 degrees); *LAD*, left anterior descending artery; *RCA*, right coronary artery; x = mean arterial pressure. Statistical comparison with control values: *p < 0.05; **p < 0.01; #p < 0.001; ^ p = 0.046 versus combined relative value of LAD and RCA flows. (From Grundeman PF, Borst C, van Herwaarden JA, et al. Vertical displacement of the beating heart by the Octopus tissue stabilizer: influence on coronary flow. *Ann Thorac Surg* 1998;65:1348–1352, with permission.)

F. Anticoagulation
   1. Heparin management
      a. Heparin anticoagulation protocols are institution specific. Similar to on-pump surgery, there are few data that recommend targeting specific activated clotting time (ACT) values.
      b. Some surgeons request full heparinization similar to on-pump procedures (i.e., ACT target greater than 400 seconds); others request lower doses of heparin, such as would be used for other vascular procedures, or some value in between.
      c. If perfusion assistance is used (PADCAB), heparinization to ACT values in excess of 300 seconds is recommended.
   2. Protamine neutralization
      a. Extracorporeal circulation induces a postoperative multifactorial defect in coagulation that may help reduce early graft thrombosis. When coagulation is reversed after OPCAB or MIDCAB, no such hypocoagulable state exists. There is evidence that the coagulation system is activated by the stress of surgery, as has been shown for other major surgical procedures [10].
      b. Rather than attempting to neutralize all of the heparin effect acutely (e.g., 200 mg of protamine), incremental doses often are given. If "full" heparinization has been used, administration of 50 mg of protamine may bring the ACT down to near 200 seconds, after which small increments (10 to 25 mg) can be given to achieve an ACT that is about 25% to 50% above control (i.e., 150 to 180 seconds).
      c. If the patient is clinically bleeding with an elevated ACT, then heparin should be completely neutralized.
      d. Prolonged OPCAB procedures may be associated with extensive blood loss and use of cell salvage devices (i.e., washing of salvaged blood so it is free of coagulation proteins and platelets). Over time, this may induce a coagulopathy similar to that seen after CPB.
   3. Antiplatelet therapy
      a. Platelet aggregation and adhesion initiate thrombosis at the site of vascular anastomoses. As with coronary angioplasty and stent procedures, antiplatelet therapy may reduce early graft thrombosis in CABG, whether done with or without CPB.
      b. Some centers administer a dose of aspirin as a suppository once the patient is anesthetized.
      c. In on-pump CABG, administration of aspirin within 4 hours after the procedure reduces graft thrombosis. This strategy also should be applied to OPCAB and MIDCAB if a preoperative dose is not given.
      d. There are no published data regarding use of newer antiplatelet drugs in this setting. As with all such therapies (including aspirin), the concern about bleeding must be balanced with the desire to prevent graft thrombosis.
   4. Antifibrinolytic therapy
      a. Use of aprotinin and lysine analogues to inhibit fibrinolysis has become common practice with on-pump CABG, as both types of therapy have been shown to reduce perioperative blood loss.
      b. There are no data indicating that clinically significant fibrinolysis is associated with OPCAB or MIDCAB. Thus, there are no data to support prophylactic use of antifibrinolytic drugs if extracorporeal circulation is not used.
      c. Most retrospective studies and the few prospective randomized studies that have been published document a significant reduction in the need for blood products after OPCAB versus on-pump CABG (without the use of antifibrinolytic drugs for the OPCAB procedures).

G. Recovery
   1. Extubation in the operating room
      a. For uncomplicated procedures, recovery from OPCAB or MIDCAB can be rapid without requiring postoperative ventilation/sedation.
      b. Normothermia, hemostasis, and hemodynamic stability must be assured.
      c. Residual anesthesia/paralysis from long-acting agents must be avoided.

    d. Extra time spent in the operating room to achieve extubation may be more costly than a few hours of postoperative ventilation/sedation.

  2. ICU management

    a. For most patients, early postoperative management can use the "fast-track" technique, where mechanical ventilation is withdrawn within 1 to 2 hours of surgery, and patients are mobilized to a chair late in the day or the evening of surgery.

    b. ICU stay is driven by institutional practice, but for patients who are undergoing straightforward, uncomplicated procedures, there may be no indication for more than a few hours in a high-intensity nursing area (i.e., the postanesthetic care unit or the ICU).

  3. Short-term outcome

    a. As mentioned earlier, recent publications report short-term vessel patency as equivalent with on-pump and off-pump techniques [11]. Limited long-term data suggest better patency rates with on-pump techniques, but these data do not yet reflect recent improvements in coronary artery stabilizing devices. Early recurrence of symptoms, quality of life, and event-free survival appear at least equivalent for multivessel OPCAB versus on-pump CABG [12,13].

    b. Most reports indicate reduced transfusion requirements as well as reduced hospital stay for MIDCAB or OPCAB [14]. Results from randomized trials of OPCAB versus on-pump CABG suggest these may be true benefits.

    c. If length of stay is reduced, cost almost certainly will be reduced. If there is no significant reduction in stay, the cost of specialized retractor systems may exceed the disposable costs for CPB.

    d. The anticipated reductions in neurologic events, renal dysfunction, pulmonary complications, dysrhythmias, and other adverse outcomes have not been definitively shown to date.

II. Minimally invasive valve surgery

  A. Introduction. Similar to MIDCAB, the premise of MIVS is that "smaller is better" for valve surgery as well: a partial sternotomy or small thoracotomy with port incisions may achieve some benefits when compared to standard median sternotomy. Similar to OPCAB, alternative approaches were explored in the late 1990s, with the first publication in 1998. Proposed [15,16] but unproved advantages to these approaches include the following:

    1. Reduced hospital length of stay and costs
    2. Quicker return to full activity
    3. Less atrial fibrillation (26% vs. 38% in one report [17])
    4. Fewer blood transfusions
    5. Equivalent functional outcomes (mortality, valve function, quality of life)
    6. Less pain
    7. Earlier ambulation

    In addition, surgeons are of the opinion that reoperation should be easier after MIVS, as the pericardium is not opened over the right ventricular outflow tract. These proposed benefits may be observed with specific surgeons in specific centers; however, there have been no rigorous or randomized studies. The limited data available suggest that pulmonary function is not affected by the use of the limited incision. Because all valve repair or replacement surgeries must be done with CPB, there may be no difference in the systemic inflammatory response between the smaller and larger surgical incisions.

  B. Surgical approaches (Fig. 13.4)

    1. Port access (Heartport) describes direct surgical visualization and operation through small openings (ports) and a small right horizontal thoracotomy incision. In order to avoid sternotomy, the Heartport system uses alternative access sites and cannulas. The aorta is cannulated through a long femoral catheter or a shorter transthoracic catheter. These devices are advanced to the ascending aorta and include an "endoaortic clamp" or inflatable balloon to achieve aortic occlusion ("cross-clamp") from within. They include a

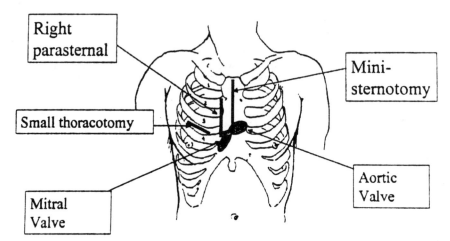

FIG. 13.4 Incisions for minimally invasive valve surgery. The most common approach is the "mini" sternotomy, which extends from the sternal notch part way to the xiphisternum but is diverted to the right at the level of the third or fourth interspace (for the aortic valve), leaving the lower sternum intact. The mitral valve can be accessed through the small right thoracotomy. (From Clements F, Glower DD. Minimally invasive valve surgery. In: Clements F, Shanewise J, eds. *Minimally invasive cardiac and vascular surgical techniques. Society of Cardiovascular Anesthesiologists monograph.* Philadelphia: Lippincott Williams & Wilkins, 2001:30, with permission.)

      cardioplegia administration port. Venous cannulation also is accomplished with a long catheter introduced via the femoral vein, supplemented with a pulmonary artery vent. A coronary sinus catheter is used to administer cardioplegia. Placement of these catheters can be time consuming and requires imaging with fluoroscopy and/or TEE. A limited number of institutions still use this approach to MIVS.

    2. Video-assisted port-assisted (using the Heartport cannulas and small incisions with video equipment to visualize and perform valve surgery). This currently is performed in a small number of institutions worldwide.

    3. Robotic (see below). This technique currently is performed in Europe but is not approved for MIVS in the United States.

    4. Direct-access (small incision—many types: anterior lateral minithoracotomy, partial sternotomy upper or lower, right parasternal, others). The choice of incision depends somewhat upon the heart valve being replaced or repaired. The right parasternal approach is preferred by some surgeons (especially for aortic valve access) because there is no sternal disruption and it is cosmetically pleasing. The avoidance of sternotomy bleeding into the pericardial sac may result in less perioperative bleeding. One associated potential problem is sacrifice of the right IMA.

    5. Reduced length skin incision with full median sternotomy can give a more cosmetic result.

  C. Preoperative assessment. In addition to understanding the valvular and associated cardiac disease, the anesthesiologist must have a good appreciation of the surgical plan. Nonsternotomy and port-access approaches require specific positioning, including having the arms extended or cephalad, and will have implications for peripheral venous, central venous, and arterial catheter placement. Port-access procedures will require planning for fluoroscopic and TEE assistance to guide and monitor placement of catheters.

D. Monitoring

1. Central venous catheter versus PAC. Because of pericardial traction and/or compression of the right atrium, pulmonary artery, or right ventricular outflow tract, pressures recorded from central venous or pulmonary artery catheters may not accurately reflect chamber volume. In addition, due to limited ability to palpate around the heart, there may be an increased risk of inadvertently including the pulmonary artery catheter in surgical sutures. These considerations must be balanced with the potential need to guide fluid and inotropic therapy perioperatively.

2. **TEE. There can be little doubt that TEE monitoring is an integral part of MIVS [18]. With limited access the surgeon cannot rely on visual cues about cardiac distension or volume status.** Thus, TEE is used in the following ways:

   a. Prepump to determine:

      1. Valve dysfunction
      2. Cardiac volume and function
      3. Arterial cannulation site
      4. Specialized cannula placement, especially for Heartport
      5. Ventricular function and regional wall-motion disturbances

   b. During CPB for Heartport, TEE is used to monitor appropriate placement of the endoaortic "clamp" and to detect intracardiac air, which can be extensive in more than 50% of MIVS cases.

   c. After CPB, TEE is used in the usual manner to assist with management of postoperative ventricular dysfunction. This is more frequent in patients with significant intracardiac air. It is also used to assess valve function and to look for aortic dissection.

E. Specific anesthesiology concerns. Regardless of the type of surgical access to MIVS, there are several common problems that require enhanced awareness:

1. Long surgical learning curve. Expect anything during this period.
2. Limited surgical access (small incision)

   a. Urgent cardiac pacing and direct current cardioversion may need to be performed transthoracically. Appropriate skin electrodes/patches must be placed before surgery is started.

   b. Big fingers, sponges, or instruments can compress vascular structures, which can cause large swings in hemodynamic parameters.

   c. "Blind" suture placement can lead to bleeding from posterior sites that can be very difficult to control. Full median sternotomy occasionally is required to control the bleeding.

   d. Inadequate valve repair or replacement. Paravalvular leaks or valve dysfunction from suture-induced valve sticking can occur.

   e. Errant suture placement may cause coronary artery compromise, leading to myocardial ischemia, or may affect the conduction system, leading to heart block or dysrhythmias.

   f. De-airing maneuvers are very difficult, even when they are guided by TEE. Residual air may embolize to the coronary arteries and result in acute cardiac decompensation.

   g. Tamponade. After chest closure, even a small amount of bleeding can lead to tamponade physiology in the mini-incision area.

F. Postoperative management. The goal is early recovery and extubation. As in MIDCAB and OPCAB, this is governed by a number of factors, including patient stability and temperature, duration of the procedure, and use of short-acting agents. Extubation in the operating room is uncommon. Certain incisions (i.e., thoracotomy) may lend themselves to the use of intercostal blocks for postoperative pain relief.

III. Robotically enhanced cardiac surgery

A. Historical perspective

1. Use of robotics in surgery initially was considered for transfer of surgical expertise to a site remote from the surgeon (e.g., battlefield, developing country).
2. Robotic enhancement of dexterity has been applied to endoscopic instruments, allowing on-site performance of complex tasks that are otherwise impossible.

   3. Computer-assisted robotic cardiac surgery in patients was first reported by
      Loulmet et al. [19] and Reichenspurner et al. [20] in 1999.
B. Introduction
   1. Taylor et al. [21] described the complementary capabilities of surgeon and
      machine.
      a. Surgeons are dexterous, adaptive, fast, and can execute motions over a
         large geometric scale. They develop judgment and experience. Limiting
         factors include geometric inaccuracy and inexact exertion of directional
         force. Performance is compromised by confined spaces or bad exposure.
         Surgeons become tired, and with age skills and vision can diminish.
      **b. Machines are precise and untiring. Computer-controlled instru-
         ments can be moved through an exactly defined trajectory with
         controlled forces, facilitating work in confined spaces.**
   2. Endoscopic surgery, by avoiding the stress, pain, and cosmetic insult of open
      procedures, improves some outcomes and increases patient satisfaction. Lapa-
      roscopic cholecystectomy illustrates rapid adaptation of surgical practice to
      endoscopic techniques. In 1999, 85% of gallbladder surgeries (approximately
      1,100,000 surgeries) were performed via this minimally invasive approach [22].
   3. Many excisional or ablative procedures lend themselves to current endosco-
      pic instrumentation. Reconstructive procedures (e.g., vascular anastomoses)
      are more difficult because of the requirement for multiple planes of fine
      motor activity.
   4. Robotic enhancement of dexterity potentially allows the use of endoscopic tech-
      niques for complex surgery. For coronary bypass surgery, the goal is to avoid
      both sternotomy and CPB. Robotic devices permit construction of coronary
      artery grafts through endoscopic portals on the beating heart [23].
C. Technologic advances permitting endoscopic surgery
   1. Development of the charge-coupling device (CCD) allowed high-resolution video
      images to be transmitted through optical scopes to the surgeon.
   2. High-intensity xenon and halogen light sources improved visualization of the
      surgical field.
   3. Improved hand instrumentation permitted procedures that previously could
      be performed only through an open incision to be executed by less invasive
      methods [24].
   4. The surgeon now can view digitally enhanced images that provide better visu-
      alization than direct viewing, owing to magnification and illumination.
   5. The major limitations of endoscopic instruments are control of fine motor
      activity and surgery in a confined space.
   6. Placement of a microprocessor between the surgeon's hand and the tip of the sur-
      gical instrument dramatically enhances control and fine movement. Table 13.2
      lists the ways in which computerized dexterity enhancement addresses limita-
      tions of conventional endoscopy.
D. Endoscopic robotic-assisted systems
   1. Robotic systems consist of three principal components (Fig. 13.5):
      a. Surgeon console. The surgeon sits at the console and grasps specially de-
         signed instrument handles. The surgeon's motions are relayed to a com-
         puter processor, which digitizes his or her hand motions.
      b. Computer control system. The digitized information from the computer
         control system is related in real time to robotic manipulators, which are
         attached to the operating room table.
      c. Robotic manipulators. These manipulators hold the endoscopic instrument
         tips, which are inserted into the patient through small ports.
   2. Currently two robotic systems are commercially available: the da Vinci sys-
      tem (Intuitive Surgical, Mountain View, CA, U.S.A.) and the Zeus system
      (Computer Motion, Goleta, CA, U.S.A.). Falk et al. [25] summarized key char-
      acteristic operating features of these robotic systems, which feature different
      manipulator technologies.
   3. A number of enhancements are required to move robotic systems toward more
      widespread acceptance.

Table 13.2 Endoscopic versus computer-enhanced instrumentation systems

	Conventional endoscopic instruments	Computer-enhanced systems
Degrees of freedom	4	6
Tremor filter	No	Yes
Motion transmission	1:1	1:1 to 5:1
Hand–eye alignment	Poor	Natural
Fulcrum effect	Reversed motion	Not effective
Force ratio (hand/tip)	Large/abnormal/not linear	Programmable/linear
Indexing	Not possible	Possible
Ergonomics	Unfavorable	Favorable

Degrees of freedom, number of different directions of movement. For instance, if something is capable of moving the x, y, and z directions, then it has three degrees of freedom. The Da Vinci can probably move in the x, y, and z directions plus it can rotate and act like forceps.
Tremor filter, image filter that filters out camera vibrations or filters out surgeon tremors at the control station.
Motion transmission, displacement amplifier to make finer movements possible. At the 5:1 setting, the robot moves 1 cm for every 5-cm movement of the surgeon at the control station.
Hand–eye alignment, assesses hand–eye coordination.
Fulcrum effect, fulcrum is the point or support on which a lever turns. The conventional instrument is said to be reversed motion, meaning that if the surgeon moves in one direction, the actual motion of the instrument is in the opposite direction.
Force ratio, feedback physical force the surgeon feels at the control station when operating.

     a. Development of endoscopic Doppler ultrasonography may aid in internal thoracic (mammary) artery harvesting, especially when the vessel is covered by fat or muscle.

     b. Although they provide articulation, the endoscopic stabilizers available via port access need refinement to permit easier placement.

     c. Multimodal three-dimensional image visualization and manipulation systems may allow modeling of the range of motion of the robotic arms to individual patient data sets (computerized tomographic scan, ECG-gated magnetic resonance imaging). This may help to optimize port placement and minimize the risk of collisions in the future.

     d. "Virtual" cardiac surgical planning platforms will allow the surgeon to examine the topology of the patient's thorax in order to plan the port placement and the endoscopic procedure.

   E. Anesthetic considerations related to robotic surgery. Robotic surgery requires the anesthesiologist to interact with the surgeon and machine to maintain ideal operating conditions as well as stable hemodynamics and rhythm in an environment that may change rapidly due to regional ischemia and cardiac manipulation. When the patient is fully instrumented and the robotic surgery is under way, direct access to the operative field is limited and likely to be delayed. Anticipation and excellent communication are especially important in situations where rapid surgical interventions are all but impossible.

     1. Preoperative preparation

        a. Similar to OPCAB or MIDCAB, the anesthesiologist must discuss the procedure with the surgeon to understand the coronary anatomy, what is planned, and what special considerations might be involved (see above).

        b. Specific to robotic surgery are considerations that may be applicable to the selected robot (e.g., site of ports, location of manipulators, electrical interference).

     2. Monitoring. Monitoring must take into account the patient's pathology, the surgeon's familiarity with the robotic technique, anticipated problems, and duration

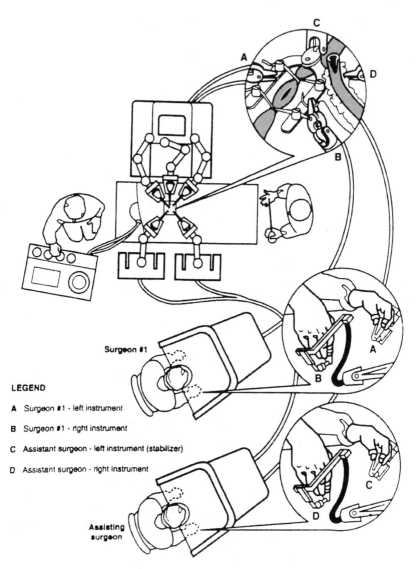

FIG. 13.5 Schematic illustration of setup for endoscopic beating heart coronary artery bypass grafting using two consoles and five manipulator arms. The surgeon at the primary console manipulates two instruments and navigates the endoscope. The assisting surgeon directs the stabilizer and an assisting tool from a second console. *A,* left tool (primary surgeon); *B,* right tool (primary surgeon); *C,* stabilizer (left hand assisting surgeon); *D,* assisting tool (right hand assisting surgeon). (From Falk V, Fann JI, Grunenfelder J, et al. Endoscopic computer-enhanced beating heart coronary artery bypass surgery. *Ann Thorac Surg* 2000;70: 2029–2033, with permission.)

of the procedure. As robotic procedures are still in the early stages of development, high-intensity monitoring probably is warranted in most patients (i.e., use of PACs and/or TEE).

3. Induction and maintenance of anesthesia
   a. Specific anesthetic techniques are similar to other cardiac surgery where rapid emergence from anesthesia is desired ("fast track").
   b. Position is critical for appropriate location of ports and access for robotic manipulators. Typically this is left arm beside the body, right arm up (suspended in a sling). There has been one case report of transitory paresthesia attributed to arm position.
   c. Deflation of the left lung is required for visualization. This can be accomplished with a double-lumen endobronchial tube or bronchial blocker.
   d. Carbon dioxide is insufflated into the left hemithorax during one-lung anesthesia. Mechanical impairment of cardiac contractility and filling may ensue. The insufflation pressure should be 6 to 8 mmHg. Absorption of CO_2 may cause respiratory acidosis, tachycardia, dysrhythmias, and pulmonary hypertension. Impaired cardiac function is rapidly reversible after release of CO_2 from the chest cavity [26].
   e. External defibrillator/pacing pads should be attached to the patient because surgical access to the heart to perform either of these functions is limited and delayed.
   f. Similar to OPCAB and MIDCAB, a multimodal approach should be taken to prevent heat loss, especially in view of the fact that robotic procedures may be lengthy. All the techniques mentioned above can be used for robotic surgery as well.

4. Anticoagulation and reversal. See discussion under "OPCAB and MIDCAB" in Section **I.F.**

5. Avoiding hemodynamic compromise. As in OPCAB, the heart may be positioned within the chest in a manner that compromises venous return or ventricular function.
   a. Keep cardiac preload high. Consider intravascular volume loading and the head-down (Trendelenburg) position.
   b. Tilt the operating table to the side to facilitate surgical exposure.
   c. Maintain coronary perfusion pressure with α-adrenergic agonists if needed.
   d. Use epicardial pacing if bradycardia occurs.
   e. Closely watch insufflation pressure and monitor end-tidal CO_2 concentration as well as periodic arterial blood gases.

6. Postoperative management
   a. Extubation in the operating room may be possible (see above for OPCAB and MIDCAB).
   b. If postoperative ventilation is anticipated, plan to change the double-lumen tube for a single-lumen endotracheal tube.
   c. Postoperative pain management will depend on the size and number of port incisions. If a thoracotomy incision was made, either intercostal or epidural analgesia should be considered.

IV. Transmyocardial laser revascularization
A. Historical perspective
   1. TMLR is a procedure for treatment of refractory angina pectoris using laser energy to create a series of channels in ischemic myocardium (Fig. 13.6).
   2. The concept dates back to 1933, when Wearn et al. [27] demonstrated direct vascular communication between the coronary arteries and the chambers of the heart via a sinusoidal network in the human heart. Use of omentopexy by Beck [28] in 1935 and implantation of the IMA directly into the myocardium by Vineberg [29] in 1954 were attempts at indirect myocardial perfusion based on Wearn's description.
   3. In 1965, Sen et al. [30] used needle acupuncture to create transmural channels through ischemic myocardium to direct blood into the myocardium from the ventricle. This concept was based on the reptile heart, in which the left ventricle is perfused directly via channels radiating from the left ventricle.

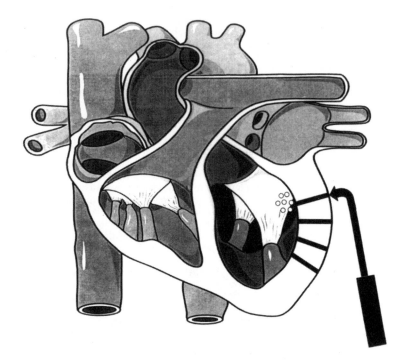

FIG. 13.6 Illustration of transmyocardial laser and epicardial position of the laser device for creating channels. The device can be placed through a left thoracotomy incision (isolated procedure) or through a standard sternotomy (supplement to coronary artery bypass graft). Full-thickness penetration is confirmed by transesophageal echocardiographic visualization of microbubbles in the left ventricular cavity.

    4. Mirhoseini and Clayton [31] in the 1980s used carbon dioxide laser energy to create transmyocardial channels.
    5. Reports of prospective randomized clinical trials [32,33] led to approval of carbon dioxide and holmium lasers for treatment of refractory angina pectoris. In addition, the safety and efficacy of both lasers used as an adjunct to CABG has been evaluated [34].
B. Laser mechanism of injury
    1. Three types of lasers are used for TMLR: carbon dioxide (CO_2), holmium (YAG), and XeCl excimer. The CO_2 and holmium lasers operate in the infrared region, whereas the excimer laser is in the ultraviolet region.
    2. **To create a channel through myocardium, tissue is ablated (chemical bonds between atoms are broken). Infrared lasers achieve ablation by vaporization of myocardium, which is followed by intense collagen deposition and scarring.**
    3. The ventricle should be filled with blood to act as a beam stop and prevent perforation of the posterior ventricular wall or damage to the chordae tendineae of the mitral valve.
    4. Ultraviolet lasers achieve ablation via radiation absorption by covalent bonds within tissue proteins. There tends to be more thermal damage to tissue surrounding the channels with infrared lasers than with ultraviolet lasers. In addition to thermal injury, mechanical injury occurs through the production of vapor bubbles and the presence of shock waves. Production of free radical molecules also causes cellular injury [35,36].

C. Mechanisms responsible for clinical benefit
   1. **The exact mechanism contributing to improved clinical outcome from TMLR remains controversial.**
   2. Direct channel patency early with subsequent endothelialization of these channels has been proposed. However, histopathologic studies have failed to confirm this hypothesis.
   3. **Another proposed theory involves neovascularization** in response to laser-induced tissue injury. TMLR may lead to vascular angiogenic growth factor-like molecules that induce neovascularization and improved regional collateral blood flow.
   4. A placebo effect has been postulated but is unlikely to account for sustained relief of angina in study patients.
   5. Sympathetic denervation has been postulated, especially to explain the immediate relief of angina experienced by some patients [37]. This would damage cardiac afferent nerve function and the sensation of angina pain. Although more studies are necessary, neovascularization and sympathetic denervation are likely mechanisms of action that may occur concurrently.
D. Patient selection
   1. The largest use of TMLR is in combination with conventional CABG, especially in reoperative patients. TMLR frequently may be used as an adjunct to bypass grafting in areas of incomplete coronary artery revascularization.
   2. TMLR is indicated in a select group of patients with severe diffuse coronary artery disease who are poor candidates for conventional angioplasty or coronary revascularization. These patients experience anginal symptoms refractory to medical therapy or cannot be weaned from intravenous antianginal medications. These patients must demonstrate reversible ischemia determined by myocardial perfusion scanning and possess a left ventricular ejection fraction greater than 25%.
   3. Additional candidates may include heart transplant recipients who develop severe coronary artery disease as a result of allograft rejection.
   4. Contraindications to TMLR include severely depressed left ventricular ejection fraction, congestive heart failure, ischemic mitral regurgitation, preexisting arrhythmias, ventricular mural thrombus, long-term anticoagulant therapy, and chronic obstructive pulmonary disease.
E. Preoperative evaluation
   1. Assessment of patients who present for TMLR is similar to that for patients who present for CABG.
   2. Standard blood chemistry, hematology, and coagulation profiles are obtained.
   3. ECG, exercise stress testing, and transthoracic echocardiography (with or without dobutamine stress) are performed to assess arrhythmias, valvular and ventricular function, the presence of ventricular thrombus, and low cardiac output states. Multiple gated scintigraphic angiography (MUGA) scanning may be used to assess ventricular function.
   4. Coronary angiography is performed to determine if the vessels can be grafted and to decide if TMLR will be performed as an isolated procedure or as an adjunct to CABG.
   5. Myocardial perfusion scanning techniques, such as thallium scintigraphy and positron emission tomography, are performed to identify areas of viable but ischemic myocardium. These tests also will serve as a baseline for comparison with postoperative results.
F. Anesthetic considerations
   1. **Laser safety**
      a. Operating room windows and outside doors must be marked with signs indicating that a laser procedure is occurring.
      b. The patient's eyes must be protected with moist gauze. All operating room personnel must wear protective goggles.
   2. **Isolated TMLR**
      a. **Preoperative preparation**
         (1) Patients selected for isolated TMLR present with inoperable severe coronary artery disease. In addition, there is a high incidence of

coexisting diseases, such as diabetes, lung disease, hypertension, prior myocardial infarction, and prior CABG. They require close hemodynamic control with focus on optimizing myocardial oxygen supply and consumption.

(2) Anticoagulant therapy should be discontinued before surgery. Antianginal, antiarrhythmic, and pulmonary medications should be continued the morning of surgery.

(3) Preoperative sedation may consist of a benzodiazepine to relieve anxiety. Consideration also should be given to the addition of an antisialagogue if one-lung ventilation is planned.

(4) In the operating room, adequate venous access is essential because many patients have undergone previous cardiac surgery and bleeding is a significant risk.

(5) These patients are prone to acute ischemic events in the perioperative period. An ECG with computerized ST-segment analysis and trending is used for ischemia detection. Pulmonary artery catheters usually are placed because these patients often have poor ventricular function.

(6) Insertion of a thoracic epidural catheter should be considered to facilitate early extubation and provide postoperative analgesia.

(7) The operating room should be warm, with every effort made to maintain patient normothermia.

b. **Induction and maintenance of anesthesia**

(1) The goals are to maintain hemodynamic stability, facilitate early extubation, and provide reliable postoperative analgesia.

(2) After induction, a left double-lumen tube or left bronchial blocker is placed for left lung collapse.

(3) A TEE probe is inserted after induction to monitor ventricular function, mitral valve competence, and gaseous bubbles in the left ventricle generated by transmyocardial laser strikes.

(4) External defibrillation patches should be placed on the patient.

(5) The patient is placed in a 45-degree right lateral decubitus position with the groin exposed in case emergency CPB or insertion of an IABP is needed.

(6) An anterior thoracotomy is performed through the left fifth intercostal space, the pericardium is opened anteriorly, and the area of ischemic myocardium is exposed.

(7) **The laser probe is placed through the chest wall and positioned against the epicardium. The laser is synchronized to the ECG signal and fired at the peak of the R wave. The laser energy is absorbed by blood in the left ventricle.**

(8) Transmyocardial laser channels are confirmed by detection of ventricular bubbles by TEE and the appearance of bright red blood from the channels.

(9) It may be beneficial to avoid nitrous oxide because of the potential for bubble expansion during laser channel creation.

c. **Recovery**

(1) After hemostasis is obtained, the incision is closed and an attempt may be made to extubate the patient in the operating room.

(2) After extubation, the patient is transported to a telemetry area for postoperative monitoring [38,39].

3. **Combined TMLR and CABG**

a. **Preoperative preparation**

(1) Preoperative preparation is similar to that for isolated TMLR.

b. **Induction and maintenance of anesthesia**

(1) Induction and maintenance are similar to on-pump CABG.

(2) The procedure is performed through a median sternotomy and uses CPB with full heparinization.

(3) After initiation of CPB, the surgeon inspects the heart. Viable myocardium that could not be revascularized with CABG is identified for TMLR.

(4) TMLR is performed initially on the beating heart (i.e., early during CPB) in an attempt to minimize laser channel bleeding as platelet function and coagulation factor levels are relatively normal. TMLR performed on the beating heart may cause arrhythmias and ventricular distension, in which case the procedure may be done after administration of cardioplegia.

(5) The remainder of the operation is performed in the usual fashion.

c. Recovery

(1) Recovery is similar to on-pump CABG.

4. Complications

a. Patients who present for isolated TMLR experience ongoing myocardial ischemia. There is no immediate physiologic benefit from the procedure; rather, there may be ventricular failure, infarction, hypotension, arrhythmias, or hypoxemia related to anesthesia or myocardial manipulation. Laser vaporization can directly damage myocardium and contribute further to myocardial failure.

b. Vasopressors, inotropes, an IABP, and CPB standby must be available to treat unexpected myocardial failure at any time in the perioperative period.

c. TMLR may induce atrial and ventricular arrhythmias. This frequently occurs during surgical manipulation of the heart by the surgeon or the laser probe. Ventricular arrhythmias are common during the creation of transmyocardial channels. Gating of the laser to the cardiac cycle has decreased the incidence of ventricular arrhythmias. Direct injury to the Purkinje conduction system may further complicate these arrhythmias.

d. Direct laser injury to the mitral valve apparatus with acute mitral regurgitation may precipitate heart failure. This risk is reduced with use of the holmium laser. A thorough TEE examination must be performed after the laser procedure (but before closing the chest) to diagnose this complication.

e. Vaporization of myocardium generates bubbles in the left ventricular cavity with risk for gaseous emboli.

f. Hemorrhage may occur secondary to surgical dissection in patients who had undergone previous coronary bypass or from the transmyocardial laser channels. Bleeding from the laser channels can be controlled by digital pressure for isolated TMLR, as systemic heparinization is not used. However, if TMLR is performed during CPB, the risk of bleeding from the laser channels may increase if TMLR is performed after bypass grafting before termination of CPB.

5. Outcome

a. Ongoing studies continue to examine the benefit and indications for isolated TMLR and combined TMLR/CABG [40,41].

b. Current literature indicates symptomatic and functional improvement 12 months after isolated TMLR in patients with angina refractory to medical treatment in the presence of inoperable coronary artery disease versus continued medical treatment only.

c. Studies in large numbers of patients will be necessary to determine the long-term benefit of combined TMLR/CABG versus CABG alone.

6. Future directions

a. Improvement of TMLR technique and avoidance of thoracotomy is on the horizon.

b. Percutaneous endocardial laser revascularization techniques with creation of the laser channels from the inside of the heart has been reported [42].

c. Augmentation of the clinical benefits of TMLR by simultaneous delivery of growth factors or gene therapy is under investigation.

References

OPCAB and MIDCAB

1. **Clements F, Shanewise J, eds. *Minimally invasive cardiac and vascular surgical techniques. Society of Cardiovascular Anesthesiologists monograph.* Philadelphia: Lippincott Williams & Wilkins, 2001.**
2. Benetti FJ, Naselli G, Wood M, et al. Direct myocardial revascularization without extracorporeal circulation. *Chest* 1991;100:312–316.
3. Cason BA, Gamperl AK, Slocum RE, et al. Anesthetic-induced preconditioning. *Anesthesiology* 1997;87:1182–1190.
4. Guyton RA, Thourani VH, Puskas JD, et al. Perfusion-assisted direct coronary artery bypass: selective graft perfusion in off-pump cases. *Ann Thorac Surg* 2000;69:171–175.
5. Zenati M, Cohen HA, Griffith BP. Alternative approach to multivessel coronary disease with integrated coronary revascularization. *J Thorac Cardiovasc Surg* 1999;117:439–446.
6. **Resano FG, Stamou SC, Lowery RC, et al. Complete myocardial revascularization on the beating heart with epicardial stabilization: anesthetic considerations. *J Cardiothorac Vasc Anesth* 2000;14:534–539.**
7. Moises VA, Mesquita CB, Campos O, et al. Importance of intraoperative transesophageal echocardiography during coronary surgery without cardiopulmonary bypass. *J Am Soc Echocardiogr* 1998;11:1139–1144.
8. Dhole S, Mehta Y, Saxena H, et al. Comparison of continuous thoracic epidural and paravertebral blocks for postoperative analgesia after minimally invasive direct coronary artery bypass surgery. *J Cardiothorac Vasc Anesth* 2001;15:288–292.
9. Grundeman PF, Borst C, van Herwaarden JA, et al. Vertical displacement of the beating heart by the Octopus tissue stabilizer: influence on coronary flow. *Ann Thorac Surg* 1998;65:1348–1352.
10. Mariani MA, Gu J, Boonstra P, et al. Procoagulant activity after off-pump coronary operation: is the current anticoagulation adequate? *Ann Thorac Surg* 1999;67:1370–1375.
11. Puskas JD, Thourani VH, Marshall J, et al. Clinical outcomes, angiographic patency, and resource utilization in 200 consecutive off-pump coronary bypass patients. *Ann Thorac Surg* 2001;71:1477–1484.
12. Cleveland JC Jr, Shroyer ALW, Chen AY, et al. Off-pump coronary artery bypass grafting decreases risk-adjusted mortality and morbidity. *Ann Thorac Surg* 2001;72:1282–1289.
13. **Van Dijk D, Nierich AP, Jansen EWL, et al., for the Octopus Study Group. Early outcome after off-pump versus on-pump coronary bypass surgery: results from a randomized study. *Circulation* 2001;104:1761–1766.**
14. Ascione R, Williams S, Lloyd CT, et al. Reduced postoperative blood loss and transfusion requirement after beating-heart coronary operations: a prospective randomized study. *J Thorac Cardiovasc Surg* 2001;212:689–696.

Minimally Invasive Valve Surgery

15. **Cosgrove DM, Sabik JF, Navia JL. Minimally invasive valve operations. *Ann Thorac Surg* 1998;65:1535–1539.**
16. Swerc MF, Benckart DH, Savage EB, et al. Partial versus full sternotomy for aortic valve replacement. *Ann Thorac Surg* 1999;68:2209–2213.
17. Asher CR, DiMengo JM, Weber MM, et al. Atrial fibrillation early postoperatively following minimally invasive cardiac valvular surgery. *Am J Cardiol* 1999;84:744–747.
18. **Secknus MA, Asher CR, Scalia GM, et al. Intraoperative transesophageal echocardiography in minimally invasive cardiac valve surgery. *J Am Soc Echocardiogr* 1999;12:231–236.**

Robotic Surgery

19. **Loulmet D, Carpentier A, d'Attellis N, et al. Endoscopic coronary artery bypass grafting with the aid of robotic assisted instruments. *J Thorac Cardiovasc Surg* 1999;118:4–10.**
20. **Reichenspurner H, Damiano RJ, Mack MJ, et al. Use of the voice-controlled and computer-assisted surgical system ZEUS for endoscopic coronary artery bypass grafting. *J Thorac Cardiovasc Surg* 1999;118:11–16.**

21. Taylor, RH, Lavallee S, Burdea GC, et al. *Computer-integrated surgery: technology and clinical applications.* Cambridge: The MIT Press, 1996.
22. **Mack MJ. Minimally invasive and robotic surgery. *JAMA* 2001;285:568–572.**
23. Damiano RJ. Endoscopic coronary artery bypass grafting—the first steps on a long journey [Editorial]. *J Thorac Cardiovasc Surg* 2000;120:806–807.
24. **Mohr FW, Falk V, Digeler A, et al. Computer-enhanced "robotic" cardiac surgery: experience in 148 patients. *J Thorac Cardiovasc Surg* 2001;121:842–853.**
25. Falk V, Diegler A, Mohr FW. Developments in robotic cardiac surgery. *Curr Opin Cardiol* 2000;15:378–387.
26. Ohtsuka T, Imanaka K, Endsh M. Hemodynamic effects of carbon dioxide insufflation under single-lung ventilation during thoroscopy. *Ann Thorac Surg* 1999;68:29–33.

Transmyocardial Laser Revascularization
27. Wearn JT, Mettier SR, Klump TG, et al. The nature of the vascular communications between the coronary arteries and the chambers of the heart. *Am Heart J* 1933;9:143–170.
28. Beck CS. The development of a new blood supply to the heart by operation. *Ann Surg* 1935;102:801–813.
29. Vineberg AM. Development of an anastomosis between the coronary vessels and a transplanted internal mammary artery. *Can Med Assoc J* 1946;55:117–119.
30. Sen PK, Udwadia TE, Kinaire SG, et al. Transmyocardial acupuncture. *J Thorac Cardiovasc Surg* 1950;50:181–189.
31. Mirhoseini M, Clayton MM. Revascularization of the heart by laser. *J Microsurg* 1981; 2:253–260.
32. **Frazier OH, March RJ, Horvath KA. Transmyocardial revascularization with a carbon dioxide laser in patients with end stage coronary artery disease. *N Engl J Med* 1999;341:1021–1028.**
33. **Allen KB, Dowling RD, Fudge TL, et al. Comparison of transmyocardial revascularization with medical therapy in patients with refractory angina. *N Engl J Med* 1999;341:1029–1036.**
34. **Allen KB, Dowling RD, DelRossi AJ, et al. Transmyocardial laser revascularization combined with coronary artery bypass grafting: a multicenter, blinded, prospective, randomized, controlled trial. *J Thorac Cardiovasc Surg* 2000;119: 540–549.**
35. Hartman RA, Whittaker P. The physics of transmyocardial laser revascularization. *J Clin Laser Med Surg* 1997;15:255–259.
36. Shehada RE, Mansour HN, Grundfest WS. Laser tissue interaction in direct myocardial revascularization. *Semin Interv Cardiol* 2000;5:63–70.
37. Sola OM, Shi Q, Vernon RB, et al. Cardiac denervation after transmyocardial laser. *Ann Thorac Surg* 2001;71:732.
38. **Grocott HP, Newman MF, Lowe JE, et al. Transmyocardial laser revascularization: an anesthetic perspective. *J Cardiothorac Vasc Anesth* 1997;11:206–210.**
39. Thrush DN. Anesthesia for laser transmyocardial revascularization. *J Cardiothorac Vasc Anesth* 1997;11:481–484.
40. **Allen KB, Shaar CJ. Transmyocardial laser revascularization: surgical experience overview. *Semin Interv Cardiol* 2000;5:75–81.**
41. Kraatz EG, Misfeld M, Jungbluth B, et al. Survival after transmyocardial laser revascularization in relation to nonlasered perfused myocardial zones. *Ann Thorac Surg* 2001;71:532–536.
42. Lauer B, Junghans U, Stahl F, et al. Catheter-based percutaneous myocardial laser revascularization in patients with end-stage coronary artery disease. *J Am Coll Cardiol* 1999;34:1663–1670.

14. ANESTHETIC MANAGEMENT FOR PATIENTS WITH CONGENITAL HEART DISEASE

Laurie K. Davies and Daniel G. Knauf

I. Introduction

The care of children undergoing cardiovascular surgery provides a remarkable challenge to the anesthesiologist. In the last decade, improvements in diagnostic capability, cardiopulmonary bypass (CPB) techniques, monitoring, and perioperative care have permitted more complicated procedures to be performed on smaller, sicker children with remarkable success. The environment is dynamic, because operative procedures and technology are being modified constantly in an effort to further improve the safety and outcome for these special children.

Each child presents a unique set of circumstances and pathophysiologic concerns. Much of the knowledge regarding appropriate management for adults undergoing cardiac surgery will not apply to these children. Anesthesiologists caring for these patients must be flexible and innovative. Rigid protocols rarely are appropriate; instead, an individualized plan for each patient is mandatory. Team effort and good communication are essential to the success of a pediatric cardiovascular surgical program. Being a part of a successful team effort and caring for these patients are among the most exciting and rewarding experiences in medicine today.

    A. Incidence. Congenital heart disease (CHD) is relatively uncommon. It is estimated to occur in fewer than 1% of all live births (Table 14.1). The true incidence probably is quite a bit higher. Much fetal wastage is thought to occur because of the presence of congenital heart defects that are incompatible with life. Also, some heart lesions [e.g., bicuspid aortic valve and patent ductus arteriosus (PDA)] may be relatively asymptomatic early in life; thus, the true incidence of CHD is unknown.

    Certain lesions are more likely to become manifest early in life than are others. With these caveats in mind, the lesions most likely to be encountered in the first year of life are ventricular septal defect (VSD), transposition of the great vessels (TGV), tetralogy of Fallot, coarctation of the aorta, and hypoplastic left heart syndrome.

    Different reference populations may demonstrate different patterns of CHD. For instance, infants who are premature and small for their gestational ages have an increased prevalence of CHD (especially VSD and PDA) compared with full-term newborns. Congenital heart defects are more common among infants of diabetic mothers than among those of nondiabetic mothers. Infants with abnormal chromosomes have an increased frequency of congenital heart defects. About 23% to 56% of children with trisomy 21 have CHD [1]. The most common defects in children

Table 14.1 Reported estimate of prevalence per 1,000 live births for specific congenital heart defects

Defect	Prevalence
Ventricular septal defect	0.38
Transposition	0.21
Tetralogy of Fallot	0.21
Coarctation of aorta	0.18
Hypoplastic left-sided heart syndrome	0.16
Patent ductus arteriosus	0.14
Atrioventricular septal defect	0.12
Pulmonary stenosis	0.19
Pulmonary atresia	0.07
Secundum atrial septal defect	0.07
Total anomalous pulmonary venous drainage	0.06
Tricuspid atresia	0.06
Aortic stenosis	0.04
Double-outlet right ventricle	0.03
Truncus arteriosus	0.03
Other	0.18

Modified from Daniels SR. Epidemiology. In Long WA, ed. *Fetal and neonatal cardiology*. Philadelphia: WB Saunders, 1990:430.

with Down syndrome appear to be VSD, atrial septal defect (ASD), PDA, and atrioventricular (AV) canal defects.

B. Prognosis. The outlook for these children today has improved considerably over that of previous years. A better understanding of the pathophysiology of individual lesions allows development of a rational treatment care plan. Earlier complete repairs are being performed successfully, often resulting in the avoidance of the long-term sequelae of unrepaired CHD. Cardiac transplantation also has become a viable option for some children whose lesions cannot be surgically repaired. For any of these options to be successful, the patient's care must be thoughtfully individualized with vigilance, anticipation, and meticulous attention to detail.

II. Physiologic considerations

A. *What is the difference between fetal and adult circulation?*

In order to develop an understanding of the clinical and anesthetic implications of CHD, one must be familiar with the fetal and the adult circulations. Three important channels characteristic of the circulation *in utero* allow preferential shunting of blood: ductus venosus, foramen ovale, and ductus arteriosus (Fig. 14.1).

1. **Ductus venosus.** Well-oxygenated blood from the placenta, with a partial pressure of oxygen of about 33 mm Hg, travels through the umbilical vein to enter the liver. The ductus venosus allows about one half of this blood to be shunted from the liver directly into the inferior vena cava.

2. **Foramen ovale.** About one third of the blood entering the right atrium from the inferior vena cava is preferentially shunted across the foramen ovale into the left atrium. On the other hand, superior vena cava blood (which is poorly oxygenated) primarily enters the right ventricle (RV), with 2% to 3% crossing the foramen ovale.

3. **Ductus arteriosus.** RV blood is largely shunted across the ductus arteriosus into the descending aorta (rather than perfusing the high-resistance pulmonary circulation).

4. **Implications.** The structure of the fetal circulation allows the well-oxygenated blood (which has a high glucose content) from the inferior vena cava to preferentially perfuse the brain, coronary circulation, and upper extremities. The lower portion of the body receives blood with a low oxygen content from the ductus arteriosus. Hence, the systemic and pulmonary circulations in the fetus function in parallel, with each ventricle receiving only a portion of the systemic cardiac output. The adult situation, in contrast, requires the two circulations to work in series, each processing the entire cardiac output.

B. *What is the transitional circulation?*

At birth, remarkable changes occur rapidly in the circulation that allow the infant to adapt to the stresses of extrauterine life. A period of transition in the neonatal circulation occurs before permanent adaptation to the normal adult pattern takes place. This transitional stage is unstable and may exist for a few hours or for many weeks, depending on the stresses imposed. Factors contributing to the instability of the transitional circulation are the state of the ductus arteriosus, foramen ovale, and pulmonary vascular bed, as well as the immaturity of the neonatal heart. Conditions that may prolong the transitional circulation include hypoxia, hypothermia, acidosis, hypercarbia, sepsis, prematurity, and CHD.

1. **Closure of the ductus arteriosus.** Functional closure of the ductus arteriosus usually occurs within a few hours of birth, but anatomic closure may not occur for several weeks. During this period, the resistance to ductus arteriosus blood flow is responsive to changes in arterial Po_2 (P_aO_2); that is, increased P_aO_2 increases resistance, and decreased P_aO_2 decreases resistance. Prostaglandin E_1 (PGE_1) infusion relaxes the ductal musculature and increases ductal flow, which may be left-to-right, right-to-left, or bidirectional. Maintenance of ductal patency may be important for the infant with cyanotic heart disease until repair or palliative surgery can be performed.

2. **Closure of the foramen ovale and ductus venosus.** The foramen ovale functionally closes when left atrial pressure exceeds right atrial pressure; this usually occurs within a few hours after birth. Anatomic closure does not occur for many months, and about 30% of adults demonstrate probe patency of the

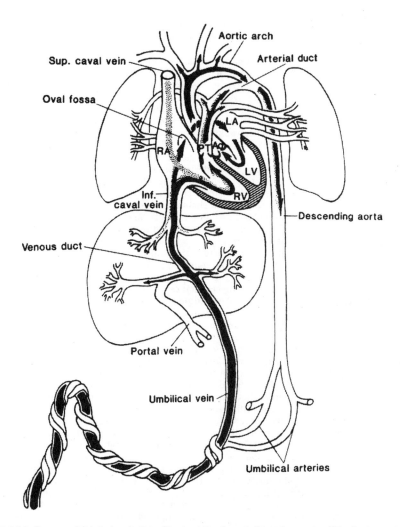

FIG. 14.1 Course of fetal circulation. See text for description. *Ao,* aorta; *DA,* ductus arteriosus; *DV,* ductus venosus; *LA,* left atrium; *LV,* left ventricle; *PA,* pulmonary artery; *PT,* pulmonary trunk; *RA,* right atrium; *RV,* right ventricle. (From Hoffman JIE. The circulatory system. In: Rudolph AM, ed. *Pediatrics,* 17th ed. Norwalk, CT: Appleton & Lange, 1982:1232, with permission.)

foramen ovale. Right-to-left intracardiac shunting may occur across this area with coughing or the Valsalva maneuver or if pulmonary hypertension develops. Umbilical arteries and veins close shortly after birth, as does the ductus venosus. The latter forms the ligamentum venosum.

3. **Pulmonary vascular resistance.** Pulmonary vascular resistance (PVR) is high *in utero* but declines rapidly after birth in the term infant. Usually, it is lower than systemic levels within 24 hours of birth. Thereafter, it falls at a moderate rate for 5 to 6 weeks and then more gradually for the next 2 to 3 years. During this period, a child's pulmonary vascular bed is more reactive than that of an adult, and a rise in pulmonary artery (PA) pressure can easily be produced

by hypoxemia, hypercarbia, acidosis, or bronchospasm. If this reaction occurs shortly after birth, it may result in shunting across the ductus arteriosus or foramen ovale or other cardiac defects. Later in life, only a patent foramen ovale or cardiac defect remains as a possible shunt site.

C. *How is a child's heart structurally different from that of an adult?*

1. **Size.** At birth, both ventricles are approximately equal in size and wall thickness. With the changeover from the fetal circulation, the left ventricle (LV) must accommodate a greater pressure and volume workload; conversely, the pressure load of the RV is reduced, and its volume work is only slightly increased. The LV hypertrophies in response to the increased workload and becomes roughly twice as heavy as the RV by about age 6 months.

2. **Ultrastructure.** The neonate's heart is ultrastructurally immature. Myofibrils are arranged in a disorderly fashion and have a smaller percentage of contractile proteins than do those in the adult (30% vs. 60%). Autonomic innervation is incomplete at birth. The sympathetic innervation to the heart is decreased, as are cardiac catecholamine stores. In contrast, the parasympathetic innervation of the neonatal heart is comparable with that of the adult heart. These observations often are cited to explain the frequent vagal predominance that occurs in infants compared with adults. Sympathetic innervation also is immature in the peripheral vasculature. Therefore, control of vascular tone and myocardial contractility in infants depends largely on adrenal function and circulating or exogenously administered catecholamines. There are differences in myocardial calcium metabolism. In the mature myocardium, the sarcoplasmic reticulum is the predominant source of calcium ion for excitation–contraction coupling, but the sarcoplasmic reticulum is poorly developed in the immature heart. Because the neonatal myocardial cell is deficient in T tubules that, in the mature myocardium, provide electrical coupling between the cell membrane and the sarcoplasmic reticulum, it is incapable of internal release and reuptake of calcium for contraction and instead depends on transmembrane calcium transport for the development of tension. These differences in calcium handling by the cell provide some explanation for the clinical observation that newborns require greater serum ionized calcium levels for optimal myocardial contractility.

3. **Compliance.** The immature heart has a functionally decreased compliance compared with the adult heart. This difference reflects, in part, the ultrastructure of the heart and the increased volume load that each ventricle must handle with the transition from a parallel fetal to an adult series circulation. The RV and LV are more intimately interrelated as a result of this decreased compliance and similarity in size. Dysfunction of one ventricle quickly leads to biventricular failure. Reduced compliance also means that the immature heart is more sensitive to volume overload. A neonate's ventricular function curve is shifted to the right and downward compared with that of an adult. Over the physiologic range of ventricular filling pressures, stroke volume changes are, in fact, small.

This relatively fixed stroke volume makes a neonate highly dependent on heart rate and sinus rhythm for optimal cardiac output. In comparison, the adult heart is much more responsive to changes in preload to effect a change in stroke volume and thereby change cardiac output. Increases in pressure work are poorly tolerated by both the right and left sides of the immature heart. The neonate, therefore, responds poorly to either volume or pressure loading, because resting cardiac function is on or near the plateau of the cardiac function curve.

D. *How are congenital cardiac lesions meaningfully characterized?*

1. **Flow pattern.** Patients with congenital heart defects are a diverse group. Rather than memorize an approach to each lesion, one should group the many anatomic varieties into a few understandable categories (Table 14.2). Most defects can be assigned to one of three groups: (i) those resulting in increased pulmonary blood flow; (ii) those resulting in decreased pulmonary blood flow; and (iii) those resulting in obstruction to blood flow. The first two groups feature an

Table 14.2 Flow characteristics of various congenital cardiac lesions

Increased pulmonary blood flow lesions	Atrial septal defect
	Ventricular septal defect
	Patent ductus arteriosis
	Endocardial cushion defect (atrioventricular canal abnormality)
	Anomalous origin of coronary arteries
	Transposition of the great arteries[a]
	Anomalous pulmonary venous drainage[a]
	Truncus arteriosus[a]
	Single ventricle[a]
Decreased pulmonary blood flow lesions	Tetralogy of Fallot
	Pulmonary atresia
	Tricuspid atresia
	Ebstein anomaly
	Truncus arteriosus[a]
	Transposition of the great arteries[a]
	Single ventricle[a]
Obstructive lesions	Aortic stenosis
	Pulmonary stenosis
	Coarctation of the aorta
	Asymmetrical septal hypertrophy

[a] Systemic hypoxemia occurs as a result of the mixing of systemic and pulmonary venous returns. Classification as an increased or decreased pulmonary blood flow lesion depends on the absence or presence within the anatomic variation of obstruction to pulmonary blood flow.
Modified from Schwartz AJ, Campbell FW. Pathophysiological approach to congenital heart disease. In: Lake CL, ed. *Pediatric cardiac anesthesia.* Norwalk, CT: Appleton & Lange, 1988:9.

abnormal shunt pathway, whereas the third group has no shunting of blood. A fourth group could include lesions in which no pulmonary–systemic exchange of blood occurs (e.g., TGV). However, infants with TGV either have naturally occurring or artificially induced mixing of systemic and pulmonary venous returns and often can be classified into one of the first two groups, depending on whether obstruction to pulmonary blood flow is present.

2. **Clinical status: Cyanosis versus heart failure.** Cyanosis and congestive heart failure (CHF) are the major manifestations of CHD. Thus, the pathophysiologic classification must be related to the clinical status. Cyanosis occurs most commonly with lesions in which pulmonary blood flow is anatomically decreased or functionally decreased as mixing of systemic and pulmonary venous blood occurs.

CHF occurs most commonly in shunt lesions with excessively increased pulmonary blood flow or obstructive lesions that stress the ventricle beyond its capacity to pump effectively. Note that a child can be cyanotic but still fall into the category of having a lesion with increased pulmonary blood flow and may even manifest CHF. Two examples of such a situation are an infant with TGV and a large VSD or a child with truncus arteriosus. Even the most complex lesions usually fall into one of the three categories, even if they are characterized by mixed features (Table 14.2).

E. *When and why do patients become symptomatic?*
Many types of CHD may not be detected immediately after birth. The age at which heart defects become manifest obviously depends on the type of lesion, its severity, and the state of the infant's transitional circulation. Increased pulmonary blood flow lesions typically become symptomatic as PVR decreases and shunt flow to the lungs increases. These changes may take days to weeks to occur. Also, if the defect is small, it may remain asymptomatic.

Decreased pulmonary blood flow lesions often are detected earlier, usually because they result in significant cyanosis. If obstruction to pulmonary blood flow is severe, patients with such lesions may be dependent on left-to-right flow across their PDA. As the PDA closes in the first few days of life, hypoxemia becomes even more pronounced and may be incompatible with survival.

Infants with TGV and inadequate intracardiac communication become extremely cyanotic as their PDA closes. On the other hand, if a large VSD or PDA is present, these patients may develop excessive pulmonary blood flow as PVR decreases during the first few weeks of extrauterine life. Cyanosis will persist, however. Left untreated, hypertrophic vascular changes and pulmonary hypertension will occur.

Left-sided obstructive lesions cause pulmonary congestion without pulmonary volume overload. They impede flow from the pulmonary venous system to the systemic arterial system and can precipitate CHF. The symptomatology and age at presentation depend on the severity of the lesion. If the ductus arteriosus is patent, it allows right-to-left shunting of blood around the lesion, improving systemic perfusion but causing cyanosis.

III. Preoperative assessment

A. *What should the anesthesiologist look for?*

In developing an anesthetic plan for these children, one must understand the pathophysiology of the individual lesion and appreciate the degree of clinical symptomatology. As in any other assessment, taking a careful history and the physical examination probably are the most important parts of the preoperative evaluation. One must remember that the infant cannot relate the symptoms experienced, and the parents often fail to understand the significance of some of their observations.

1. **Age at presentation.** The age at presentation often provides a clue to the severity of the lesion. Infants with decreased pulmonary blood flow or inadequate mixing may be persistently cyanotic or may have intermittent episodes that often are associated with agitation, crying, or exercise. If a child is older, cyanotic episodes may be associated with "squatting" [which increases systemic vascular resistance (SVR) and promotes increased pulmonary blood flow]. This change in pulmonary blood flow dynamics may partially alleviate the cyanosis. However, particularly severe episodes can result in loss of consciousness or seizures.

2. **Frequency of episodes.** The frequency of episodes suggests the severity of the lesion. Knowledge that cyanotic episodes are intermittent confirms the dynamic nature of the shunt and should alert one to the fact that the same scenario is probable during anesthesia and surgical manipulations. Alterations in SVR and PVR may result in profound changes in the magnitude of the right-to-left shunt.

3. **Cyanosis.** During the physical examination, an important consideration is that clinical cyanosis depends on the absolute concentration of deoxygenated hemoglobin in the blood rather than on the oxygen saturation. More than 3 g/dL of deoxygenated arterial blood hemoglobin should make central cyanosis recognizable. The oxyhemoglobin saturation at which central cyanosis becomes clinically apparent varies from about 62% when the hemoglobin level is 8 g/dL to about 88% in the polycythemic infant whose hemoglobin level is 24 g/dL. Therefore, cyanosis is detected more easily when the infant's hematocrit is elevated. However, recognition of cyanosis is more difficult if a newborn has a significant proportion of fetal hemoglobin because it is more highly saturated at a given Po_2 (Fig. 14.2). Therefore, the newborn with a high proportion of fetal hemoglobin may have a large reduction in Po_2 before central cyanosis is clinically apparent.

   Infants with a preductal coarctation of the aorta may demonstrate cyanosis that is restricted to the lower half of the body, because the RV supplies the descending aorta with deoxygenated blood via the PDA.

4. **Respiration.** Infants with cyanotic heart disease often have an increased tidal volume. Clubbing of the fingers may occur but may not be evident early in life. Children with decreased pulmonary blood flow usually have exercise intolerance. These patients also have a blunted ventilatory response to hypoxia.

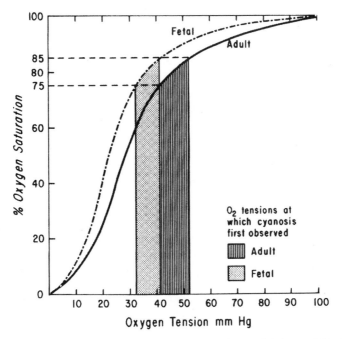

FIG. 14.2 Hemoglobin–oxygen dissociation curves for fetal and adult hemoglobin. Note that an infant with a high proportion of fetal hemoglobin will have a low P_aO_2 (33 to 42 mm Hg) before cyanosis is observed. (From Lees MH, King DH. Heart disease in the newborn. In: Adams FH, Emmanouilides GC, Riemenschneider TA, eds. *Heart disease in infants, children and adolescents.* Baltimore: Williams & Wilkins, 1989:844, with permission.)

5. **Congestive heart failure.** Infants with too much pulmonary blood flow present with CHF early in infancy when PVR decreases. A history of feeding difficulties and failure to thrive are characteristic of CHF in infancy. Other features include tachypnea, tachycardia, irritability, inappropriate sweating (often with feeding), nasal flaring, sternal and intercostal retractions, cardiomegaly, and hepatomegaly. A history of wheezing, frequent respiratory infections, and pneumonia is common. The distinction between left-sided and right-sided heart failure in the newborn is less obvious than in the adult. Peripheral edema and rales are rarely present in the young infant. Systemic perfusion may be compromised, as evidenced by decreased pulses, pallor, and poor capillary refill. A severely compromised infant may be apathetic and have a weak cry and little spontaneous movement.

   Left-sided obstructive lesions may cause CHF with clinical manifestations that are similar to those of pulmonary volume overload. Note, however, that the symptoms are a result of pulmonary venous congestion without abnormal shunting. If the lesion is located so that LV *outflow* is obstructed, LV hypertrophy will develop. If the site of obstruction involves the *inflow* to the LV, LV hypertrophy does not occur, and LV end-diastolic pressure is normal.

6. **Associated anomalies.** Look carefully for associated congenital anomalies, because they are common in newborns with cardiac disease. Other problems peculiar to the newborn or premature infant include difficulty with temperature regulation, impaired nutrition, susceptibility to dehydration and hypoglycemia, respiratory difficulties, coagulation abnormalities, and central nervous system disorders.

B. *Which preoperative laboratory studies are helpful?*

Laboratory studies of particular interest include hematocrit, white blood cell count, coagulation profile, and electrolyte and serum glucose determinations. Sickle cell screening and measurement of digoxin level should be included when applicable.

1. **Hematocrit.** The hematocrit progressively rises as hypoxemia becomes more profound. In fact, periodic checks of the hematocrit provide a simple method to follow the patient's level of hypoxemia. Increasing hematocrit may serve as a cue for the appropriate timing of surgery for patients with complex cyanotic lesions. However, poor nutrition and iron deficiency in a hypoxemic child can prevent this increase in hematocrit and may mislead the clinician into thinking the hypoxemia is less severe than it really is. A high hematocrit can result in increased blood viscosity, which can lead to spontaneous thrombosis and resultant cerebral, renal, or pulmonary infarctions. This process may be aggravated by the relative dehydration produced by a long period without oral intake. If the polycythemia is sufficiently severe (i.e., hematocrit is greater than 60% to 65%), phlebotomy may be required. Patients with cyanotic CHD are prone to develop coagulopathies because of platelet dysfunction and hypofibrinogenemia.

2. **White blood cell count.** Elevations in white blood cell count and a white blood cell shift in the differential should raise the suspicion of a systemic infection. Fever and upper respiratory infection must be ruled out. Children with elevated white blood cell counts should not be electively anesthetized, because immunologic function is compromised by CPB. Also, prosthetic material frequently is used in the surgical repair; if this material is inadvertently seeded by a bacteremia, the consequences may be disastrous.

3. **Coagulation studies.** Results of coagulation studies must be normal before CPB can be performed. A family history of bleeding tendencies should be sought. Unsuspected factor deficiencies have manifested and caused uncontrollable bleeding after surgery, when it may be difficult to identify the source of the problem.

4. **Electrolytes.** Electrolyte problems may be present in the newborn, especially if the child is receiving medication or total parenteral nutrition. Hypokalemia, hypomagnesemia, hypocalcemia, and hypoglycemia should be ruled out. Hypocalcemia is common in children with DiGeorge syndrome (a congenital disorder of the third and fourth branchial arches that is associated with thymic hypoplasia and congenital heart defects, especially aortic arch abnormalities or left-sided obstructive lesions).

5. **Glucose.** Hypoglycemia is especially common in infants with hypoplastic left-sided heart syndrome. The newborn's myocardium has an increased glucose dependence compared with the adult myocardium; thus, hypoglycemia may aggravate myocardial failure. As an aside, infant donor hearts for transplantation are best maintained with a high-glucose environment, before and after harvest. Hypoglycemia can occur because of reduced synthetic function, decreased glycogen stores, or reduced systemic perfusion resulting in compromised hepatic function. Under anesthesia, hypoglycemia will be masked and may be missed unless the clinician looks for it. Conversely, these children often come to the operating room with concentrated dextrose in their hyperalimentation solution. Steroids are commonly administered on CPB, and this combination can result in significant hyperglycemia. Substantial literature exists showing the detrimental effect of hyperglycemia during complete, incomplete, and focal cerebral ischemia in animals and adult humans. Specific data are lacking in children, although Steward et al. [2] suggested a worse neurologic outcome with hyperglycemia in a retrospective review of 34 children undergoing deep hypothermic circulatory arrest (DHCA). However, the Boston Circulatory Arrest Study suggested that normal blood glucose levels during reperfusion were associated with poorer neurologic outcome, whereas hyperglycemic levels appeared associated with better outcome [3]. It has been speculated that substrate deficiency in the immature brain may be an issue and that normal blood glucose levels during the reperfusion period after cerebral ischemia in infants may be insufficient for complete cerebral recovery.

6. **Digoxin.** Many children scheduled for heart surgery are receiving digoxin. After CPB, both a rebound increase in digoxin level and an increased sensitivity to the drug have been reported. Perioperative dysrhythmias are common and may be related to digoxin toxicity. Other factors may play a role in this enhanced toxicity, including hypokalemia, calcium fluxes, hypomagnesemia, and decreased creatinine clearance. Therefore, verify that the digoxin level is within the normal range and withhold digoxin preoperatively.

7. **Sickling test.** A sickling test should be performed in appropriate children. Hypothermia, acidosis, and anemia, as induced by CPB, decreased perfusion, and the bypass circuit itself enhance sickling if hemoglobin S is present. If the sickling test result is positive, hemoglobin electrophoresis should be performed to delineate the type of hemoglobinopathy. Depending on the type of defect, exchange transfusion may be indicated before or at the initiation of CPB.

8. **Electrocardiography.** The electrocardiogram shows great variability, especially during the first 24 hours of life. In some instances, the electrocardiogram is diagnostically helpful. For example, extreme left- or right-axis deviation with counterclockwise frontal vector and RV hypertrophy suggests a form of endocardial cushion defect.

9. **Echocardiography and cardiac catheterization.** Two-dimensional echocardiography with quantitative Doppler and color flow mapping has revolutionized the diagnosis of CHD. In many institutions, the technology has become so refined that most surgical procedures are performed on the basis of this study alone. Cardiac catheterization is used to confirm the diagnosis and to provide information concerning vascular resistance, the magnitude of shunts, and coronary anatomy.

10. **Chest radiography.** Chest radiography serves to evaluate the type and severity of the heart disease. It also is used to identify simulators of heart disease (e.g., meconium aspiration, mediastinal masses, pneumothorax, hyaline membrane disease, and diaphragmatic hernia) and to rule out significant pulmonary pathology.

C. *What should the anesthesiologist tell the family about risk?*

1. **Neurologic sequelae.** Morbidity and mortality vary with the lesion being repaired or palliated and with the institution involved. Ironically, as mortality has decreased, important morbidities have become more prominent. Neurologic sequelae remain one of the most common and potentially devastating complications of CHD and its repair. Early postoperative neurologic dysfunction may occur in as many as 25% of these children, with seizures occurring in approximately 20% of neonates after CPB. The seizures generally are self-limited, and some early series reported no long-term adverse sequelae. However, the group from Boston was the first to prospectively study a relatively homogeneous group of infants with TGV undergoing repair using either a predominantly low-flow CPB or DHCA strategy. They demonstrated that seizures are an important prognostic indicator of neurodevelopmental outcome [4]. The study also showed that there was a significantly higher incidence of seizures among infants randomized to circulatory arrest compared to those randomized to low-flow bypass. Follow-up of these children has shown a continuing important association between postoperative seizures and outcome, with an important decrement in cognitive and verbal skills assessments as well as motor skills [5]. Avoidance of circulatory arrest is not the entire solution to the problem, however, because the Boston group showed that there was a risk of seizures and suboptimal neurodevelopmental outcome even when continuous bypass was used.

Multiple factors contribute to the risk for neurodevelopmental sequelae. A complex interaction of preoperative, perioperative, and postoperative events can conspire to produce brain injury. Many children with CHD have preexisting brain malformations. Multiple chromosomal anomalies with combined cardiac and neurologic features have been described, the best known being Down syndrome (trisomy 21) and the catch–22 spectrum of conditions associated with microdeletions in the 22q11 region of chromosome 22. Neurologic manifestations of the catch–22 spectrum may be subtle early in life but become more apparent over time. The potential impact of this chromosomal anomaly is enormous, because monosomy 22q11 has an estimated prevalence of 5% to 10% in the population of children with CHD. Brain injury also may be acquired in the preoperative period. Abnormal cardiovascular function may be associated with poor brain growth, embolic infarction, cerebrovascular thrombosis, and abscess formation. Hopefully, earlier repair of children with CHD will limit this mechanism of brain injury. Hypoxic-ischemic/reperfusion or embolic injury are thought to be the principal mechanisms of brain injury occurring in the intraoperative period [6]. Injury also can occur in the postoperative period, during which unstable hemodynamics and increased cerebral energy needs may result in a mismatch of oxygen supply and demand to the brain. Intensive research is ongoing in this area of brain injury to try to prevent this devastating problem.

D. *When should oral intake stop?*

Nil per os (NPO) guidelines used for other infants and children generally can be used in patients with CHD. Recent evidence suggests that clear liquids can be continued until 2 to 4 hours before surgery. In children with *cyanotic* heart disease, meticulous attention must be paid to the patient's state of hydration. Specifically, orders must be written to awaken the child 2 hours before surgery to offer clear liquids. If uncertainty exists concerning the precise time of surgery, place an intravenous catheter and begin an infusion to prevent dehydration in patients with cyanotic heart disease.

E. *Which sedation is appropriate?*

The need for sedation must be individualized, but certain guidelines can be offered. A thorough explanation to the patient and family is in order, because the parents' anxiety often is transmitted to the child. Neonates and infants younger than 6 months rarely require any sedation, because separation anxiety is not an issue. In older children, if intravenous access already is established and the child's parents are allowed to accompany him or her to the preoperative holding area, additional sedation may be unnecessary, because incremental intravenous agents can be titrated before transfer to the operating room.

Children between the ages of 1 and 5 years benefit most from judicious sedation. A variety of agents and routes can be used. I prefer to avoid intramuscular injections and use either intravenous or oral midazolam. If given intravenously, I titrate in 0.1- to 0.25-mg increments; if given orally, I give 0.5 mg/kg. Patient acceptance is improved if the drug is offered in sweetened apple juice. An oral dose of 0.5 mg/kg typically results in easy separation from the parents at 15 to 30 minutes. If given intranasally, 0.2 mg/kg will be effective at about 10 to 15 minutes. These patients must be monitored when sedation is given. Pulse oximetry and careful observation are mandatory, because the hemodynamic status may be adversely and unpredictably affected if hypercarbia or hypoxemia occurs.

Some physicians routinely administer anticholinergics preoperatively. Others give atropine in the operating room only if clinically necessary. Keep in mind that slow heart rates often are not tolerated in infants whose stroke volume is relatively fixed.

F. *When does the patient need intravenous infusions?*

Children who require vasoactive infusions preoperatively come to the operating room with such access already available. For others, the timing of intravenous access is strictly up to the anesthesiologist involved. For many cases, a gentle inhalation induction with subsequent expeditious venous catheter placement before intubation is appropriate. Again, if the timing of surgery is uncertain, preoperative intravenous catheter placement is desirable to avoid dehydration, especially in children with cyanotic heart disease.

G. *When is prostaglandin E_1 indicated?*

PGE_1 is indicated whenever it is thought that maintaining, reopening, or enlarging an existing ductus arteriosus will benefit the neonate. Common situations in which it is used include the presence of (a) lesions with decreased pulmonary blood flow; (b) TGV; and (c) left-sided heart outflow obstruction.

With TGV, the response to PGE_1 is variable, but in some infants, mixing of systemic and pulmonary circulation improves sufficiently to reduce hypoxemia slightly and to relieve acidosis. With left-sided heart outflow obstruction (e.g., hypoplastic left-sided heart syndrome, coarctation) PGE₁ will open the ductus and allow right-to-left flow across it, improving systemic perfusion and perhaps even coronary blood flow. It also may dilate the pulmonary vascular bed.

Stabilization of the infant before surgical intervention and improved outcome often result from PGE₁ infusion. Side effects include apneic spells, seizures, systemic hypotension, inhibition of platelet aggregation, peripheral edema, and unexplained fever. Cortical proliferation in long bones can occur with chronic use. Because PGE₁ is metabolized rapidly, it must be infused continuously, usually at a dose of 0.05 to 0.1 µg/kg/min. As much as 80% of circulating PGE₁ is metabolized in one pass through the lungs; thus, the ductal response diminishes within minutes after its discontinuation.

IV. Equipment and infusions
A. *What is required?*

Care for an infant undergoing heart surgery demands meticulous attention to detail and extreme vigilance. A well-thought-out plan should be developed before induction so that all equipment needed is available and in working order (Table 14.3).

1. **Anesthetic and surgical considerations.** The anesthesia machine and circuit should be checked as for all procedures. Multiple sizes of endotracheal tubes, masks, and laryngoscope blades must be available. Appropriate equipment to keep the infant warm may be needed, including a heating/cooling blanket, radiant warming lights, a fluid warmer, and a heated humidifier. A working operating room table that allows optimal positioning to facilitate surgical exposure is required. A defibrillator with both nonsterile (external) and sterile (internal) paddles, a dual-chamber pacemaker generator, a cardiac output computer, and a coagulation analyzer must be operational. A fibrillator frequently is needed intraoperatively to induce ventricular fibrillation during open chamber procedures.

2. **Monitoring.** Equipment needed to monitor the patient includes a pulse oximeter, a hemodynamic monitor, appropriate catheters for arterial and venous cannulation, transducers (zeroed and calibrated to mercury), a blood pressure cuff, a stethoscope, thermistors, and a mixed venous oxygen saturation monitor. Equipment used to monitor central nervous system function may include electroencephalography (EEG), transcranial Doppler (TCD), jugular venous saturation monitoring, and near-infrared spectroscopy. Transesophageal echocardiography has become an extraordinarily valuable tool for diagnostic purposes (confirmation and delineation of anatomy, detection of unsuspected defects or residual defects after repair) and for ventricular function and volume monitoring.

3. **Intravenous fluids.** Two intravenous fluid sets should be prepared, and all air bubbles should be removed from the tubing. This task is made easier if one begins with warm fluid; microbubble formation seems to occur less frequently than if cold fluid is allowed to warm when the room temperature is raised. All

Table 14.3 Equipment used during pediatric cardiac surgery

Heating/cooling blanket
Radiant warming lights
Fluid warmer
Heated humidifier
Defibrillator (external, internal)
Pacemaker generator
Cardiac output computer
Coagulation analyzer
Fibrillator
Infusion pumps
Transesophageal echocardiography

From Davies LK. Anesthesia for pediatric cardiovascular surgery. In: Kirby RR, Gravenstein N, Lobato EB, et al., eds. *Clinical anesthesia practice*. Philadelphia: WB Saunders, 2002:1219, with permission.

intravenous and monitoring tubing must be bubble-free whenever a potential shunt is present, because intracardiac shunts can be bidirectional and may become right-to-left during surgery. Air filters can be used, but the same amount of effort must be expended to remove air from intravenous tubing, because air filters cannot be relied on to trap all air. Another drawback to air filters is that they slow down intravenous infusions significantly and may make it difficult to keep up with volume replacement.

A method to carefully control and limit intravenous fluid intake is important, because many patients have barely compensated excess pulmonary blood flow and volume. Infusion using a limited amount in a buret chamber and a minidripper, use of infusion pumps with set volumes, or administration of fluid via syringe in bolus increments are methods that can be used to limit intake. At least three infusion pumps that allow accurate titration of vasoactive drugs should be available.

4. **Preparation of infusions.** Appropriate intravenous solutions for mixing infusions (e.g., normal saline and 5% dextrose in water) and cassettes for the pumps should be on hand. Common infusions to be available on short notice include sodium nitroprusside, epinephrine, isoproterenol, dopamine, and amrinone or milrinone.

Some thought should be given to the appropriate concentrations for the patient's body size so that fluid overload can be minimized. In general, I find it useful to mix the infusions such that a starting dose infuses at about 2 to 3 mL/hour. In the following example for sodium nitroprusside, I solve for "concentration" so that my infusion pump rate is approximately 2 to 3 mL/hour.

$$\text{Rate (2–3 mL/hr)} = \frac{\mu g/kg/min \times weight\ (kg) \times 60\ min/hr}{\text{Concentration } (\mu g/mL)}$$

If the patient weighs 10 kg and a starting dose of 1 $\mu g/(kg \cdot min)$ is desired, the formula is:

$$3\ mL/hr = \frac{1\ \mu g/kg/min \times 10\ kg \times 60\ min/hr}{200\ \mu g/mL}$$

Therefore, I would mix 50 mg of sodium nitroprusside in 250 mL of diluent for a final concentration of 200 μ/mL and begin my infusion at 3 mL/hour. Table 14.4 lists commonly used drugs and bolus doses or initial infusion rates.

In general, infusions are not prepared unless they are needed. Instead, commonly needed drugs are mixed in syringes so that a small bolus can be given if required. If needed repetitively, an infusion is mixed. Table 14.5 lists drugs that should be available in syringes at the beginning of each pediatric cardiac surgical case. A narcotic, a benzodiazepine, and a muscle relaxant also should be on hand for ready use.

5. **Blood and blood products.** Blood products appropriate to the particular procedure and patient size should be readied in advance. Preparation may range from typing and screening for simple procedures to typing and cross-matching of multiple units of blood or platelets (or both) and fresh frozen plasma for complex pump cases. At the University of Florida, infants younger than 4 months undergo typing and screening and then preferentially receive type O blood without a cross-match because the risk of transfusion reaction is low.

Transfusion-acquired cytomegalovirus infection generally is a benign entity in immunocompetent patients who receive blood. However, immunologically immature patients (especially low-birth-weight infants) can become symptomatic if infected. Therefore, our routine is to use cytomegalovirus-negative blood products in children younger than 4 months. For infants with aortic arch abnormalities, blood products should be irradiated, because these cardiac lesions may be associated with DiGeorge syndrome. Such patients may have an absent thymus and increased susceptibility to graft-versus-host disease after transfusion.

Table 14.4 Nonanesthetic drugs and dosages[a]

	Drug	Dose
Inotropic infusions	Epinephrine	0.01–0.1 µg/kg/min
	Isoproterenol	0.01–0.1 µg/kg/min
	Norepinephrine	0.01–0.1 µg/kg/min
	Dopamine	2–10 µg/kg/min
	Dobutamine	2–10 µg/kg/min
	Amrinone[b]	2–2.5 mg/kg bolus divided over 30–60 min, followed by 5–20 µg/kg/min infusion
	Milrinone	50 µg/kg bolus, followed by 0.4–0.8 µg/kg/min infusion
Vasodilator infusions	Nitroglycerin	1–2 µg/kg/min
	Nitroprusside	1–5 µg/kg/min
	Aminophylline	0.5 mg/kg slowly, followed by 0.5–1 mg/kg/h infusion[c]
	Prostaglandin E_1	0.05–0.1 µg/kg/min
	Labetalol	10–100 mg/h
Antiarrhythmic drugs	Lidocaine	1 mg/kg bolus 0.03 mg/kg/min infusion
	Adenosine	0.15 mg/kg bolus
	Procainamide	2 mg/kg over 5 min
	Dilantin	2–4 mg/kg over 5 min
	Bretylium	5 mg/kg bolus
	Amiodarone	5 mg/kg over 1 hr., then 5 mg/kg over 12 hours. Repeat as needed.
β-Blocking drugs	Propranolol	0.01–0.1 mg/kg
	Esmolol	0.5–1 mg/kg bolus 100–300 µg/kg/min infusion
Others	Calcium chloride	10–20 mg/kg
	Sodium bicarbonate	1 mEq/kg (or as determined by base deficit)
	Phenylephrine	1–10 µg/kg
	Ephedrine	0.05–0.2 mg/kg
	Heparin	≥3 mg/kg (300 U/kg)
	Protamine	≥3 mg/kg

[a] The dose of each drug varies with the clinical context.
[b] Cannot be mixed in dextrose-containing solutions.
[c] Maintenance rate determined by plasma levels.
From Davies LK. Anesthesia for pediatric cardiovascular surgery. In: Kirby RR, Gravenstein N, Lobato EB, et al., eds. *Clinical anesthesia practice.* Philadelphia: WB Saunders, 2002:1220, with permission.

V. Anesthetic induction and maintenance
A. *Which monitors are needed before induction?*
No absolute rule exists for determining the amount of monitoring necessary before induction. In some patients, particularly if a "steal" induction is ideal, anesthesia can be started with just a pulse oximeter and a precordial stethoscope. Then, as the patient is induced, electrocardiography and blood pressure monitoring can be quickly established. In others, it may be preferable to begin with all monitors (even invasive ones) in place. Generally, arterial and central venous catheters are placed after induction, although occasionally they may need to be placed before the procedure.
B. *When does a patient need intravenous access before induction?*
The timing of intravenous access, as noted previously, often is a matter of personal preference. However, polycythemic patients must be well hydrated either by

Table 14.5 Bolus drugs available in syringes

Drug	Syringe concentration	Bolus dose
Calcium chloride	100 mg/mL	10–20 mg/kg
Epinephrine	10 µg/mL	0.2–1 µg/kg (inotropy)
	100 µg/mL	10–100 µg/kg (cardiac arrest)
Isoproterenol	20 µg/mL	1–10 µg
Phenylephrine	100 µg/mL	1–10 µg/kg
Lidocaine	20 mg/mL	1 mg/kg
Esmolol[a]	10 mg/mL	0.5–1 mg/kg
Heparin	1,000 U/mL	300 U/kg (cardiopulmonary bypass)
		100 U/kg (vascular nonpump)
Atropine	0.4 mg/mL	0.01–0.02 mg/kg
Succinylcholine	20 mg/mL	1–2 mg/kg
Ephedrine	5 mg/mL	0.05–0.2 mg/kg
Sodium thiopental	25 mg/mL	3–5 mg/kg
Pancuronium	1 mg/mL	0.1–0.15 mg/kg (intubation)

[a] Available for treatment of hypercyanotic spells in patients with tetralogy of Fallot.
From Davies LK. Anesthesia for pediatric cardiovascular surgery. In: Kirby RR, Gravenstein N, Lobato EB, et al., eds. *Clinical anesthesia practice.* Philadelphia: WB Saunders, 2002:1220, with permission.

mouth or intravenously. Children with extremely poor cardiac function who require inotropes may not tolerate an inhalation induction; thus, an intravenous induction is preferred. Most other pediatric patients tolerate a judicious inhalation induction with subsequent placement of intravenous catheters.

If myocardial reserve is impaired, a high-dose inhalation technique cannot be used for long; once catheters are placed, a transition is made either to a completely intravenous narcotic technique or to a combination of intravenous and inhalation techniques. If the anesthesiologist is uncertain about his or her ability to place an intravenous catheter rapidly during an inhalation induction, it should be inserted before induction.

C. *How does cardiac disease affect the rate of induction?*
  1. **Inhalation agents.** Intracardiac shunting can alter the uptake of inhalation anesthetics. The final effect on rate of induction depends on the size and direction of the shunt and the patient's cardiac output. A right-to-left intracardiac shunt prolongs induction, because the uptake of anesthetic into the blood occurs more slowly. If high concentrations of agents are used to speed induction and a relative anesthetic overdose occurs, it is difficult to remedy, because the inhalation agents are slow to be eliminated. A left-to-right shunt generally has a negligible effect on the speed of induction if the systemic perfusion is preserved at a normal level.
  2. **Intravenous agents.** Response to intravenously administered drugs is faster with a right-to-left shunt because the dilution effect and the pulmonary transit time are reduced in proportion to the magnitude of the shunt. A left-to-right shunt has a minimal effect on the response to intravenous drugs if systemic perfusion is preserved.
D. *What problems are likely to occur during induction?*
  Any number of untoward events can occur during induction of anesthesia in pediatric patients with heart disease.
  1. **Airway obstruction.** Airway obstruction is poorly tolerated in these patients, especially small infants or those with cyanotic heart disease. The margin for error is extremely small and minor problems can quickly become life threatening. Airway obstruction that causes hypoxemia or hypercarbia increases PVR. A reversal of a left-to-right intracardiac shunt or aggravation of

a right-to-left shunt may result, exacerbating the problem and creating a vicious cycle.

2. **Dysrhythmias.** The patient may become bradycardic or develop a nodal rhythm with induction. Because stroke volume is relatively fixed, cardiac output suffers in this context. Acidosis can occur quickly when perfusion is marginal; this further depresses myocardial contractility, increasing PVR and decreasing SVR.

Dysrhythmias can result from many causes, including light anesthesia, hypoxemia, hypercarbia, drugs, and electrolyte abnormalities.

Significant potential problems may occur during central venous access acquisition. The drapes or patient position may serve to kink the endotracheal tube as it warms to body temperature. Dysrhythmias during this phase generally are induced mechanically from the catheter or guidewire. Familiarity with the lengths of the catheter kit components makes insertion to excessive depth less likely. Mechanically induced dysrhythmias respond better to removal of the stimulus than to pharmacologic therapy.

E. *Which anesthetic technique should the anesthesiologist use?*

The choice of drug(s) is not as important as an understanding of the lesion's pathophysiology. Of help is the development of hemodynamic goals for each patient in terms of heart rate, contractility, preload, SVR, and PVR (Table 14.6). In several lesions, overriding considerations dominate. An appropriate approach for a patient with aortic insufficiency may be completely different than that for a patient with tetralogy of Fallot. Once the goals are defined, appropriate agents, dosages, and routes of administration can be selected. Many agents can be used so long as they are administered in a thoughtful fashion.

F. *How should the patient be positioned?*

Data are scarce regarding the safest way to position a patient for heart surgery. The major issues are prevention of brachial plexus injury and optimal patient access. I find it useful to place the patient in a supine position on a heating blanket

Table 14.6 Cardiac grid for common congenital heart diseases (desired hemodynamic changes)

	Preload	PVR	SVR	HR	Contractility
Atrial septal defect	↑	↑	↓	N	N
Ventricular septal defect (right-to-left)	N	↓	↑	N	N
Ventricular septal defect (left-to-right)	↑	↑	↓	N	N
Idiopathic hypertrophic subaortic stenosis	↑	N	N–↑	↓[a]	↓[a]
Patent ductus arteriosus	↑	↑	↓	N	N
Coarctation	↑	N	↓	N	N
Valvular pulmonic stenosis	↑	↓	N	↓	↑
Infundibular pulmonary stenosis	↑	↓	N	↓	↓[a]
Aortic stenosis	↑	N	↑[a]	↓[a]	N–↑
Mitral stenosis	↑	N–↓	N	↓[a]	N–↑
Aortic regurgitation	↑	N	↓	N–↑	N–↑
Mitral regurgitation	↑	N–↓	↓	N–↑	N–↑

[a] An overriding consideration.

HR, heart rate; N, normal or no change; PVR, pulmonary vascular resistance; SVR, systemic vascular resistance.

From Moore RA. Anesthesia for the pediatric congenital heart patient for noncardiac surgery. *Anesthesiol Rev* 1981;8:27, with permission.

covered with a thin sheet and to abduct the upper arms 90 degrees with the hands above the head to allow easy access to, and inspection of, arterial and venous cannulation sites. The shoulders and elbows are supported at an angle of about 30 degrees above the table by a "wedge" cushion in order to lessen the danger of any stretch on the brachial plexus.

Access to the patient's head is crucial for visual inspection to rule out superior vena cava syndrome, for pupil evaluation, and for airway manipulation. A piece of eggcrate foam can be placed under the patient's head to minimize the chance of pressure necrosis; many heart surgery cases are lengthy, and low perfusion pressure occurs during CPB. However, because infants have such large occiputs, elevation of the head in this way occasionally may result in encroachment on the surgical field.

VI. Monitoring

Anesthetic induction generally proceeds with noninvasive monitors. A five-lead electrocardiograph is used to facilitate detection of rhythm disturbances and myocardial ischemia. An esophageal lead also can be used to more easily diagnose dysrhythmias, especially when tachycardia is present. Lead V_5 can be placed in its normal position and covered with an adhesive drape to protect it from the surgical scrub solutions. The monitor mode of the electrocardiograph will minimize baseline drift, whereas the diagnostic mode allows better resolution of the P and T waves.

A. *When is an arterial catheter indicated?*

An indwelling arterial catheter is required whenever continuous monitoring of arterial pressure or frequent blood sampling is necessary. All procedures using CPB require placement of an arterial catheter, because noninvasive methods are not useful if no pulsatile flow is present. Most closed heart procedures also benefit from beat-to-beat monitoring of arterial pressure.

The arterial catheter is placed after intubation, preferably percutaneously in the nondominant radial artery. Other sites commonly used include the dorsalis pedis, posterior tibial, femoral, and, occasionally, temporal arteries. A surgical cutdown is used only as a last resort because of the disproportionately high incidence of thrombosis and infection. For coarctation repairs, the arterial catheter must be placed in the right radial artery; if this is unsuccessful, the catheter can be placed in a temporal artery. In patients with a Blalock–Taussig shunt, the catheter must be placed on the side opposite the Blalock–Taussig shunt or in a lower extremity artery. A 22- or 24-gauge catheter is used, depending on the child's size.

B. *When is central venous access needed?*

1. **Central venous catheters.** Central venous access is established routinely when knowledge of right-sided heart filling pressure trends or the need to administer vasoactive drugs rapidly is desirable. Access to the central circulation also allows placement of PA or pacing catheters. The decision as to which type and size of catheter should be used depends on the type of operation performed and on the size and clinical status of the patient.

   A central venous catheter is used routinely in patients undergoing CPB. Monitoring superior vena caval pressure during extracorporeal circulation is useful for assessing adequacy of venous drainage, particularly when two venous cannulas are used. A central catheter with at least two lumens allows drug and fluid delivery via one lumen and uninterrupted central venous pressure measurements via the other.

   My guidelines for catheter length and size are listed in Table 14.7. Follow-up verification of appropriate catheter position occurs on review of the postoperative chest film.

2. **PA catheters.** Monitoring of PA pressure is helpful when PVR is problematic. Placement of the PA catheter can be accomplished percutaneously or by the surgeon using a direct transthoracic approach. If the patient's size is too small to accept a balloon flotation catheter, a combined percutaneous and direct intraoperative approach can be used. In this scenario, the catheter is placed through a sterility sheath into the introducer and advanced into the superior vena cava. When the chest and heart are open, the surgeon can advance the catheter into the proximal PA. In complex cardiac anomalies with shunts, the

Table 14.7 Guidelines for central venous pressure catheter size and length in relationship to patient size

Patient weight (kg)	Internal jugular catheter size[a]	CVP catheter length (cm)
<2.5	3 Fr SL or 4 Fr DL	5
2.5–5.0	4 Fr DL or 5 Fr DL	5
5–10	5 Fr DL or 5 Fr introducer	8
10–20	5 Fr DL or 6 Fr introducer	8–12
>20	5–7 Fr DL or 6 Fr introducer	12–15

[a] Catheter size also is influenced by operative procedure. If significant blood loss is anticipated and peripheral venous access is limited, a larger size central venous pressure (CVP) catheter may be preferred.
DL, double-lumen; Fr, French; SL, single-lumen.
From Davies LK. Anesthesia for pediatric cardiovascular surgery. In: Kirby RR, Gravenstein N, Lobato EB, et al., eds. *Clinical anesthesia practice*. Philadelphia: WB Saunders, 2002:1222, with permission.

surgeon generally will thread the percutaneously placed PA catheter into position at the end of the surgical procedure, because the catheter often is in the field of repair.

Continuous mixed venous oximetry is available with selected PA catheters and may be helpful in titrating vasoactive infusions, in providing an early warning of deteriorating cardiac output, and in assessing residual shunts. The patient's size must be large enough to accommodate a 5 to 6 Fr introducer to facilitate percutaneous placement of a PA catheter.

Smaller infants requiring PA pressure monitoring will have transthoracic PA catheters placed at the close of surgery. The PA catheter also is useful postoperatively to assess pressure gradients by carefully measuring pullback pressures upon its removal. Some PA catheters allow measurement of cardiac output by thermodilution; however, this method is not used often in small children because of the significant fluid load it imposes on the patient.

3. **Left atrial catheters.** Left atrial pressure monitoring commonly is used in patients with CHD because disparities in left- and right-sided heart function often are present. This catheter is inserted by the surgeon at the end of repair, usually via the right superior pulmonary vein. One must be careful with its use; the risk of systemic embolization of clot or air is real because the catheter is in the left side of the heart. The risk of bleeding and cardiac tamponade is present when the catheter is removed.

C. *Where should temperature be measured?*

The optimal site for temperature monitoring during cardiac cases is controversial; remember that gradients exist between various sites (Fig. 14.3). Commonly used are the esophagus, nasopharynx, rectum, tympanic membrane, blood, and bladder. Temperature monitoring is important because the rate of cooling and rewarming appears to be important in the production of brain injury. Monitoring in at least two sites is advisable to ensure that the temperature gradient between inflow (blood temperature) and bladder or rectal temperature does not exceed 10°C and that uniform cooling and warming has occurred.

D. *How do end-tidal and arterial carbon dioxide pressures correlate?*

Monitoring of end-tidal carbon dioxide partial pressure ($P_{ET}CO_2$) is useful to corroborate tracheal intubation. The arterial to end-tidal carbon dioxide partial pressure difference [$P_{(a-ET)}CO_2$] can be increased in patients with cardiopulmonary disease. It also may be increased in small children, depending on the sampling site and ventilatory pattern. Patients with CHD have altered ventilation/perfusion ratios; this produces abnormalities of both the physiologic dead space to tidal volume ratio (VDS/VT) and venous admixture (Qs/Qt).

In patients with cyanotic heart disease, in which Qs/Qt can be large, $P_{ET}CO_2$ significantly underestimates P_aCO_2. Because intracardiac shunting often is dynamic, the $P_{(a-ET)}CO_2$ is ever changing; thus, even $P_{ET}CO_2$ trends are not reliable in these

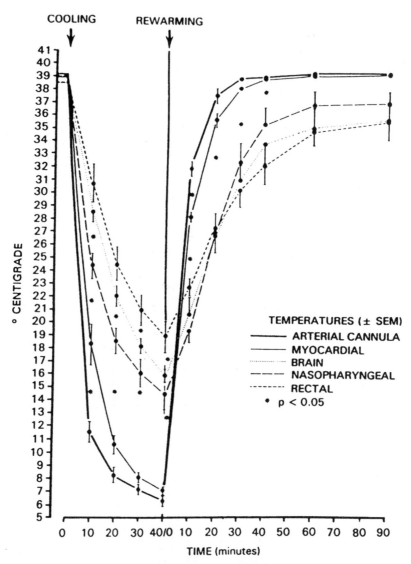

FIG. 14.3 Average temperature (± SEM) of arterial cannula, myocardium, cerebral cortex, nasopharynx, and rectum during 40 minutes of cooling and 90 minutes of rewarming during cardiopulmonary bypass in six pigs. (From Stefaniszyn HJ, Novick RJ, Keith FM, et al. Is the brain adequately cooled during deep hypothermic cardiopulmonary bypass? *Curr Surg.* 1983;40:294, with permission.)

patients. Periodic measurement of P_aCO_2 is necessary to document adequate ventilation. $P_{ET}CO_2$ monitoring during PA banding reflects the decrease in pulmonary blood flow. As the band is tightened, the $P_{(a-ET)}CO_2$ gradient increases.

E. *How should blood gases be managed on cardiopulmonary bypass?*

The strategy of management of the pH has received considerable attention over the past few years. Blood gas management strategy may be more important in children because greater degrees of hypothermia are used, resulting in more profound differences in blood carbon dioxide levels. Briefly, there are two schools of thought regarding carbon dioxide management. In the alpha-stat strategy, no carbon dioxide is added to the circuit, and electrochemical neutrality is maintained with the blood gas measurement not corrected to temperature (i.e., reported at 37°C). Enzymatic function is well maintained in this milieu. In contrast, with the pH-stat strategy, carbon dioxide is added to the system to maintain a constant pH over varying temperatures. Blood gases are temperature corrected and reported at actual body temperature. In this scenario, hydrogen ions accumulate, total carbon dioxide stores are elevated, and the microcirculatory pH becomes increasingly acidotic at deep hypothermic temperatures. It initially was believed that intracellular pH also became increasingly acidotic, but more recent data have shown that the intracellular pH changes only slightly [7].

Evidence in adults suggests that either carbon dioxide management on CPB does not matter or that an alpha-stat strategy is advantageous. Recently, randomized prospective studies of adults using moderate hypothermia showed that postoperative neurologic or neuropsychologic outcome is slightly, but consistently, better with alpha-stat management [8].

Although acid–base management probably is not as important when moderate hypothermic temperatures are used, it may be critical in the setting of deep hypothermia. Investigations have been performed to try to understand the correct acid–base management approach in children, but controversy remains. Proponents of the alpha-stat method suggest that the luxuriously high blood flows seen with pH-stat management may put the brain at risk for damage due to microemboli, cerebral edema, or high intracranial pressure, or it may predispose to an adverse redistribution of blood flow ("steal") away from marginally perfused areas in patients with cerebrovascular disease. On the other hand, proponents of the pH-stat strategy suggest that enhanced CBF may be helpful in improving cerebral cooling before the initiation of circulatory arrest. Total CBF is increased, global cerebral cooling is enhanced, and a redistribution of brain blood flow occurs during pH-stat management. An increased proportion of CBF is distributed to deep brain structures (thalamus, brainstem, and cerebellum) when pH-stat management is used [9]. However, other data suggest that cerebral metabolic recovery after circulatory arrest may be better with the alpha-stat method than with the pH-stat mode. This variation in results has led some authors to advocate a crossover strategy, that is, using a pH-stat approach during the first 10 minutes of cooling to provide maximal cerebral metabolic suppression followed by a change to alpha-stat strategy to remove the severe acidosis that accumulates during profound hypothermia with the use of pH-stat. This approach appears to offer maximal metabolic recovery in animals (Fig. 14.4) [10]. Choice of acid–base management may be particularly important in the subgroup of patients with aortopulmonary collaterals where cerebral cooling is problematic. It appears that addition of carbon dioxide during cooling enhances cerebral perfusion and improves cerebral metabolic recovery [11]. A recent, randomized, single-center trial in human infants younger than 9 months found that those managed with a pH-stat strategy generally had better outcomes than those in the alpha-stat group [12]. The pH-stat infants had a significantly shorter recovery time to first EEG activity and a tendency to fewer EEG-manifested seizures. In the subset of transposition babies, those assigned to pH-stat tended to have a higher cardiac index despite a lower requirement for inotropic agents, less frequent acidosis and hypotension, and a shorter duration of mechanical ventilation and intensive care unit stay. The data suggest that pH-stat management may enhance systemic and cerebral protection in this group of patients.

Why the apparent difference in outcome between adults and children relative to pH management? It may be related to differences in the mechanism of brain injury on CPB. In adults, emboli appear to play a prominent role in adverse neurologic outcome. It is postulated that the decrease in CBF associated with alpha-stat management might be protective by limiting cerebral microemboli. On the other hand, the mechanism of injury in children may relate more to hypoperfusion or activation of excitotoxic pathways [13]. If a pH-stat strategy is used, the increase in

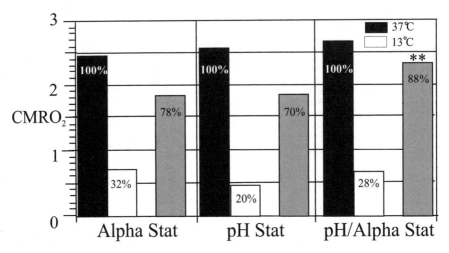

FIG. 14.4 Effects of three different cooling strategies: α-stat, pH-stat, and a cross-over of pH-stat followed by α-stat on cerebral metabolic suppression before deep hypothermia and circulatory arrest (DHCA) and recovery of cerebral metabolism after DHCA. The pH-stat strategy provides better metabolic suppression before DHCA than α-stat, but cerebral metabolic recovery after DHCA is poor. Initial cooling with a pH-stat strategy followed by conversion to α-stat before DHCA results in the greatest cerebral metabolic recovery after DHCA. *Solid black bar*, 37°C; *white bar*, 13°C; *gray bar*, after DHCA. (From Kern FH, Greeley WJ. pH-stat management of blood gases is not preferable to α-stat in patients undergoing brain cooling for cardiac surgery. *J Cardiothorac Vasc Anesth* 1995;9:215, with permission.)

CBF may be beneficial in ensuring complete brain cooling and slowing oxygen consumption, thus increasing the brain's tolerance for DHCA.

F. *How should the central nervous system be monitored?*

Central nervous system insults associated with cardiac surgery remain an unsolved problem. Brain damage can occur as a result of global hypoxia-ischemia or focal emboli. EEG has been used to try to provide a measure of cerebral electrical activity and function during cardiac surgery. Unfortunately, the EEG may not be reliable in predicting or preventing brain ischemia during CPB because of the effects of hypothermia and anesthetic agents and because of the likelihood of focal embolic injury. Newer, computerized, processed EEG monitors are less cumbersome and allow easier recognition of trends and abrupt changes. The advantage of EEG is that it can be obtained in patients of any age or size with no risk and may be effective in detecting catastrophic events causing global ischemia. EEG also can be useful for assessing adequacy of cerebral cooling by ensuring electrocerebral silence before circulatory arrest.

CBF has been measured using the Fick principle and xenon Xe 133 clearance. Unfortunately, this technique does not provide continuous measurement of CBF and is more applicable to the research setting rather than clinical care. TCD sonography uses the Doppler principle to detect shifts in frequency of reflected signals from blood in motion to calculate flow velocity. Because it is thought that the diameters of the large cerebral arteries insonated are relatively constant, trends in flow velocity should pattern those of CBF. Thus, even though quantitative measurement of CBF cannot be made from TCD, qualitative inferences may be appropriate. TCD can provide an indirect measure of cerebral vascular resistance (which is increased with elevated intracranial pressure or markedly elevated central venous pressure). TCD can be helpful in detecting suboptimally placed cannulae, because distortion of the superior vena cava can result in an impediment to cerebral venous drainage. TCD also is useful for detecting cerebral emboli. At present, the technology does not allow determination of emboli type (air vs. particulate) or size.

Cerebral metabolism has been estimated by monitoring jugular venous bulb saturation, the cerebral equivalent of "mixed venous" blood. A low saturation suggests an elevation in cerebral metabolism outstripping the cerebral oxygen provided. However, this blood is the effluent from many areas of the brain and regional areas of cerebral hypoperfusion can easily be missed. Near-infrared spectroscopy is a noninvasive method of monitoring brain oxygen saturation (cerebral oximetry). Its noninvasiveness is appealing, but it also suffers from the drawback that it only reflects global perfusion.

Because neurologic morbidity is such an issue, I believe neurologic monitoring will become more prevalent and techniques will be refined over the next decade. Anesthesiologists will become more skilled in "pattern recognition" of scenarios that require intervention.

G. *What is the role of echocardiography?*

Perioperative echocardiography is increasingly used in many centers for pediatric cardiac surgery. Both epicardial and, more recently, transesophageal studies have been performed to better define cardiac anatomy and assess surgical repair. Technologic improvements allow better imaging, smaller probe size, and multiplane capability, thereby substantially increasing the information provided by this modality. Several studies have demonstrated that two-dimensional and Doppler color flow imaging can demonstrate previously unappreciated anatomic details and allow assessment of quality of repair and ventricular function after bypass. The ultimate role of echocardiography in the operating room and intensive care unit is still evolving and will hinge on demonstration of improvement in outcome in these patients.

VII. Cardiopulmonary bypass

A. *How does it differ in children?*

The physiology of extracorporeal circulation is similar in adults and children. However, significant differences in technique are applied to infants and small children (Table 14.8). Smaller cannulas are used in children, but proportionally they may be so large that they obstruct venous drainage into the heart or arterial outflow

Table 14.8 Differences in adult versus pediatric cardiopulmonary bypass

Parameter	Adult	Pediatric
Hypothermic temperature	Rarely below 25°–32° C	Commonly 15°–20°C
Use of total circulatory arrest	Rare	Common
Pump prime		
Dilution effects on blood volume	25%–33%	200%–300%
Additional additives in pediatric primes		Blood, albumin
Perfusion pressures	Typically 50–80 mm Hg	20–50 mm Hg
Influence of pH management strategy	Minimal at moderate hypothermia	Marked at deep hypothermia
Measured P_aCO_2 differences	30–45 mm Hg	20–80 mm Hg
Glucose regulation		
Hypoglycemia	Rare; requires significant hepatic injury	Common; reduced hepatic glycogen stores
Hyperglycemia	Frequent; generally easily controlled with insulin	Less common; rebound hypoglycemia may occur

Modified from Kern FH, Schulman SR, Lawson DS, et al. Extracorporeal circulation and circulatory assist devices in the pediatric patient. In Lake C, ed. *Pediatric cardiac anesthesia,* 3rd ed. Stamford, CT: Appleton & Lange, 1998:219–257.

from it before institution of bypass or after its discontinuation. Almost all cardiac repairs in children necessitate the use of dual venous cannulas so that all venous blood can be diverted to the bypass circuit and the heart can be opened to allow repair of the intracardiac defect.

1. **Profound hypothermia and total circulatory arrest.** An alternative method used in very small children with complex heart disease is profound hypothermia and total circulatory arrest. This technique uses a single venous drainage cannula during the period of cooling. When a core temperature of about 15° to 20°C is reached, the pump is stopped and the venous cannula removed. The major advantage of this technique is that it provides excellent exposure without cannulas or blood in the operative field. Deep hypothermia also enhances myocardial protection, decreases CPB time, and decreases blood trauma. The Boston Circulatory Arrest Study showed that the use of circulatory arrest is associated with a higher risk of seizures. There was a strong correlation between duration of circulatory arrest and the occurrence of seizures. Seizures in the perioperative period significantly increased the risk of both lower IQ scores and neurologic abnormalities [14]. Based on this study, most centers have minimized the use of DHCA; when it must be used, make every effort to limit its duration to less than 35 to 40 minutes.

2. **Venous drainage.** Venous drainage problems are more common in children than in adults. The inferior vena cava is quite short, and inadvertent cannulation of the hepatic veins is possible. If this occurs, marked engorgement of the splanchnic vessels can result in mesenteric ischemia. Problems with superior vena cava drainage are possible, especially if a left superior vena cava is present. Occlusion of this vessel causes significant venous hypertension; it must be cannulated or cerebral ischemia may result. Careful attention should be paid to superior vena cava pressure by frequent inspection of the head. The upper venous cannula can easily be kinked or drainage otherwise impaired with retraction of the heart.

3. **Systemic-to-PA shunt occlusion.** When CPB is first initiated, the surgeon must quickly occlude any systemic-to-PA shunts (e.g., PDA or Blalock–Taussig shunt). Otherwise, continued perfusion of these shunts will lead to underperfusion of the systemic circulation, possible hemorrhagic edema of the lungs, and continued pulmonary venous return with possible overdistention of the left side of the heart.

4. **Perfusion flow and pressure.** CPB flow rates are proportionately higher in infants and children than in adults, ranging from 80 to 150 mL/(kg · min). Adult rates usually range from about 1.8 to 2.2 L/(min · m²) or about 50 mL/(kg · min). Perfusion pressures tend to be lower in children (20 to 50 mm Hg) when adequate oxygenation and perfusion are apparent. The optimal pressure or flow is unclear, and significant interinstitutional variation exists.

5. **Moderate hypothermia and ventricular fibrillation.** Moderate hypothermia combined with ventricular fibrillation is used often in pediatric cardiac repair. With this technique, the patient is cooled to about 28° to 30°C, and the heart is fibrillated but continues to be perfused because an aortic cross-clamp is not placed. The surgeon can open the cardiac chambers without risking entrainment of air into the left side of the heart and subsequent ejection into the arterial circulation.

Deliberate fibrillation often is used during work on the right side of the heart or for relatively simple repairs such as ASD closure. The advantages of deliberate fibrillation with moderate hypothermia include a favorable myocardial supply/demand ratio, decreased risk of air embolus to the brain, and avoidance of aortic cross-clamping and cardioplegia. However, surgical exposure is limited because of the significant amount of blood in and continued motion of the heart. Therefore, aortic cross-clamping and cardioplegic protection of the heart are necessary for more complex intracardiac repairs, especially in small children.

6. **Bypass circuit volume.** The bypass circuit volume is large relative to the blood volume in infants. In pediatric CPB circuits, the priming volume may be as much as 700 mL, whereas the estimated blood volume of a 3-kg neonate is

250 to 300 mL. Accordingly, the hematocrit is reduced by approximately 70%. In contrast, an adult CPB circuit is primed with 1,500 mL for a patient with an estimated blood volume of 5 L; a drop in hematocrit of less than 25% results. Small infants undergoing complex repairs often require transfusion of red blood cells, platelets, and fresh frozen plasma to offset the dilutional reduction of hematocrit and clotting factors. More recently, technologic improvements have allowed miniaturization of the circuit with priming volumes of about 150 to 200 mL. Although these values represent an improvement, it still results in a significant degree of hemodilution in these small children.

B. When should blood be added to the bypass circuit?

In general, hemodilution during bypass is desirable and tolerated, because microcirculatory perfusion is improved and metabolic needs are reduced by hypothermia. However, if the hematocrit is lowered too far, oxygen-carrying capacity is diminished and anaerobic metabolism results. The ideal hematocrit during CPB is unknown. However, for most complex repairs, a hematocrit of 20% to 25% during CPB is used.

The CPB circuit must be primed. Each circuit has an obligatory volume that is required to fill the tubing, filters, pumps, and oxygenator. Therefore, it may be necessary to add red blood cells to the priming solution to reach the desired hematocrit. Calculation of the hematocrit on bypass is quite simple, as follows.

1. Determine the patient's estimated blood volume.
2. Multiply the estimated blood volume by the measured hematocrit (Hct) to yield the patient's red blood cell mass (RBCM).
3. Ask the perfusionist what the circuit priming volume is.
4. Add the estimated blood volume to the priming volume to obtain the total volume on bypass (CPBV).
5. Predicted Hct on bypass = RBCM/CPBV
6. If the predicted Hct on bypass is less than desired, the quantity of red blood cells that must be added is calculated as follows:

CPBV × Desired hematocrit = Required RBCM
Required RBCM – Patient's RBCM = RBCM to be added

C. How is anticoagulation managed?

Heparin is given to prevent initiation of the coagulation cascade by contact of blood with the bypass circuit. A dose of 300 units/kg generally is sufficient, although 400 units/kg sometimes is recommended for neonates. This dose is given through a central catheter after aspiration to verify blood return.

1. **Activated clotting time.** Measuring activated clotting time about 3 to 5 minutes after heparin administration can allow documentation of its effect. A value of about 400 seconds appears adequate to prevent clotting on bypass. Activated clotting time is relatively simple to determine and is reasonable to monitor, because occasionally a patient does exhibit marked heparin resistance. The activated clotting time also can signal a potentially catastrophic drug administration error when a substance other than heparin is injected. If the patient remains normothermic, the activated clotting time generally is rechecked every 20 to 30 minutes. With significant hypothermia, heparin effect is prolonged.

D. Should antifibrinolytics be used?

In an effort to minimize transfusion requirements, many groups have focused on preservation of platelet function and prevention of fibrinolysis, using drugs such as ε-aminocaproic acid and aprotinin. Although the data supporting the decreased transfusion requirement in redo operations in adults are fairly convincing, the data are not as clear in infants. Some groups have reported dramatic decreases in blood loss, whereas others have shown no difference in donor exposures to banked blood [15,16]. Many of the studies on aprotinin usage in children are difficult to interpret because of wide variations in dosage regimens, patient age, type of operation, and other factors. When aprotinin is dosed according to patient weight or body surface area, much lower plasma concentrations than those found in the adult population result [17]. It appears that the large volume of the pump prime relative to the patient's small blood volume leads to a greater dilution of the drug during bypass. In order to compensate for the hemodilution, more aprotinin may need to be added to the prime to achieve plasma levels sufficient to inhibit activation of the coagulation cascade.

E. *How are patients weaned?*

Success in weaning from bypass is critically dependent on the surgeon's ability to completely repair the defect. Residual shunts, obstruction, or valvular dysfunction are tolerated poorly after bypass.

1. **Preparation.** Be certain the patient is optimally prepared before attempting discontinuation of bypass (Table 14.9). Near the end of the surgical repair, gradual rewarming is begun. Temperature gradients are common; be sure that the patient is thoroughly and evenly rewarmed. The speed and method of rewarming may be critical. Postischemia hyperthermia is particularly deleterious in the setting of altered cerebral energy metabolism. On the other hand, mild degrees of hypothermia have been shown to be protective. Infusion of afterload-reducing agents, such as sodium nitroprusside, given during rewarming may be helpful to dilate the vascular bed and promote uniform rewarming. Allowing time for reperfusion of the heart after the cross-clamp is removed makes possible dissipation of "evil humors" (cardioplegia) and reestablishment of aerobic metabolism.

2. **Heart rate and rhythm.** Sinus rhythm is essential, because ventricular function typically is impaired after bypass and ischemia. Optimal heart rate also is important in improving cardiac output, because stroke volume may be less than ideal. A heart rate of 120 to 160 beats/min is desirable. The atrium may be paced if the patient has a slower sinus rate, or sequential AV pacing may be required if a rhythm other than sinus exists. New electrocardiographic ST changes may indicate the presence of air in the coronary arteries or ongoing myocardial ischemia. A transient increase in coronary perfusion pressure (as occurs with application of a partial occlusion clamp to the aorta distal to the aortic cannula) promotes clearance of this air.

3. **Other monitored parameters.** Hemodynamic monitors should be rechecked and transducers re-zeroed. The surgeon may elect to insert a left atrial pressure catheter to assess ventricular filling and function. Laboratory values, including hematocrit, potassium, ionized calcium, arterial blood gas partial pressures, and pH, should be rechecked after aortic cross-clamp release and before discontinuation of bypass is attempted.

4. **Vasoactive drugs.** Vasodilator and inotropic drugs should be available for infusion by calibrated pumps, especially after intracardiac repair. Significant hemodynamic compromise may result from hypoxic-ischemic reperfusion injury that is superimposed on marginal baseline ventricular function. Ventricular performance usually is readily improved by inotrope or combined inotrope and vasodilator support. Impaired postoperative cardiac performance is clearly associated with higher morbidity and mortality.

Table 14.9 Checklist for discontinuation of bypass

---

1. Complete rewarming (core temperature $\geq 35°C$)
2. Complete reperfusion of heart after cardioplegia
3. Sinus rhythm with appropriate heart rate
4. Evaluate ST changes
5. Check electrolytes, blood gases, and hematocrit
6. Optimize pulmonary function
7. Check hemodynamic monitors
8. Prepare vasodilator or inotropic drugs, if indicated
9. Prepare platelets and fresh frozen plasma, if indicated

From Davies LK. Anesthesia for pediatric cardiovascular surgery. In: Kirby RR, Gravenstein N, Lobato EB, et al., eds. *Clinical anesthesia practice.* Philadelphia: WB Saunders, 2002:1227, with permission.

5. **Cardiovascular changes.** Arterial pressure may be normal or above normal when cardiac output is high, normal, or low; thus, knowing the arterial pressure is not helpful with regard to diagnosis of cardiac dysfunction. After CPB, SVR generally is high in both adults and children because of circulating catecholamines and antidiuretic hormone as well as other influences. In the neonate, this response may be amplified, leading to uninhibited vasoconstriction.

6. **Afterload reduction.** Children poorly tolerate an increased pressure workload. Therefore, afterload reduction (generally with sodium nitroprusside) may be useful to improve cardiac output. When cardiac output still is impaired after vasodilator therapy, a combination of afterload reduction, volume expansion, and inotropic support is warranted.

F. **Measurement of blood pressure.** If the blood pressure is low during attempted weaning from bypass, another method of blood pressure measurement must be available to check the accuracy of the peripheral data. The surgeon can easily place an exploring needle into the ascending aorta (often at the site of the previous cardioplegia infusion) and connect it to a pressure transducer. A noninvasive (cuff) blood pressure measurement also can be obtained.

In small children, a significant difference in blood pressure measurements often is present between central aortic and peripheral arterial sites. The reason for this discrepancy is not clear, but it usually resolves over time. Before starting administration of inotropes or vasopressors, be certain that the pressure measurement is accurate. If the discrepancy persists, placement of a femoral arterial catheter helps to guide therapy.

G. *How is increased pulmonary vascular resistance managed?*
Pulmonary function must be optimized before discontinuation of bypass is attempted. Increased PVR results from increased lung water, complement activation, catecholamines, and atelectasis.

1. **Lung expansion and oxygenation.** The lungs must be vigorously reexpanded to increase functional residual capacity (Fig. 14.5). The endotracheal tube is not

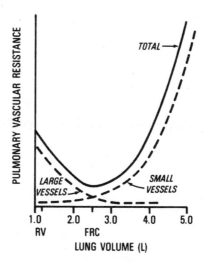

FIG. 14.5 Asymmetrical U-shaped curve relates total pulmonary vascular resistance to lung volume. The trough of the curve occurs when lung volume equals function residual capacity (*FRC*). Total pulmonary resistance is the sum of resistance in small vessels (increased by increasing lung volume) and in large vessels (increased by decreasing lung volume). *RV,* residual volume. (From Benumof JL. Respiratory physiology and respiratory function during anesthesia. In: Miller RD, ed. *Anesthesia,* 2nd ed. New York: Churchill Livingstone, 1986:1122, with permission).

Table 14.10 Alteration of pulmonary vascular resistance

Increase resistance	Decrease resistance
Hypoxia	Oxygen
Hypercarbia	Hypocarbia
Acidosis	Alkalosis
Hyperinflation	Normal functional residual capacity
Atelectasis	Blocking sympathetic stimulation
Sympathetic stimulation	Low hematocrit
Surgical constriction	Modified ultrafiltration
High hematocrit	Nitric oxide
	Phosphodiesterase inhibitors

Modified from Hickey PR, Wessel DL. Anesthesia for treatment of congenital heart disease. In: Kaplan JA, ed. *Cardiac anesthesia,* 2nd ed. Orlando: Grune & Stratton, 1987:656.

routinely suctioned, as suctioning may precipitate bleeding in anticoagulated patients. Any wheezing is treated vigorously with inhaled bronchodilators. I prefer albuterol 2.5 mg, administered via a nebulizer attached between the endotracheal tube and the circle system. If secretions prevent appropriate deflation of the lungs, careful suctioning with a soft red rubber catheter is indicated.

Vigorous hyperventilation without positive end-expiratory pressure (PEEP) is one of the most powerful tools available to decrease PVR. The pulmonary vascular responsiveness to hypercarbia is accentuated in the postbypass period; thus, even small increases in P_aCO_2 are associated with significant increases in resistance. High inspired oxygen concentrations should be used, and metabolic acidosis should be avoided.

2. **Pharmacologic interventions.** α-Stimulation causes pulmonary vasoconstriction, whereas β-stimulation causes vasodilation. Many pharmacologic agents have been used with only marginal success in an attempt to selectively decrease PVR. The agents most commonly used include sodium nitroprusside, nitroglycerin, isoproterenol, aminophylline, amrinone, milrinone, PGE_1, and perhaps adenosine. Inhaled nitric oxide offers promise as a truly selective pulmonary vasodilator, but its use is prohibitively expensive and typically it is not readily available.

Factors that increase or decrease PVR are summarized in Table 14.10.

VIII. **Postbypass issues**

A. *What is modified ultrafiltration and when is it used?*

The inflammatory response on bypass is significant and may be responsible for much of the morbidity seen in these children. Endothelial injury can cause an increase in total body water and increased capillary permeability, with resultant multiorgan failure. Conventional ultrafiltration on CPB has been used to try to prevent tissue edema, but its effectiveness has been limited. It is difficult to remove much water during bypass and still maintain a safe acceptable reservoir volume. In 1993, the technique of modified ultrafiltration (MUF) performed in the immediate postbypass period was described [18]. The aortic cannula is left in place and approximately 10 to 30 mL/kg/min of blood is siphoned from the aorta, pumped through a hemoconcentrator (dialysis membrane), and returned to the right atrium (Fig. 14.6). Volume is infused from the reservoir as necessary to maintain hemodynamic stability. Multiple studies have documented the effectiveness of MUF in ameliorating many of the adverse effects of CPB. MUF improves hemodynamics, reduces total body water, and decreases the need for blood transfusions compared with nonfiltered controls [19]. It is associated with significant increases in hematocrit, fibrinogen, and total plasma protein levels, but no change in platelet count [20]. MUF has been shown to improve intrinsic LV systolic function, improve diastolic compliance, increase blood pressure, and decrease

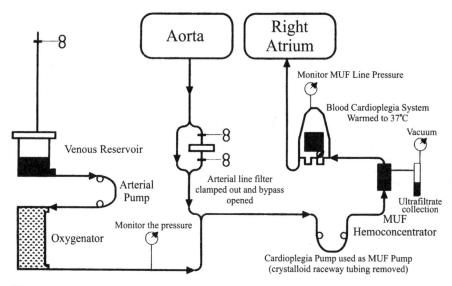

FIG. 14.6 Diagram of a modified ultrafiltration system. After cardiopulmonary bypass (CPB), modified ultrafiltration proceeds using the blood cardioplegia roller pump from the CPB circuit. Blood is pumped from the aortic cannula through the ultrafilter and heat exchanger and is reinfused into the patient through the venous cannula. (From Kern FH, Shulman SR, Lawson DS, et al. Extracorporeal circulation and circulatory assist devices in the pediatric patient. In: Lake CL, ed. *Pediatric cardiac anesthesia,* 3rd ed., Stamford, CT: Appleton & Lange, 1998:219, with permission.)

inotropic drug use in the early postoperative period [21]. It has been shown to decrease levels of the lung vasoconstrictor endothelin-1, significantly decrease the pulmonary/systemic pressure ratio after CPB, and may help prevent pulmonary hypertensive crises [22]. It improves lung compliance, reduces cytokine levels, and removes activated complement (C3a and C5a) [23]. After DHCA, MUF also improves the brain's ability to use oxygen [24]. The data summarizing its beneficial effects are listed in Table 14.11.

B. *How should protamine be administered?*

Protamine is given after termination of CPB to neutralize the effects of heparin. It is not administered until MUF is complete and the venous cannula has been removed. Generally, a dose of 3 to 4.5 mg/kg (1 to 1.5 mg for every 100 units of heparin) is given. Satisfactory reversal of heparin is suggested by return of the activated clotting time to baseline value. Protamine can cause serious adverse reactions in some patients. These reactions include systemic hypotension, pulmonary hypertension, and allergic reactions. The mechanism for these events is not entirely clear, but it may involve antibody-mediated immune responses, complement activation, and histamine release.

Histamine release is provoked by rapid administration of large doses of protamine. Slow administration with a controlled infusion is effective in ameliorating this side effect. Pretreatment with antihistamine or administration into the left atrium also has been proposed. Catastrophic pulmonary hypertension is less common and probably occurs because of complement activation and thromboxane release. Allergic reactions to protamine can occur, usually in patients with prior exposure to protamine-containing insulin preparations.

Fortunately, serious reactions to protamine appear to be less common in neonates and children than in adults. If the drug is administered slowly after removal of the

Table 14.11 Summary of effects of modified ultrafiltration

Feature	Effect	Reports
Total body water accumulation	⇓	*a*
Hematocrit	⇑	*a, b, c*
Blood loss	⇓	*a, c, d*
Blood transfusion requirement	⇓	*a, c, d*
Colloid osmotic pressure	⇑	*b, e*
Cardiac output	⇑	*a, f*
Heart rate	⇓	*f*
Arterial blood pressure	⇑	*a, f*
Systemic vascular resistance	⇔	*g*
Pulmonary vascular resistance	⇓	*g,h*
Diastolic compliance	⇑	*f*
Inotropic drug use	⇓	*f*
Renal function	⇔	*a*
Cerebral recovery from Deep hypothermic circulatory arrest	⇑	*b, i*
Plasma endothelin-1	⇓	*h*
Lung compliance	⇑	*j*
Cytokine levels	⇓	*k*
Activated complement levels	⇓	*l*
Heparin concentration	⇑	*m*

a Naik SK, Knight A, Elliott MJ. A prospective randomized study of a modified technique of ultrafiltration during pediatric open-heart surgery. *Circulation* 1991;84:III422–431.

b Daggett CW, Lodge AJ, Scarborough JE, et al. Modified ultrafiltration versus conventional ultrafiltration: a randomized prospective study in neonatal piglets. *J Thorac Cardiovasc Surg* 1998;115:336–341.

c Draaisma AM, Hazekamp MG, Frank M, et al. Modified ultrafiltration after cardiopulmonary bypass in pediatric cardiac surgery. *Ann Thorac Surg* 1997;64:521–525.

d Friesen RH, Campbell DN, Clarke DR, et al. Modified ultrafiltration attenuates dilutional coagulopathy in pediatric open heart operations. *Ann Thorac Surg* 1997;64:1787–1789.

e Ad N, Snir E, Katz J, Birk E, et al. Use of the modified technique of ultrafiltration in pediatric open-heart surgery: a prospective study. *Isr J Med Sci* 1996;32:1326–1331.

f Davies MJ, Nguyen K, Gaynor JW, et al. Modified ultrafiltration improves left ventricular systolic function in infants after cardiopulmonary bypass. *J Thorac Cardiovasc Surg* 1998;115:361–369.

g Naik SK, Balaji S, Elliott MJ. Modified ultrafiltration improves haemodynamics after cardiopulmonary bypass in children. *J Am Coll Cardiol* 1992;19:37A.

h Bando K, Vijay P, Turrentine MW, et al. Dilutional and modified ultrafiltration reduces pulmonary hypertension after operations for congenital heart disease: a prospective randomized study. *J Thorac Cardiovasc Surg* 1998;115:517–525.

i Skaryak LA, Kirshbom P, DiBernardo LR, et al. Modified ultrafiltration improves cerebral metabolic recovery after circulatory arrest. *J Thorac Cardiovasc Surg* 1995;109:744–752.

j Meliones JN, Gaynor JW, Wilson BG, et al. Modified ultrafiltration reduces airway pressure and improves lung compliance after congenital heart surgery. *J Am Coll Cardiol* 1995;25:271A.

k Millar AB, Armstrong L, van der Linden J, et al. Cytokine production and hemofiltration in children undergoing cardiopulmonary bypass. *Ann Thorac Surg* 1993;56:1499–1502.

l Andreasson S, Gothberg S, Berggren H, et al. Hemofiltration modifies complement activation after extracorporeal circulation in infants. *Ann Thorac Surg* 1993;56:1515–1517.

m Williams GD, Ramamoorthy C, Totzek FR, et al. Comparison of the effects of red cell separation and ultrafiltration on heparin concentration during pediatric cardiac surgery. *J Cardiothorac Vasc Anesth* 1997;11:840–844.

Modified from Elliott MJ. Recent advances in paediatric cardiopulmonary bypass. *Perfusion* 1999;14:237–246.

venous cannula but with the aortic cannula still in place, CPB can be reinstituted quickly if a catastrophic reaction occurs.

C. *What are the causes of low cardiac output?*

Low cardiac output can have many causes but is categorized according to its major determinants: heart rate, rhythm, contractility, preload, and afterload.

1. **Heart rate.** Infants and children have a relatively fixed cardiac stroke volume and therefore modify cardiac output by heart rate changes. Therefore, cardiac output is considered to be rate dependent. Heart rates of at least 120 beats/min should be sought in an effort to optimize cardiac output. A lower heart rate should be treated either pharmacologically or by pacing. Pacing often is preferred, because it has negligible side effects.

2. **Dysrhythmias.** Dysrhythmias after CPB often are tolerated poorly and may require electrical conversion. Sinus rhythm at a reasonable rate is crucial to maximize cardiac output. Do not hesitate to use electrical pacing to optimize myocardial performance. Unfortunately, arrhythmias caused by abnormal automaticity may occur that are difficult to treat. Junctional ectopic tachycardia (JET) is an uncommon but life-threatening arrhythmia seen almost exclusively in neonates and infants after congenital heart surgery [25]. JET is of special significance for the anesthesiologist because it usually manifests intraoperatively or in the immediate postoperative period. JET remains among the more difficult tachycardias to control, leading to severe hemodynamic instability and death. It is thought to result from abnormal automaticity, with the focus of active discharge located at the AV node or the proximal bundle of His, yet the atrial tissue is not directly involved in the arrhythmia mechanism. Therefore, an important characteristic of this tachyarrhythmia is a lack of response to cardioversion, overdrive pacing, and conventional medications.

JET is classically recognized as a narrow QRS tachycardia with AV dissociation and an atrial rate that is slower than the ventricular rate. Typically, peak JET rates range from 170 to 300 beats/min. The onset ("warmup") and termination are gradual (Fig. 14.7). Retrograde conduction and retrograde P waves

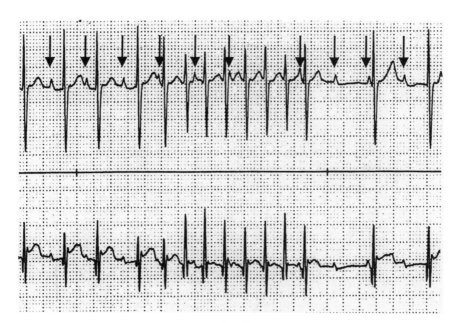

FIG. 14.7 Junctional ectopic tachycardia (JET) at 280 beats/min. Note atrioventricular dissociation as JET warms up with no change in atrial rate (*arrows*).

can be seen on the ECG. Interestingly, a wide QRS may be seen if there is an associated bundle branch block that occurs either as a rate-dependent aberration or as a fixed abnormality due to surgical damage of the bundle branch.

Postoperatively, JET has been generally refractory to most conventional antiarrhythmic drugs. If the chest still is open, topical cooling with cold saline may be helpful. Remarkably, it usually resolves on its own within the first 3 days of presentation. Therapy should be directed toward decreasing the junctional rate to allow atrial pacing with AV synchrony to reestablish hemodynamic stability.

3. **Decreased contractility.** Poor contractility can occur due to surgical trauma (as from a ventriculotomy incision), preexisting volume or pressure overload condition, injury or malperfusion of a coronary artery, residual effects of myocardial ischemia and reperfusion, metabolic and acid–base derangements, hypoxemia, and drug effects.

4. **Decreased preload.** Decreased preload may occur from hypovolemia, cardiac tamponade, positive airway pressure, and increased PVR that causes diminished return to the left side of the heart.

5. **Increased afterload.** Increased afterload can be a major problem for both the left and right sides of the heart. Many congenital lesions are associated with pulmonary vascular changes and pulmonary hypertension. Thus, control of RV function and afterload is crucial to maintain adequate cardiac output.

D. **What are the causes and treatment of excessive bleeding?**

1. **Causes.** Most commonly, patients bleed postoperatively as a result of inadequate surgical hemostasis. Inadequate heparin neutralization also can be a factor. Thrombocytopenia or platelet dysfunction is the next most common cause. Platelets are sequestered in the bypass circuit and become dysfunctional because of surface exposure and hypothermia.

Patients with cyanotic heart disease and significant polycythemia have a baseline abnormality of platelet function and clotting factors. They often demonstrate a decrease in factors II, V, VII, VIII, and IX; hypofibrinogenemia; and an increase of fibrin split products, all of which may lead to excessive bleeding.

2. **Treatment.** While a source of bleeding is sought, the patient must be aggressively treated with volume replacement. Crystalloid solutions are the mainstay of therapy, but their administration should be tempered by the knowledge that a total body inflammatory response after bypass leads to problems with increased vascular permeability and edema. Decreased colloid oncotic pressure can be a problem after CPB because of hemodilution and destruction of serum proteins. Judicious use of albumin-containing solutions may be warranted.

If continuing red blood cell loss is a problem, packed red blood cell transfusion is indicated. Typically, a hematocrit of 25% to 30% in acyanotic children and 30% to 40% in cyanotic children seems reasonable. In children with good cardiac reserve after simple repairs, an even lower hematocrit of 18% to 20% may be well tolerated. If no surgical source is found and the activated clotting time is normal, an empiric platelet transfusion often is used. Only after prolonged, deep hypothermic cases in small infants should transfusion with fresh frozen plasma be necessary.

E. **What metabolic problems are likely?**

1. **Potassium disorders.** Metabolic derangements are relatively common. Hyperkalemia and hypokalemia are the most common electrolyte abnormalities. Hyperkalemia commonly is seen immediately after the cross-clamp is removed if large amounts of cardioplegic solution have been used. If cardiac output is poor, hyperkalemia may remain problematic. Typically, hypokalemia evolves because patients exhibit a marked kaliuresis after bypass. Unless the serum potassium value is at least 4.5 mEq/L or renal function is impaired, I almost routinely begin a potassium chloride infusion of approximately 0.25 mEq/kg/hour after CPB. Remember that dysrhythmias associated with digitalis toxicity are enhanced by hypokalemia.

2. **Calcium abnormalities.** Hypocalcemia occurs frequently, especially after rapid transfusion of blood products. A decrease in the ionized fraction can lead to decreased myocardial contractility and decreased vascular smooth muscle tone.

3. **Miscellaneous problems.** Hypomagnesemia can occur and can enhance ventricular irritability. Hyperglycemia is common after CPB and is relatively resistant to treatment with insulin. Although hyperglycemia occurs somewhat less frequently in children than in adults, maintenance of normoglycemia often is difficult. Sodium changes typically do not present a major problem after bypass, although hypernatremia can occur if large quantities of sodium bicarbonate have been given.

F. *When should the patient be extubated?*

Most patients undergoing complex repairs remain intubated and mechanically ventilated for several hours to days after surgery. This approach allows heavy sedation, recovery of myocardial function, and stabilization of hemodynamic status. For simple repairs (e.g., ASD, simple VSD, and coarctation), extubation may be considered at the end of the procedure if the patient is stable and awake and if bleeding is controlled. Obviously, all normal criteria for extubation, including reversal of muscle relaxation, good spontaneous ventilation, and the ability to maintain and protect the airway, should be present.

IX. **Specific lesions**

The following section reviews some of the more common lesions encountered in practice. Although separated into categories based on manifestation of cyanosis or CHF, it is important to remember that these divisions are arbitrary. For some lesions [transposition of the great arteries (TGA) is a good example], the patient may be cyanotic, may be in CHF, or both, depending on other associated lesions. The consequences of these lesions vary from patient to patient, so one must be careful to individualize care to each child.

A. **Lesions likely to cause cyanosis**
   1. **Tetralogy of Fallot**
      a. **General considerations**
         (1) The four basic abnormalities are infundibular pulmonary stenosis, VSD, RV hypertrophy, and overriding aorta (Fig. 14.8).
         (2) Spectrum of disease ranges from "pink tet" (mild stenosis, large VSD with predominant left-to-right shunt) to pulmonary atresia with obliteration of the outflow tract and marked cyanosis.
         (3) Classic tet will have decreased pulmonary blood flow and increased blood flow to the body. Variations in the physiology are dependent on the degree of infundibular stenosis.
         (4) Occurs equally in males and females.
         (5) In 10% of patients with tetralogy of Fallot, the left anterior descending coronary artery (LAD) arises from the right rather than the left coronary artery.
         (6) Rarely overtly cyanotic at birth unless the RV outflow tract (RVOT) is atretic. Cyanosis may not develop for several months but then becomes progressively more severe.
         (7) X-ray film shows decreased pulmonary markings. Right aortic arch occurs in about 25% of cases.
         (8) Squatting increases SVR, helping to shunt more blood to the lungs.
         (9) Tet spells are spells or episodes of paroxysmal hyperpnea that occur in 20% to 70% of patients, with a peak frequency at age 2 to 3 months. The spells usually are initiated by crying, feeding, or defecation. Although the etiology is uncertain, spells probably are initiated by events that result in increased oxygen demand associated with decreasing arterial P_aO_2 and pH and increasing P_aCO_2. As the hypoxia continues, SVR decreases further and the right-to-left shunt increases. Some suggest that the spells may be initiated or exacerbated by infundibular hypercontractility or "spasm." Transient cerebral ischemia can occur, leading to paleness, limpness, and unconsciousness.
      b. **Surgical procedures**
         (1) Complete repair
            (a) Ligate previous Blalock–Taussig (BT) shunt if present
            (b) Infundibular resection of excess muscle in RVOT
            (c) Patch closure of VSD

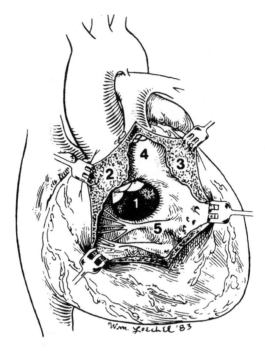

FIG. 14.8 Tetralogy of Fallot showing ventricular septal defect (VSD) with overriding aorta (*1*) and right ventricular parietal (*2*) and septal (*3*) bands of myocardial hypertrophy. The infundibular septum (*4*) is hypoplastic and deviated anteriorly. The papillary muscle of the conus (*5*) inserts along the lower margin of the VSD. (From Arciniegas E, ed. *Pediatric cardiac surgery*. Chicago: Year Book, 1985:204, with permission.)

> **(d)** Patch the RVOT (subannular or transannular) to enlarge that area
>
> **(e)** RV to PA conduit may be necessary if patient has pulmonary atresia or an anomalous LAD coursing across the RVOT.
>
> **(2)** Systemic pulmonary shunts. These procedures may be indicated to palliate cyanotic children who are not candidates for complete repair, such as patients with small PAs or annulus, pulmonary atresia, or anomalous LAD coursing across the pulmonary outflow tract. The resulting increased pulmonary blood flow is thought to stimulate growth of small PAs, allowing subsequent complete repair.
>
> > **(a)** Subclavian artery to PA anastomosis (Blalock–Taussig shunt), either native or modified
> >
> > **(b)** Central shunt: Anastomosis between aorta and PA with tube graft
> >
> > **(c)** Waterston: Ascending aorta to right PA; no longer performed because of kinking of the right PA and difficulty controlling the amount of pulmonary blood flow
> >
> > **(d)** Potts: Descending aorta to left PA; no longer performed because of difficult takedown at later surgery and difficulty in controlling shunt size.
>
> **c. Anesthetic considerations.** Knowing the patient's anatomy is crucial in developing a rational anesthetic plan. It is particularly critical to know whether there is anterograde flow across the RVOT or if the patient is totally dependent on a BT shunt for pulmonary circulation. Patients with

anterograde flow across the RVOT have the potential for dynamic obstruction and the possibility for therapeutic interventions to change the caliber of the outflow tract.

(1) Preoperative. Preoperative evaluation should center around assessment of degree of cyanosis. One should seek evidence of hypercyanotic spells and their frequency. A spot check of O_2 saturation may be helpful. It also is helpful to follow the hematocrit over time, because increasing cyanosis will provoke an increase in red blood cells in an attempt to maintain O_2-carrying capacity. Other laboratory values that may be useful are coagulation studies, because hypercyanotic patients often have a coexisting coagulopathy.

   (a) NPO status. It is important to keep the patient with tetralogy of Fallot well hydrated for two reasons. (i) If the patient is polycythemic, a prolonged NPO period may put the patient at risk for dehydration with increased viscosity and sludging. If the degree of polycythemia is too extreme, preoperative phlebotomy may even be indicated. (ii) Hypovolemia will exacerbate the RV outflow obstruction if the patient has infundibular stenosis. I like to think of tetralogy of Fallot as a right-sided version of idiopathic hypertrophic subaortic stenosis. Keeping the patient euvolemic or even a bit hypervolemic will help "stent open" the RVOT and improve pulmonary blood flow.

   (b) Premedication. The goal in approaching the anesthetic is to have a calm, relaxed child. Good preoperative interactions with the parents and child are crucial. Premedication can be a valuable aid, but it is important that the patient not be sedated to the point of hypercarbia, which can increase PVR and precipitate increased right-to-left shunting. Intramuscular injections are best avoided, because the anxiety and stress they cause can lead to a "tet" spell. Careful monitoring of S_pO_2 after premedication is indicated because the response may be variable.

   (c) Subacute bacterial endocarditis (SBE) prophylaxis is essential. See American Heart Association guidelines for appropriate drugs and timing [26].

(2) Intraoperative. Choice of anesthetic should be individualized. Many different drugs have been used successfully. It is imperative to maintain or even augment intravascular volume. Hemodynamic goals are a deep anesthetic (to avoid sympathetic surges) with maintenance of normal-to-high SVR and low PVR. Meticulous attention must be paid to airway management, because airway obstruction can quickly result in the triggering of a "tet spell." Hypercarbia with a further decrease in oxygenation will cause an increase in PVR, triggering a vicious cycle of further desaturation and decreased pulmonary blood flow. Inhalational induction has been used successfully in children with tetralogy of Fallot. Halothane is an ideal drug because it maintains SVR and relaxes the RV infundibulum, increasing pulmonary blood flow. One must be cautious with inhalational induction, however, because the baseline decreased pulmonary blood flow results in a slow change in blood anesthetic tension. Induction of anesthesia may be slowed, but, more importantly, if a relative overdose of halothane results, it is difficult to remove agent from the body because of the limited pulmonary blood flow. If intravenous induction is preferred, one should choose a technique that maintains SVR and minimizes PVR.

   One should be watchful for problems with RV dysfunction after repair. Typically the surgical repair involves a significant right ventriculotomy and a patch across the RVOT. The surgeon usually tries to spare the pulmonary valve, but this may result in some residual obstruction across that area. Conversely, if the valve must be sacrificed, the patient will be left with significant pulmonary insufficiency.

Fortunately these patients usually do not have baseline elevated PVR, because their preoperative situation is characterized by decreased pulmonary blood flow. However, the patient may have small PAs, which will exacerbate any RV dysfunction. If aortic cross-clamp time is prolonged, one might anticipate myocardial dysfunction on that basis. Therapeutic interventions should revolve around efforts to support RV function and decrease PVR. Afterload reduction and/or an inotrope may be beneficial, especially if a right ventriculotomy was performed.

- (a) Problems and complications
  - (i) Hemorrhage
  - (ii) Residual RVOT obstruction
  - (iii) RV failure (especially if RV/LV peak pressure is greater than 0.7 after repair)
  - (iv) Heart block
  - (v) Residual VSD
  - (vi) Late arrhythmias and sudden death

2. **Transposition of the great arteries**
   a. **General considerations**
      (1) TGA is the most common severe congenital cardiac abnormality diagnosed during infancy. Males predominate over females by a ratio of almost 3:1. Additional cardiac or noncardiac anomalies are rare. These infants usually are of normal birth weight.

      (2) Left and right circulations are arranged in separate parallel circuits rather than the usual series configuration (Fig. 14.9). Thus, the aorta arises from the right side of the heart, which pumps deoxygenated blood to the body, which then returns back to the right atrium. The PA arises from the LV, which pumps oxygenated blood back to the lungs. After birth, the patient must retain some method that allows mixing of the pulmonary and systemic circulations to sustain life. Typically, an ASD, VSD, or PDA allows that mixing. If the patient does not have adequate mixing, a Rashkind balloon atrial septostomy is performed in the cardiac catheterization laboratory to improve the patient's clinical condition.

      (3) Clinical presentation. The diagnosis of TGA is generally made shortly after birth. The patient will be cyanotic and, if mixing is inadequate, will develop marked metabolic acidosis. If the patient has an associated VSD, cyanosis will be less severe. The patient can develop pulmonary overload and signs of CHF if the VSD is large. If a patient has a PDA, differential cyanosis of the upper and lower body may be observed. This occurs because oxygenated blood is pumped from the LV to the PA and ductus arteriosus into the descending aorta. In this situation, the upper part of the body will be more cyanotic than the trunk and lower extremities.

   b. **Surgical procedures**
      (1) Atrial switch operations (Senning and Mustard procedures) are designed to reroute the blood coming into the atrium using an intra-atrial baffle. Therefore, systemic venous blood (deoxygenated) goes to the LV (and then to the PA and the lungs) while the oxygenated pulmonary venous return is redirected to the RV (and then to the aorta and the systemic circulation). In the case of the Senning procedure, the baffle is configured using a right atrial flap, whereas the Mustard procedure uses a pericardial baffle. Both of these procedures result in a physiologic correction of the problem but not an anatomic correction, because the RV remains the ventricle that pumps to the systemic circulation.

      (2) Arterial switch operation (Jatene). The arterial switch operation has become the procedure of choice since it provides both a physiologic and anatomic correction of the problem (Fig. 14.10). Basically, the great vessels are transected above the valves and moved to their op-

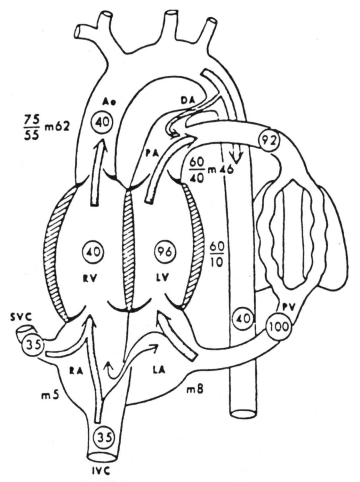

FIG. 14.9 Transposition of the great arteries. Systemic venous blood returns to the right heart and is pumped to the body through the transposed aorta. Similarly, left heart blood is pumped to the lungs. Survival after birth is possible only if mixing occurs between the two circulations (e.g., atrial septal defect, patent foramen ovale, ventricular septal defect, patent ductus arteriosus). *Ao,* aorta; *DA,* ductus arteriosus; *IVC,* inferior vena cava; *LA,* left atrium; *LV,* left ventricle; *PA,* pulmonary artery; *PV,* pulmonary vein; *RA,* right atrium; *RV,* right ventricle; *SVC,* superior vena cava. (From Rudolph AM. Aortopulmonary transposition. In: *Congenital diseases of the heart.* Chicago: Year Book, 1974:475, with permission.)

posite ventricles. The origins of the left and right coronary arteries are dissected off as individual buttons that are rotated into place and reimplanted into the neoaorta. The new PA is reconstructed where the coronary artery buttons were removed. When the procedure is complete, the LV receives oxygenated blood from the lungs, which it then pumps to the body. The RV pumps the systemic venous return to the lungs in the usual fashion.

(3) The Rastelli procedure may be an appropriate choice for patients with TGA, VSD, and LV outflow tract obstruction. In that situation,

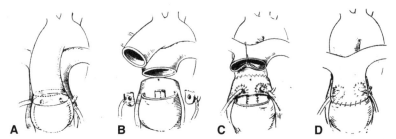

FIG. 14.10 The arterial switch operation repairs transposition of the great arteries **(A)** by dividing the great arteries and excising the coronary ostial buttons **(B)**, transferring the coronary arteries to the neoascending aorta, and anastomosing the neoascending aorta to the distal ascending aorta **(C, D)** and the neomain pulmonary artery to the distal main pulmonary artery. (From Arciniegas E, ed. *Pediatric cardiac surgery.* Chicago: Year Book, 1985:275, with permission.)

the VSD is closed so that LV blood is directed to the aorta and a conduit is created between the RV and the PAs.

c. Anesthetic considerations

    (1) Preoperative. Medical management initially is used to stabilize the patient and improve perfusion. If mixing is inadequate, the patient will develop profound metabolic acidosis. PGE$_1$ can be infused to maintain or reopen the ductus arteriosus. The patient may require an emergent Rashkind atrial septostomy to facilitate adequate mixing. Cardiac catheterization may be helpful if there are concerns regarding variations of normal coronary artery anatomy.

    The timing of surgical intervention is dictated by the patient's particular anatomy. If the child has TGA with intact ventricular septum, it is important to perform the Jatene procedure during the first month of life while the LV mass still is adequate. If surgery is delayed too long, the LV will decondition because it is working against the relatively low-resistance pulmonary circuit. On the other hand, if the patient has TGA with a VSD, the LV will remain "loaded" and the ventricular mass will not decrease. Thus, if necessary, surgery can be delayed for a few months to optimize the patient's condition.

    (2) Intraoperative. These patients typically come to the operating room for their arterial switch operation with an intravenous catheter in place and PGE$_1$ infusing. It is critical that the PGE$_1$ infusion not be interrupted in order to maintain patency of the ductus arteriosus. Premedication is not necessary. An intravenous induction usually is used with a predominant narcotic technique. Because the mixing occurs at the atrial level, few strategies exist to improve mixing if the patient becomes even more hypoxemic. Volume loading occasionally will improve the situation, and ensuring adequate depth of anesthesia may be helpful to decrease oxygen consumption. Neonates undergoing the Jatene procedure have the potential to manifest both left and right heart dysfunction. LV dysfunction can occur secondary to coronary artery insufficiency or prolonged cross-clamp time. During the Jatene procedure, the coronary arteries undergo significant dissection and manipulation. Careful attention must be paid to the ST-segment patterns, because myocardial ischemia can occur in these infants. A nitroglycerin infusion at a rate of about 1 to 2 μg/kg/min can aid in relaxation of these vessels. On occasion, surgical revision of one of the coronary artery implantations may be necessary if there is too much stretch or kinking of the vessel. Right heart dysfunction also can be a problem, because these children typically are operated on in the first few weeks of life. PVR during this time period often is high and dynamic. CPB during this time frame increases the PVR, putting an increased workload on the right heart. If the patient has been receiving PGE_1 for a prolonged period of time (more than 2 weeks), it may be advisable to keep a low dose infusing after the repair and wean off it over about 3 days. Abrupt discontinuation of the drug may result in exacerbation of pulmonary hypertension.

d. Problems and complications

    (1) Mustard or Senning operation

        (a) Arrhythmias, especially related to sinus node dysfunction

        (b) Caval obstruction, particularly the superior vena cava

        (c) Pulmonary vein obstruction

        (d) Tricuspid insufficiency

        (e) RV (systemic) failure

        (f) Residual atrial shunt

    (2) Arterial switch (Jatene) operation

        (a) Hemorrhage

        (b) Coronary insufficiency

        (c) Myocardial infarction and LV failure

        (d) Narrowing of the reconstructed PA (late)

    (3) Rastelli

        (a) Conduit narrowing or obstruction

        (b) Residual atrial shunt

3. Tricuspid atresia

a. General considerations. Tricuspid atresia is the third most common cyanotic lesion after tetralogy of Fallot and TGA. There is an absence of the tricuspid valve with no direct communication between the right atrium and the RV. The right atrium is enlarged and thickened, and an obligatory right-to-left shunt at the atrial level is essential to maintain left heart filling. Often this will be a secundum ASD or a stretched foramen ovale. The left side of the heart becomes volume overloaded because it must accept both the systemic and pulmonary blood flow. The RV generally is severely hypoplastic and a VSD is present. Extracardiac anomalies are present in 20% of patients with tricuspid atresia.

Clinical presentation depends on the type of tricuspid atresia (Fig. 14.11). In the most common form of tricuspid atresia, the great arteries are related normally and there is some degree of obstruction to pulmonary blood flow. Over time, the cyanosis will increase as the VSD closes or the infundibular obstruction increases. In about one third of cases, the great arteries are transposed. In this situation, the patient may have normal or increased pulmonary blood flow and manifest signs of CHF. As well, the VSD can become restrictive, resulting in significant subaortic obstruction.

b. Surgical procedures. The goal in caring for these patients is to optimize their physiologic state so that the Fontan operation can be performed by about age 2 to 4 years. Typically, these patients require a multistaged approach to accomplish this goal. Symptomatic neonates may require palliation for either severe cyanosis or CHF. Most commonly, the infant will have decreased pulmonary blood flow and require a systemic-to-PA shunt. On the other hand, about 10% to 15% of patients with tricuspid atresia have markedly increased pulmonary blood flow and may require PA banding to protect the pulmonary vascular tree. If the ASD is restrictive, the patient will require a balloon atrial septostomy.

At about age 6 to 18 months, a bidirectional cavopulmonary anastomosis is created by performing either a bidirectional Glenn procedure (Fig. 14.12) or a hemi-Fontan operation (Fig. 14.13). Both of these procedures result in the same physiologic outcome. Superior vena caval blood passes directly into the PA. These procedures will decrease the volume load on the heart and lower the PA pressures, making the patient a better candidate for the

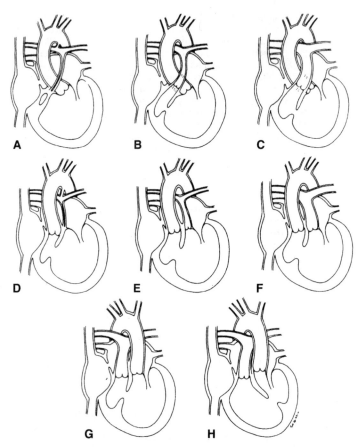

FIG. 14.11 Type I tricuspid atresia, without transposition of the great arteries. **A:** Type Ia, pulmonary atresia with virtual absence of the right ventricle. **B:** Type Ib, pulmonary hypoplasia with subpulmonary stenosis, diminutive right ventricle, and small ventricular septal defect **C:** Type Ic, no pulmonary hypoplasia. There is a diminutive right ventricle. Type II tricuspid atresia, with D-transposition of the great arteries. **D:** Type IIa, pulmonary atresia, aorta arises from the right ventricle. **E:** Type IIb, pulmonary or subpulmonary stenosis. **F:** Type IIc, normal or enlarged pulmonary artery. Type III tricuspid atresia, with L-transposition of the great arteries. **G:** Type IIIa, pulmonary or subpulmonary stenosis. **H:** Type IIIb, subaortic stenosis. There is ventricular inversion. (From Arciniegas E, ed. *Pediatric cardiac surgery.* Chicago: Year Book, 1985:298–300, with permission.)

final operation, the Fontan procedure. Cavopulmonary anastomoses cannot be performed in the neonatal period because PVR is too high. Because blood flow to the lung becomes passive, resistance must be minimal or flow will not occur.

At about age 2 to 4 years, the completion Fontan procedure is performed (Fig. 14.14). It is accomplished by channeling the remaining systemic venous return in the inferior vena cava to the PAs, often by using a lateral tunnel technique with a Gore-Tex tube graft. Usually a fenes-

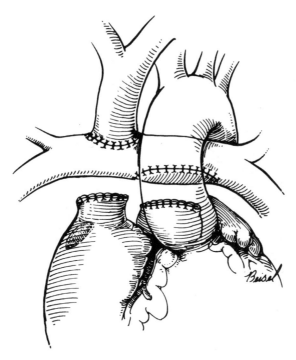

FIG. 14.12 Bidirectional cavopulmonary anastomosis. The divided main pulmonary artery (PA) is seen behind the aorta with patch closure of the distal main PA, and the proximal main PA is oversewn. The superior vena cava has been divided. The cardiac end is oversewn, whereas the cephalic end is sewn end-to-side to the right PA. Superior vena caval blood can flow bidirectionally into both the right and left PAs.

tration also is placed in this baffle, which allows some venous blood to shunt into the left atrium and improves left heart filling. However, this deoxygenated blood can cause some mild desaturation. The fenestration typically will close spontaneously in the first year postoperatively. If it does not or hypoxemia becomes problematic, the patient can be taken to the cardiac catheterization laboratory and an ASD device closure used to resolve it.

Patient selection is extremely important in determining the success of the Fontan procedure. Ideally, PVR should be low (less than 4 Woods units) and the mean PA pressure less than 15 mm Hg. Adequately sized PAs, no systemic AV valve dysfunction, reliable sinus rhythm, and preserved LV function also are important.

c. Anesthetic considerations

    (1) Preoperative. It is imperative to determine the patient's primary physiologic impairment by examining the chest x-ray film, echocardiogram, and cardiac catheterization data. If a neonate has reduced pulmonary blood flow, PGE_1 is given to maintain ductal patency. A balloon atrial septostomy may be necessary if the ASD is small. If the patient has ventricular dysfunction on the basis of chronic volume overload, inotropic support may be needed. In the older patient undergoing a completion Fontan procedure, judicious use of premedication may be beneficial as long as hypoventilation is avoided. If the patient

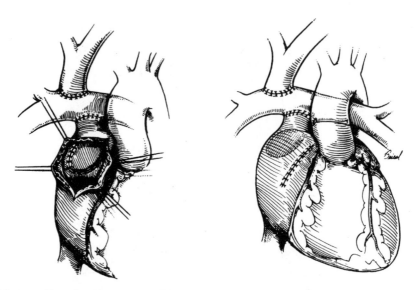

FIG. 14.13 Hemi-Fontan operation. The superior vena cava is divided and each end is anastomosed to the right pulmonary artery. The right atrium is opened, and a Gore-Tex patch is sewn over the orifice of the superior vena cava as it enters the right atrium. Physiologically, this repair is the same as the bidirectional cavopulmonary anastomosis (see Fig. 14.12). The Hemi-Fontan simplifies subsequent surgery to complete the Fontan operation. To complete the Fontan procedure, the Gore-Tex patch is excised and a rectangular piece of Gore-Tex is used to fashion a tunnel from the inferior to the superior vena caval orifice (not shown).

is polycythemic due to hypoxemia, care should be taken to avoid a prolonged NPO status.

(2) Intraoperative. Care of the patient undergoing either a systemic-to-PA shunt or a PA band is covered elsewhere. In general, the goal in caring for children undergoing a bidirectional Glenn, hemi-Fontan, or Fontan procedure is to optimize PVR to promote pulmonary blood flow. An inhalational induction can be used as long as care is taken to maintain airway patency and minimize PVR. If the patient's pulmonary blood flow is ductal dependent, hypotension should be avoided because ductal flow depends on arterial pressure. If ventricular dysfunction is an issue, careful intravenous induction with agents with minimal depressant effects may be preferable.

After the repair, pulmonary blood flow becomes passive and depends on the caval pressure to be able to overcome PVR. Measurement of filling pressures on both the right and left sides of the heart can be helpful in optimizing therapy for patients after the Fontan procedure. A right atrial pressure greater than 10 mm Hg more than the left atrial pressure suggests obstruction to pulmonary blood flow, and therapy should be directed toward decreasing PVR. These maneuvers include optimizing functional residual capacity, hyperventilation, increasing F_{IO_2}, and avoiding acidosis. If the patient is bronchospastic, treatment with inhaled β-agonists may be beneficial. Nitric oxide at a dose of 10 to 40 ppm can be given. Typically, a CVP of about 12 to 15 mm Hg will be necessary to drive blood through the lungs. If a CVP greater than 20 mm Hg is necessary, the prognosis for survival is poor. Fenestrating the Fontan has become the norm, because blood

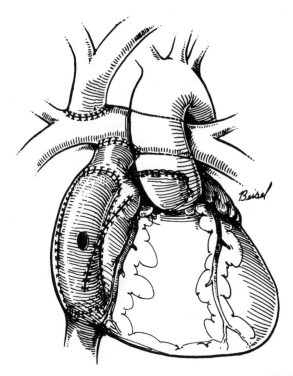

FIG. 14.14 The fenestrated Fontan operation. The superior vena cava is divided and each end is sewn to the right pulmonary artery. The right atrium is opened and a rectangular piece of Gore-Tex is used to fashion a tunnel (lateral baffle) to direct all the inferior vena caval blood flow to the superior vena caval orifice and into the pulmonary arteries. A fenestration (3 or 4 mm in diameter) is placed in the midportion of the Gore-Tex baffle.

which right-to-left shunts helps load the LV and preserve cardiac output. Patients generally tolerate the resultant mild hypoxemia well as long as cardiac output is maintained.

The bidirectional Glenn or hemi-Fontan procedure is tolerated well because inferior vena caval blood continues to be connected to the systemic ventricle. This blood, even though it is desaturated, allows adequate filling of the ventricle, maintaining cardiac output. Attention must be paid to minimizing PVR to ensure adequate pulmonary blood flow and oxygenation.

Increased intrathoracic pressure will limit pulmonary blood flow after a Fontan procedure. Spontaneous ventilation is preferable for optimizing flow. However, hypercarbia will increase PVR and counteract any positive effect of spontaneous ventilation. Ideally it is best to have a limited time of positive-pressure ventilation and to tailor the anesthetic so that the patient can begin spontaneous ventilation and be extubated as soon as possible. Infusion of a short-acting narcotic after bypass may facilitate that goal.

d. **Problems and complications**
   (1) Systemic venous hypertension (with resultant pleural or pericardial effusions, hepatomegaly, ascites, and peripheral edema)

(2) Decreased cardiac output

(3) Atrial arrhythmias

(4) Hypoxemia secondary to residual right-to-left shunt

(5) Thrombosis along the conduit

(6) Pulmonary arteriovenous fistulas

4. **Total anomalous pulmonary venous return**

   a. **General considerations.** In this lesion, all of the pulmonary venous blood drains into the right atrium either directly or indirectly. There is an obligatory interatrial communication by which pulmonary venous blood enters the left atrium and then the LV and aorta. There are four basic types of total anomalous pulmonary venous return (TAPVR) (Fig. 14.15): (i) *supracardiac*—the common pulmonary vein drains through a vertical vein into either a left or right superior vena cava; (ii) *intracardiac*—the common pulmonary vein drains into the coronary sinus and then into the

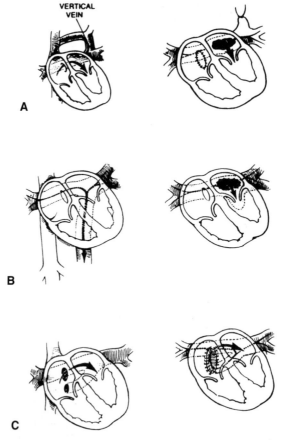

FIG. 14.15 Total anomalous pulmonary venous return. **A:** Supracardiac type **(left)** and surgical correction **(right)**. **B:** Infracardiac type **(left)** and surgical correction **(right)**. **C:** Intracardiac type **(left)** and surgical correction **(right)**. (From Waldhausen JA, Pierce WS, eds. *Johnson's surgery of the chest,* 5th ed. Chicago: Year Book, 1985:355, 357, 359, with permission.)

right atrium; (iii) *infracardiac*—the pulmonary venous blood drains into a descending vein, which traverses the diaphragm and enters the inferior vena cava, portal vein, or ductus venosus; and (iv) *mixed type*—the different pulmonary segments drain to separate sites in the systemic venous system. The most important factor in evaluating these patients is whether or not there is any obstruction to the pulmonary venous drainage. The presence or absence of obstruction is the main determinant of the patient's clinical presentation and prognosis. It should be noted that TAPVR is associated with other complex cardiac lesions in a significant percentage of patients.

The patient with obstruction to drainage will be severely symptomatic in the first week of life. The patient will be markedly cyanotic with respiratory distress. The chest x-ray film is remarkable for a nearly normal heart size but shows a pulmonary interstitial pattern characteristic of pulmonary venous obstruction. Severe obstruction is most likely in patients with the infracardiac type but can occur in patients with any of the types of TAPVR. Infants with severe obstruction have severe pulmonary hypertension and require surgical intervention within the first few days of life.

Patients without pulmonary venous obstruction will have a much more subtle clinical presentation. In this scenario, the patient may be relatively asymptomatic early but has a pulmonary overload situation. Mild cyanosis with oxygen saturations of about 85% to 90% may be difficult to appreciate. These patients are at risk for early development of pulmonary vascular obstructive disease.

b. Surgical procedures. Patients with TAPVR with obstruction must be surgically repaired expeditiously because medical management is not effective. Their condition can rapidly deteriorate and they can die. The goal of the correction is to connect the pulmonary venous system back into the left atrium, eliminate the anomalous connection to the systemic venous system, and close the ASD. Hypothermic CPB with circulatory arrest is commonly used. In the supracardiac type, the common pulmonary trunk is connected directly to the posterior left atrium, the ASD is closed, and the vertical vein is ligated. With the intracardiac type, the coronary sinus is "unroofed" and a patch is used to divert the pulmonary venous return (and the coronary sinus blood) into the left atrium across the ASD. For the infracardiac type, the common pulmonary vein is directly anastomosed to the left atrium, the descending vein is ligated, and the ASD is closed.

c. Anesthetic considerations

(1) Preoperative. Neonates with TAPVR and obstruction represent a true surgical emergency. The only therapy that may be considered preoperatively would be a balloon or blade atrial septostomy in the cardiac catheterization laboratory if the ASD is restrictive. This intervention will increase flow into the left atrium and potentially improve systemic perfusion. This is only a temporizing measure, and surgical intervention should occur as soon as possible. These neonates typically present with severe pulmonary hypertension, cyanosis, and poor perfusion. They often are already intubated and receiving inotropic support. PGE_1 may decompress a hypertensive PA system and even open a ductus venosus, relieving a degree of pulmonary venous obstruction.

(2) Intraoperative. A technique should be used to minimize myocardial depression, typically with intravenous narcotics and paralytics. Inhalational anesthetics generally are not tolerated in the sick neonate but may be acceptable in the older child without obstruction and minimal symptoms.

Two issues arise when planning therapy for separation from CPB. First, these children have reactive pulmonary vascular beds, and efforts must center around decreasing PVR to improve right heart function. Therefore, high oxygen levels, hyperventilation, alkalosis, nitrates, isoproterenol, PGE₁, and nitric oxide may be considered. Second, because the left heart has been chronically underloaded, it may be relatively hypoplastic, noncompliant, and poorly functional. Inotropes and vasodilators may be helpful in improving systemic perfusion. Thus, these patients are at risk for significant dysfunction of both the LV and RV.

  d. Problems and complications
   (1) Pulmonary venous obstruction
   (2) Pulmonary hypertension and increased reactivity
   (3) RV failure
   (4) LV failure
   (5) Arrhythmias, predominantly supraventricular
 5. Truncus arteriosus
  a. General considerations. These patients have a single arterial vessel, the truncus, arising from the base of the heart (Fig. 14.16). A high VSD invariably is present under the truncal valve. PAs arise either from a common stem (90% of the time) or separately from the truncus. A right aortic arch occurs in about 25% of cases. The truncal valve usually consists of three or four cusps, although this can vary from two to six cusps. In about half of patients, the valve is dysplastic and insufficient. Extracardiac anomalies are common. Fortunately, this defect is relatively uncommon.

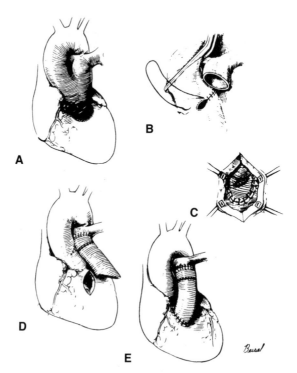

FIG. 14.16 A: Truncus arteriosus. **B:** The pulmonary trunk is separated. **C:** The ventricular septal defect is closed with a prosthetic patch. **D:** A valved conduit (usually pulmonary allograft) is used to establish right ventricle to pulmonary artery continuity. **E:** The complete repair. (From Waldhausen JA, Pierce WS, eds. *Johnson's surgery of the chest,* 5th ed. Chicago: Year Book, 1985:397, with permission.)

These patients are symptomatic early in infancy, with a picture of CHF. These infants have markedly increased pulmonary blood flow, and arterial saturation is dependent on the ratio of pulmonary blood flow to systemic blood flow. Even though mixing of the two circulations occurs, cyanosis may be only minimal. Because of the high flow and pressures going to the lungs, damage to the pulmonary vascular bed occurs early. Untreated, the majority of children will die in the first 6 months of life.

b. Surgical procedures. Palliation with PA banding can be done, but it is not effective and is associated with a high mortality. More commonly, complete repair is performed in infants younger than 6 months. In this procedure, the VSD is patched so as to direct blood from the LV out the aorta (truncus). The PAs are disconnected from the truncus and an RV-to-PA conduit is placed. If the truncal valve is severely insufficient, it must be repaired or replaced.

c. Anesthetic considerations

(1) Preoperative. Care of these patients is similar to any other critically ill neonate. Preoperative sedation is not necessary. These patients may already be intubated on positive-pressure ventilation. If CHF is severe, they may be receiving positive inotropic drugs.

Some of these patients have DiGeorge syndrome with absent thymus and immunologic deficiency. If so, they are susceptible to graft-versus-host disease and require irradiated blood products. They also are prone to infection and require regular antibiotic prophylaxis. Until the diagnosis is known with certainty, one should assume the worst and take appropriate precautions. If a thymus is found at operation, then the diagnosis has been excluded.

(2) Intraoperative. The anesthetic technique must account for the fact that the child is in a tenuous hemodynamic state. The goal should be to preserve systemic blood flow while minimizing pulmonary blood flow. High-dose narcotics are used most often. One must take care not to hyperventilate the patient, because that will lower PVR and shunt more blood to the lungs. Maneuvers to try in an attempt to limit pulmonary blood flow include limiting inspired oxygen concentration, maintaining normocarbia or even hypercarbia, and using PEEP. The surgeon also can put a tourniquet around the PAs to constrict flow. This is especially important during CPB to ensure that systemic perfusion is adequate. One must be careful not to lower SVR too much, especially if the truncal valve is insufficient. In that case, diastolic pressure may already be low, which predisposes the baby to coronary insufficiency.

After the repair, therapy should be directed toward increasing pulmonary blood flow. These children have an incredibly reactive pulmonary vasculature and often benefit from sedation for several days postoperatively to minimize pulmonary vascular crises. Inotropic therapy usually is necessary for separation from bypass.

d. Problems and complications

(1) LV dysfunction

(2) Pulmonary hypertensive crises and RV failure

(3) Truncal valve regurgitation

(4) Heart block

(5) Conduit stenosis due to growth

6. Hypoplastic left heart syndrome

a. General considerations. Hypoplastic left heart syndrome is a term used to describe a spectrum of diseases, with the common denominator being underdevelopment of the left side of the heart (Fig. 14.17). The patient may have mitral atresia, aortic atresia, and/or a hypoplastic aortic arch. With all of these lesions, the LV is small. All blood flow returning to the heart from the lungs passes from the left atrium to the right atrium, where it mixes with the systemic venous return. The RV then becomes the pumping

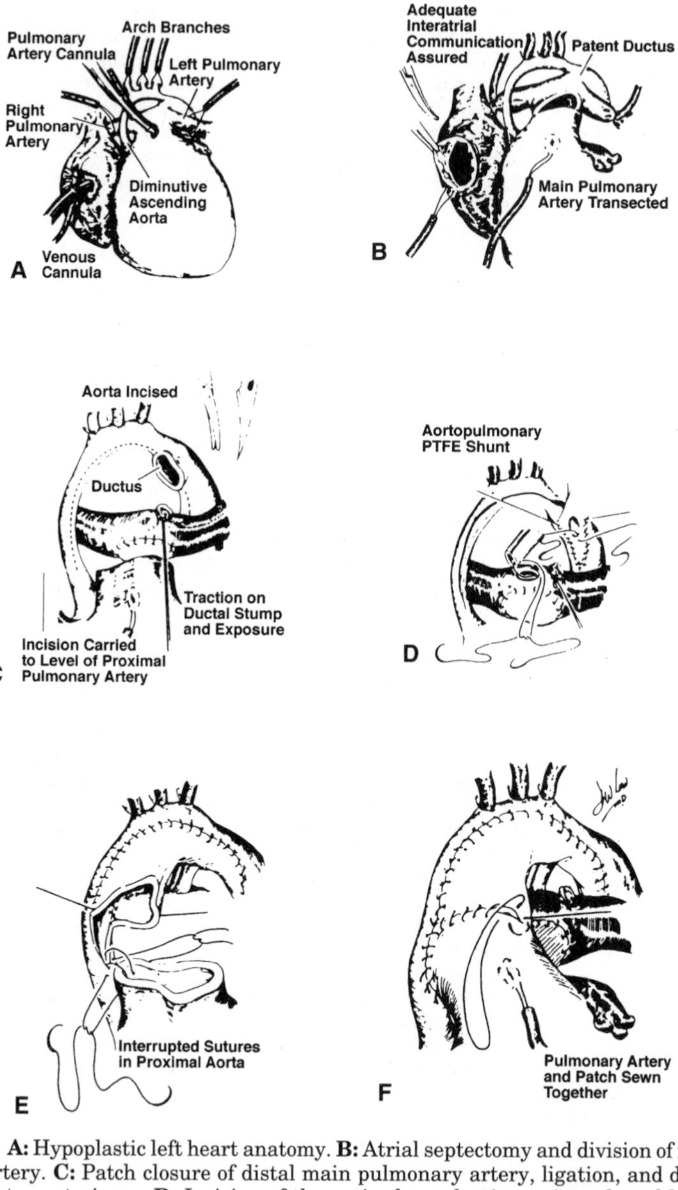

FIG. 14.17 A: Hypoplastic left heart anatomy. B: Atrial septectomy and division of main pulmonary artery. C: Patch closure of distal main pulmonary artery, ligation, and division of patent ductus arteriosus. D: Incision of the entire hypoplastic aortic arch and homograft patch enlargement and central aortopulmonary shunt. E: Anastomosis of proximal main pulmonary artery and reconstructed aortic arch. F: Completed repair. (From Edwards LH, Norwood W, eds. *Atlas of cardiothoracic surgery*. Philadelphia: Lea & Febiger, 1989, with permission.)

chamber for both the pulmonary and systemic circulation. Blood entering the PA goes to the lungs and across the PDA to the body. Perfusion to the cerebral and coronary circulation is dependent on retrograde flow through the hypoplastic aortic arch.

These infants often may appear healthy at birth as long as the ductus arteriosus is widely patent. Within a few hours to a few days, the patient's condition rapidly deteriorates as the ductus arteriosus begins to close and systemic perfusion becomes inadequate. These infants manifest tachypnea, tachycardia, cardiomegaly, poor peripheral pulses, and what has been termed "gray cyanosis" (a result of both systemic desaturation and low cardiac output). Without therapy, the average age at death is 4 to 5 days. Extracardiac anomalies (usually minor genitourinary malformations) occur in about 15% to 25% of cases.

b. Surgical procedures. There are basically two surgical options for these infants. They can undergo either orthotopic cardiac transplantation or a staged reconstructive procedure as first described by Norwood. Although transplantation is an attractive option, it is not generally performed, primarily because of limited availability of donor organs. The Norwood procedure has been refined over the years, but it still consists of the following important components (Fig. 14.17B–F): (a) atrial septectomy; (b) anastomosis of the proximal PA to the diminutive aorta, with homograft augmentation of the aorta and aortic arch; and (c) an aortopulmonary shunt. The first stage of a Norwood procedure is a palliative operation whose purpose is to create a more stable physiology. By augmenting the aorta and anastomosing it to the PA, systemic perfusion then comes directly from the RV and is no longer dependent on the PDA. The main pulmonary trunk is disconnected from the PAs, and pulmonary blood flow is provided via the aortopulmonary shunt. The Norwood procedure generally is performed in the first month of life. Then, at about 6 months, the child undergoes the second stage of palliation, either a bidirectional Glenn shunt or a hemi-Fontan. This interim procedure is necessary in order to take some of the volume load off the RV, which allows remodeling and helps preserve its function. Later, at about 18 to 24 months, the final completion Fontan is performed.

c. Anesthetic considerations. The following discussion centers on care of the infant undergoing the first stage of the Norwood procedure. Anesthetic considerations for stage 2 (cavopulmonary connection) or stage 3 (Fontan) have been covered elsewhere.

(1) Preoperative. There are two major goals that must be accomplished to successfully care for these critically ill neonates. First, the PDA must be kept patent to allow systemic perfusion. Second, the balance between SVR and PVR must be maintained in order to optimize blood flow to each circuit. PGE_1 is infused to maintain patency of the ductus arteriosus. These neonates typically present with profound metabolic acidosis at the time of diagnosis. This abnormality should be aggressively treated to improve cardiac function. The children typically are intubated and sedated to minimize oxygen consumption. Mild hypercarbia (PCO_2 45 to 55 mm Hg), low oxygen concentrations, and PEEP are helpful in restricting pulmonary blood flow. It is important to remember that oxygen is a powerful pulmonary vasodilator and can cause excessive pulmonary blood flow and inadequate systemic perfusion. These children commonly are maintained on room air. If PVR is too low, a mildly hypoxic (FIO_2 18%) mixture also can be considered. When the pulmonary and systemic circuits are well balanced, one would expect to see S_pO_2 values of about 75% to 80%. Higher values imply inadequate systemic perfusion and pulmonary overload. Transfusion often is necessary to keep the hematocrit about 45% to ensure adequate oxygen delivery to the tissues. The children may require inotropic support, and dopamine may be advantageous if PVR is low.

(2) **Intraoperative.** All of the preoperative strategies must be continued in the operating room. Anesthesia usually is accomplished with narcotics to minimize myocardial depression. Inotropic agents may be required to maintain stability during dissection. After repair, individual management is dictated by how large the aortopulmonary shunt is and how much pulmonary blood flow results. The same physiology exists after repair, with emphasis on balancing the systemic and pulmonary blood flows. One must be sure to fully expand the lungs to avoid atelectasis. Then, the degree of ventilation and the oxygen concentration used depends on the patient's oxygen saturation. Some centers advocate adding CO_2 to the circuit to allow vigorous ventilation and maintenance of functional residual capacity without causing respiratory alkalosis. As previously mentioned, one would expect to see a S_pO_2 of about 75% to 80% when the pulmonary and systemic flows are ideally matched. These children may benefit from heavy postoperative sedation to avoid pulmonary hypertensive crises.

d. **Problems and complications**
   (1) Too much or too little pulmonary blood flow
   (2) Inadequate systemic perfusion
   (3) Myocardial dysfunction
   (4) AV valvular regurgitation
   (5) Myocardial ischemia
   (6) Pulmonary hypertensive crisis

B. **Lesions likely to cause CHF**
1. **Ventricular septal defect**
   a. **General considerations.** Ventricular septal defect occurs commonly, either in conjunction with other cardiac defects or as an isolated lesion. VSDs can be categorized into four types (Fig. 14.18): (i) *supracristal defect* just under the pulmonary valve; (ii) *infracristal perimembranous defect,* the most common type; (iii) *canal or inlet-type defect,* a form of partial AV canal; and (iv) *muscular defects* in the trabecular portion of the ventricular septum. The size of the defect and the PVR determine the amount of blood flow that passes left-to-right to the pulmonary bed. A small VSD, termed "restrictive," often will cause minimal symptoms and may close

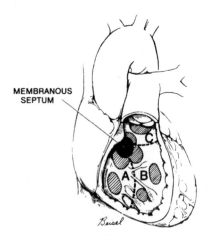

FIG. 14.18 The location of ventricular septal defects in the membranous inlet (*A*), trabecular (*B*), and infundibular (*C*) septa. (From Waldhausen JA, Pierce WS, eds. *Johnson's surgery of the chest,* 5th ed. Chicago: Year Book, 1985:335, with permission.)

spontaneously in the first 5 years of life. Large defects are nearly equal in cross-sectional-area to the area of the aortic annulus and allow free communication between the two ventricles. The pressures in both ventricles will be equal and, because PVR usually is about one sixth of SVR, pulmonary blood flow will be greater than systemic blood flow. This excess flow will cause dilation of the left atrium, LV, and usually the RV. If the defect is large, the patient will develop symptoms of CHF at about age 1 month as the PVR falls. The child generally manifests tachypnea, tachycardia, failure to thrive, and frequent respiratory infections. The child may have mild cyanosis if he or she has a respiratory infection or pulmonary overload, but this hypoxemia improves with oxygen. If a large VSD remains unrepaired, the high pressure and flow to the lungs will result in irreversible pulmonary vascular damage. As this situation develops, the patient will become less symptomatic as the pulmonary blood flow decreases. The terminal stage of this process results in a reversal of the shunt so that the flow becomes right-to-left, the so-called "Eisenmenger complex." If the process has advanced to this point, surgical repair can no longer be performed. The time course for the development of this pulmonary vascular damage is variable. Because of this problem, most centers plan repair of large defects within the first year of life.

b. Surgical procedures

   (1) Complete repair using CPB typically is the operation of choice for most patients. Patch closure of the defect usually is accomplished by approaching it through the right atrium and tricuspid valve. On occasion, a right ventriculotomy may be necessary to visualize defects in the ventricular apex or RVOT.

   (2) PA banding was formerly the procedure of choice for infants in order to limit the excessive pulmonary blood flow and allow growth, then complete repair was performed later at about age 4 years. Today a one-stage complete repair is done more commonly, even in infancy. However, PA banding still may play a role in patients with multiple muscular VSDs or other complex lesions associated with VSD and excess pulmonary perfusion.

c. Anesthetic considerations

   (1) Preoperative. Children who require surgery early in life have large VSDs and excessive pulmonary blood flow. Initial medical management includes digitalis, diuretics, and often antibiotics (because the children typically present with respiratory infections). The choice of whether or not premedication is indicated depends on the age of the child and the degree of ventricular dysfunction. Most children younger than about 10 months will not need any preoperative sedation. On the other hand, an older child may benefit from judicious sedation, keeping in mind the importance of avoiding hypercarbia so that pulmonary hypertension is not exacerbated.

   (2) Intraoperative. Choice of anesthetic agents depends on the clinical status of the patient. If the patient has limited cardiac reserve, a primary narcotic technique may be beneficial. If the child is less symptomatic, inhalational induction can be used, with a switch toward a balanced technique when intravenous access is secured.

      One must be meticulous in de-airing the intravenous fluids whenever there is an abnormal connection between the left and right sides of the heart. Even when the patient has a predominant left-to-right shunt, the direction of flow can easily change at any time. If air ends up on the left side of the heart, it can be pumped to the brain and cause a stroke.

      If the VSD is nonrestrictive, care must be taken not to overventilate the child after intubation. Hypocarbia and hyperoxia will lower PVR and make the left-to-right shunt even more profound, often at the expense of systemic perfusion. Using a lower inspired oxygen concentration and normocarbia can help to balance the circulations. Application of 5 to 10 cm H_2O PEEP can help limit the excessive pulmonary flow by diverting more to the body.

Separation from CPB generally is straightforward for most patients. However, if the patient has preexisting pulmonary vascular disease, RV dysfunction can be problematic. In that case, efforts should be directed toward decreasing PVR and optimizing cardiac output. A combination of vasodilators and inotropes often can be beneficial. Phosphodiesterase inhibitors may be particularly helpful because of their pulmonary vasodilatory properties.

  d. **Problems and complications**
    (1) Pulmonary hypertension and RV dysfunction
    (2) Residual left-to-right shunt
    (3) LV dysfunction, especially if the cross-clamp time is prolonged
    (4) Heart block, usually due to swelling along the patch suture line. Usually it resolves over several days; however, it can be permanent if the conduction system is inadvertently damaged during the repair.
    (5) Respiratory insufficiency and slow weaning from the ventilator if the patient had increased lung water preoperatively
    (6) Aortic insufficiency only occurs rarely if the VSD was supracristal and sutures distort the septal cusp

2. **Atrial septal defect**
  a. **General considerations.** There are three types of ASDs (Fig. 14.19): (i) *ostium secundum* (the most common type) is located centrally at the area of the fossa ovalis; (ii) *sinus venosus type* occurs at the junction of the superior vena cava and right atrium and usually is associated with partial anomalous pulmonary venous return; and (iii) *ostium primum defect* occurs low in the septum and often is associated with a cleft mitral valve. Ostium primum defects sometimes are referred to as partial AV canals, and the patient may have some associated mitral insufficiency. ASDs occur more commonly in females than in males.

  ASDs will result in an atrial level left-to-right shunt causing increased volume to the right side of the heart. The size of the defect and the ratio of LV and RV compliance determine the amount of flow. These defects often can be large and the pulmonary blood flow can be three to four times the systemic blood flow. Patients usually are asymptomatic, especially if it is a secundum defect. If CHF symptoms occur early in infancy, one should be

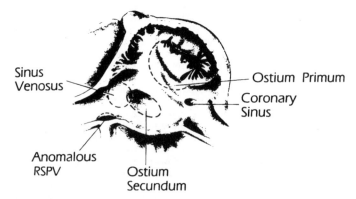

FIG. 14.19 Artist's depiction of the opened right atrium showing the anatomic location of atrial septal defects. *RSPV,* right superior pulmonary vein. (From Doty DB. *Cardiac surgery.* Chicago: Year Book, 1985:1, with permission.)

suspicious that the patient has another coexisting defect. PVR changes do not develop early, and the Eisenmenger physiology usually does not occur until after the second decade of life, if at all. It is not unusual for a patient to reach the fourth decade of life and have an undiagnosed ASD. Patients may first come to medical attention due to occurrence of a stroke or because of development of symptomatology during pregnancy. Closure of ASDs typically is recommended in order to prevent paradoxical emboli and pulmonary vascular disease.

b. Surgical procedures. Repair most commonly is performed with CPB and mild hypothermia. The procedure can be done using fibrillation, or the aorta can be cross-clamped. The defect is visualized through a right atriotomy. If it is a secundum defect, it often can be closed primarily. If it is large, a patch may be necessary. For a sinus venosus defect, a patch is positioned to redirect flow from the partial anomalous pulmonary venous return to the left atrium. If the pulmonary veins enter the superior vena cava, a rather elongated patch may be necessary to tunnel the veins over to the left atrium. Repair of an ostium primum defect requires a patch and attention to the cleft mitral valve. If necessary, sutures are used to restore competency to the mitral valve, taking care not to make it stenotic. Because the AV conduction system runs right along the inferior rim of the defect, particular attention must be paid to the placement of these stitches in order to avoid heart block.

Device closure of ASDs in the cardiac catheterization laboratory may be an option for some patients, depending on the size and location of the defect. As more experience is gained and the technology of the device improves, transcatheter ASD closure may become more common, thus obviating the need for surgery in some patients.

c. Anesthetic considerations. These children typically are healthy and usually undergo surgery at about age 4 to 5 years. Just about any anesthetic technique can be used successfully. Premedication often is helpful to facilitate separation from their parents and a smooth induction. Typically, the CPB time is relatively short and weaning from bypass is uneventful. The anesthetic technique should be tailored toward a goal of extubation at the end of the procedure if no complications arise. Therefore, we usually limit the amount of narcotics used and rely more heavily on inhaled anesthetics. As with any lesion involving an intracardiac communication, one must be sure to avoid any air in the intravenous catheters.

One interesting thing to keep in mind is that central venous pressure in these patients can be misleading postoperatively. The right atrium has become accustomed to handling a high volume and often is dilated and compliant. Subsequently, when the ASD is closed, the volume in the right atrium decreases acutely. If one relies on the CVP measurement with a goal of replacing volume to a "normal" value of 8 to 10 mm Hg, it is likely that the patient will be markedly overhydrated and liable to fall off the back of the Frank–Starling curve. It is much better to visually inspect the surgical field to determine adequacy of volume replacement.

d. Problems and complications
   (1) Atrial arrhythmias, especially atrial fibrillation or paroxysmal atrial tachycardia
   (2) Complete heart block in ostium primum repairs
   (3) Mitral insufficiency or stenosis after cleft repair with ostium primum defects
   (4) Persistent left-to-right shunt
   (5) Pulmonary edema if patient is overtransfused

3. AV canal defects
   a. General considerations. This defect, also known as endocardial cushion defect, represents a spectrum of disease resulting from failure of the endocardial cushions, which form the central part of the heart, to develop and fuse properly. The result is a defect in lower atrial and upper ventricular

septa and deficiencies in the mitral and tricuspid valves (Fig. 14.20). The defect can be partial or complete. In the partial type, there may be just an interatrial communication (an ostium primum defect) or just an interventricular communication. A cleft in the mitral valve usually is present, causing varying degrees of mitral valve insufficiency. In the complete type of AV canal, the entire central portion of the cardiac septum is absent and there is a single AV valve with free communication among the four cardiac chambers. The common AV valve may be relatively competent or freely insufficient. This lesion occurs with equal frequency in males and females. It is the most common cardiac anomaly seen in children with Down syndrome.

The patient's clinical condition depends on the anatomic variation present. In general, AV canal physiology results from a large left-to-right shunt with pulmonary overload and CHF. These children normally manifest early in life, with the typical features of excessive pulmonary blood flow. Generally, the larger the ventricular defect and the greater the mitral insufficiency, the sicker the infant. Cyanosis is rare, unless the child has superimposed pulmonary stenosis, a respiratory infection, or high PVR. Some patients with AV canal have LV outlet tract obstruction, which alters their prognosis.

Infants with complete AV canal develop irreversible pulmonary vascular disease early in life. Therefore, most centers plan surgical repair within the first 6 months of life.

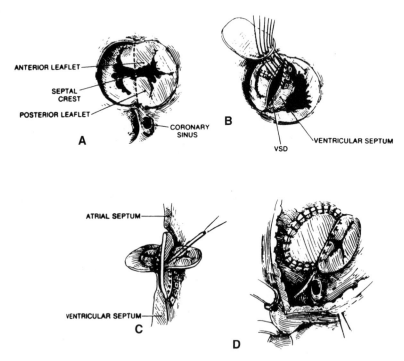

FIG. 14.20 A: Artist's depiction of complete atrioventricular canal as viewed from above. **B:** The pericardial patch is attached to the rightward aspect of the ventricular septum. *VSD,* ventricular septal defect. **C:** The valve leaflets are attached to the pericardial patch. **D:** The completed repair from the right atrial view. (From Waldhausen JA, Pierce WS, eds. *Johnson's surgery of the chest,* 5th ed. Chicago: Year Book, 1985:349, with permission.)

b. Surgical procedures. The practice of PA banding as a palliative step before complete repair has largely been abandoned, except in infants with complex anatomy that precludes complete repair at an early age. Results from PA banding have been disappointing, and the results of early complete repair have steadily improved. PA banding still may be indicated in patients with an unbalanced AV canal in order to limit the pulmonary blood flow and protect the vasculature for future interventions.

Complete repair is accomplished using CPB with moderate hypothermia or occasionally DHCA. The defects are visualized through a right atriotomy. Careful inspection of the defects must be carried out, because there is significant variability among patients. The septal defects are closed with either one or two patches and the AV valves are reconstructed and attached to the patch. When reconstructing the AV valves, it is important to make them as competent as possible without creating AV valve stenosis. Extreme care must be taken when suturing the VSD patch to avoid the conduction system, which lies close to the defect.

c. Anesthetic considerations

   (1) Preoperative. Infants with complete AV canal generally have been managed medically with digitalis and diuretics before surgery. It is important to check for electrolyte abnormalities. One may consider holding the morning digitalis dose. These infants typically do not require preoperative sedation, especially if they have Down syndrome.

   (2) Intraoperative. Choice of anesthetic agents depends on the patient's clinical condition. If the child has severe CHF, intravenous induction with predominantly narcotics may be advisable. With lesser degrees of symptomatology, an inhalational technique may be appropriate. The goals in managing these patients are to minimize myocardial depression and to maintain or even slightly increase PVR while preventing increases in SVR. One must be careful to keep the patient normocapnic after intubation, with consideration for decreasing inspired oxygen concentration and perhaps using PEEP to limit pulmonary blood flow.

   Complete repair of an AV canal requires a lengthy period of CPB. One should anticipate difficulty with elevated PVR as well as ventricular dysfunction and possibly AV valve insufficiency upon separation from bypass. Typically both inotropic and vasodilator therapy are required. Because of the dysplastic nature of the AV valves, early inotropic support is begun in an effort to allow the heart to operate more efficiently at a lower filling pressure. The goal is to avoid ventricular distention and annular dilation, which is likely to exacerbate AV valve insufficiency. Thus, it is ideal to try to keep the left atrial pressure around 10 to 12 mm Hg. If AV conduction problems occur, AV pacing may be necessary. Because of the reactivity of these infants' pulmonary vasculature, they typically are deeply sedated and ventilated for a variable period of time postoperatively to facilitate their recovery.

d. Problems and complications

   (1) Pulmonary hypertension and RV failure

   (2) LV dysfunction and low systemic output

   (3) Mitral and/or tricuspid insufficiency

   (4) Heart block

   (5) Ventricular and atrial arrhythmias

   (6) Residual shunt

4. Patent ductus arteriosus

   a. General considerations. This lesion is one of the more common lesions encountered, especially in conjunction with other cardiac anomalies. The ductus arteriosus is a normal fetal vessel between the aorta and the left PA, which serves *in utero* to allow most of the blood from the RV to bypass the nonaerated lungs. Normally, this vessel functionally closes within hours after birth. Patency beyond the first few days of life can occur and may result in significant hemodynamic consequences if the lumen is large and the PVR is low. Rubella, prematurity, and hypoxemia are known risk factors associated with nonclosure of the ductus arteriosus.

Typically, the clinician is likely to encounter two distinct populations with isolated PDA. It is noted commonly in the premature neonatal intensive care unit group, often causing pulmonary overload with respiratory distress and inability to wean from the ventilator. These children often can be successfully medically treated with indomethacin to promote closure of the PDA. However, on occasion, surgical therapy may be necessary if indomethacin is contraindicated or not successful. Older children, often asymptomatic, represent the other group of patients in whom a heart murmur is detected on their routine physical examination before school. The degree of symptomatology depends on the amount of flow to the lungs. One would expect to see a wide pulse pressure with bounding pulses and a continuous murmur heard both on the front and back of the chest. Of course, one must remember that PDA commonly occurs in association with other more complex lesions and, in those cases, the manifestations will be more dependent on the associated anatomy.

   b. **Surgical procedures.** The classic surgical approach for repair involves a limited left thoracotomy. The vessel is located and can be ligated with suture or clamped with vascular clips. Many surgeons doubly ligate and divide the vessel to ensure that it will not recanalize. Recently, many centers have advocated a thoracoscopic approach to the procedure. As well, many interventional cardiologists perform catheter closure of PDAs, using a variety of closure devices. These have included disk devices, coils, and buttons. Although there is a learning curve to all of the newer procedures, improvement in the design of the equipment has resulted in excellent results with minimal complications.

   c. **Anesthetic considerations.** Most of the patients will be tiny premature infants. In addition to the usual considerations for these types of children, one must pay particular attention to respiratory care, temperature, and fluid management. Because of the increased pulmonary blood flow, these neonates usually will come to the operating room already intubated. They may benefit from the judicious application of continuous positive airway pressure to help improve oxygenation and manage the excess lung water. During the thoracotomy, the nondependent lung will be compressed and not ventilated, and hypoxemia can become an issue. One must balance the need to ventilate aggressively enough to maintain oxygenation while trying to avoid using airway pressures that may injure these immature lungs. It is important and can be a challenge to keep these children warm, especially if the infant must be transported to the operating room for the procedure. One should try to restrict the fluids administered, because these neonates already are fluid overloaded and in CHF.

   Management of the older child is straightforward. The surgical procedure is short, and invasive monitoring generally is not required. It is important to be sure to obtain adequate venous access because there is a chance of significant blood loss, although this complication is rare. These patients may benefit from preoperative sedation to facilitate separation from their parents. Any anesthetic technique is acceptable, tailoring it toward a goal of extubation at the end. The pain from a thoracotomy is significant, so judicious use of intravenous or epidural narcotics is advisable.

   d. **Problems and complications**
       (1) Ligation of the incorrect vessel (descending aorta or left PA) can cause systemic hypoperfusion or hypoxemia
       (2) Recurrent laryngeal nerve damage
       (3) Ductal recanalization
       (4) LV dysfunction caused by the acute increase in afterload due to removal of the low-resistance pulmonary circuit

5. Coarctation of the aorta

   a. General considerations. The typical aortic coarctation is a localized narrowing of the aorta just distal to the left subclavian artery and just proximal
   to, opposite, or distal to the insertion of the ductus arteriosus. This lesion
   is likely to become symptomatic during two periods of life. Infants with
   severe obstruction can develop symptoms of CHF early in life. Others remain asymptomatic until adolescence or adulthood. Often the lesion is discovered at a routine physical examination because of a heart murmur, with
   diminished distal pulses and a pressure gradient between the upper and
   lower limbs. These children often exhibit upper extremity hypertension,
   and rib notching on chest x-ray film occurs after about age 8 years due to
   the development of collateral circulation (Fig. 14.21).

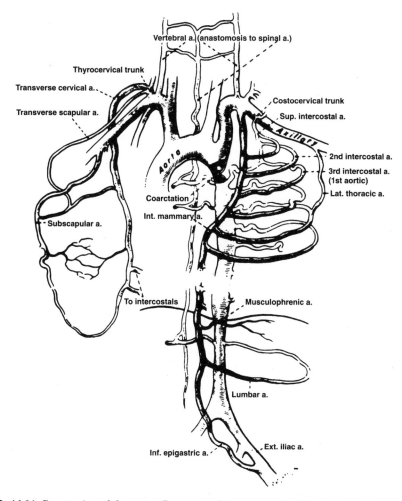

FIG. 14.21 Coarctation of the aorta. Depiction of the course of collateral circulation in patients with coarctation of the aorta. (From Edwards JE, et al. The collateral circulation in
coarctation of the aorta. *Mayo Clin Proc* 1948;23:334, with permission.)

The symptomatic neonate with coarctation demonstrates LV failure, with distal hypoperfusion and metabolic acidosis. If the child has a preductal coarctation and pulmonary hypertension, flow across the ductus can be right-to-left, causing "differential cyanosis" of the upper (pink) and lower (blue) body. In the first few days of life, the discrepancy in pressures in the upper versus lower extremities may be difficult to appreciate, especially if the ductus is open and ventricular function is poor. Many neonates with this lesion require preoperative inotropic support.

Associated cardiovascular malformations are common, especially bicuspid aortic valve (occurring in about 50% of patients as a coexisting lesion). In the extreme form of aortic isthmus narrowing, complete interruption of the aorta occurs. In that case, a large VSD almost invariably is present. The lower part of the body then is perfused by the ductus arteriosus.

b. **Surgical procedures.** Surgical repair is through a left thoracotomy. Several different surgical techniques have been used. For infants, a subclavian flap angioplasty often is used. In older children, the affected area is resected and an end-to-end anastomosis is done. Occasionally, interposition grafts are required if the coarctation segment is long. Patch augmentation of the aorta has generated concern because of the high incidence of aneurysm formation at the site of repair. Balloon angioplasty of the coarctation is another option, but its use has been associated with a high incidence of residual or recurrent stenosis. There may be a place for its use, however, in situations of recurrent stenosis after surgical repair.

c. **Anesthetic considerations.** Although the surgical approach is similar, anesthetic technique will be markedly different between an infant with coarctation and CHF and an older child with relatively asymptomatic coarctation. The critically ill neonate typically will come to the operating room with PGE_1 infusing to allow postductal flow. This infant will require a high-dose narcotic technique to minimize hemodynamic embarrassment. The older child typically has LV hypertrophy and hypertension and can benefit from volatile anesthetics that provide some myocardial depression. Either an inhalational technique or an intravenous induction is acceptable in the older child. Both groups require antibiotic prophylaxis.

The site for monitoring blood pressure is important. A right radial arterial catheter should be placed. The left arm is avoided, because the subclavian artery often must be clamped or ligated to facilitate repair. When the aorta is cross-clamped, the upper body blood pressure will rise. One must be careful not to try to lower this pressure back to "normal," because spinal cord perfusion is critically dependent on this pressure head. Inadequate perfusion to the spinal cord can result in paraplegia. Some centers monitor the spinal cord with somatosensory evoked potentials. If so, one must design a plan to provide a steady-state anesthetic with agents that only minimally affect the evoked potentials. A continuous infusion of narcotics with a low concentration of volatile agent works well.

After removal of the cross-clamp, aggressive control of the blood pressure is indicated. The neonates typically do not manifest hypertension, but the older patients often exhibit a paradoxical increase in blood pressure to levels even higher than beginning levels. Initial control can be obtained with sodium nitroprusside, but prolonged use of this drug is associated with tachyphylaxis. Combination agents such as labetalol, which provide both α- and β-blockade, are ideal. It can be initially infused intravenously and later switched to oral use when the patient is taking fluids by mouth.

Adequate pain control can help to control the hypertension. Thoracic epidural infusions of local anesthetics and narcotics are effective and well tolerated. Intravenous patient-controlled analgesia is another alternative in the older population. Intercostal nerve blocks may not be a good choice because of the prominent collateral vessels in that area, which increase the potential for significant bleeding.

In the older group, extubation at the end of the surgical procedure is desirable. Early extubation aids in blood pressure control. It also allows one to perform a thorough neurologic examination. The neonatal population usually benefits from continued intubation, ventilation, and diuresis, at least overnight.

d. Problems and complications

(1) Paraplegia, although rare (a reported incidence of 0.4%), occurs unpredictably. It seems to be associated with poor collateralization and prolonged distal hypotension.

(2) Hemorrhage

(3) Paradoxical hypertension, often requiring treatment for weeks to months

(4) Mesenteric arteritis with abdominal pain, thought to be secondary to reactive vasoconstriction and ischemia

(5) Damage to adjacent structures, including the left recurrent laryngeal nerve (resulting in vocal cord paralysis), phrenic nerve (causing diaphragm paralysis), sympathetic trunk (causing Horner syndrome), and thoracic duct (causing a chylothorax)

C. Miscellaneous procedures

1. Vascular rings

a. General considerations. Although the specific anatomy can vary, these anomalies of the aortic arch and its branches result in the presence of a blood vessel on each side of the trachea and esophagus. Encirclement of these structures generally causes significant symptoms that appear in infancy. These children may present with severe inspiratory stridor, dyspnea, wheezing, dysphagia, and a cough. Frequent respiratory infections are common, resulting from airway obstruction and aspiration from esophageal compression. Three types of vascular rings are likely (Fig. 14.22): (i) *double aortic arch* (from persistence of the primitive double arch), (ii) *right aortic arch with left ductus arteriosus,* and (iii) *retroesophageal right subclavian artery* (resulting in an incomplete ring). PA sling is a rarer type of vascular ring that occurs when the left PA comes off the right PA and encircles the right main stem bronchus and distal trachea before going to the left lung.

b. Surgical procedures. The surgical approach depends on the particular vascular anatomy. Repair usually is performed through a left thoracotomy. It is important to define the anatomy carefully, to determine which vessel of the rings is expendable. This vessel is ligated and divided, and the ductus or ligamentum is divided to provide as much mobility as possible. Repair of a PA sling usually requires a median sternotomy and CPB. The left PA is divided from the right PA and reimplanted into the main PA anterior to the trachea. Many of these children will have complete tracheal rings and will require tracheoplasty.

c. Anesthetic considerations. These children typically are small, with varying degrees of respiratory distress. Careful airway management is critical. Vascular rings can behave similarly to an anterior mediastinal mass, with tracheal compression during induction of anesthesia. An inhalational induction is preferred, with neuromuscular blocking agents given only after the airway is secured. Multiple sizes of endotracheal tubes should be available.

Monitoring should include an arterial line; in some cases, a central line may be advisable. Adequate venous access is mandatory, because significant bleeding occasionally occurs during this type of procedure. In infants with this lesion, intraoperative transesophageal echocardiography probably is contraindicated. It contributes little to the management of these patients, and limited space within the vascular ring may precipitate an airway crisis with probe placement.

Many of these children have tracheomalacia from the vascular ring, and the condition often persists even after the ring is released. They often have significant secretions in their airways, because their cough has been ineffective due to the ring. In small children with preoperative respiratory distress, one should anticipate postoperative mechanical ventilation.

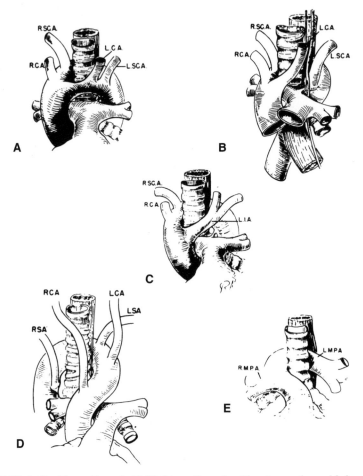

FIG. 14.22 A: Double aortic arch. **B:** Right aortic arch with retroesophageal left subclavian artery. **C:** Right aortic arch with mirror-image branching and left ligamentum arteriosum. **D:** Left aortic arch with retroesophageal right subclavian artery and right ligamentum arteriosum. **E:** Anomalous left pulmonary artery from right pulmonary artery. *LCA,* left carotid artery; *LMPA,* left main pulmonary artery; *LSCA (LSA),* left subclavian artery; RCA, right carotid artery; RMPA, right main pulmonary artery; RSCA (RSA), right subclavian artery. (From Arciniegas E, ed. *Pediatric cardiac surgery.* Chicago: Year Book, 1985:119, 122, 123, with permission.)

Older children with incomplete rings and minimal symptoms often can be extubated at the end of the procedure. Effective pain management with either an epidural or patient-controlled analgesia can help facilitate postoperative management.

   d. Problems and complications

      (1) Hemorrhage

      (2) Injuries to adjacent structures (phrenic nerve, recurrent laryngeal nerve, thoracic duct)

      (3) Prolonged respiratory support

2. PA banding

    a. General considerations. PA banding is performed when an infant has a cardiac lesion causing excessive pulmonary blood flow and pressures that is not amenable to primary repair. PA banding now is rarely performed, but it still has a place for patients in whom total repair is not technically feasible. It is important to palliate the situation with a PA band so that the lungs are not subjected to high flow and pressure for a long period, thus preventing permanent damage to the vasculature. The child can undergo a more definitive repair of the lesion at a later time. Infants scheduled for PA banding may have a wide variety of lesions, but the objective is the same: to limit PA flow and avoid irreversible PA hypertension. Application of the band will decrease some of the left-to-right shunt (without causing it to flow right-to-left) and improve systemic perfusion.

    b. Surgical procedure. PA banding is performed through a small left anterior thoracotomy. A Silastic band is passed around the main PA and then a clip is used to tighten the band (Fig. 14.23). The goal is to limit the flow without causing hypoxemia. We generally measure pressures distal to the band and progressively tighten the band until the pressure distally is half the systemic pressure. As the band is tightened, one would expect to see an increase in systemic pressure as more blood is diverted from the lungs to the body.

    c. Anesthetic considerations. This procedure usually is performed in infants with failure to thrive and complex cardiac anatomy. Premedication usually is not necessary. Both inhalational and intravenous inductions have been used successfully. The goals of therapy include keeping PVR high and SVR low, and minimizing myocardial depression. It is a good idea to avoid hyperoxia and hyperventilation to prevent pulmonary blood flow from increasing even more than baseline. The procedure typically is short,

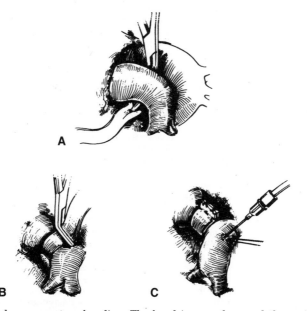

FIG. 14.23 Pulmonary artery banding. The band is passed around the main pulmonary artery (**A**) and is snugged down (**B**). Pulmonary artery pressure measurements are obtained (**C**) to verify proper "tightness" of the band. (From Waldhausen JA, Pierce WS, eds. *Johnson's surgery of the chest.* Chicago: Year Book, 1985:345, with permission.)

and if the child was not in respiratory distress preoperatively, extubation at the end of the case often can be accomplished.

Careful attention must be paid to pulse oximetry and capnography during the banding. Typically, the patient's saturation decreases, but rarely below 85%. A significant drop in end-tidal CO_2 can be an early warning sign that the band is too tight.

   d. Problems and complications
      (1) Inappropriate sizing of the band, either too loose or too tight
      (2) Migration of the band causing interference with blood flow to the right or left lung
      (3) Distortion and possible stenosis of the branch PAs

   3. Systemic-to-PA shunts
      a. General considerations. Children who are cyanotic because of inadequate pulmonary blood flow can be palliated with systemic-to-PA shunts. The partially saturated systemic arterial blood picks up more oxygen on its second pass through the lungs but then mixes with desaturated systemic venous return before being ejected into the systemic circulation. The resulting systemic saturation depends on the ratio of pulmonary-to-systemic blood flow and the degree of desaturation of the mixed venous blood. In addition to improving systemic oxygen saturation, these shunts often are used to stimulate PA growth in children whose PAs are too small for definitive repair.

      Because the pulmonary blood flow exceeds the systemic blood flow, ventricular volume overload can result. The shunt size must be chosen carefully to prevent excessive pulmonary blood flow and systemic hypoperfusion. Long-term systemic-to-PA shunts can cause pulmonary vascular obstructive changes.

      b. Surgical procedures. There are several different surgical procedures that have been used to deliver more blood to the lungs in children with inadequate pulmonary blood flow (Fig. 14.24). These include the Blalock–Taussig shunt, the modified Blalock–Taussig shunt, Potts, Waterston, and central shunt. The Blalock–Taussig shunt (or the modified shunt) is used most commonly. The surgical approach is through a thoracotomy, usually on the side opposite the aortic arch. In this procedure, the subclavian artery is identified, ligated, and anastomosed to the PA. In the modified version, the subclavian artery is left *in situ,* and a tube graft is sewn from the subclavian artery to the PA. Various shunts and their connections are listed in Table 14.12.

      c. Anesthetic considerations. Some of these infants have pulmonary blood flow that is totally ductal dependent (e.g., pulmonary atresia) and come to the operating room on PGE_1. Clearly it is important to ensure that infusion is not interrupted. Others will have more dynamic obstruction (e.g., tetralogy of Fallot) and may benefit from judicious sedation to prevent anxiety and crying. Oral midazolam at a dose of approximately 0.5 mg/kg works well. Inhalational induction usually is well tolerated and may help to relax the dynamic infundibular obstruction, if present.

      One should use maneuvers to try to decrease PVR and promote pulmonary blood flow. High oxygen concentration, hyperventilation, and avoidance of metabolic acidosis are helpful. One must recognize that end-tidal CO_2 will underestimate arterial P_aCO_2 during this procedure because the branch PA is clamped and not perfused. Measurement of arterial blood gases can be helpful in guiding management. The arterial catheter must be placed in the arm opposite the surgical procedure during a Blalock—Taussig shunt because the subclavian artery will be clamped.

      After the shunt is complete and open, the lung should be reexpanded and ventilated. The shunt size can be assessed by temporarily clamping and unclamping the shunt and watching the hemodynamics. One should expect to see a drop in systemic blood pressure when the shunt is open. A decrease in mean arterial blood pressure of more than 10 mm Hg suggests that the shunt is too large. Excessive pulmonary blood flow can cause systemic hypoperfusion, pulmonary edema, and metabolic acidosis. Difficulty

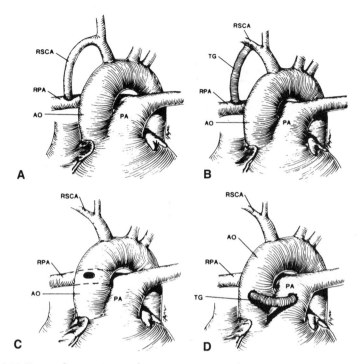

FIG. 14.24 Types of systemic-to-pulmonary artery anastomoses. **A:** Classic Blalock–Taussig anastomosis. **B:** Modified Blalock–Taussig shunt using prosthetic graft. **C:** Direct aorto-pulmonary (Waterston) anastomosis. **D:** Central aortopulmonary shunt with prosthetic graft. *AO,* aorta; *PA,* main pulmonary artery; *RPA,* right pulmonary artery; *RSCA,* right subclavian artery; *TG,* tube graft. (From Hickey PR, Wessel DL. Anesthesia for treatment of congenital heart disease. In: Kaplan JA, ed. *Cardiac anesthesia,* 2nd ed. Philadelphia: Grune & Stratton, 1987:683, with permission.)

weaning from the ventilator might occur. On the other hand, one would like to use a shunt as large as the child can tolerate in order to promote PA growth. Getting the right balance is critical.

It may be feasible to extubate older infants at the end of the procedure. Smaller neonates may benefit from overnight mechanical ventilation and diuresis.

d. Problems and complications

(1) Inappropriate size shunt, either too large or too small

(2) Problems specific to the type of shunt used (listed in Table 14.12)

X. Noncardiac surgery

The care of patients with CHD undergoing noncardiac surgery often is more challenging than caring for them during corrective repair. Likely scenarios for which these patients will require an anesthetic include the following:

1. Diagnostic workup before planned cardiac repair. These children may require an anesthetic for cardiac catheterization, magnetic resonance imaging, or transesophageal echocardiography. It is ideal to provide an anesthetic that replicates their baseline condition as closely as possible so that measurements of pressures and resistances will be representative. It is particularly important to deliver an inspired oxygen concentration close to room air with a normal P_aCO_2.

Table 14.12 Systemic-to-pulmonary shunts

Shunt	Anastomosis	Complications
Classic Blalock–Taussig	Right subclavian artery to right pulmonary artery (with left aortic arch)	Kinking of right pulmonary artery, right arm ischemia, excessive pulmonary flow
Modified Blalock–Taussig	Tube graft from right (or left) subclavian artery to right (or left) pulmonary artery	Kinking of right pulmonary artery, tube graft does not allow for growth, chylothorax
Waterston	Ascending aorta to right pulmonary artery	Kinking of right pulmonary artery, amount of blood flow difficult to control
Potts	Descending aorta to left pulmonary artery	Rarely used, difficult to control shunt size, and difficult takedown at later repair
Central (aortic-pulmonary shunt)	Anastomosis between aorta and pulmonary artery with tube graft	Distortion of main pulmonary artery, excessive pulmonary flow
Glenn	Superior vena cava to right pulmonary artery	Thrombosis, superior vena cava syndrome, insufficient pulmonary blood flow, pulmonary arteriovenous fistula

2. Dental procedures before planned cardiac repair. Removal of carious or infected teeth with dental restoration may be indicated before cardiac surgery in order to remove a potential source of infection. This may be particularly important if synthetic material is to be implanted during the cardiac repair.
3. After surgical palliation or correction for elective noncardiac surgery. In this situation, it is imperative that the team has access to the old records and cardiology follow-up to ensure that the patient's condition is optimized. Knowing the patient's physiology and anatomy is necessary to develop a rational anesthetic plan. Not all patients are left with a perfect cardiac surgical repair, and one must understand what residual problems exist. Occasionally it is appropriate to delay elective surgery until further cardiac surgery is performed.
4. Emergent noncardiac surgery. This situation is particularly problematic because there may be no time to obtain old medical records or ensure that the patient is in optimal condition.
5. Pregnancy with labor and delivery or cesarean section. As more children have undergone successful cardiac repair, many of them are reaching childbearing age. Understanding their particular physiology allows one to individualize their care.
6. Surgery for the patient with inoperable cardiac disease. Occasionally patients with this problem (for example, intracardiac shunt with pulmonary vascular disease and Eisenmenger physiology) will present for noncardiac surgery. The risks in this scenario are tremendous, and the patient and family should be informed of the prognosis and participate in the decision-making process as to whether the surgery should go forward. Careful monitoring and postoperative management are required for even the most superficial cases.

Preoperative testing before noncardiac surgery is somewhat dependent on the type and extent of the planned procedure. A hematocrit and coagulation profile is particularly important in patients who are cyanotic. Echocardiographic and cardiac catheterization data should be reviewed to assess the (a) type and severity of the lesion; (b) ventricular function; (c) status of the pulmonary vasculature; and (d) response to pulmonary vasodilators. Most patients will require bacterial endocarditis prophylaxis as dictated by the American Heart Association [26] (Table 14.13).

Table 14.13 Antibiotic endocarditis prophylaxis

Prophylaxis recommended	Prophylaxis not required
Prosthetic valves	6 months following surgical repair if no residua (consider for secundum atrial septal defect, ventricular septal defect, or patent ductus arteriosus)
Previous bacterial endocarditis	Orotracheal intubation
Systemic-to-pulmonary artery shunts	Cardiac catheterization
Most cardiac structural abnormalities	

One issue of concern regarding monitoring is that the end-tidal CO_2 measurement often is inaccurate as an estimate of P_aCO_2, particularly in cyanotic children. The extremity in which the blood pressure is taken also may be important. One should avoid the arm on the side of a Blalock–Taussig shunt, because the subclavian artery is no longer supplying blood to that arm. In a patient with coarctation of the aorta, blood pressure should be measured in the right arm, since the other extremities may be distal to the obstruction. The patient with supravalvar aortic stenosis will have an artifactually elevated right arm blood pressure.

Care of the patient undergoing noncardiac surgery should be similar to that provided during cardiac surgery. It is critically important to understand the patient's individual physiology and to develop hemodynamic goals for the particular lesion.

References

1. Hoffman JIE. Incidence of congenital heart disease: I. Postnatal incidence. *Pediatr Cardiol* 1995;16:103–113.
2. Steward DJ, DaSilva CA, Flegel T. Elevated glucose levels may increase the danger of neurological deficit following profoundly hypothermic cardiac arrest. *Anesthesiology* 1988; 68:653.
3. Burrows FA. Neurologic protection in pediatric cardiac surgery. In: Society of Cardio-vascular Anesthesiologists 20th Annual Meeting 1998 Workshops, Seattle, WA, April 25–29, 1998.
4. **Newburger JW, Jonas RA, Wernovsky G, et al. A comparison of the periopera-tive neurologic effects of hypothermic circulatory arrest versus low flow cardio-pulmonary bypass in infant heart surgery.** *N Engl J Med* 1993;329:1057–1064.
5. Bellinger DC, Wypij D, Kuban KCK, et al. Developmental and neurological status of children at 4 years of age after heart surgery with hypothermic circulatory arrest or low-flow cardiopulmonary bypass. *Circulation* 1999;100:526–532.
6. **DuPlessis AJ. Mechanisms of brain injury during infant cardiac surgery.** *Semin Pediatr Neurol* **1999;6:32–47.**
7. Swain JA, McDonald TJ, Robbins RC, et al. Relationship of cerebral and myocardial intracellular pH to blood pH during hypothermia. *Am J Physiol* 1991;260:H1640–H1644.
8. Murkin JM, Martzke JS, Buchan AM, et al. A randomized study of the influence of per-fusion technique and pH management strategy in 316 patients undergoing coronary artery bypass surgery. II. Neurologic and cognitive outcomes. *J Thorac Cardiovasc Surg* 1995;110:349–362.
9. Aoki M, Nomura F, Stromski ME, et al. Effects of pH on brain energetics after hypo-thermic circulatory arrest. *Ann Thorac Surg* 1993;55:1093–1103.
10. Skaryak LA, Chai PJ, Kern FH et al. Blood gas management and degree of cooling: effects on cerebral metabolism before and after circulatory arrest. *J Thorac Cardiovasc Surg* 1995;110:1649–1657.
11. Kirshbom PM, Skaryak LA, DiBernardo LR, et al. pH-stat cooling improves cerebral metabolic recovery after circulatory arrest in a piglet model of aorto-pulmonary collat-erals. *J Thorac Cardiovasc Surg* 1996;111:147–157.
12. **DuPlessis AJ, Jonas RA, Wypij D, et al. Perioperative effects of alpha-stat ver-sus pH-stat strategies for deep hypothermic cardiopulmonary bypass in infants.** *J Thorac Cardiovasc Surg* **1997;114:990–1001.**

13. Vannucci RC. Mechanisms of perinatal ischemic brain damage. In: Jonas RA, Newburger JW, Volpe JJ, eds. *Brain injury and pediatric cardiac surgery*. Boston: Butterworth-Heinemann, 1996:201–214.
14. Jonas R. Neurological protection during cardiopulmonary bypass/deep hypothermia. *Pediatr Cardiol* 1998;19:321–330.
15. Boldt J, Knothe C, Zickmann B, et al. Comparison of two aprotinin dosage regimens in pediatric patients having cardiac operations: influence on platelet function and blood loss. *J Thorac Cardiovasc Surg* 1993;105:705–711.
16. D'Errico CC, Shayevitz JR, Martindale SJ, et al. The efficacy and cost of aprotinin in children undergoing reoperative open heart surgery. *Anesth Analg* 1996;83:1193–1199.
17. Mossinger H, Dietrich W. Activation of hemostasis during cardiopulmonary bypass and pediatric aprotinin dosage. *Ann Thorac Surg* 1998;65:S45–S51.
18. **Elliott MJ. Ultrafiltration and modified ultrafiltration in pediatric open-heart operations. *Ann Thorac Surg* 1993;56:1518–1522.**
19. Naik SK, Knight A, Elliott MJ. A prospective randomized study of a modified technique of ultrafiltration during pediatric open-heart surgery. *Circulation* 1991;84:III-422–III-431.
20. Friesen RH, Campbell DN, Clarke DR, et al. Modified ultrafiltration attenuates dilutional coagulopathy in pediatric open-heart operations. *Ann Thorac Surg* 1997;64:1787–1789.
21. Davies MJ, Nguyen K, Gaynor JW, et al. Modified ultrafiltration improves left ventricular systolic function in infants after cardiopulmonary bypass. *J Thorac Cardiovasc Surg* 1998;115:361–370.
22. Bando K, Vijay P, Turrentine MW, et al. Dilutional and modified ultrafiltration reduces pulmonary hypertension after operations for congenital heart disease: a prospective randomized study. *J Thorac Cardiovasc Surg* 1998;115:517–527.
23. Andreasson S, Gothberg S, Berggren H, et al. Hemofiltration modifies complement activation after extracorporeal circulation in infants. *Ann Thorac Surg* 1993;56:1515–1517.
24. Skaryak LA, Kirshbom P, DiBernardo LR, et al. Modified ultrafiltration improves cerebral metabolic recovery after circulatory arrest. *J Thorac Cardiovasc Surg* 1995;109:744–752.
25. Botero M and Davies LK. Diagnosis and management of arrhythmias in children after cardiac surgery. *Semin Cardiothorac Vasc Anesth* 2001;5:122–133.
26. Dajani AS, Taubet KA, Wilson W, et al. Prevention of bacterial endocarditis: recommendations by the American Heart Association. *Circulation* 1997; 97:358–366.

15. ANESTHETIC MANAGEMENT FOR CARDIAC TRANSPLANTATION

Anne L. Rother and Charles D. Collard

Cardiac transplantation is an established treatment option for end-stage heart disease. Since the first human cardiac transplant by Barnard in 1967, more than 55,000 cardiac transplants have been performed worldwide [1]. Despite the increasingly high-risk patient population selected for cardiac transplantation, survival rates remain satisfactory due to continuing advances in therapeutic immunosuppression, surgical techniques, and the diagnosis and treatment of allograft rejection. Cardiac transplantation in the United States is limited to member centers of the United Network for Organ Sharing (UNOS), the central agency responsible for coordinating organ procurement and allocation. In order to maintain UNOS membership, centers must perform a minimum of 12 cardiac transplants annually and achieve a 1-year survival rate of at least 70% [2].

I. End-stage heart failure
The majority of patients awaiting cardiac transplantation have end-stage cardiac failure. In the United States alone, more than 4.5 million people are affected by cardiac failure, with more than 500,000 new cases diagnosed each year [3]. The 5-year mortality rate for end-stage heart disease with congestive heart failure (CHF) is approximately 70%, with sudden death occurring at six to nine times the rate of the general population.

A. Etiology
Coronary artery disease (CAD) and cardiomyopathy are the most common causes of end-stage cardiac failure in adults, accounting for approximately 90% of patients undergoing cardiac transplantation (Fig. 15.1). Congenital and valvular heart disease also account for a small percentage of adult cardiac failure patients [1]. Irrespective of the etiology, end-stage cardiac failure has a poor prognosis, with the 1-year mortality of patients with New York Heart Association (NYHA) class IV symptoms exceeding 50% [4].

B. Pathophysiology
End-stage cardiac failure is characterized by irreversible, severe ventricular dysfunction resulting in low cardiac output (CO), poor end-organ perfusion, and activation of compensatory neurohumoral pathways. In the initial stages of ventricular failure, stroke volume (SV) is maintained by increases in left ventricular (LV) end-diastolic volume and myocardial fiber length. Eventually this results in cardiac

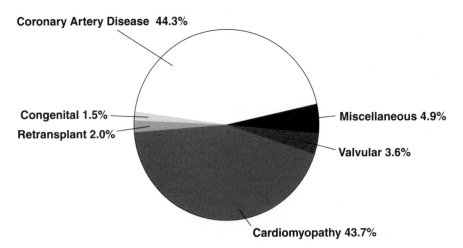

FIG. 15.1 Primary diagnoses of adult cardiac transplant recipients in 1999. (From Hosenpud JD, Bennett LE, Keck BM, et al. The Registry of the International Society for Heart and Lung Transplantation: Seventeenth official report—2000. *J Heart Lung Transplant* 2000;19: 909–931, with permission.)

dilation, increased LV and pulmonary venous pressures, and pulmonary hypertension (HTN). Together, these processes result in cardiomegaly, severe dyspnea, and peripheral edema. Other organ systems, such as the liver and kidneys, are compromised by persistent decreases in end-organ perfusion and elevated venous pressures. In an attempt to restore CO and end-organ perfusion, compensatory neurohumoral mechanisms lead to sympathetic nervous system activation with persistent elevations in circulating catecholamines. Preload and peripheral vascular tone are maintained by activation of the renin-angiotensin-aldosterone system resulting in increased sodium and water retention. However, with continued progression of cardiac failure, SV becomes "fixed" and unresponsive to increases in preload. Additionally, increases in afterload are poorly tolerated (Fig. 15.2). Chronic circulating catecholamine elevations may result in myocardial β_1-adrenergic receptor down-regulation, making the heart less responsive to positive inotropic therapy [5].

C. Medical management of end-stage heart disease

1. Therapeutic aims

The therapeutic goals for cardiac failure are to increase CO, reduce myocardial afterload, decrease sodium and water retention, and prevent thromboembolism. Combination therapy with positive inotropes, diuretics, vasodilators, β-receptor antagonists and anticoagulants has an established role in the treatment of cardiac failure. However, it is important to note that although pharmacologic treatment often provides symptomatic relief, short- and medium-term mortalities are only decreased by approximately 20% [6].

a. Inotropes

Inotropic agents commonly used to treat cardiac failure include digitalis, sympathetic amines, and phosphodiesterase-III inhibitors. Digitalis often is used to treat CHF complicated by atrial fibrillation. Effective orally, digitalis exerts a positive inotropic effect by inhibiting the myocardial cell sodium pump and increasing cytosolic calcium concentrations. Digitalis also prolongs atrioventricular conduction time by increasing parasympathetic tone, leading to a decrease in heart rate (HR). Digitalis blood levels

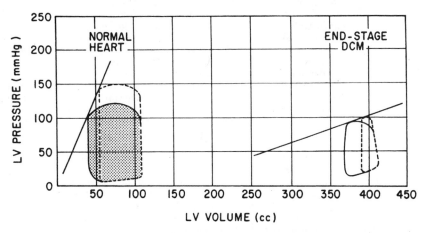

FIG. 15.2 Pressure-volume (P-V) relationships in a normal heart and a heart with end-stage, dilated cardiomyopathy (DCM). Shown are the left ventricular (LV) P-V loops *(dotted lines)* obtained from a normal heart and a heart with end-stage DCM after an increase in afterload. The slope of the *straight lines* depicts the LV end-systolic P-V relationship. Note that the myopathic heart SV is markedly decreased by increases in afterload. (From Clark NJ, Martin RD. Anesthetic considerations for patients undergoing cardiac transplantation. *J Cardiothorac Anesth* 1988;2:519–542, with permission.)

should be monitored because significant side effects, such as atrial and ventricular arrhythmias, can occur, particularly in the presence of hypokalemia. Myocardial β_1-adrenergic receptor stimulation by catecholamines, such as epinephrine, norepinephrine, dobutamine, or dopamine, often is used to improve myocardial contractility and ventricular diastolic relaxation. However, prolonged catecholamine therapy may result in myocardial β_1-adrenergic receptor down regulation and increase the risk of arrhythmias. Phosphodiesterase-III inhibitors, such as amrinone and milrinone, commonly are referred to as inodilators, because they combine both positive inotropic and vasodilatory activity by inhibiting cyclic adenosine monophosphate (cAMP) metabolism. Phosphodiesterase-III inhibitor administration may be particularly useful for treatment of acute CHF exacerbations. However, the benefits of long-term treatment with phosphodiesterase-III inhibitors are not established, and an increased incidence of hypotension and atrial and ventricular arrhythmias has been reported [5].

b. Diuretics

Diuretics commonly are used in the management of end-stage heart failure to decrease pulmonary and peripheral venous pressures by reducing intravascular volume. Spironolactone is an aldosterone antagonist and potassium-sparing diuretic that has been shown to reduce end-stage heart failure mortality. In addition to reducing sodium and water retention, spironolactone has vasodilator activity. Prolonged diuretic use may be complicated by ventricular arrhythmias resulting from electrolyte abnormalities such as hypokalemia and hypomagnesemia.

c. Vasodilators

Vasodilators are used in the treatment of CHF to reduce myocardial preload and afterload, thereby reducing myocardial work and oxygen demand. In the last decade, angiotensin-converting enzyme (ACE) inhibitors have become central to the management of chronic CHF. Combining both venous and arteriole dilator activity, ACE inhibitors have been shown to improve the prognosis of CHF. Although the exact mechanisms by which they exert their protective effects are unclear, ACE inhibitors have been demonstrated to attenuate many of the neuroendocrine processes associated with cardiac failure. Side effects of ACE inhibitors include hypotension, hyperkalemia, and renal insufficiency. The nitrates (e.g., nitroglycerine and sodium nitroprusside) may be useful for relieving the symptoms of pulmonary edema by reducing ventricular filling pressures and afterload.

d. β-Adrenergic receptor blockade

Although once thought contraindicated, β-adrenergic receptor blockade has become standard treatment for end-stage cardiac failure. Long-term therapy of CHF with β-adrenergic receptor antagonists has been shown to improve hemodynamics and increase survival [2]. Although the exact mechanisms by which β-adrenergic receptor antagonists produce their favorable effects are unclear, it is thought to be due in part to attenuation of the cardiac failure-associated neurohumoral response.

e. Anticoagulants

Patients with CHF are at increased risk for thromboembolism as a result of low CO and a high incidence of coexistent atrial fibrillation. Long-term prophylactic anticoagulation with agents such as warfarin is common and may contribute to perioperative bleeding at the time of cardiac transplantation.

D. Mechanical circulatory assist devices

The growing number of cardiac transplant candidates, combined with a static number of donors, has significantly increased the use of mechanical circulatory assist devices for patients who decompensate or otherwise might die before a suitable donor can be procured. Cardiac transplant candidates with hemodynamic decompensation who fail to respond to maximal medical therapy may require placement of an intraaortic balloon pump or ventricular assist device (VAD) as a "bridge-to-cardiac transplantation" [7]. However, potential VAD recipients must meet the

Table 15.1 Indications for adult cardiac transplantation

New York Heart Association Class III or IV congestive heart failure symptoms unrelieved
  despite maximal therapy and *at least* one of the following:
  1. Requiring continuous mechanical or inotropic support
  2. Peak O_2 uptake (VO_2 max) <14 mL/kg/min
  3. Left ventricular ejection fraction ≤20%
Refractory angina pectoris due to inoperable coronary artery disease
Life-threatening, refractory ventricular arrhythmias
Cardiac tumor confined to the myocardium without evidence of metastases

same cardiac transplantation inclusion and exclusion criteria as medically managed patients. Currently, two implantable VADs are approved by the U.S. Food and
Drug Administration for bridge to transplantation: the Novacor N100 (Baxter
Novacor Division, Oakland, CA, USA) and HeartMate Ventricular Assist Systems
(Thermo Cardiosystems Inc., Woburn, MA, USA). Approximately 70% of patients
receiving a VAD for bridge to transplantation subsequently undergo successful cardiac transplantation [8].

II. The cardiac transplant recipient
The last decade has witnessed a significant increase in the number of eligible cardiac transplant candidates. Advances in immunosuppressive therapy and surgical technique have led
to improved outcomes for many patients who previously would not have been considered eligible for cardiac transplantation. In particular, there has been a large increase in recipients
at the extremes of age, with the number of recipients older than 65 years quadrupling in the
past decade. However, donor numbers have remained static, with transplantation waiting
times increasing steadily. In 1999, there were only 2,316 donors for 7,546 patients on the
UNOS cardiac transplantation waiting list [9].

A. Cardiac transplantation indications
UNOS selection guidelines for cardiac transplantation include patients with
end-stage heart failure with a life expectancy of less than 1 year, severe inoperable angina, refractory ventricular arrhythmias, or unresectable cardiac tumors
(Table 15.1). Potential cardiac transplant candidates must have all reversible causes
of cardiac failure excluded and have exhausted all other surgical options. Although
many patients qualify for cardiac transplantation, actual donor heart allocation
is based on UNOS priority status (Table 15.2), ABO blood group compatibility,
body-size match, and distance from the donor center.

B. Cardiac transplantation contraindications
There has been a gradual relaxation in the conventional cardiac transplantation exclusion criteria as experience with increasingly complex cases has grown.

Table 15.2 Medical urgency status codes for adult donor heart allocation

1A Inpatient with *at least one* of the following:
  a. Assisted mechanical circulatory support for acute, hemodynamic decompensation
  b. Assisted mechanical circulatory support for >30 days with significant device-related
     complications
  Mechanical ventilation
  Continuous infusion of a single high-dose intravenous inotrope or multiple inotropes
  Life expectancy without transplantation of <7 days
1B Assisted mechanical circulatory support for >30 days
  Continuous infusion of intravenous inotropes
2 Patient of any age who does not meet the criteria for status 1A or 1B
7 Temporarily inactive

From *1999 annual report of the U.S. Scientific Registry of Transplant Recipients and the Organ Procurement
and Transplantation Network: transplant data 1989–1998.* Rockville, VA: United Network for Organ Sharing.

Exclusion criteria include severe, irreversible, end-organ disease and conditions incompatible with immunosuppression (Table 15.3). In particular, evaluation of pulmonary vascular resistance (PVR) and its reversibility is critical in the preoperative evaluation of cardiac transplant candidates, as pulmonary HTN is a predictor of postoperative right ventricular (RV) failure and mortality [10]. Methods used to quantify the severity of pulmonary HTN include calculation of PVR and the transpulmonary gradient [mean pulmonary artery (PA) pressure – pulmonary capillary wedge pressure (PCWP)]. In general, patients are not considered potential orthotopic cardiac transplant recipients if they demonstrate a PVR greater than 6 Woods units or transpulmonary gradient greater than 12 mm Hg, without evidence of pharmacologic reversibility. Reversibility of pulmonary HTN is evaluated by vasodilator administration, including intravenous sodium nitroprusside and inhaled nitric oxide (NO). Options for patients with severe irreversible pulmonary HTN include heterotopic cardiac or combined heart-lung transplantation.

III. The cardiac transplant donor
A. Donor selection
The primary factor limiting cardiac transplantation is the shortage of donors. Over the past decade, the median waiting time for cardiac transplantation has increased in all age groups, with approximately 30% of patients dying before cardiac transplantation [11]. Therefore, in an attempt to increase donor numbers, the criteria for cardiac organ donation have been relaxed in recent years with an increased acceptance of older donors with and without evidence of CAD. However, the risk of failed transplantation increases with donor age and the presence of concomitant disease [12]. Absolute and relative contraindications for heart donation are listed in Table 15.4.

Acceptance of a potential organ donor requires confirmation of brain death and organ viability. Echocardiographic evaluation of cardiac function and coronary angiography for male donors older than 45 years and female donors older than 50 years are recommended [4]. Although cardiac transplant recipients are screened preoperatively for the percentage of reactive antibodies, donors and recipients are matched only on ABO blood group and weight ratio unless the percentage of reactive antibodies is greater than 20% [5]. For recipients with an elevated PVR, a higher donor-to-recipient weight ratio may be associated with a better post-transplantation outcome as small donor hearts are at increased risk for RV failure due to an inability to overcome even mild elevations in PVR in large recipients.

B. Determination of brain death
The declaration of brain death of a potential donor is the first step in the process of procuring a heart for transplantation. The Uniform Determination of Death Act defines death as either irreversible cessation of (a) circulatory and respiratory

Table 15.3 Contraindications to heart transplantation

Absolute contraindications
Severe, irreversible pulmonary hypertension (>6 Wood units/m^2)
Terminal malignancy
Irreversible, severe hepatic, renal, or pulmonary disease
Active infection
HIV-positive serology
Alcohol or intravenous drug abuse

Relative contraindications
Advanced age (>65 years)
Severe cerebral or peripheral vascular disease
Insulin-dependent diabetes mellitus
Pulmonary infarction
Morbid obesity (>130% ideal body weight)
Major psychiatric disorder

HIV, human immunodeficiency virus.

Table 15.4 Contraindications to heart donation

Absolute contraindications
Positive serology for syphilis, HTLV-4, and HIV
Presence of malignancy with extracranial metastatic potential
Left ventricular ejection fraction <40%
Significant valvular abnormality
Significant coronary artery disease
Relative contraindications
Sepsis
Hepatitis B surface antigen positive
Hepatitis C antibody positive
Repeated need for cardiopulmonary resuscitation
High-dose inotropic support exceeding 24 hours

HIV, human immunodeficiency virus; HTLV-4, human T-cell lymphotropic virus-4.

function or (b) all brain function, where the determination of death is made in accordance with accepted standards. For the diagnosis of brain death to be made, the loss of brain function must be irreversible, the patient's core body temperature must be greater than 32.5°C, and no drug with the potential to alter neurologic or neuromuscular function should be present [13].

C. **Pathophysiology of brain death**

Brain death significantly alters the body's homeostatic mechanisms and, if improperly managed, can preclude the individual from organ donation. Approximately 25% of potential cardiac donors are lost due to suboptimal medical management [11].

1. **Cardiovascular function**

In an attempt to maintain cerebral blood flow, a "sympathetic storm" resulting in HTN, tachycardia, and electrocardiogram (ECG) changes consistent with ischemia is common in the 1 to 2 hours before brainstem coning. Although this period of autonomic hyperactivity usually is brief and generally requires no treatment, occasionally severe systemic HTN may result in acute LV failure and pulmonary edema. The period after the sympathetic storm frequently is characterized by hypotension, which may be due to neurogenic shock, hypovolemia, or ventricular dysfunction. However, noxious stimuli may induce hypertensive responses mediated by intact spinal sympathetic reflexes. Arrhythmias are common and result from electrolytic disturbances, hypothermia, myocardial ischemia, or trauma. Despite optimal donor support, terminal cardiac arrhythmias usually occur within 48 to 72 hours of brain death [14].

2. **Fluid and electrolyte disturbances**

Common electrolyte abnormalities observed after brain death include hypernatremia, hypokalemia, hypomagnesemia, and hypocalcemia. Diabetes insipidus (DI) and hyperglycemia are common after brain death and frequently lead to hypovolemia and electrolyte disturbances. DI is due to a deficiency of antidiuretic hormone (ADH) that results in a massive diuresis characterized by serum hypernatremia and low urinary sodium. Increased circulating catecholamine levels and injudicious administration of glucose-containing fluids contribute to hyperglycemia.

3. **Pulmonary function**

Hypoxemia resulting from lung trauma, infection, or pulmonary edema frequently occurs after brain death. Although adult respiratory distress syndrome is the most common cause of pulmonary edema, pulmonary edema also may be neurogenic or cardiogenic in origin.

4. **Temperature**

Hypothermia due to a reduction in metabolic rate, an inability to shiver or vasoconstrict, and the injudicious administration of nonwarmed intravenous fluids is common after brain death. Adverse consequences of hypothermia include decreased tissue oxygen delivery, coagulopathy, and cardiovascular instability.

5. Coagulation

Coagulopathy may result from hypothermia and dilution of clotting factors after massive transfusion. Additionally, tissue factor release from the ischemic brain can lead to disseminated intravascular coagulation.

D. Perioperative management of the cardiac transplant donor

Posttransplant cardiac function is directly dependent on donor care before organ harvesting. Thus, the goal of medical management after brain death is to ensure optimal myocardial and end-organ perfusion.

1. Cardiovascular function

Donor systemic blood pressure (BP) and central venous pressure (CVP) should be monitored continuously. Hemodynamic goals include maintenance of systemic BP greater than 100 mm Hg and a CVP of 8 to 12 mm Hg. Inotropic support should be commenced only after hypotension has been treated with adequate intravenous fluid replacement. Prolonged inotropic support of the donor heart may result in myocardial β_1-adrenergic receptor down-regulation, thus increasing the posttransplantation inotropic drug requirement. Dopamine, epinephrine, and norepinephrine commonly are used for donor cardiovascular support. High-dose α-adrenergic receptor agonists should be used with caution, as peripheral and splanchnic vasoconstriction may result in acidosis and decreased perfusion of other potential donor organs, such as the liver and pancreas. Intravenous corticosteroid or thyroxine administration should be considered for treatment of refractory hypotension [14].

2. Fluid and electrolytes

DI is treated with 1-desamino-8-D-arginine vasopressin (DDAVP) and warmed intravenous fluids to replace urinary losses. Sodium and glucose administration should be limited. Hyperglycemia should be treated with an insulin infusion, and electrolyte/acid–base status monitored frequently and corrected as necessary.

3. Pulmonary function

Arterial blood gases should be maintained within normal limits with a P_aO_2 greater than 100 mm Hg and P_aCO_2 of 35 to 40 mm Hg. Efforts to prevent pulmonary aspiration, atelectasis, and infection are warranted. Pulmonary edema should be managed with positive end-expiratory pressure (PEEP) ventilation and diuretic therapy.

4. Temperature

Core temperature monitoring is mandatory because hypothermia adversely affects coagulation, cardiac rhythm, and oxygen delivery. Use of warmed intravenous fluids, warming blankets, and heated humidifiers may prevent hypothermia.

5. Coagulation

Blood product replacement should be guided by repeated donor platelet and clotting factor measurements. The donor should be transfused with packed red blood cells (RBC) as necessary to maintain a hematocrit of 25% to 30%. Antifibrinolytic administration to control donor bleeding is not recommended because of the risk of microvascular thromboses.

E. Anesthetic management of the donor during organ harvest

Anesthetic management of the donor during organ harvesting is an extension of preoperative management, with continued monitoring of volume status, and systemic arterial and central venous pressures. An inspired oxygen concentration (F_iO_2) of 1.0 is optimal for organ viability, unless the lungs are to be harvested. To decrease the possibility of oxygen toxicity in the case of donor lung harvest, the lowest possible F_iO_2 that will maintain the P_aO_2 greater than 100 mm Hg should be used. Although intact spinal reflexes still may result in HTN, tachycardia, and muscle movement, these signs do not indicate cerebral function or pain perception. Nondepolarizing muscle relaxants commonly are used to prevent spinal reflex-mediated muscle movement in response to noxious stimuli.

F. Organ harvest technique

After initial dissection, the patient is fully heparinized. The perfusion-sensitive organs (kidneys and liver) are removed before cardiectomy. The donor heart is excised *en bloc* via median sternotomy after dissection of the pericardial attach-

ments. The superior and inferior venae cavae are ligated first, allowing exsanguination. The aorta is cross-clamped and cold cardioplegia administered. The
aorta and pulmonary arteries are transected, leaving the native donor arterial
segments as long as possible. Finally, the pulmonary veins are individually divided
after lifting the donor organ out of the thoracic cavity. Hypothermia is the principal means of donor heart preservation. Thus, the donor heart is placed in a plastic
bag containing ice-cold saline and transported in an ice-filled cooler. Optimal myocardial function after transplantation is achieved when the donor heart ischemic
time is less than 4 hours.

IV. Surgical techniques for cardiac transplantation
  A. Orthotopic cardiac transplantation
    More than 98% of cardiac transplants currently performed are orthotopic [9].
    The recipient is placed on standard cardiopulmonary bypass (CPB) and, if present,
    the PA catheter withdrawn into the superior vena cava. The femoral vessels often
    are selected for arterial and venous CPB cannulation in patients undergoing re-
    peat sternotomy. Otherwise, the distal ascending aorta is cannulated and bicaval
    cannulas with snares placed, completely excluding the heart from the native cir-
    culation. The aorta and pulmonary arteries are clamped and divided. Depending
    on the implantation technique (Fig. 15.3), either both native atria or a single left
    atrial cuff containing the pulmonary veins is preserved. The native atrial appendages
    are discarded because of the risk of postoperative thrombus formation.
    The donor heart is first inspected for the presence of a patent foramen ovale. If
    patent, the foramen ovale is surgically closed, as right-to-left interatrial shunting
    and hypoxemia may occur in the presence of elevated right-sided pressures after
    transplantation. The donor and recipient left atria are anastomosed first, followed
    by the right atria, or cavae when a bicaval anastomotic technique is chosen. The
    subsequent order of anastomoses varies depending on the donor heart ischemic
    time and the experience of the surgeon. The donor and recipient aortas are joined
    and the aortic cross-clamp removed with the patient in Trendelenburg position to

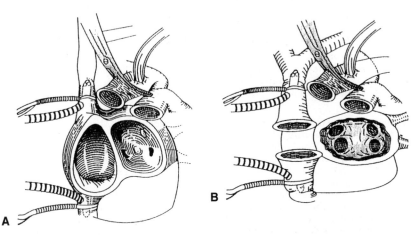

FIG. 15.3 Surgical techniques for cardiac transplantation. **A: Biatrial technique.** The
donor heart is anastomosed to the main bulk of the recipient's native right and left atria.
B: Bicaval technique. The donor heart left atrium is anastomosed to a single left atrial cuff,
including the pulmonary veins, in the recipient. (From Aziz TM, Burgess MI, El Gamel A, et al.
Orthotopic cardiac transplantation technique: a survey of current practice. *Ann Thorac Surg*
1999;68:1242–1246, with permission.)

decrease air embolism. After completion of the PA anastomosis and placement of temporary epicardial pacing wires, the heart is de-aired and the patient weaned from CPB.

1. Biatrial implantation

The biatrial implantation technique preserves portions of the recipient's native atria to create two atrial anastomoses (Fig. 15.3A). Biatrial implantation was the original technique described for cardiac transplantation and has been performed successfully for more than 3 decades [12].

2. Bicaval implantation

The bicaval implantation technique is a modification of the classic biatrial technique [15]. In this technique, only a single, small, left atrial cuff containing the pulmonary veins is preserved in the recipient, and bicaval and left atrial anastomoses are performed (Fig. 15.3B). Potential advantages of the bicaval technique include the following:

   a. Decreased distortion of the tricuspid valve annulus
   b. Decreased incidence and severity of tricuspid valve regurgitation
   c. Preserved synchronous atrial contraction
   d. Improved right heart function
   e. Lowered risk of thromboembolism

B. Heterotopic cardiac transplantation

Heterotopic transplantation accounts for less than 1% to 2% of cardiac transplantation procedures performed each year [9]. In this technique, the recipient's heart is not excised. Instead, the donor heart is placed within the right anterior thorax and anastomosed to the recipient's native heart such that a parallel circulation is established. The recipient and donor atria are anastomosed, followed by the aortas. An artificial conduit usually joins the pulmonary arteries, with the native and donor RVs ejecting into the native PA. Similarly, both the native and donor LVs eject into the native aorta. Thus, the recipient's RV, which is conditioned to eject against elevated pulmonary arterial pressures, will provide most of the right-sided ventricular output, whereas the healthy donor LV will make the major contribution to left-sided ventricular output [16]. Situations in which heterotopic cardiac transplantation may be advantageous include the following:

1. Recipients with severe pulmonary HTN
2. Small donor-to-recipient size ratio
3. Prolonged donor heart ischemic time

Disadvantages of heterotopic cardiac transplantation include the following:

1. High operative mortality rate
2. Requirement for continued medical treatment of the failing native heart
3. Potential for the native heart to be a thromboembolism source
4. Compromised pulmonary function due to placement of donor heart in the right chest

V. Preoperative management of the cardiac transplant patient

A. Personnel timing and coordination

In order to avoid prolonged donor heart ischemic times, close communication between the transplant center and the organ retrieval team must be maintained. Anesthetic induction of the recipient should be timed so that CPB is commenced immediately upon donor heart arrival.

B. Preoperative evaluation of the cardiac transplant patient

The anesthesiologist usually has limited time for preoperative assessment of the cardiac transplant recipient. However, the recipient in most instances will have been under the care of a medical team experienced in the management of end-stage cardiac failure, and the patient's medical therapy will have been optimized. The preoperative anesthetic evaluation of the cardiac transplant recipient should include a thorough history, physical examination, and review of the patient's medical record. The ECG, echocardiogram, chest X-ray film, and cardiac catheterization results should be noted, and all hematologic, renal and liver function tests should be reviewed.

1. **Concomitant organ dysfunction**

   Chronic systemic hypoperfusion and venous congestion in the recipient may produce reversible hepatic and renal dysfunction. Mild-to-moderate elevations of hepatic enzymes and bilirubin and prolongation of prothrombin time are common. Preoperative hepatic dysfunction and anticoagulant medication may contribute to the abnormal coagulation profile frequently observed in cardiac transplant recipients. Blood urea nitrogen (BUN) commonly is elevated in patients with end-stage heart disease due to chronic hypoperfusion and the concomitant prerenal effects of high-dose diuretics.

2. **Preoperative medications**

   Preoperative inotropic support should be continued throughout the pre-CPB period. Patients receiving digitalis–diuretic combinations have an increased risk of dysrhythmias in the presence of hypokalemia. Anticoagulants such as warfarin may increase the need for perioperative blood product administration. For patients who have undergone prior cardiac surgery, previous exposure to the antifibrinolytic aprotinin should be noted, as reexposure is associated with an increased anaphylaxis risk.

3. **Preoperative monitoring and circulatory support**

   The position, function, and duration of insertion of invasive monitoring catheters should be noted. Similarly, the function and settings of intraaortic balloon pumps and VADs should be reviewed. Patients with invasive monitoring lines and mechanical circulatory support require extra personnel and vigilance to ensure safe transport from the intensive care unit (ICU) to the operating room.

VI. **Anesthetic management of the cardiac transplant recipient**

A. **Premedication**

   The patient with end-stage cardiac failure has elevated levels of circulating catecholamines and is preload-dependent. Even a small sedative dose of medication may result in vasodilation and hemodynamic decompensation. Therefore, premedication should be avoided or carefully titrated intravenously, together with the administration of supplemental oxygen.

B. **Importance of aseptic technique**

   Perioperative immunosuppressive therapy places the cardiac transplant recipient at increased risk for infection. Therefore, it is essential that the anesthesia equipment is clean and that all invasive procedures are carried out using aseptic technique. Administration of a broad-spectrum antibiotic, such as cephazolin, for the first 24 hours after anesthetic induction is common.

C. **Monitoring**

   Noninvasive monitoring should include a standard five-lead ECG, noninvasive BP measurement, pulse oximetry, capnography, nasopharyngeal temperature, and urinary output. Large-bore peripheral and central venous access for rapid infusion of fluids and vasoactive drugs should be obtained. Invasive monitoring should include systemic arterial and central venous and/or PA pressures [5]. If intraoperative transesophageal echocardiography (TEE) is planned, monitoring of CVP alone may be adequate. However, a PA catheter frequently is helpful in the post-CPB period, permitting monitoring of CO and ventricular filling pressures, and calculation of systemic vascular resistance and PVR. These indices are particularly useful for assessment and treatment of post-CPB pulmonary HTN and RV dysfunction. Traditionally, catheterization of the right internal jugular vein is avoided to preserve this route for the multiple postoperative endomyocardial biopsies routinely performed to screen for myocardial rejection. Nonetheless, difficulty with endomyocardial biopsy (EMB) by alternative routes has not been reported in circumstances where the right internal jugular vein was used for central access.

D. **Considerations for repeat sternotomy**

   Many cardiac transplant recipients will have undergone previous cardiac surgery and are at increased risk for inadvertent trauma to the great vessels or preexisting coronary artery bypass grafts during repeat sternotomy. Therefore, patients undergoing repeat sternotomy should have external defibrillation pads placed, and cross-matched, irradiated, packed RBCs should be available in the operating room before anesthetic induction. Additionally, the potential for a prolonged surgical dissection time in patients undergoing repeat sternotomy often necessitates that anesthesia be induced at an earlier than usual time to coordinate with donor heart arrival. Other considerations for repeat sternotomy include the potential for increased perioperative bleeding and the need for femoral or axillary CPB cannulation.

E. Anesthetic induction

1. **Hemodynamic goals**

   Cardiac transplant recipients typically have hypokinetic, noncompliant ventricles sensitive to alterations in myocardial preload and afterload. Hemodynamic goals for anesthetic induction are to maintain HR and contractility, avoid acute changes in preload and afterload, and prevent increases in PVR. Inotropic support often is required during anesthetic induction and throughout the pre-CPB period.

2. **Aspiration precautions**

   Patients presenting for cardiac transplantation should be considered to have a "full stomach," because most surgical procedures are performed at short notice. In addition, commencement of oral cyclosporine or azathioprine preoperatively increases the risk of aspiration on induction by increasing stomach content volume. Thus, administration of oral sodium citrate and/or intravenous metoclopramide may be useful to promote gastric emptying. In addition, a rapid or modified rapid sequence anesthetic induction with maintenance of cricoid pressure during positive-pressure ventilation should be considered.

3. **Anesthetic agents**

   Due to the slow circulation time in patients with end-stage cardiac failure, a delayed response to administered anesthetic agents on induction is common. Intravenous anesthetics commonly used for anesthetic induction of the cardiac transplant recipient include etomidate (0.2 to 0.3 mg/kg) in combination with fentanyl (5 to 10 µg/kg) or sufentanil (5 to 8 µg/kg). High-dose narcotic regimens have been used successfully. Bradycardia occurring in response to high-dose narcotics should be treated promptly, as CO in patients with end-stage heart disease is HR dependent. Small doses of midazolam, ketamine, or scopolamine help ensure amnesia, but they should be used cautiously as they may synergistically lower systemic vascular resistance and induce hypotension.

4. **Muscle relaxants**

   Due to its vagolytic and mild sympathomimetic properties, the muscle relaxant pancuronium commonly is used to counteract high-dose narcotic-induced bradycardia. Muscle relaxants with minimal cardiovascular effects (e.g., cisatracurium or vecuronium) may be more appropriate for patients who present with tachycardia secondary to preoperative inotropic support.

F. Anesthetic maintenance

During the pre-CPB period, anesthetic goals include maintenance of hemodynamic stability and end-organ perfusion. Most anesthetic maintenance regimens are narcotic based, with supplemental inhalational agents and benzodiazepines administered as required. Although most inhalational agents have negative inotropic effects, low concentrations of these agents usually are well tolerated and decrease the risk of awareness. Anesthetic depth can be difficult to assess in this patient population because the sympathetic response to light planes of anesthesia often is blunted. Furthermore, the use of narcotic-based anesthetic regimens may increase the incidence of awareness during anesthesia. Thus, benzodiazepine supplementation often is warranted to prevent intraoperative recall.

Antifibrinolytics such as tranexamic acid, ε-aminocaproic acid, and aprotinin commonly are administered after anesthetic induction to prevent postoperative bleeding. Aprotinin, a polypeptide protease inhibitor with platelet-preserving properties, has been shown to decrease perioperative blood loss in patients undergoing repeat sternotomy [17]. A small test dose of aprotinin should always be administered because of the risk of anaphylaxis with reexposure.

G. Cardiopulmonary bypass

CPB for cardiac transplantation is similar to that normally used for routine cardiac surgical procedures. Femoral venous and arterial cannulation sites frequently are chosen in patients undergoing repeat sternotomy because of the risk of injury to the heart and great vessels. Moderate hypothermia (28° to 30°C) commonly is used during CPB to improve myocardial protection. In addition, hemofiltration and/or mannitol administration are common during CPB, because patients with CHF often have a large intravascular blood volume and coexistent renal impairment. Although immunosuppressive regimens vary among transplantation centers, high-dose intravenous glucocorticoids such as methylprednisolone frequently are administered before aortic cross-clamp release to reduce the likelihood of hyperacute rejection.

VII. Termination from cardiopulmonary bypass and the post–coronary bypass period

Before CPB termination, the patient should be normothermic, and all electrolyte/acid–base abnormalities corrected. Complete de-airing of the heart before aortic cross-clamp removal is essential because intracavitary air may pass into the coronary arteries, resulting in significant ventricular dysfunction. TEE may be particularly useful for assessing the efficacy of cardiac de-airing maneuvers. Inotropic agents should be commenced before CPB termination. An HR of 90 to 110 beats/min, a mean systemic arterial BP greater than 65 mm Hg, and ventricular filling pressures of approximately 12 to 16 mm Hg (CVP) and 14 to 18 mm Hg (PCWP) often are required in the immediate post-CPB period. Cardiovascular support and the prevention of rejection and infection are the focus of therapy in the immediate postoperative period. Triple immunosuppressive agent therapy commonly is commenced in the ICU. Although inotropic support usually is required for several days, patients often are extubated within 24 hours and discharged from the ICU by postoperative day 3. Clinical considerations in the immediate postoperative period include the following:

A. Autonomic denervation of the transplanted heart

During orthotopic cardiac transplantation, the cardiac autonomic plexus is transected, leaving the transplanted heart without autonomic innervation. The newly denervated heart does not respond to direct autonomic nervous system stimulation or to drugs that act indirectly through the autonomic nervous system (e.g., atropine). Instead, the denervated transplanted heart only responds to direct-acting agents such as catecholamines. Because transient, slow nodal rhythms are common after aortic cross-clamp release, a direct-acting β-adrenergic receptor agonist commonly is commenced before CPB termination to achieve an HR of 90 to 110 beats/min. Isoproterenol, a potent β-adrenergic receptor agonist with chronotropic, inotropic, and vasodilatory activity, is used in many transplantation centers. Infusions of dopamine, dobutamine, or epinephrine also are effective. The choice of agent will depend on the clinical situation and need for inotropic support, or renal or pulmonary vasodilation. Newly transplanted hearts unresponsive to pharmacologic stimulation may require temporary epicardial pacing. Although most initial dysrhythmias resolve, 5% to 10% of cardiac transplant recipients require a permanent pacemaker [10].

B. Right ventricular dysfunction

RV failure is a significant cause of early morbidity and mortality, accounting for nearly 20% of early deaths [2]. Therefore, prevention, diagnosis, and aggressive treatment of RV dysfunction after CPB is essential. Acute RV failure after cardiac transplantation may be due to preexistent pulmonary HTN in the recipient, transient pulmonary vasospasm, tricuspid or pulmonic valve insufficiency secondary to early postoperative RV dilation, and donor–recipient size mismatch. Additional factors that may contribute to postoperative RV dysfunction include a prolonged donor heart ischemic time, inadequate myocardial protection, and surgical manipulation of the heart. RV distension and hypokinesis may be diagnosed by TEE or direct observation of the surgical field. Other findings suggesting RV failure include elevations in CVP, PA pressure, and transpulmonary gradient (greater than 15 mm Hg).

The goal of therapy for RV dysfunction is a PVR less than 6 Woods units or a transpulmonary gradient less than 5 to 10 mm Hg. Increased F_iO_2, correction of acid–base abnormalities, and hyperventilation (P_aCO_2 of 25 to 30 mm Hg) may reduce PVR. RV function may be improved by inotropic support and pulmonary vasodilation. Pharmacologic agents commonly used for pulmonary vasodilation include the nitrates, prostacyclin [prostaglandin I_2 (PGI_2)], prostaglandin E_1 (PGE_1), phosphodiesterase-III inhibitors, and inhaled NO [18]. In contrast to nonselective vasodilators such as nitroglycerin and sodium nitroprusside that typically produce systemic hypotension, inhaled NO (20 to 80 ppm) selectively reduces PVR and improves ventilation/perfusion (VQ) mismatch. NO activates guanylate cyclase in vascular smooth muscle cells, producing an increase in cyclic guanosine monophosphate and smooth muscle relaxation. NO has little systemic effect because it is inactivated by hemoglobin and has a 5- to 10-second half-life. NO administration results in the formation of nitrogen dioxide and methemoglobin, and the levels of these toxic metabolites should be monitored. In the presence of severe LV dysfunction, selective dilation of the pulmonary vasculature by NO may lead to an increase in PCWP and pulmonary edema. Thus, agents producing both pulmonary and systemic vasodilation may be a better choice in this setting. Intravenous or inhaled PGI_2 produces pronounced decreases in RV and LV outflow impedence and increases systemic perfusion. Thus, PGI_2 is useful for treating pulmonary HTN in the presence of biventricular dysfunction. RV failure refractory to medical treatment may require insertion of a VAD.

C. Left ventricular dysfunction

Post-CPB LV dysfunction may be a result of a prolonged donor heart ischemic time, inadequate myocardial perfusion, intracoronary embolization of intracavitary air, or surgical manipulation. The incidence of post-CPB LV dysfunction is greater in donors requiring prolonged, high-dose inotropic support before organ harvest. Continued postoperative inotropic support with dobutamine, epinephrine, or norepinephrine may be required.

D. Coagulation

Coagulopathy after cardiac transplantation is common, and perioperative bleeding should be treated early and aggressively to avoid morbidity associated with mediastinal reexploration. Potential etiologies include hepatic dysfunction secondary to chronic hepatic venous congestion, preoperative anticoagulation, CPB-induced platelet dysfunction, hypothermia, and hemodilution of clotting factors. After ruling out surgical bleeding, blood product administration should be guided by repeated measurements of platelet count and clotting factors. Due to an increased risk of infection and graft-versus-host disease, all administered blood products should be cytomegalovirus (CMV) negative, and irradiated or leukocyte depleted. RBCs and platelets should be administered through leukocyte filters. The efficacy of DDAVP for the treatment of postoperative bleeding in this setting has not been proven.

E. Renal dysfunction

Renal dysfunction, as evidenced by increased serum creatinine and oliguria, is common in the immediate postoperative period. Contributing factors include preexisting renal impairment, cyclosporine-associated renal toxicity, perioperative hypotension, and CPB. Treatment of renal dysfunction includes diuretics and optimization of CO and systemic BP. Significant renal dysfunction may require dose adjustment or substitution of nephrotoxic drugs, such as cyclosporine. Although commonly used, the efficacy of dopamine for the treatment of postoperative renal dysfunction has not been established.

F. Pulmonary dysfunction

Postoperative pulmonary complications, such as atelectasis, pleural effusion, and pneumonia, are common and may be reduced by PEEP ventilation, regular endobronchial suctioning, and chest physiotherapy. Bronchoscopy to clear pulmonary secretions often is useful. Pulmonary infection in the immunosuppressed recipient should be treated early and aggressively.

G. Hyperacute allograft rejection

Cardiac allograft hyperacute rejection is caused by preformed anti–human leukocyte antigen (HLA) antibodies present in the recipient. Although extremely rare, hyperacute rejection results in severe cardiac dysfunction and death within hours of transplantation. Assisted mechanical circulatory support until cardiac retransplantation is the only therapeutic option.

VIII. The role of intraoperative transesophageal echocardiography

Intraoperative TEE is an invaluable tool for the management of the cardiac transplant recipient. In addition to monitoring ventricular function, TEE in the pre-CPB period may be used to identify intracavitary thrombus, estimate recipient PA pressures, and evaluate the aortic cannulation and cross-clamp sites for the presence of atherosclerotic disease [19]. TEE also may be used in the post-CPB period to evaluate the efficacy of cardiac de-airing, cardiac function, and surgical anastomoses. Stenosis of the main PA should be excluded by continuous-wave Doppler measurement of the pressure gradient across the anastomosis. After orthotopic cardiac transplantation, the long axis of the left atrium often appears larger than usual because of joining of the donor and recipient left atria. Occasionally, excess donor atrial tissue may obstruct the mitral valve orifice, resulting in pulmonary HTN and RV failure. TEE findings in the immediate post-CPB period frequently include impaired ventricular contractility, decreased diastolic compliance, and acute mild-to-moderate tricuspid, pulmonic, and mitral valve regurgitation. Although LV size and function typically are normal on long-term echocardiographic follow-up of healthy cardiac transplant recipients, RV enlargement and tricuspid valve regurgitation persists in up to 66% of patients [10]. Persistent tricuspid valve regurgitation may result from geometrical alterations of the right atrium or ventricle, asynchronous contraction of the donor and recipient atria, or valvular damage occurring during EMB.

IX. Cardiac transplantation survival and complications

Survival after cardiac transplantation continues to improve, with 1- and 3-year survival rates approaching 86% and 80%, respectively [1]. Greater than 90% of patients surviving 5 years will have NYHA class I activity levels. Infection and acute rejection are the most common causes of death in the first year after cardiac transplantation. However, after the first year, annual mortality is relatively constant at approximately 4%, with allograft CAD being the most common cause of death (Fig. 15.4). Factors associated with increased post–cardiac transplantation mortality include elevated recipient PVR, increased donor age, and prolonged donor heart ischemic time. Complications of cardiac transplantation include the following:

A. Infection

Bacterial respiratory infections are more common than viral infections in the first month after transplantation. However, CMV is the most common infection after the

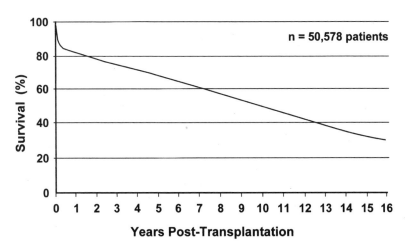

FIG. 15.4 Cardiac transplant survival. The overall 1-year survival for cardiac transplantation is 81%. After 1 year, mortality is nearly constant at a rate of 4% per year. (From Hosenpud JD, Bennett LE, Keck BM, et al. The Registry of the International Society for Heart and Lung Transplantation: Seventeenth official report—2000. *J Heart Lung Transplant* 2000;19: 909–931, with permission.)

first month. Infection should be diagnosed and treated aggressively because of the increased risk of morbidity and mortality in these immunocompromised patients.

B. Acute allograft rejection

Despite a significant reduction in the overall incidence of acute allograft rejection by current immunosuppressive regimens, rejection still occurs frequently during the first year after cardiac transplantation. Risk factors for acute rejection include implantation of a female donor heart in a male recipient, a prolonged donor heart ischemic time, previous allograft rejection, and extremes of age [10]. Although new-onset fatigue, dysrhythmias, or CHF suggest the diagnosis, EMB remains the gold standard for confirming acute allograft rejection. Percutaneous EMB usually is performed through the right internal jugular vein at regular internals after transplantation. Repeated EMB is associated with an increased incidence of tricuspid valve regurgitation. Low-grade or clinically asymptomatic acute allograft rejection may be treated by increasing the oral corticosteroid dose. However, acute rejection associated with hemodynamic decompensation requires additional immunosuppressive therapy with agents such as intravenous OKT-3 or antithymocyte globulin.

C. Systemic Hypertension

More than 90% of cardiac transplant patients will develop systemic arterial HTN. Although the precise mechanisms for this process are unclear, a number of different factors are thought to contribute to its etiology [20]. After cardiac transplantation, immunosuppressive therapy and cardiac denervation commonly lead to neuroendocrine activation, increased sympathetic nervous system activity, and renal impairment. Cyclosporine increases thromboxane production and renal vascular resistance, and its long-term administration in particular is linked to the development of HTN. Additionally, corticosteroid mineralocorticoid activity leads to sodium and water retention and is implicated in the pathogenesis of HTN. HTN occurs more commonly in older cardiac transplant recipients with preexisting HTN and contributes to the incidence of allograft CAD and adverse cardiovascular events. Treatment of HTN after cardiac transplantation often is difficult and usually requires dietary sodium restriction as well as combination medical therapy using calcium channel antagonists and ACE inhibitors.

D. Allograft coronary artery disease

Accelerated allograft CAD is the major factor limiting long-term cardiac transplantation survival and is the leading cause of death after 1 year [4]. A diffuse, concentric myointimal distribution often not adequately imaged by coronary angiography is pathognomonic for allograft CAD. Factors thought to contribute to the pathogenesis of allograft CAD include a prolonged donor heart ischemic time, older age of recipient, hyperlipidemia, HTN, and CMV infection. Denervation of the transplanted heart often results in "silent" myocardial ischemia that may go unrecognized until the development of severe cardiac dysfunction. Treatment options for allograft CAD include percutaneous transluminal coronary angioplasty and coronary artery bypass graft surgery. However, the success of these procedures usually is limited because of the diffuse nature of the disease. Retransplantation is the only definitive therapeutic option. However, with the current shortage of donor hearts the decision to proceed with cardiac retransplantation must be considered carefully, as retransplantation has a poorer prognosis than the primary procedure [6].

E. Immunosuppressive drug side effects

Cardiac transplant recipients require lifelong immunosuppression. Although immunosuppressive protocols vary among transplant centers, most regimens include triple therapy combinations of azathioprine, cyclosporine, and corticosteroids. Newer drugs such as tacrolimus (FK506) and mycophenolate mofetil (MMF) may be substituted for cyclosporine and azathioprine, respectively [2]. In addition to placing the patient at increased risk of infection, immunosuppressants are associated with numerous acute side effects (Table 15.5). Further, chronic immunosuppression increases the risk of malignancies such as lymphoma, Kaposi sarcoma, renal cell carcinoma, and hepatobiliary and skin tumors.

X. Pediatric cardiac transplantation

Cardiac transplantation for pediatric end-stage heart disease accounts for 10% of cardiac transplants [16]. The primary indications for pediatric cardiac transplantation are complex

Table 15.5 Immunosuppressive agents

Agent	Mechanism of action	Side effects
Cyclosporine	Inhibits T-cell proliferation Inhibits interleukin-2 expression	Nephrotoxicity, hypertension, tremors, headache, paresthesias, hyperkalemia, hypomagnesemia, hepatotoxicity, gingival hyperplasia
Azathioprine	Inhibits DNA synthesis Inhibits lymphocyte proliferation	Leukopenia, thrombocytopenia, anemia, infection, hepatotoxicity, pancreatitis, nausea, vomiting, diarrhea
Corticosteroids	Decrease T-cell activation Inhibit cytokine production Inhibits leukocyte chemotaxis	Infection, hyperglycemia, hypertension, osteoporosis, adrenal suppression, myopathy, peptic ulcer disease, hyperlipidemia, psychological disturbances
Mycophenolate mofetil	Inhibits DNA synthesis Inhibits lymphocyte proliferation	Nausea, abdominal cramps, diarrhea, neutropenia, rarely hepatic and bone marrow toxicity
Tacrolimus (FK506)	Inhibits T-cell activation	Nephrotoxicity, anemia, hyperkalemia, hyperglycemia, hypertension, nausea, vomiting
OKT3	Opsonizes and lyses T cells	Fever, chills, hypotension, bronchospasm, pulmonary edema, aseptic meningitis, seizures, nausea, vomiting, diarrhea
Antilymphocyte globulin	Opsonizes and lyses T cells	Anaphylaxis, leukopenia, thrombocytopenia, hypotension, infection, fever, chills, hepatitis, serum sickness

congenital heart disease (e.g., hypoplastic left heart syndrome) in infants younger than 1 year and cardiomyopathy [21]. At present, more than 50% of pediatric cardiac transplant recipients are younger than 5 years. Survival rates for pediatric cardiac transplantation are comparable to those of adult recipients, although long-term results of cardiac transplantation for complex congenital heart disease are unknown. Rejection accounts for approximately 30% of deaths after pediatric cardiac transplantation [21]. Interestingly, rejection as a cause of death is lowest in infants younger than 1 year when cardiac transplant recipients of all age groups are compared, suggesting a decreased immune response in this age group [2]. Similar to adult programs, pediatric cardiac transplant programs face a severe donor heart shortage. The lack of available donor hearts is further compounded by the fact that the use of totally implantable VADs as a bridge to transplantation is limited to patients with a body surface area greater than 1.5 m² [16]. Thus, long-term mechanical circulatory support until the time of transplantation is not an option for many children.

A. Perioperative considerations

The pediatric patient presenting for cardiac transplantation presents a number of unique anesthetic challenges. Many patients will have undergone previous palliative or corrective cardiac surgery that may make intravenous and arterial access more difficult to obtain and increase the risk of repeat sternotomy-associated morbidity. Additionally, the hemodynamic goals of anesthesia induction and maintenance will be dictated not only by the presence of end-stage heart failure, but also by the unique pathophysiology of underlying complex congenital heart disease. The presence and severity of preoperative pulmonary HTN in neonates and infants must be carefully assessed, as additional increases in PVR in the post-CPB period may rapidly lead to failure of the newly implanted, thin-walled RV. It is for this reason that the use of undersized pediatric donors (less than 75% of the recipient's weight) is avoided, because of the increased risk of posttransplantation RV failure and mortality [16].

Surgical and CPB time for pediatric cardiac transplantation often is prolonged and requires deep hypothermic circulatory arrest. These factors significantly contribute to the post-CBP coagulopathy that frequently occurs despite routine antifibrinolytic administration. Blood product administration often is required after CPB. Immunosuppressive therapy is commenced early in the perioperative period. However, due to the high incidence of complications associated with long-term corticosteroid therapy in pediatric cardiac transplant recipients, steroids often are discontinued and replaced with tacrolimus. Similar to adults, acute allograft rejection is monitored by EMB. However, the role of echocardiography and other noninvasive methods of detecting myocardial allograft rejection are being evaluated to prevent and reduce the morbidity of repeated EMB in pediatric patients.

XI. Anesthesia for the previously transplanted patient

As increasing numbers of patients undergo and survive cardiac transplantation, many of these patients will undergo additional surgical procedures in their lifetime. Common surgical procedures after cardiac transplantation are listed in Table 15.6. Many of these subsequent surgical procedures are directly attributable to sequelae of atherosclerosis, cardiac transplantation, or immunosuppression [22]. Understanding the unique physiologic and pharmacologic features of the previously transplanted patient is essential to ensure optimal anesthetic management.

A. Physiology of the cardiac transplant patient

The cardiac autonomic plexus is transected during orthotopic cardiac transplantation, leaving the transplanted heart completely denervated. It now is known that partial efferent sympathetic neuronal reinnervation commences within 12 months of cardiac transplantation [23]. The degree of reinnervation varies considerably between individuals and is of uncertain functional significance. Parasympathetic neu-

Table 15.6 Common surgical procedures after cardiac transplantation

Reexploration for mediastinal bleeding
Infectious complications
  Laparotomy
  Craniotomy
  Thoracotomy
  Abscess drainage
  Bronchoscopy
Steroid-related complications
  Hip arthroplasty or pinning
  Laparotomy for perforated viscus
  Cataract excision
  Vitrectomy
  Scleral buckle
Aortic or peripheral vascular surgery and amputation
Pancreatic and biliary tract surgery
Retransplantation

Modified from Wyner J, Finch EL. Heart and heart-lung transplantation. In: Gelman S, ed. *Anesthesia and organ transplantation*. Philadelphia: WB Saunders, 1987:111–137.

ronal reinnervation is much less extensive, resulting in a characteristic high resting HR (90 to 110 beats/min) and absent reflex bradycardic response after carotid sinus massage or a Valsalva maneuver. In contrast to the normal heart, which increases CO primarily by increasing HR, the transplanted heart increases CO primarily by increasing SV. As acute changes in CO, HR, and SV in the transplanted heart are mediated mainly by adrenal secretion and circulation of direct-acting catecholamines, the response to stressful stimuli (e.g., laryngoscopy and tracheal intubation), hypovolemia, and exercise may be delayed or blunted [10]. Although most previously transplanted patients have near-normal ventricular contractility at rest, exercise or physiologic stress may uncover a reduction in functional reserve.

Although autonomic reinnervation is variable, the intrinsic control systems of the heart remain intact, and cardiac impulse formation and conduction are normal. Right bundle branch block is the most common conduction abnormality after cardiac transplantation and is thought to result from prolonged donor heart ischemia and elevated recipient PVR [10]. Sinus bradyarrhythmias occur in 20% of cardiac transplant patients and may result from prolonged donor heart ischemia. The late onset of atrial arrhythmias, however, should raise the suspicion of allograft CAD or acute rejection. Ventricular arrhythmias are uncommon unless advanced allograft CAD is present.

B. Pharmacology of the cardiac transplant patient

Autonomic denervation of the transplanted heart significantly alters the pharmacodynamic activity of many drugs (Table 15.7). Drugs that mediate their actions through the autonomic nervous system generally are ineffective in altering HR and contractility, although partial autonomic reinnervation may explain individual variation among cardiac transplant patients. In contrast, drugs that act directly on the heart are effective. The β-adrenergic response of the transplanted heart to direct-acting catecholamines, such as epinephrine and norepinephrine, often is increased, whereas the response to α-adrenergic agents may be reduced [22]. Reflex bradycardia or tachycardia in response to changes in systemic arterial BP is absent. Narcotic-induced decreases in HR frequently are diminished in the transplanted heart. Drugs with mixed activity (e.g., dopamine and ephedrine) will mediate an effect only through their direct actions. Parasympathomimetics such as atropine and glycopyrrolate will not alter HR, although their peripheral anticholinergic activity remains unaffected. Although anticholinesterase administration (e.g., neostigmine) will have little effect on HR, anticholinergic coadministration still is warranted to counteract peripheral muscarinic effects.

C. Preoperative evaluation

A thorough medical history, physical examination, and review of medical record should be undertaken for all patients undergoing anesthesia. Current medications

Table 15.7 Drug effects on the denervated heart

Drug	Action	Heart rate	Blood pressure
Atropine	I	—	—
Digoxin	D	$-/\downarrow$	–
Dopamine	B	$\uparrow$	$\uparrow$
Ephedrine	B	$-/\uparrow$	$-/\uparrow$
Fentanyl	I	–	–
Isoproterenol	D	$\uparrow$	$-/\uparrow$
Neostigmine	I	$-/\downarrow$	–
Norepinephrine	D	$\uparrow$	$\uparrow$
Pancuronium	I	–	–
Phenylephrine	I	–	$\uparrow$
Verapamil	D	$\downarrow$	$\downarrow$

B, indirect and direct; D, direct; I, indirect; $\uparrow$, increased; $\downarrow$, decreased; –, no effect.

should be noted. Particular attention should be paid to determining cardiac allograft function, evidence of rejection or infection, complications of immunosuppression, and end-organ disease. Systemic HTN is common, and a significant proportion of patients will have allograft CAD within 1 year of cardiac transplantation. The absence of angina pectoris symptomatology does not exclude significant CAD, because denervation of cardiac pain afferents frequently results in silent myocardial ischemia [24]. The patient's activity level and exercise tolerance are good indicators of allograft function. Symptoms of dyspnea and CHF suggest significant CAD or myocardial rejection. The presentation of infection may be atypical in immunosuppressed patients, with fever and leucocytosis often absent. The patient's airway should be examined carefully, because lymphoproliferative disease and soft tissue changes secondary to corticosteroid administration may increase the potential for airway obstruction. Hematocrit, coagulation profile, electrolytes, and creatinine should be checked, because immunosuppressive therapy commonly is associated with anemia, thrombocytopenia, electrolyte disturbances, and renal dysfunction. Recent chest x-ray films, ECGs, and coronary angiograms should be reviewed. More than one P wave may be seen on the ECG from patients in whom cardiac transplantation was performed using a biatrial technique (Fig. 15.5). Although seen on the ECG, the P wave originating in the native atria does not conduct impulses across the anastomotic line.

D. Anesthesia management

1. Clinical implications of immunosuppressive therapy

All cardiac transplant patients are immunosuppressed and consequently at higher risk for infection. All anesthetic equipment should be clean, and all vascular access procedures should be carried out using aseptic technique. Antibiotic prophylaxis should be considered for any procedure with the potential to produce bacteremia. Oral immunosuppressive medication should be

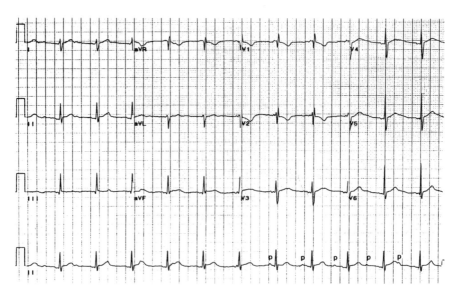

FIG. 15.5 Transplanted heart electrocardiogram is commonly characterized by two sets of P waves, right-axis deviation, and incomplete right bundle branch block. The donor heart P waves are small and precede the QRS complex, whereas P waves originating from the recipient's atria (labeled *p*) are unrelated to the QRS complex. (From Fowler NO. *Clinical electrocardiographic diagnosis.* Philadelphia: Lippincott Williams & Wilkins, 2000:225, with permission.)

continued without interruption or given intravenously to maintain blood levels within the therapeutic range. Intravenous and oral doses of azathioprine are approximately equivalent. Administration of large volumes of intravenous fluids will decrease blood levels of immunosuppressants; therefore, levels should be checked daily. Immunosuppressant nephrotoxicity may be exacerbated by coadministration of other potentially renal toxic medications, such as nonsteroidal antiinflammatory agents or gentamicin [22]. Chronic corticosteroid therapy to prevent allograft rejection may result in adrenal suppression. Thus, supplemental "stress" steroids should be administered to critically ill patients or patients undergoing major surgical procedures. The intravenous dose of methylprednisolone is equivalent to the oral dose of prednisolone.

2. Monitoring

Standard anesthetic monitors should be used, including five-lead ECG, to detect ischemia and dysrhythmias. Cardiac transplant patients frequently have fragile skin and osteoporotic bones secondary to chronic corticosteroid administration. Care with tape, automated BP cuffs, and patient positioning is essential to avoid skin and musculoskeletal trauma. As for all patients undergoing anesthesia, invasive monitoring should be considered only for situations in which the benefits outweigh the risks. Importantly, cardiac transplant patients have an increased risk of developing catheter-related infections with a high associated morbidity and mortality. Intraoperative TEE permits rapid evaluation of volume status, cardiac function, and ischemia, and may be a useful substitute for invasive monitoring. Should central venous access be required, alternative routes usually are taken to preserve the right internal jugular vein for EMB. Careful monitoring of neuromuscular blockade with a peripheral nerve stimulator is recommended in the previously transplanted patient, because cyclosporine has been reported to prolong neuromuscular blockade after administration of nondepolarizing neuromuscular blocking agents [22]. In contrast, an attenuated response to nondepolarizing muscle relaxants has been reported in patients receiving azathioprine.

3. Techniques of anesthesia

Both general and regional anesthesia techniques have been used safely in cardiac transplant patients. In the absence of significant cardiorespiratory, renal, or hepatic dysfunction, there is no absolute contraindication to any anesthetic technique. For any selected anesthetic technique, maintenance of ventricular filling pressures is essential as the transplanted heart increases CO primarily by increasing SV.

a. General anesthesia

General anesthesia frequently is preferred over regional anesthesia for cardiac transplant patients, because alterations in myocardial preload and afterload may be more predictable. Cyclosporine and tacrolimus decrease renal blood flow and glomerular filtration via thromboxane-mediated renal vasoconstriction [4]. Thus, renally excreted anesthetics and muscle relaxants should be used with caution in patients receiving these medications. Cyclosporine and tacrolimus also lower the seizure threshold, and hyperventilation should be avoided. Elevations in the resting HR and a delayed sympathetic response to noxious stimuli in cardiac transplant recipients may make anesthetic depth difficult to assess.

b. Regional anesthesia

Many immunosuppressants cause thrombocytopenia and alter the coagulation profile. Both the platelet count and coagulation profile should be within normal limits if spinal or epidural regional anesthesia is planned. Ventricular filling pressures should be maintained after induction of central neural axis blockade to prevent hypotension caused by the delayed response of the denervated transplanted heart to a rapid decrease in sympathetic tone. Volume loading, ventricular filling pressure monitoring, and careful titration of local anesthetic agents may prevent hemodynamic instability. Hypotension should be treated with vasopressors that directly stimulate the heart.

4. Blood transfusion

The cardiac transplant recipient is at increased risk for blood product transfusion complications. Adverse reactions include infection, graft-versus-host disease, and immunomodulation. Use of irradiated, leukocyte-depleted, CMV-negative blood products and white blood cell filters for blood product administration reduces the incidence of adverse transfusion reactions. The blood bank should receive early notification if the use of blood products is anticipated, as the presence of reactive antibodies delaying cross-match is not infrequent.

E. Pregnancy after cardiac transplantation

Despite an increased incidence of preeclampsia and preterm labor, increasing numbers of cardiac transplant recipients are successfully carrying pregnancies to term. In general, the transplanted heart is able to adapt to the physiologic changes of pregnancy [25]. Due to an increased sensitivity to the β-adrenergic effects of tocolytics such as terbutaline and ritodrine, use of alternative drugs such as magnesium and nifedipine may be considered. Although pregnancy does not adversely affect cardiac allografts, the risk of acute cardiac allograft rejection may be increased post partum. All immunosuppressive drugs used to prevent cardiac allograft rejection cross the placenta, although most are not thought to be teratogenic [22].

XII. Future directions

Continuing therapeutic advances for the management of end-stage cardiac failure will influence the selection and management of future cardiac transplant recipients. Development of noninvasive methods to diagnose myocardial rejection and novel immunosuppressive agents will further improve cardiac transplantation morbidity and mortality. Surgical alternatives such as xenotransplantation and the total artificial heart currently are being evaluated and, if successful, may greatly alleviate the current donor heart shortage problem. Finally, advances in myocardial gene therapy eventually may eliminate the need for cardiac transplantation.

References

1. **Hosenpud JD, Bennett LE, Keck BM, et al. The registry of the international society for heart and lung transplantation: seventeenth official report—2000. *J Heart Lung Transplant* 2000;19:909–931.**
2. **Miniati DN, Robbins RC, Reitz BA. Heart and heart-lung transplantation. In: Braunwald E, Zipes DP, Libby P, eds. *Heart disease: a textbook of cardiovascular medicine,* 6th ed. Philadelphia: WB Saunders, 2001:615–634.**
3. Givertz MM, Wilson SC, Braunwald E. Clinical aspects of heart failure: high-output failure; pulmonary edema. In: Braunwald E, Zipes DP, Libby P, eds. *Heart disease: a textbook of cardiovascular medicine,* 6th ed. Philadelphia: WB Saunders, 2001:534–561.
4. Argenziano M, Goldstein DJ, Oz MC, et al. Cardiac transplantation for end-stage heart disease. *Cardiol Rev* 1999;7:349–355.
5. **McGowan FX, Bailey PL. Heart, lung and heart-lung transplantation. In: Cook DR, Davis PJ, eds. *Anesthetic principles for organ transplantation.* New York: Raven Press, 1994:85–157.**
6. Costanzo MR. Current status of heart transplantation. *Curr Opin Cardiol* 1996;11: 161–165.
7. Hunt SA, Frazier OH. Mechanical circulatory support and cardiac transplantation. *Circulation* 1998;97:2079–2090.
8. Edwards NM, Rajasinghe HA, John R, et al. Cardiac transplantation in over 1000 patients: a single institution experience from Columbia University. *Clin Transplant* 1999: 249–261.
9. 1999 Annual report of the US Scientific Registry of Transplant Recipients and the Organ Procurement and Transplantation Network: transplant data 1989–1998. Rockville, MD: United Network for Organ Sharing, 2000.
10. Taylor AJ, Bergin JD. Cardiac transplantation for the cardiologist not trained in transplantation. *Am Heart J* 1995;129:578–592.
11. Dabol R, Edwards NM. Cardiac transplantation and other therapeutic options in the treatment of end-stage heart disease. *Compr Ther* 2000;26:109–113.
12. Nisco SJ, Reitz BA. Developments in cardiac transplantation. *Curr Opin Cardiol* 1994; 9:237–246.
13. **Wijdicks EF. The diagnosis of brain death. *N Engl J Med* 2001;344:1215–1221.**

14. **Scheinkestel CD, Tuxen DV, Cooper DJ, et al. Medical management of the (potential) organ donor.** *Anaesth Intens Care* **1995;23:51–59.**

15. Aziz TM, Burgess MI, El-Gamel A, et al. Orthotopic cardiac transplantation technique: a survey of current practice. *Ann Thorac Surg* 1999;68:1242–1246.

16. Addonizio LJ. Current status of cardiac transplantation in children. *Curr Opin Pediatr* 1996;8:520–526.

17. Goldstein DJ, Oz MC, Smith CR, et al. Safety of repeat aprotinin administration for LVAD recipients undergoing cardiac transplantation. *Ann Thorac Surg* 1996;61:692–695.

18. Schmid ER, Burki C, Engel MH, et al. Inhaled nitric oxide versus intravenous vasodilators in severe pulmonary hypertension after cardiac surgery. *Anesth Analg* 1999;89: 1108–1115.

19. **Suriani RJ. Transesophageal echocardiography during organ transplantation.** *J Cardiothorac Vasc Anesth* **1998;12:686–694.**

20. Jenkins GH, Singer DRJ. Hypertension in thoracic transplant recipients. *J Hum Hypertens* 1998:12;813–823.

21. **Boucek MM, Faro A, Novick RJ, et al. The Registry of the International Society for Heart and Lung Transplantation: fourth official pediatric report—2000.** *J Heart Lung Transplant* **2001;20:39–52.**

22. **Kostopanagiotou G, Smyrniotis V, Arkadopoulos N, et al. Anesthetic and perioperative management of adult transplant recipients in nontransplant surgery.** *Anesth Analg* **1999;89;613–622.**

23. Murphy DA, Thompson GW, Ardell JL, et al. The heart reinnervates after transplantation. *Ann Thorac Surg* 2000;69:1769–1781.

24. Toivonen, HJ. Anaesthesia for patients with a transplanted organ. *Acta Anaesthiol Scand* 2000;44:812–833.

25. Riley ET. Obstetric management of patients with transplants. *Int Anesthiol Clin* 1995; 33:125–141.

John L. Atlee

An arrhythmia, any rhythm other than normal sinus rhythm at an appropriate rate, may be associated with mechanical cardiac dysfunction or heart failure. Treatment with drugs or devices is indicated when arrhythmias produce destabilizing hemodynamic imbalance consequent to bradycardia, tachycardia, or atrioventricular (AV) dissociation. Drug therapy today is no longer empirical. Rather, drugs are selected based on modification of specific molecular targets important to the genesis and maintenance of arrhythmias. Increased awareness of proarrhythmia, the provocation of new or worse arrhythmias by antiarrhythmic drugs, has influenced selection of drugs as treatment. Thus, electrical therapies have gained wider acceptance in acute rhythm management and have an important role in cardiac surgery. For similar reasons, electrical, catheter, and surgical ablation therapies have achieved increased importance in the management of recurring or chronic arrhythmias. The emphasis in this chapter is on device therapy and perioperative management for patients with implanted devices. Electrocardiographic (ECG) diagnosis is not discussed. Whereas concepts of arrhythmogenesis, antiarrhythmic action, and drug selection are discussed, the reader is referred to Chapter 2 for discussion of specific antiarrhythmic drugs and indications.

I. Concepts of arrhythmogenesis

A. Normal electrophysiology.
Two types of fibers can be distinguished based on their resting membrane potential (i.e., working atrial and ventricular muscle fibers) or maximum diastolic potential [MDP; i.e., automatic sinoatrial (SA) and AV node (AVN) fibers] [1–3]. The former are "fast response" fibers. Their action potential (AP) upstrokes are largely dependent on rapid influx of Na^+ (Fig. 16.1) and AP propagation is fast. However, in SA node (SAN) or AVN cells with low MDPs (–60 to –70 mV), AP upstroke and propagation are slow due to reduced Na^+ influx through partially inactivated Na^+ channels, hence the term "slow response" fiber.

1. **Automaticity.** The SAN serves as the primary pacemaker for the heart. Cells normally exhibiting automaticity also are found along the sulcus terminalis and in the coronary sinus ostium (i.e., subsidiary atrial pacemakers) and within the AV junction and His–Purkinje system. Due to overdrive suppression of automaticity, the SAN normally suppresses these lower pacemakers. However, they may assume control of the heart if the SAN defaults or if imbalance enhances their discharge rate relative to the SAN. Automaticity is explained by a net gain of intracellular positive charges during diastole. The ionic mechanism depends on the MDP. At reduced MDP of SAN cells (–50 to –60 mV), the pacemaker current I_f, which is carried by a channel that is relatively selective for monovalent cations, contributes only about 20% to the pacemaker current. A decline in outward K^+ current I_K (Fig. 16.1) and increased inward Ca^{2+} current $I_{Ca,L}$ (Fig. 16.1) are largely responsible for SAN automaticity. However, in secondary pacemaker fibers with higher MDP (–70 to –90 mV), I_f assumes greater importance.

2. **Conduction.** AP upstroke velocity, which is determined by the magnitude of inward current flowing during phase 0 (Fig. 16.1), and effective axial resistivity are the most important determinants of conduction velocity. The latter is the resistance to current flow in the direction of propagation. The extent and distribution of gap junctions between adjacent cardiac fibers has a profound influence on axial resistance and conduction velocity. Longitudinal axial resistance is lower than transverse axial resistance. Thus, conduction in cardiac muscle is anisotropic. A reduction in gap junctional conductance due to ischemia-mediated intracellular Ca^{2+} accumulation or to aging may be the cause for slowed conduction.

B. Abnormal electrophysiology.
Abnormal cardiac electrophysiology often is a consequence of partial depolarization of fast response fibers. Causes include ischemia, hypoxia, myocardial injury, and acute electrolyte imbalance, especially hyperkalemia. Reduced AP upstroke velocity and slow conduction in partially depolarized fibers comes from incomplete recovery from inactivation of Na^+ channels (depressed fast response). Membrane depolarization to –50 mV inactivates all the Na^+ channels. At potentials positive to –55 mV, Ca^{2+} inward current is activated to generate the AP upstroke. With loss of membrane potential and depressed fast response, electrophysiologic (EP) changes often are heterogeneous due to varying degrees of Na channel inactivation among fibers. This produces uneven conduction and refractoriness, which are conducive to reentry.

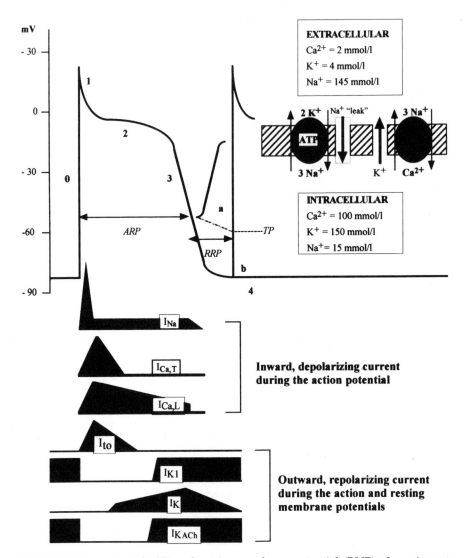

FIG. 16.1 Action potential (AP) and resting membrane potential (RMP) of a quiescent Purkinje fiber. Extracellular and intracellular ion concentrations during phase 4, and the active and passive ion exchangers that restore intracellular ion concentrations during phase 4 are shown to the right of the AP. Inward depolarizing and outward repolarizing currents are shown below the AP. The adenosine triphosphate (ATP)-dependent Na/K pump maintains steep outwardly and inwardly directed gradients (*arrows*) for K^+ and Na^+, respectively, and generates small net outward current. The passive Na/Ca exchanger generates small net inward current. A small, inward "leak" of Na^+ keeps the RMP slightly positive to the K equilibrium potential (–96 mV). AP phase 0 is the upstroke, phase 1 is initial rapid repolarization, phase 2 is the plateau, and phase 3 is final repolarization. The cell is unresponsive to propagating AP or external stimuli during the absolute refractory period (*ARP*). A small electrotonic potential (*a*) occurs in response to a propagating AP or external stimulus during the relative refractory period (*RRP*). It is incapable of self-propagation. A normal AP is generated at the end of the RRP (*b*), when the Na channels have fully recovered from inactivation. It is capable of propagation. Note that threshold potential (*TP*) for excitation is more positive during the RRP.

1. **Abnormal automaticity.** Depressed fast response fibers may exhibit abnormal automaticity. This is spontaneous phase 4 depolarization that occurs in fibers that do not normally exhibit automaticity (atrial or ventricular muscle) or at a reduced level of maximum diastolic membrane potential in automatic Purkinje fibers. Abnormal automaticity is a likely mechanism for escape rhythms and slow monomorphic VT with acute myocardial infarction (AMI).

2. **Afterpotentials and triggered arrhythmias.** Small depolarizing potentials may occur before [early afterdepolarization (EAD)] or after full AP repolarization [delayed afterdepolarization (DAD)]. If these reach threshold for regenerative depolarization, they may initiate triggered tachyarrhythmias. DADs result from oscillatory release of Ca^{2+} from overloaded sarcoplasmic reticulum and may be the cause for ventricular arrhythmias with AMI, and atrial or ventricular arrhythmias with digitalis excess. EADs occur with acquired or congenital QT interval prolongation. The latter involves defects in genes encoding Na and K channels affecting repolarization. EADs are the likely inciting mechanism for torsades de pointes ventricular tachycardia (VT) and any polymorphic VT in association with QT interval prolongation.

3. **Reentry.** Impulses originating in the SAN normally continue until the entire heart has been activated and becomes refractory. Reentry of excitation can occur if some fibers are not activated and the propagating impulse returns by another pathway to excite them. For reentry to occur, there must be (a) an area of unidirectional conduction block, (b) an alternate pathway for conduction, and (c) sufficient delay of the propagating impulse to permit tissue proximal to the site of unidirectional block to recover from refractoriness. Slowed conduction may be caused by delayed recovery from excitation after premature beats, reduced Na^+ channel availability in depressed fast response fibers, or changes in gap junctional resistance brought about by aging or disease processes. Unidirectional block of conduction may occur as the result of nonuniform recovery of excitability due to regional differences in refractoriness or geometric factors. It now is possible to map tachycardia circuits during EP studies and to interrupt reentry circuits by surgical or radiofrequency (RF) catheter techniques.

4. **Types of reentry.** *Anatomic reentry* requires a fixed, anatomically defined circuit. Such circuits might occur in fibrotic regions of the atria or ventricles, or in surviving muscle fibers with healed infarction. Anatomically defined circuits are involved in VT due to bundle branch reentry, atrial flutter resulting from reentry confined to the right atrium, and paroxysmal supraventricular tachycardia (SVT) due to reentry involving the AVN or AVN and accessory AV pathways. *Functional reentry* occurs in contiguous fibers with discordant EP properties. Disparate excitability and refractoriness and anisotropic distribution of intercellular resistance allow initiation and maintenance of reentry.

C. **Substrates and triggers.** Myocardial remodeling consequent to disease provides a substrate for arrhythmias. However, arrhythmias may not occur without inciting imbalance. For example, patients with healed infarction may have zones of fibrous scar tissue intermingled with surviving normal fibers. These provide potential pathways for anatomic reentry. However, they may require a trigger provided by atrial or ventricular extrasystoles generated by an automatic or triggered focus in response to a catecholamine surge or other imbalance. In contrast, with ischemia, there is no fixed anatomic substrate. Conduction and refractoriness are nonuniform due to varying degrees of Na channel inactivation and altered gap junctional conductance. These changes are conducive to reentry. Once again, extrasystoles with some inciting imbalance may be the trigger for arrhythmias. The concept of substrates and imbalance suggests that remedial intervention for tangible imbalance is key to effective antiarrhythmia strategies.

D. **Etiology of clinical arrhythmias.** It has long been held that a mechanistic approach to arrhythmia management is most advantageous. However, determining specific EP mechanisms of clinical arrhythmias often may not be possible, especially in the critical care and perioperative arena, where effects of multiple drugs, physiologic imbalance, and underlying myocardial disease interact to initiate and sustain arrhythmias. For example, consider the origin of new-onset atrial fibrillation after cardiopulmonary bypass in a patient with coronary artery disease, hypertension, and chronic pulmonary disease. Any of these conditions may provide the substrate for anatomic or functional reentry. The inciting factor might be DAD-induced atrial extrasystoles due to Ca^{2+} overload secondary to inadequate atrial protection, ischemia, and/or elevated catecholamines. Alternatively, such imbalance might partially depolarize some fibers so that abnormal automaticity is the mechanism for extrasystoles. Confirmed or postulated mechanisms for clinical arrhythmias are listed in Table 16.1.

   E. Drugs as treatment for arrhythmias. The emphasis on treatment for arrhythmias, especially ventricular arrhythmias in patients with structural heart disease, has moved from drugs to electricity (pacing; cardioverter–defibrillator). Although drugs have proved safe and effective in normal heart, their safety and efficacy have been modest in structurally abnormal heart. Chronic drug therapy in patients with structural heart disease is associated with increased mortality due to proarrhythmia (defined below). Nonetheless, drugs remain an important adjunct to electrical therapy for acute management of ventricular tachyarrhythmias and are a mainstay for both acute and long-term treatment for atrial tachyarrhythmias.

II. Pacing, cardioversion, and defibrillation: indications and technology. Today, more than 500,000 patients in the United States have implanted pacemakers, and up to 115,000 new devices are implanted each year [4,5]. The number of internal cardioverter–defibrillators (ICD) implanted has steadily increased, reaching 50,000 new implants yearly worldwide in 1999. Because of technologic advances, pacemakers have become smaller but increasingly complex. Although this complexity has greatly expanded therapeutic opportunities, at the same time it has increased potential for malfunction in the perioperative setting. Similarly, ICD have undergone explosive evolution. Except in infants and small children, a formal thoracotomy no longer is used for implantation. Contemporary devices are much smaller (i.e., suitable for pectoral implantation), use biphasic shocks (substantially reduced shock current requirements), and incorporate all features of modern pacemakers, including dual-chamber pacing and adaptive-rate pacing (ARP). Finally, ICDs with dual-chamber tachycardia discrimination and either cardioversion or defibrillation now are available.

   A. Temporary pacing. Compared to drugs for treating cardiac rhythm disturbances, temporary pacing has several advantages. The effect is immediate, control is precise, and there is reduced risk of untoward effects and proarrhythmia.

Table 16.1 Confirmed or postulated electrophysiologic mechanisms for clinical arrhythmias

Mechanism	Arrhythmias
Altered normal automaticity	Sinus bradycardia and tachycardia; wandering atrial pacemaker; AV junctional and ventricular escape rhythms
Abnormal automaticity	Slow monomorphic VT, junctional or idioventricular rhythms in acute MI; some ectopic atrial tachycardia
Triggered activity (DAD)	VT in first 24 hours of acute MI; atrial or VT with digitalis toxicity; catecholamine-mediated VT
Triggered activity (EAD)	Long QT interval with polymorphic VT (i.e., torsades de pointes)
Anatomic reentry	Paroxysmal SVT due to reentry involving the sinoatrial node, atria, AV node, or accessory AV pathways; VT with healed infarction; atrial flutter
Functional reentry	Atrial fibrillation; monomorphic or polymorphic VT with acute MI; ventricular fibrillation

AV, atrioventricular; DAD, delayed afterdepolarization; EAD, early afterdepolarization; MI, myocardial infarction; SVT, supraventricular tachycardia; VT, ventricular tachycardia.

1. **Indications.** Temporary pacing is indicated for rate support in patients with disadvantageous bradycardia or escape rhythms. Prophylactic or stand-by pacing is indicated for patients at increased risk for sudden high-degree AV heart block (AVHB). Temporary pacing can be used to overdrive or terminate atrial or ventricular tachyarrhythmias. The endpoint for temporary pacing is resolution of the indication or implantation of a permanent pacemaker for a continuing indication. Usual and less established indications for temporary pacing are listed in Table 16.2.

2. **Technology.** Transvenous endocardial or epicardial leads usually are used for temporary pacing. Either route is suitable for single- or dual-chamber pacing. The noninvasive transcutaneous and transesophageal routes also are available. Transcutaneous pacing produces simultaneous ventricular and atrial or global ventricular capture and thus does not preserve optimal hemodynamics in patients with intact AV conduction. With available technology for transesophageal pacing, only atrial pacing is possible. Thus, the method is not suitable for patients with advanced AVHB or atrial fibrillation.

B. **Permanent pacing.** Permanent pacemakers are no longer prescribed simply for rate support. They have become an integral part of treatment, along with drugs and other measures, to prevent arrhythmias and improve quality of life in patients with heart failure.

1. **Indications.** The presence or absence of symptoms directly attributable to bradycardia has an important influence on the decision to implant a permanent pacemaker [6]. There is increasing interest in multisite pacing as part of the management for patients with structural heart disease and heart failure. In the past, pacemakers were prescribed to treat reentrant tachyarrhythmias. Today, this capability can be programmed for either the atrium or ventricle as part of "tiered therapies" with an ICD.

   a. **AV heart block.** Patients may be asymptomatic or have symptoms related to bradycardia, ventricular arrhythmias, or both. There is little evidence that pacing improves survival with isolated first-degree AV block, even though marked first-degree block may be symptomatic without higher degree block due to the close proximity of atrial systole to the preceding ventricular systole. With type I, second-degree AV block due to AVN conduction

Table 16.2 Usual and less-established indications for temporary cardiac pacing

Usual indications	Less-established indications
• Sinus bradycardia or escape rhythm with symptoms or hemodynamic compromise • As bridge to permanent pacing with advanced second- or third-degree AV heart block, regardless of etiology • During AMI: asystole; new bifascicular block with first-degree AV heart block; alternating BBB with disadvantageous bradycardia not responsive to drugs; or type II, second-degree AVHB • Bradycardia-dependent tachyarrhythmias (e.g., torsades de pointes with LQTS)	• During AMI: new or age-indeterminate right BBB with LAFB, LPFB, or first-degree AV heart block, or with left BBB; recurrent sinus pauses refractory to atropine; overdrive pacing for incessant VT • During AMI: new or age-indeterminate bifascicular block or isolated right BBB • Heart surgery: (i) to overdrive hemodynamically disadvantageous AV junctional and ventricular rhythms; (ii) to terminate reentrant SVT or VT; (iii) to prevent pause- or bradycardia-dependent tachydysrhythmias; (iv) insertion of pulmonary artery with left BBB

AMI, acute myocardial infarction; AV, atrioventricular; AVHB, atrioventricular heart block; BBB, bundle branch block; LAFB, left anterior fascicular block; LPFB, left posterior fascicular block; LQTS, long QT syndrome; SVT, supraventricular tachycardia; VT, ventricular tachycardia.

delay, progression to higher degree block is unlikely, and pacing usually is not indicated. With type II, second-degree AV block within or below the His bundle, symptoms are frequent, prognosis is poor, and progression to third-degree AV block is common. Nonrandomized studies strongly suggest that pacing improves survival in patients with third-degree AVHB and symptoms.

   b. Bifascicular and trifascicular block. Syncope is common in patients with bifascicular block but usually not recurrent or associated with an increased incidence of sudden death. Bifascicular block with periodic third-degree AV block and syncope is associated with an increased incidence of sudden death. Prophylactic permanent pacing is indicated in this circumstance. Although third-degree AV block most often is preceded by bifascicular block, the rate of progression is slow (years). Further, there is no credible evidence for acute progression to third-degree AV block during anesthesia and surgery.

   c. AVHB after AMI. Pacing indications after AMI are mostly related to the presence of intraventricular conduction defects, not necessarily to symptoms. The requirement for temporary pacing with AMI by itself does not constitute an indication for permanent pacing. The long-term prognosis for survivors of AMI is related primarily to the extent of myocardial injury and nature of intraventricular conduction defects, rather than to AV block itself. With the exception of isolated left anterior fascicular block, AMI patients with intraventricular conduction disturbances have unfavorable short- and long-term prognoses, with increased risk of sudden death. This prognosis is not necessarily due to the development of high-grade AV block, although the incidence of such block is higher in these patients.

   d. Sinus node dysfunction. Sinus node dysfunction (SND) may manifest as sinus bradycardia, pause, or arrest, or sinoatrial block, with or without escape rhythms. It often occurs in association with paroxysmal supraventricular tachyarrhythmias (bradycardia–tachycardia syndrome). Patients with SND may have symptoms due to bradycardia, tachycardia, or both. Correlation of symptoms with arrhythmias is essential and is established by ambulatory monitoring. SND also presents as chronotropic incompetence (inability to increase rate appropriately). An adaptive-rate pacemaker may benefit these patients by restoring more physiologic heart rates. Although SND often is the primary indication for a pacemaker, pacing does not necessarily improve survival, but it may improve quality of life and reduce risk of subsequent atrial fibrillation and thromboembolic events.

   e. Hypersensitive carotid sinus syndrome or neurally mediated syndrome. Hypersensitive carotid sinus syndrome is syncope/presyncope due to an exaggerated response to carotid sinus stimulation. It is an uncommon cause of syncope. The relative contribution of cardioinhibitory (bradycardia, asystole, heart block) and vasodepressor components (vasodilation) must be determined before a pacemaker is prescribed. A hyperactive response is defined as asystole for longer than 3 seconds due to sinus arrest or heart block, an abrupt decrease in blood pressure, or both. With only an inordinate inhibitory response, pacing effectively relieves symptoms. However, with a mixed response, attention to both components is essential for effective therapy. Neurally mediated syndrome accounts for 10% to 40% of patients with syncope, usually a self-limited episode of bradycardia and hypotension. Vasovagal syncope is a common presentation, but the role of permanent pacing is controversial.

   f. Pacing in children and adolescents. Indications for pacing are similar in children and adults, but there are additional considerations. For example, what is the optimal rate for the patient's age? Further, what is optimal given ventricular dysfunction or altered circulatory physiology? Hence, pacing indications are based more on correlation of symptoms with bradycardia, rather than arbitrary rate criteria, and include the following:

   1. Bradycardia only after other causes (e.g., seizures, breath holding, apnea or neurally mediated mechanisms) are excluded

2. Symptomatic patients with congenital third-degree AVHB
3. Patients with persistent advanced second- or third-degree AVHB after cardiac surgery. However, for patients with residual bifascicular block and intermittent AVHB, the need is less certain.
4. Use along with β-blockers in patients with congenital long QT syndrome, especially with pause-dependent VTs.

   g. Miscellaneous pacing indications. A dual-chamber pacemaker with short AV delay reduces left ventricular outflow tract obstruction, alleviates symptoms in *obstructive hypertrophic cardiomyopathy,* and improves functional status. Also, there is functional improvement after institution of dual-chamber pacing with short AV delay with dilated cardiomyopathy. Multisite atrial and/or ventricular pacing to improve AV synchronization may provide even more benefit. *Bradyarrhythmias after cardiac transplantation* are mostly due to SND. Because of symptoms and delayed rehabilitation, some centers are more aggressive with pacing as treatment. However, half of patients show improvement by 1 year so that long-term pacing is unnecessary. Pacing can *terminate many tachyarrhythmias* and today is usually part of tiered ICD therapy. Finally, pacing and β-blockers may be *prophylaxis for tachyarrhythmias* (paroxysmal SVT, paroxysmal atrial fibrillation, and torsades de pointes with congenital long QT syndrome).

2. **Technology.** Contemporary single- and dual-chamber pacemakers are sophisticated devices, with multiple programmable features, including automatic mode-switching and programmable lead configuration [4,5]. In addition, ARP automatically adjusts the paced rate to meet changing metabolic needs in patients with chronotropic incompetence. Pacemakers are powered by lithium iodide batteries, with an expected service life of 5 to 12 years, depending on device capabilities, need for pacing, and programmed stimulus parameters. Most systems use transvenous leads. Lead configuration is programmable. With the unipolar configuration, the pacemaker housing (can) serves as anode (+) and the distal electrode of the bipolar pacing lead as cathode (–). With the bipolar configuration, proximal and distal lead electrodes serve as anode and cathode, respectively. The ability to program unipolar pacing is necessary if lead insulation or conductor failure occurs in a bipolar lead system. Also, it permits exploitation of either configuration while minimizing its disadvantages (e.g., oversensing with unipolar leads). A dual-chamber pacemaker with automatic mode-switching is optimal for patients with AVHB and susceptibility to paroxysmal atrial tachycardia. Algorithms detect fast, nonphysiologic atrial rates and automatically switch the pacing mode to one that excludes atrial tracking and the associated risk of upper rate ventricular pacing.

C. **External cardioversion–defibrillation.** External direct-current (DC) cardioversion differs from defibrillation only in that the former incorporates a time delay circuit for shock synchronization to the R or S waves of the surface ECG.
   1. **Indications.** Synchronized shocks are used for all tachyarrhythmias amenable to cardioversion, except ventricular fibrillation (VF) or VT when the QRS complex cannot be distinguished from T waves [7]. Automatic rhythm disturbances (e.g., accelerated AV junctional or idioventricular rhythms) are not amenable to DC cardioversion.
   2. **Technology.** Improvements in technology include availability of automated external defibrillators and increasing trend to use of biphasic shocks, which can lower shock current requirements for DC cardioversion and defibrillation.
   3. **Procedure.** *Cardioversion.* Synchronization with the largest R or S wave on the ECG will prevent triggering of VF. Resynchronization should be checked after each discharge. Improper synchronization may occur when there is bundle branch block with a tall R wave, when the T wave is highly peaked, and with pacing artifacts from a malfunctioning pacemaker (i.e., failure to capture). Electrodes are placed in either an anterolateral or an anteroposterior position. Current should pass though the heart's long axis, depolarize the bulk of myocardium, and minimize flow through high-impedance bony tissue. Electrode

paste or gel is used to reduce transthoracic impedance. Bridging of the electrodes by conductive paste or gel should be avoided, because this will reduce the amount of energy delivered to the heart. Energy titration (initially use only the lowest possible energies) reduces both energy use and complications. Initial settings of 5 to 10 J may be successful for atrial flutter or stable VT.

D. Internal cardioverter–defibrillator. Contemporary ICDs are multiprogrammable, are longer lived, use transvenous leads, and may incorporate *all* capabilities of a modern dual-chamber pacemaker [4,5]. Additionally, ICDs have multiple tachycardia detection zones, with programmable detection criteria and "tiered therapy" for each (antitachycardia pacing → cardioversion shocks → defibrillatory shocks if necessary). ICDs also store arrhythmia event records and treatment results. Early clinical experience with internal atrial (atrioverter) and dual-chamber cardioverter–defibrillators has been reported. Future devices will be tailored to meet all nonpharmacologic aspects of cardiac rhythm management for individual patients. Finally, ICDs have undergone significant downsizing (50 mL or smaller) and are suitable for pectoral implantation.

1. **Indications.** ICD are used for *secondary* or *primary prevention* of sudden death [6]. Whereas an atrial ICD (atrioverter) may be prescribed for patients with susceptibility to paroxysmal atrial tachyarrhythmias or a dual-chamber ICD for patients with susceptibility to atrial and ventricular tachyarrhythmias, there is no consensus as to indications for these latter devices at this time.

    a. **Secondary prevention.** ICDs are used for *secondary prevention* in patients with coronary artery disease and history of sudden death, or documented/inducible, sustained ventricular tachyarrhythmias. ICDs are widely accepted for improving outcomes in these patients. ICDs also are indicated for patients with the long QT syndrome and recurrent syncope, sustained ventricular arrhythmias, or sudden cardiac death despite drug therapy. ICD plus class IA drugs are prescribed for patients with idiopathic VF or the Brugada syndrome, or right bundle-branch block plus ST-segment elevation (leads V_1 to V_3) plus sudden death without confirmed heart disease. Other indications are (a) sudden death survivors with hypertrophic cardiomyopathy; (b) prophylaxis for syncope and sudden death with drug-refractory arrhythmogenic right ventricular dysplasia; and (c) children with malignant tachyarrhythmias or sudden death and congenital heart disease, cardiomyopathies, or primary electrical disease (e.g., long QT syndrome).

    b. **Primary prevention.** ICDs are used for *primary prevention* of sudden death in patients with asymptomatic coronary artery disease and nonsustained ventricular tachyarrhythmias. They also may be used after coronary artery bypass surgery in patients with severe left ventricular dysfunction (ejection fraction less than 35%) and an abnormal signal-averaged ECG, or in some patients awaiting heart transplantation.

2. **Technology.** The ICD pulse generator is a self-powered minicomputer with one or two (in series) 3.2-V Li-SVO (lithium–silver vanadium oxide) batteries to power the pulse generator, circuitry, and aluminum electrolytic storage capacitors [4,5]. A major challenge in ICD design is the large range of voltages within a very small package. Intracardiac signals may be as low as 100 μV, and therapeutic shocks approach 750 V. Further, because ICD batteries contain up to 20,000 J, a potential hazard exists if the charging and firing circuits were to electrically or thermally unload all this energy into the patient in a brief time period. The number of shocks delivered during treatment usually is limited to five or six per arrhythmia. The expected service life is 5 to 8 years.

III. Device function, malfunction, and interference

A. **Pacemakers.** A single-chamber pacemaker stimulates the atria or ventricles based on programmed timing intervals [4]. By sensing spontaneous atrial or ventricular depolarizations, it can be inhibited from delivering unnecessary or inappropriate stimuli. Dual-chamber devices time delivery of ventricular stimuli relative to sensed atrial depolarizations to maintain proper AV synchrony. Figure 16.2 illustrates how a pacemaker might be configured to pace in patients with SND or AVHB. In Figure 16.2 and throughout this chapter, the North American Society for Pacing

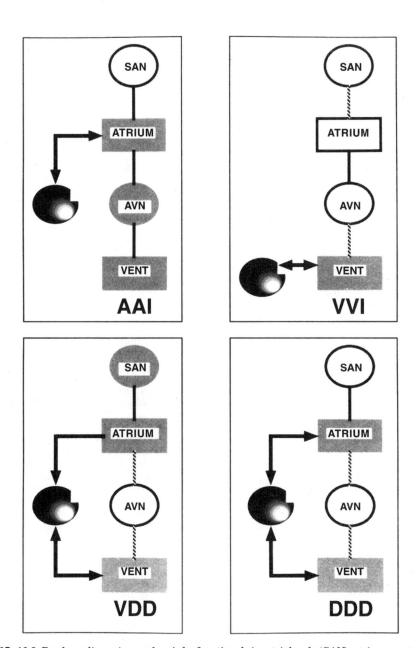

FIG. 16.2 Bradycardia pacing modes. A dysfunctional sinoatrial node (*SAN*), atrium, or atrioventricular node (*AVN*) is indicated by *open circles* or *rectangles*. Normal impulse transmission between these structures and the ventricles (*VENT*) is indicated by *solid lines,* with blocked or ineffective conduction indicated by *hashed lines.* An *arrow* pointing toward the pulse generator indicates sensing, whereas one pointing toward the atrium or ventricle indicates pacing in that chamber. **Top left:** AAI pacing for sinus arrest or bradycardia. There is a single atrial lead for both sensing and pacing. Atrial pacing occurs unless inhibited by a sensed spontaneous atrial depolarization. **Top right:** VVI pacing for AV heart block with atrial fibrillation. There is a single ventricular lead for both sensing and pacing. Ventricular pacing occurs unless inhibited by a sensed spontaneous ventricular depolarization. **Bottom left:** VDD pacing for atrioventricular (AV) heart block with normal SAN and atrial function. The atrial lead is for sensing only, and the ventricular lead is for both pacing and sensing. After a sensed atrial depolarization, the ventricle is paced after the programmed AV interval [i.e., atrial-triggered ventricular pacing (VAT)], unless first inhibited by a sensed ventricular depolarization (i.e., the VVI component of the VDD mode). **Bottom right:** Dual-chamber sequential or AV universal (*DDD*) pacing for sinus bradycardia with AV heart block. Both atrial and ventricular leads are for sensing and pacing. This mode incorporates all of the preceding pacing capabilities (*AAI, VVI,* and *VAT*).

and Electrophysiology–British Pacing and Electrophysiology Group (NASPE/BPEG) pacemaker code (also known as the NBG code) is used as a shorthand to describe pacing modes (Table 16.3).

1. **Function.** Today, most U.S. pacemakers are conventional or adaptive-rate, dual-chamber (DDD or DDDR) devices. However, with normal conduction and sinus node function, they may operate as a single-chamber device in the AAI (AAIR) or VVI (VVIR) modes (Fig. 16.2).

   a. **Single-chamber pacemaker.** These devices have a single timing interval, the atrial or ventricular escape interval, between successive stimuli in the absence of sensed depolarization. In the AAI or VVI mode (Fig. 16.3), pacing occurs at the end of the programmed atrial or ventricular escape interval unless a spontaneous atrial or ventricular depolarization is sensed first, resetting these intervals. If the device has rate hysteresis as a programmable option, then the atrial or ventricular escape interval after a sensed depolarization is programmed longer than that after a paced depolarization to encourage emergence of intrinsic rhythm and prolong battery life.

   b. **Dual-chamber pacemaker.** A DDD ("AV universal") pacemaker can pace and sense in both the atrium and the ventricle. It has two basic timing intervals whose sum is the pacing cycle duration (Fig. 16.4). The first is the AV interval, which is the programmed interval from a paced or sensed atrial depolarization to ensuing ventricular stimulation. Some devices offer the option of programmable AV interval hysteresis. If so, the AV interval after paced atrial depolarization is longer than that after sensed depolarization to maintain greater uniformity between atrial and ventricular depolarizations. The second interval is the VA interval, the interval between sensed or paced ventricular depolarization and the next atrial stimulus. During atrial and ventricular refractory periods (Fig. 16.4), sensed events do not reset the device escape timing. During the ventricular channel blanking period (Fig. 16.4), ventricular sensing is disabled to avoid overloading of the ventricular sense amplifier by voltage generated by the atrial stimulus, thereby inappropriately resetting the VA interval. Sensing during the alert periods outside the ventricular blanking and postventricular atrial and ventricular refractory periods initiates new AV or VA intervals (Fig. 16.4). Operationally, depending on sensing patterns, a DDD pacemaker can provide atrial, ventricular, dual-chamber sequential, or no pacing (Fig. 16.4).

Table 16.3 NASPE/BPEG (NBG) pacemaker code used as shorthand to designate pacing modes

I Chamber paced	II Chamber sensed	III Response to sensed event	IV Programmability/ rate response[b]	V Antitachycardia functions[c]
O = none	O = none	O = none	O = none	O = none
A = atrium	A = atrium	I = inhibit	R = adaptive rate	P = ATP
V = ventricle	V = ventricle	T = triggered		S = shock
D = dual		D = dual		D = dual
(A & V)	D = dual (A & V)	(I & T)		(P + S)
S = single[a]	S (single)[a]			

[a] Single-chamber device that paces either the atrium or ventricle.
[b] In current terminology, only the adaptive rate response (R) is indicated by the fourth position. All current pacemakers have full programming and communicating capability; therefore, the letters P (programmable), M (multiprogrammable), and C (communicating) are no longer used.
[c] Implantable cardioverter–defibrillator with antibradycardia and antitachycardia pacing capabilities. ATP, antitachycardia pacing.

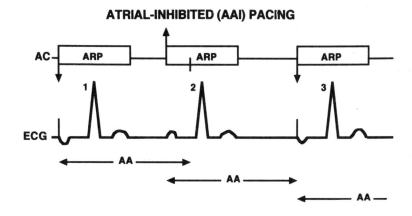

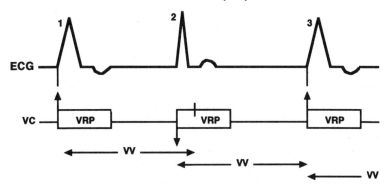

FIG. 16.3 Top: AAI pacing, as for a patient with sinus bradycardia and intact atrioventricular *(AV)* conduction. The atrium is paced (beats *1* and *3*)—*arrow* pointing toward the electrocardiogram *(ECG)* in the atrial channel *(AC)* timing diagram—unless inhibited by sensed spontaneous atrial depolarization (beat *2*)—*arrow* pointing away from the ECG in the AC timing diagram. The atrial refractory period *(ARP)* prevents R and T waves from being sensed by the AC and inappropriately resetting the atrial escape timing *(AA* interval). Note that spontaneous atrial depolarization (beat *2*) occurs before the AA interval times out, resetting the AA interval. The *short vertical line* in the AC timing diagram above beat 2 shows where the stimulus would have occurred had the previous AA interval timed out. In the absence of subsequent spontaneous atrial depolarization (beat *3*), the AA interval times out with delivery of a stimulus. **Bottom:** VVI pacing, as for a patient with atrial fibrillation and AV heart block. Beats 1 and 3 are paced, and beat 2 is spontaneous. The latter resets the ventricular escape interval *(VV)*, which otherwise would have timed out with delivery of a stimulus, indicated by the *short vertical line* in the ventricular channel *(VC)* timing diagram above beat 2. The new VV interval times out with stimulus delivery (beat *3*), because there is no sensed ventricular depolarization to reset the timing. *VRP,* ventricular refractory period.

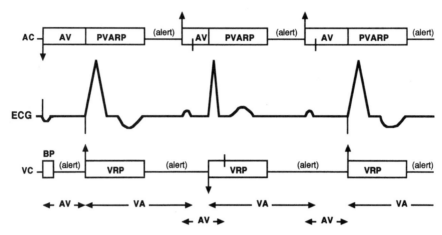

FIG. 16.4 Atrioventricular (*AV*) universal (*DDD*) pacing, as for a patient with sinus node dysfunction and AV heart block. The atrium is paced (beat *1*)—*arrow* pointing toward the electrocardiogram (*ECG*) in the atrial channel (*AC*) timing diagram above beat 1—unless inhibited by sensed atrial depolarization (beats *2* and *3*)—*arrows* pointing away from the ECG in the AC timing diagram. The AC is refractory during the AV interval and from delivery of the ventricular stimulus until the end of the postventricular atrial refractory period (*PVARP*). This prevents atrial sensing from resetting the escape timing (i.e., AV interval). The ventricular channel (*VC*) blanking period (*BP*) prevents sensing of the atrial pacing stimulus, thereby resetting the AV interval and delaying ventricular stimulus delivery. However, sensed ventricular depolarization or noise (e.g., electrocautery) in the alert period (*VC*) after the blanking period also could inhibit ventricular stimulation. As shown, this does not occur, so the AV interval times out with delivery of a ventricular stimulus. The ventricular refractory period (*VRP*) prevents sensed T waves from inappropriately resetting the VA interval. However, sensing during the alert periods after the PVARP or VRP will reset basic timing, initiating new AV and VA intervals, respectively. Because the first beat is fully paced, it is an example of asynchronous AV sequential pacing (i.e., DOO). With the second beat, a sensed spontaneous atrial depolarization initiates a new AV interval, inhibiting the atrial stimulus that would have occurred, indicated by the *short vertical line* in the AC timing diagram. Subsequently, there is spontaneous ventricular depolarization before the AV interval times out. The ventricular stimulus that otherwise would have occurred at the end of the AV interval is indicated by the *short vertical line* in the VC timing diagram below beat 2. The third beat begins with a sensed atrial depolarization. As with the beat 2, this also occurs before the VA interval times out. In the absence of sensed ventricular depolarization (beat 3), the new AV interval times out with ventricular stimulus delivery. Beat 3 is an example of atrial-inhibited, ventricular-triggered pacing (i.e., VDD).

      c. Adaptive-rate pacing. A 1996 U.S. survey indicated that ARP was a programmable feature in 83% of all implanted devices. In patients with chronotropic incompetence, ARP has been shown to improve exercise capacity and quality of life. Activity-based sensors are used most commonly. These are piezoelectric crystals that sense vibration (up-and-down motion) or acceleration (forward-backward movement). However, they do not provide feedback proportional to physiologic need. Better is the QT interval, but this is affected by changes in rate and catecholamines. Therefore, a QT-sensing device measures the stimulus to T wave interval during ventricular pacing. Minute ventilation sensors measure changes in transthoracic impedance with respiration (i.e., increase with inspiration and decrease with expiration) and provide an estimate of metabolic need that is more proportional to exercise. However, they increase current drain on the device. Other sensors in use or under development measure O_2 saturation, pH, stroke volume, or temperature. Finally, because ARP sensors may have a disproportionate response time at the beginning of exercise versus steady-state exercise, a dual-sensor ARP device may provide a more proportional response. Obviously, such complexity increases the potential for device malfunction in the perioperative setting.

2. **Malfunction.** Primary pacemaker malfunction is rare (less than 2% of all device-related problems) [5]. Pacing malfunction can occur with ICDs, because all ICDs today can pace at least the ventricle. Some devices have programmed behavior that simulates malfunction, termed pseudomalfunction. For example, failure to pace may be misdiagnosed with programmed rate hysteresis. Also, apparent device malfunction in response to electromagnetic interference (EMI) may be normal device operation (see later). Pacemaker malfunction is classified as failure to pace, failure to capture, pacing at abnormal rates, failure to sense, oversensing, and malfunction unique to dual-chamber devices (Table 16.4). Among the causes for failure to capture are drugs or conditions that affect pacing thresholds (Table 16.5). To diagnose malfunction, it is necessary to obtain a 12-lead ECG and chest x-ray film and to interrogate the device for pacing and sensing thresholds, lead impedances, battery voltage, and magnet rate. Malfunctions unique to dual-chamber devices are crosstalk inhibition and pacemaker-mediated tachycardia (PMT).

a. **Crosstalk inhibition.** Crosstalk is the unexpected appearance in the atrial or ventricular sense channel or circuit of electrical signals present in the other sense channel or circuit. For example, polarization potentials after atrial stimulus delivery may be sensed in the ventricular channel during unipolar atrial pacing. If interpreted as spontaneous ventricular events, they can inhibit ventricular output. Such crosstalk inhibition is prevented by increasing the ventricular sensing threshold, decreasing atrial output, or programming a longer ventricular blanking period (Fig. 16.4), so long as these provide adequate safety margins for atrial capture and ventricular sensing. If crosstalk cannot be prevented, many dual-chamber devices have a feature referred to as nonphysiologic AV delay or ventricular safety pacing. Whenever the ventricular channel senses anything early during the AV interval, a ventricular stimulus is triggered after an abbreviated AV interval. This either will depolarize ventricular myocardium or will fail to do so if myocardium is refractory due to spontaneous depolarization. The premature timing of the triggered ventricular stimulus prevents it from occurring during the vulnerable period of the T wave.

b. **Pacemaker-mediated tachycardia.** PMT is undesired rapid pacing caused by the device or its interaction with the patient. PMT includes runaway pacemaker; sensor-driven tachycardia; tachycardia during magnetic resonance imaging (MRI) or due to tracking myopotentials or atrial tachyarrhythmias; and pacemaker reentrant tachycardia (PRT). *Sensor-driven tachycardia* may occur with adaptive-rate devices that sense vibration, impedance changes, or the QT interval if they sense mechanical or physiologic interference to cause inappropriate high-rate pacing. Thus, it is advised that ARP be disabled in perioperative settings. ***Magnetic resonance imaging.*** Powerful forces exist in the MRI suite, including static and gradient magnetic fields, and RF fields. The static magnetic field may exert a torque effect on the pulse generator or close the magnetic reed switch to cause asynchronous pacing. The gradient magnetic field may induce voltage large enough to inhibit a demand pacemaker but is unlikely to cause pacing. The RF field may generate enough current in the leads to cause pacing at the frequency of the pulsed energy (60 to 300 beats/min). *Tachycardia due to myopotential tracking* occurs when the atrial channel of a unipolar, dual-chamber device programmed to VAT, VDD, or DDD modes senses myopotentials from muscle beneath the pulse generator, with triggered ventricular pacing up to the maximum atrial tracking rate. Tachycardia due to *tracking **atrial tachyarrhythmias*** has a similar explanation. Medication to suppress the

Table 16.4 Categories of pacemaker malfunction, ECG appearance, and likely cause for malfunction

Category of malfunction	ECG appearance	Cause for malfunction
Failure to pace	For one or both chambers, either no pacing artifacts will be present on the ECG, or artifacts will be present for one but not the other chamber	Oversensing; battery failure; open circuit due to mechanical problems with leads or system component malfunction; fibrosis at electrode–tissue interface; lead dislodgment; recording artifact
Failure to capture	Atrial and/or ventricular pacing stimuli are present, with persistent or intermittent failure to capture	Fibrosis at electrode–tissue interface; drugs or conditions that increase pacing thresholds (Table 16.5)
Pacing at abnormal rates	1. Rapid pacing rate (upper rate behavior) 2. Slow pacing rate (below lower rate interval) 3. No stimulus artifact; intrinsic rate below lower rate interval	1. Adaptive rate pacing; tracking atrial tachycardia; pacemaker-mediated tachycardia; oversensing 2. Programmed rate hysteresis, or rest or sleep rates; oversensing 3. Power source failure; lead disruption; oversensing
Failure to sense	Pacing artifacts in middle of normal P waves or QRS complexes	Inadequate intracardiac signal strength; component malfunction; battery depletion; misinterpretation of normal device function
Oversensing	Abnormal pacing rates with pauses (regular or random)	Far-field sensing with inappropriate device inhibition or triggering; intermittent contact between pacing system conducting elements
Malfunction unique to dual-chamber devices	Rapid pacing rate (i.e., upper rate behavior)	Cross-talk inhibition; pacemaker-mediated tachycardia (see text)

arrhythmia (often atrial fibrillation) or cardioversion may be necessary. Placing a magnet over the pulse generator to disable sensing in most instances (see response to magnet, later) will terminate high-rate atrial tracking. Newer dual-chamber devices with automatic mode-switching detect fast, nonphysiologic atrial tachycardia and automatically switch the device to a nontracking mode. Finally, ***pacemaker-reentrant tachycardia*** can occur in a device programmed to an atrial tracking mode. Up to 50% of patients with dual-chamber devices are susceptible to PRT because they have retrograde (VA) conduction via the AVN or an accessory AV pathway. PRT occurs when spontaneous or paced ventricular beats are conducted back to the atria to trigger ventricular pacing. To prevent PRT, a longer post postventricular atrial refractory period is programmed (Fig. 16.4). Also, placing a magnet over the pulse generator will terminate PRT in most devices by disabling sensing. However, PRT may recur after the magnet is removed.

Table 16.5 Drugs and conditions that affect or have no proven effect on pacing thresholds

Effect	Drugs	Conditions
Increase pacing threshold	Bretylium, encainide, flecainide, moricizine, propafenone, sotalol	Myocardial ischemia and infarction; progression of cardiomyopathy; hyperkalemia; severe acidosis or alkalosis; hypoxemia; hypothermia; irradiation; after cardioversion or defibrillation (implantable cardioverter–defibrillator or external)
Possibly increase pacing threshold	β-Blockers, lidocaine, procainamide, quinidine, verapamil	Myxedema; hyperglycemia
Possibly decrease pacing threshold	Atropine, catecholamines, glucocorticoids	Pheochromocytoma; hyperthyroid or other hypermetabolic states
No proven effect on pacing threshold	Amiodarone; anesthetic drugs, both inhalation and intravenous	Hyperthermia

3. **Response of pacemaker to magnet application.** Most devices respond to magnet application by a device-specific single- or dual-chamber asynchronous pacing mode. For example, Thera DR or D devices (Medtronic, Minneapolis, MN, USA) pace SOO or DOO at 85 beats/min. However, with impending power source depletion, the magnet rate may differ because it becomes the end-of-life or elective replacement indicator (Table 16.6). The end-of-life or elective replacement indicator rate is characteristic for specific devices (e.g., VOO at 65 beats/min for the Thera DR and D devices). Furthermore, the first few paced beats after magnet application may occur at a rate or output other than that seen later, providing device identification data on the strip-chart ECG recording, as well as information regarding integrity of the pulse generator and leads. In a patient whose intrinsic rhythm inhibits the device, magnet application may serve to identify the programmed mode when the correct programmer is not available for telemetry. Also, with device malfunction due to malsensing, magnet-initiated asynchronous pacing may temporarily correct the problem, confirming the presence of far-field sensing, crosstalk inhibition, T-wave sensing, or PMT. Finally, in pacemaker-dependent patients, magnet application may ensure pacing if EMI inhibits output (e.g., surgical electrocautery). However, if the device has reverted to an asynchronous interference mode (see later), the magnet response may not be the same as when the device is not in the interference mode.

Table 16.6 Elective replacement indicators that may affect the nominal rate of pacing

- **Stepwise change in pacing rate:** pacing rate changes to some predetermined fixed rate or some percentage decrease from the programmed rate
- **Stepwise change in magnet rate:** magnet-pacing rate decreases in a stepwise fashion related to the remaining battery life
- **Pacing mode change:** DDD and DDDR pulse generators may automatically revert to another mode, such as VVI or VOO, to reduce current drain and extend battery life

4. Interference. Pacemakers and ICD are subject to interference from non-biologic electromagnetic sources. In general, devices in service today are effectively shielded against EMI. Increasing use of bipolar sensing has further reduced the problem. EMI frequencies above 10^9 Hz (i.e., infrared, visible light, ultraviolet, x-rays, and gamma rays) do not interfere with pacemakers or ICDs, because the wavelengths are much shorter than the device or lead dimensions. High-intensity therapeutic x-rays and irradiation can directly damage circuitry. EMI enters a device by conduction (direct contact) or radiation (leads acting as an antenna). Devices are protected from EMI by (a) shielding the circuitry, (b) using a bipolar versus unipolar lead configuration for sensing to minimize the antenna, and (c) filtering incoming signals to exclude noncardiac signals. If EMI does enter the pulse generator, noise protection algorithms in the timing circuit help reduce its effect on the patient. However, EMI signals between 5 and 100 Hz are not filtered, because these overlap the frequency range of intracardiac signals. Therefore, EMI in this frequency range may be interpreted as intracardiac signals, giving rise to abnormal behavior. Possible responses include (a) inappropriate inhibition or triggering of stimulation, (b) asynchronous pacing (Fig. 16.5), (c) mode resetting, (d) direct damage to the pulse generator circuitry, and (e) triggering of unnecessary ICD shocks (Table 16.7). Finally, with EMI and inappropriate device behavior, it is widely assumed that placing a magnet over a pulse generator invariably will cause asynchronous pacing as long as the magnet remains in place. Not so. Whereas some devices will pace asynchronously as long as the magnet remains in place, others will cease pacing after a programmed number of intervals. In some devices, the magnet response may be programmed off. In others a variety of magnet responses may have been programmed, some of which do not provide immunity to EMI sensing. Thus, if possible, one should determine before EMI exposure what pulse generator is present and what must be done to provide protection. If this is not possible, then one must observe the magnet response during EMI to ascertain whether there is protection from EMI sensing. If, for example, electrocautery EMI causes inappropriate inhibition or triggering of output in a pacemaker-dependent patient, then it must be limited to short bursts.

B. **Internal cardioverter–defibrillator.** An ICD consists of a pulse generator and leads for tachyarrhythmia detection and therapy [4]. Modern ICDs use transvenous lead systems for sensing, pacing, and biphasic shock delivery. Epicardial leads are still used in infants and small children. Use of biphasic compared to monophasic shocks greatly lowers defibrillation energy requirements and was critical to development of smaller ICDs suitable for pectoral implantation.

1. **Sensing ventricular depolarizations.** Reliable sensing is essential. The sense amplifier must respond quickly and accurately to rates of 30 to 360 beats/min or greater, and to the varying amplitude and morphology of intracardiac signals during VT or VF. Unfiltered intracardiac electrograms are sent to the sense amplifier. This has a band-pass filter to reject low-frequency T waves and high-frequency noise, automatic gain control (auto-gain), a rectifier to eliminate polarity dependency, and a fixed or auto-adjusting threshold event detector. The sense amplifier produces a set of R-R intervals for the VT/VF detection algorithms to use.

2. **Ventricular fibrillation detection.** ICDs use rate criteria as the sole method for detecting VF. Due to the circumstances of VF, the detection algorithms must have high sensitivity and low specificity. If criteria for detection are too aggressive, the ICD likely will oversense T waves during sinus rhythm, leading to spurious shocks. If too conservative, it likely will undersense some VF but work very well during sinus rhythm. An ICD X/Y detector triggers when X of the previous Y sensed ventricular intervals are shorter than the VF detection interval. Typically, this is 70% to 80% of intervals in a sliding window of 10 to 24. This approach is very good at ignoring the effect of a small number of undersensed events due to the small amplitude of VF intracardiac signals. Any tachycardia with a cycle length less than the VF detection interval will

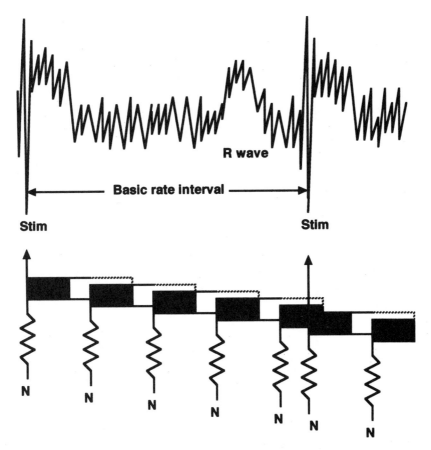

FIG. 16.5 VVI pacemaker to continuous electromagnetic interference (EMI). Temporary asynchronous pacing stimulation (*Stim*) occurs at the programmed basic rate interval. The ventricular refractory period (*rectangles*) begins with the noise (N) sampling period (*black rectangle*), during which time there is no sensing. During the remainder of this refractory period, repeated noise (N) sensing above a specified minimal frequency (e.g., 7 Hz) is interpreted as EMI. This restarts the ventricular refractory period. Portions of the previous refractory period preempted by the newly initiated ventricular refractory period are indicated by *hashed rectangles*. Therefore, so long as interference persists, the pacemaker remains refractory and escape timing is determined entirely by the programmed basic rate interval. In this example, the second paced R wave falls in the noise sampling period. It is not sensed, but it initiates a new ventricular refractory period. The spontaneous R wave is not sensed and does not affect escape timing.

initiate VF therapy. After capacitor charging but before shock delivery, an algorithm confirms the presence of VF. After shock delivery, redetection and episode-termination algorithms determine whether VF has terminated, continued, or changed.
3. **Tachycardia detection and discrimination (single-chamber ICD).** Most VT algorithms require a programmable number of consecutive R-R intervals shorter than the VT detection interval. A longer R-R interval, as might occur

Table 16.7 Perioperative EMI sources and their potential effects on implanted pacemakers or implantable cardioverter–defibrillators

EMI source	Generator damage	Complete inhibition	One-beat inhibition	Asynchronous pacing	Rate increase	Spurious shocks
Electrocautery	Yes	Yes	Yes	Yes	Yes[a,b]	Yes
External DC/DF	Yes	No	No	Yes	Yes	No
Magnetic resonance imaging scanner	Possible	No	Yes	Yes	Yes	Yes
Lithotripsy	Yes[b]	Yes[c]	Yes[c]	Yes[c]	Yes[d]	Yes
Radiofrequency ablation	Yes	Yes	No	No	Yes	Yes
Electroconvulsive therapy	No	Yes	Yes	Yes	Yes[b]	Yes
Transcutaneous electrical nerve stimulation	No	Yes	No	Yes	Yes	Unlikely
Radiation therapy	Yes	No	No	No	Yes	Yes
Diagnostic radiation	No	No	No	No	Yes	No

[a] Impedance-based adaptive-rate (AR) pulse generators.
[b] Piezoelectric crystal-based AR pulse generators.
[c] Remote potential for interference.
[d] DDD mode only.
DC/DF, direct-current cardioversion or defibrillation; EMI, electromagnetic interference.

during atrial fibrillation, would reset the VT counters. In patients with both supraventricular and ventricular tachyarrhythmias, up to 45% of ICD discharges may be inappropriate if rate is used as the sole criterion for VT therapy. To increase specificity, VT detection algorithm enhancements are programmed for one or more VT zones in single-chamber ICDs, including criteria for stability of rate, suddenness of onset, and intracardiac QRS morphology. The *rate stability criterion* is used to distinguish sustained monomorphic VT with little cycle length variation from atrial fibrillation with much greater cycle length variation. Such enhancement criteria are not available in the VF zone, where maximum sensitivity is required. Also, they are programmed only in rate zones that correspond to VT hemodynamically tolerated by the patient. The *suddenness of onset criterion* is used to distinguish sinus tachycardia from VT, because VT has a more sudden rate increase. Finally, *morphology algorithms* discriminate VT from SVT based on morphology of intracardiac electrograms.

4. **Tachycardia detection and discrimination (dual-chamber ICD).** Inadequate specificity of VT detection algorithms, despite enhancements, has been a significant problem with single-chamber ICDs. Dual-chamber ICDs use an atrial lead, which is used for bradycardia pacing and sensing for tachycardia discrimination. Detection algorithms use atrial and ventricular timing data to discriminate SVT from VT. For example, the algorithm in devices of one manufacturer has several key elements: (a) the pattern of atrial and ventricular events; (b) atrial and ventricular rates; (c) regularity of R-R intervals; (d) presence or absence of AV dissociation; and (e) atrial and ventricular pattern analysis.

5. **Tiered therapy.** Treatment options for VT include antitachycardia pacing, cardioversion, or defibrillation. Up to 90% of monomorphic VTs can be terminated by a critical pacing sequence, reducing the need for painful shocks and conserving battery life. With antitachycardia pacing, trains of stimuli are delivered at a fixed percentage of the VT cycle length. Repeated and more aggressive trains result either in termination of VT or progression to cardioversion or defibrillation.

6. **ICD malfunction.** Malfunctions specific to ICD include inappropriate shock delivery, failure to deliver therapy, ineffective shocks, and interactions with drugs or devices affecting the efficacy of therapy. There is potential for pacing malfunction as well (see earlier) [5].

   a. **Inappropriate delivery of shocks.** Artifacts consequent to lead-related malfunction may be interpreted as tachycardia, with inappropriate shock delivery. Electrocautery artifact may be similarly misinterpreted. Rapid SVT or nonsustained VT may be misdiagnosed as sustained VT or VF, especially if rate-only criteria are used for diagnosis. R- and T-wave oversensing during bradycardia pacing has led to inappropriate shocks.

   b. **Failure to deliver therapy or ineffective shocks.** Especially after repeated shocks for VF, tachyarrhythmias may be undersensed with failure to deliver therapy. Exposure to diagnostic x-rays or computed tomographic scans does not adversely affect shock delivery. AMI, severe acute acid–base or electrolyte imbalance, or hypoxia may increase defibrillation thresholds, leading to ineffective shocks. Any of these also could affect the rate or morphology of VT and the ability to diagnose VT. Finally, isoflurane and propofol do not affect defibrillation thresholds. The effect of other anesthetics or drugs used to supplement anesthesia is unknown.

   c. **Drug–device interactions affecting efficacy of ICD therapy.** Antiarrhythmic drugs are used along with ICD to suppress (a) recurring sustained VT and the need for shocks; (b) nonsustained VT that triggers unnecessary shocks; and (c) atrial fibrillation with inappropriate shocks. Also, they may be used to slow VT to make it better tolerated or more amenable to termination by antitachycardia pacing and to slow AV nodal conduction with atrial fibrillation. Possible adverse effects of combined drug and ICD therapy are (a) slowing of VT to below the programmed rate-detection threshold; (b) proarrhythmia, increasing the need for shocks;

(c) increased defibrillation thresholds; (d) reduced hemodynamic tolerance of VT; (e) increase in PR, QRS, or QT intervals, causing multiple counting and spurious shocks; and (f) altered morphology or reduced amplitude of intracardiac electrograms and failure to detect VT/VF. Lidocaine, chronic amiodarone, class IC drugs (e.g., flecainide), and phenytoin increase defibrillation thresholds. Class IA drugs (e.g., quinidine) and bretylium do not affect defibrillation thresholds.

   d. **Device–device interactions affecting efficacy of therapy.** In the past, pacemakers were used for bradycardia and antitachycardia pacing in ICD patients. Today, ICD incorporate both pacing capabilities, but there still may be occasional patients with an ICD and a pacemaker. Possible adverse interactions between the two devices include (a) sensed pacing artifacts or depolarizations may lead to multiple counting, misdiagnosis as VT/VF, and spurious shocks; and (b) ICD shocks may reprogram a pacemaker or cause failure to capture or undersensing.

   7. **Response of an ICD to magnet application.** Depending on the manufacturer and model of the ICD and how it is programmed (e.g., magnet switch inactivated), tachycardia sensing and delivery of therapy *may be* inactivated during exposure to a magnet. However, except for CPI devices (Cardiac Pacemakers Inc., St. Paul, MN, USA), sensing is inhibited only while the magnet is directly over the pulse generator. With CPI devices, magnet application for less than 30 seconds temporarily disables sensing, whereas application for longer than 30 seconds requires magnet reapplication for longer than 30 seconds to reactivate sensing.

   8. **Interference and ICD.** Reports of inappropriate ICD shocks due to EMI oversensing are infrequent. EMI initially might be misinterpreted as VF, but spurious shocks will not occur unless it continues beyond the capacitor charging period (see Section **III.A.4** and Table 16.7).

IV. Perioperative considerations for the patient with a pacemaker or ICD device [5]

   A. **Preoperative patient evaluation.** Patients with pacemakers or ICDs, especially the latter, often have serious cardiac functional impairment. Many have debilitating coexisting systemic disease as well. Special attention is paid to progression of disease and functional status, current medications, and compliance with treatment. No special testing is required because the patient has an implanted device. However, results of a recent 12-lead ECG and laboratory testing (i.e., electrolyte status) should be available.

   B. **Device identification and evaluation.** Unless the planned surgery is truly emergent or poses little risk of EMI-related device malfunction (e.g., bipolar cautery will be used; the surgical field is far removed from the device, leads and grounding plate), it is imperative to (a) identify the device, (b) determine the date and indication(s) for its implantation, and (c) to check its function. Most surgical facilities today have an onsite pacemaker/ICD clinic or service (or access to one) that should be consulted to provide this service. If not, the next best strategy is to identify the device and contact the manufacturer for advice (Table 16.8). All patients should carry a card that identifies the model and serial numbers of the device, the date of implantation, and the implanting physician or clinic. If not, an x-ray film of the pulse generator area *may* reveal a unique radiopaque code ("signature") that identifies the manufacturer and model of the device. These are listed in generic reference guides available from the manufacturers (Table 16.8). Finally, if the surgery is truly *emergent* and it is not possible to identify the device, the basic function of most suppressed pacemakers is confirmed by placing a magnet over the pulse generator to cause asynchronous pacing, provided the magnet function has not been programmed off. Cholinergic stimulation (e.g., Valsalva maneuver, carotid sinus massage, adenosine, or edrophonium) might be considered to slow the intrinsic rate sufficiently for release of pacing stimuli.

   C. **Device management.** For pacemaker-dependent patients, if EMI is likely to cause device malfunction (e.g., unipolar cautery in the vicinity of the pulse generator or leads), the device should be programmed to an asynchronous mode. For

Table 16.8 North American manufacturers of pacemakers and implantable cardioverter–defibrillators

Biotronik, Inc. 6024 Jean Road Lake Oswego, OR 97035-5369 1-800-547-9001 (24-hour hotline) 1-503-635-9936 (fax) *www.biotronik.com*	Medtronic Corporation 7000 Central Avenue NE Minneapolis, MN 55432 1-800-328-2518 (24-hour hotline) 1-800-824-2362 (fax) *www.medtronic.com*
Guidant Corporation CRM (CPI, Intermedics)[a] 4100 Hamline Avenue North St. Paul, MN 55112-5798 (CPI, Intermedics) 1-800-227-3422 (24-hour hotline) 1-800-582-4166 (fax) *www.guidant.com*	St. Jude Medical[a] Cardiac Rhythm Management Division (Pacesetter, Ventritex)[a] 15900 Valley View Court Sylmar, CA 91342 1-800-777-2237 (24-hour hotline) 1-800-756-7223 (fax) *www.sjm.com*

[a] Recently acquired or merged companies by parent company.

patients with adaptive-rate pacemakers (including some ICDs), this capability should be programmed off if EMI might cause malfunction (Table 16.7). Magnet-activated testing and tachycardia sensing (ICD) should be programmed off. If an ICD patient is pacemaker dependent, an asynchronous pacing mode should be programmed if EMI might cause undesired function. After the procedure, device function must be tested, with reprogramming or replacement if necessary.

D. **Precautions: surgery unrelated to device.** The chief concern is to reduce risk of hemodynamic instability due to inappropriate inhibition or triggering of output (pacing stimuli or shocks), or upper rate pacing behavior (adaptive-rate devices). If EMI is likely to cause device malfunction and the patient does not have an adequate intrinsic rhythm, a pacemaker should be programmed to an asynchronous mode and tachycardia sensing disabled for ICD. If the device features ARP, this should be programmed off. If ICD sensing is disabled, an external cardioverter–defibrillator must be available.

1. **Surgical electrocautery.** Locating the grounding plate as far as possible from the cautery tool reduces EMI from unipolar cautery. The pulse generator and leads should not be between the Bovie tool and grounding plate (i.e., in the current pathway). Pacing function is confirmed by monitoring heart sounds or the pulse waveform. Only the lowest possible energies and brief bursts of electrocautery should be used, especially with instability due to device malfunction. If cautery must be used in the vicinity (less than 15 cm) of the pulse generator or leads and there is significant hemodynamic instability due to EMI, then it is reasonable to place a magnet directly over the pulse generator of a pacemaker. This will cause most devices to pace asynchronously until the magnet is removed, unless the magnet mode has been programmed off. With an ICD, without knowing what device it is, how it is programmed, or what the magnet response is, a magnet should *not* be placed over an ICD pulse generator unless EMI is unavoidable and it triggers antitachycardia pacing or repeated shocks that destabilize the patient.

2. **External cardioversion or defibrillation.** Shocks probably will cause at least temporary inhibition. Transient loss of capture or sensing should be anticipated, and the stimulus amplitude may need to be increased. This is done automatically by the ICD, with a backup bradycardia pacing capability, in almost all ICDs in service today. Pulse generator damage is related to the distance of the external paddles from the pulse generator. All device manufacturers recommend the anteroposterior paddle configuration, with the paddles located at least 10 cm from the pulse generator. Further, it is advised that the lowest possible energies be used for cardioversion or defibrillation. After

cardioversion or defibrillation, the device must be interrogated to assure proper function. Reprogramming and/or lead replacement may be necessary.

E. Management for system implantation or revision. Except in infants and small children, in whom epicardial leads are widely used, most pacemaker and ICD systems use transvenous leads. The pulse generator and leads often are implanted using local anesthesia and sedation. A thoracotomy and general anesthesia are needed for epicardial lead placement. General anesthesia or monitored anesthesia care with heavy sedation may be requested for ICD system implantation or revision in adults, especially if the procedure involves repeated induction of tachyarrhythmias and shocks. With regard to management, for procedures requiring general anesthesia or monitored anesthesia care, consider the following. (a) Most patients with symptomatic bradycardia will have temporary pacing. Otherwise, chronotropic drugs with backup external pacing should be available. (b) Reliable pulse waveform monitoring is necessary. Some centers require direct arterial blood pressure monitoring. (c) Select the best surface ECG leads for P waves and ischemia diagnosis. (d) Pulmonary artery catheters, formerly advised, are seldom used today because of the widespread use of nonthoracotomy lead systems and smaller pulse generators. They also interfere with ICD lead positioning. (e) Contemporary inhalation and intravenous anesthetics are not known to increase defibrillation thresholds and are selected more with a view to hemodynamic tolerance. Inhalation agents and propofol may affect the morphology of sensed intracardiac electrograms and inducibility of tachyarrhythmias, which is a consideration during EP testing. Contemporary inhalation anesthetics (sevoflurane, desflurane) and small amounts of lidocaine for vascular access are not known to affect defibrillation thresholds. Older agents and larger amounts of lidocaine or bupivacaine for field blocks may do so. (f) An external cardioverter–defibrillator must be available and functioning. (g) With an ICD, tachycardia sensing should be disabled when unipolar electrocautery is used.

V. Catheter or surgical modification of arrhythmia substrates [8–13]. RF catheter ablation has replaced antiarrhythmic drug therapy for treatment of many types of chronic or recurring cardiac tachyarrhythmias. Tachyarrhythmias amenable to this form of treatment include those shown at EP study to have a focal origin (triggered or automatic) or are sustained by fixed, defined reentry circuits. Surgical ablation may be performed for these same arrhythmias if catheter ablation has failed or is not feasible. Additionally, a catheter or surgical maze procedure may be used to interrupt multiple reentry circuits with atrial fibrillation.

A. Radiofrequency catheter ablation. RF catheter ablation procedures are performed in an EP laboratory using conscious sedation. Usually, both tachyarrhythmia diagnosis and RF ablation can be performed in a single session. Three or four electrode catheters are inserted percutaneously into the femoral, internal jugular, or subclavian vein, or via a retrograde aortic or transseptal approach, and positioned within the heart to allow pacing and recording at key sites. The efficacy of RF catheter ablation depends on accurate identification of the site of origin of the arrhythmia. Once this site has been identified and the electrode catheter is positioned in direct contact with the site, RF energy is delivered through the catheter to destroy it. Arrhythmias that can be "cured" by RF catheter ablation and the success rates are listed in Table 16.9. RF ablation or modification of the AVN is effective in controlling the ventricular rate in severely symptomatic patients with atrial fibrillation or multifocal atrial tachycardia when drug therapy has failed or is poorly tolerated. All patients after AVN ablation and approximately 25% after AVN modification require a permanent pacemaker because of AV block. Finally, a RF catheter maze procedure has been described for patients with atrial fibrillation, in whom attempts are made to duplicate the effects of the surgical maze procedure (see later) by creating RF energy lesions in the atria. However, this procedure is time consuming and associated with risk of serious complications. At present, it is considered experimental.

B. Arrhythmia surgery. The potential morbidity of open chest surgery, as well as associated high costs, length of hospitalization, and delayed functional recovery, fostered the development of percutaneous RF catheter ablation. Nonetheless, direct surgical approaches continue to have an important role for patients with arrhyth-

Table 16.9 Tachyarrhythmias that can be "cured" by catheter radiofrequency ablation

- Paroxysmal SVT due to AV nodal reentry (success rate for fast or slow pathway ablation 82%–96% and 98%–100%, respectively)
- Paroxysmal SVT due to orthodromic AV reciprocation[a] (success rate 85%–100%)
- Paroxysmal SVT arising in the atria and due to reentry, abnormal automaticity, or triggered activity (success rate ≥92%)
- Paroxysmal SVT due to orthodromic or antidromic[b] AV reciprocation in WPW syndrome (success rate ≥95%)
- Type I atrial flutter[c] (success rate >90%)
- Focal atrial fibrillation with triggered focus in pulmonary veins or right atrium (success rate unknown due to limited experience with RF ablation)
- Idiopathic, monomorphic VT arising in the right ventricular outflow tract or verapamil-responsive left ventricular tachycardia (success rate >90%)
- Monomorphic VT in patients with coronary artery disease to reduce need for drugs or as adjunct to ICD to reduce shocks (success rate 67%–96%[d])
- Miscellaneous tachyarrhythmias: nonphysiologic sinus tachycardia (success rate for relief of symptoms 90%); automatic junctional tachycardia (success rate 82%); bundle branch reentry, wide QRS tachycardia (nearly 100% without associated myocardial VT)

[a] Atrioventricular (AV) node serves as the anterograde limb of the reentry circuit, and a concealed accessory pathway (i.e., does not manifest as delta wave during normal sinus rhythm) as the retrograde limb.
[b] Manifest accessory pathway serves as the anterograde limb (causing a preexcited, wide QRS tachycardia), and the AV node serves as the retrograde limb of the reentry circuit.
[c] Atrial rate <340 beats/min.
[d] Particular ventricular tachycardia (VT) targeted for ablation.
ICD, implantable cardioverter–defibrillator; RF, radiofrequency; SVT, supraventricular tachycardia; WPW, Wolff–Parkinson–White.

mogenic conditions refractory to catheter ablation or with associated surgical abnormalities. Surgical procedures have been designed for almost all supraventricular tachyarrhythmias but today have application primarily to the treatment of atrial fibrillation.

   1. **Surgical approaches to therapy of atrial fibrillation [10–12].** The first approach was *left atrial isolation* in conjunction with mitral valve operations. Although 70% of patients were in sinus rhythm at long-term follow-up, persistent atrial fibrillation in the isolated atrium did not reduce the risk for thromboembolic events. Next, Guiraudon et al. isolated a band of tissue connecting the sinus and AVNs. This was termed the "corridor" operation. More than 75% of patients were arrhythmia free without medications after 40 months of follow-up. However, a significant limitation was persistent impulse conduction outside the corridor (via coronary sinus fibers) leading to the recurrence of symptomatic atrial arrhythmias and the need to perform His-bundle ablation. Furthermore, the corridor operation did not reduce the risk of thromboembolism. Finally, to maintain atrial contraction and AV synchrony, preserve sinus node function, and provide symptomatic relief, Cox et al. devised the *maze procedure*. With this procedure, both atrial appendages are excised and an arrangement of incisions are made in the right and left atria. The maze procedure (a) eliminates most opportunities for reentry; (b) reduces the likelihood of fibrillation in any remaining tissue segment due to myocardial mass reduction; (c) allows the sinus impulse to be conducted to the AVN in proper sequence via tissue strips joining adjacent segments (i.e., preserves atrial transport function); and (d) eliminates blood stasis to reduce the risk of thromboembolism. One problem with the original procedure was sinus node chronotropic insufficiency, believed due to damage to the sinus node complex or its innervation (up to 40% of patients required pacemakers). The maze III procedure reduces this risk by removing the atrial incision above the superior vena cava. As an isolated procedure for treating atrial fibrillation, the maze procedure has the limitation of requiring cardiopulmonary bypass and cardioplegic

circulatory arrest. However, it has been used in conjunction with other cardiac operations, notably mitral valve surgery. The most recent modification of the procedure uses minimally invasive surgery and cryoablation, resulting in fewer atriotomies.

2. **Accessory AV pathways [11].** There are essentially two surgical approaches to division of accessory AV pathways: the endocardial and epicardial approaches. Both require a median sternotomy. With the aid of multiple electrode recording, EP mapping of the pathways is accomplished off cardiopulmonary bypass. This is particularly attractive when the epicardial approach is to be used for division of the accessory pathway, because this technique is feasible off pump. The *endocardial approach* involves a supra-annular incision within the left atrium for left-sided pathways (requires aortic cross-clamping and cold cardioplegia) and from within the right atrium for pathways crossing the tricuspid annulus (requires only cardiopulmonary bypass). Accessory pathways are divided using sharp dissection. The *epicardial approach* does not require opening the atria. It is carried out on a normothermic beating heart without cardiopulmonary bypass. Lesions are created by cryoablation. No clear-cut superiority has been demonstrated for the endocardial or epicardial approach, at least in terms of clinical results.

3. **Other supraventricular and ventricular arrhythmias [11–13].** For other *supraventricular arrhythmias* amenable to cure by focal ablation, surgery is reserved for patients with associated cardiac surgical abnormalities, intractable arrhythmias after failed RF catheter ablation, or arrhythmias not amenable to RF catheter ablation. For patients with *ventricular arrhythmias*, the role of surgery must be reconsidered in view of the dramatic advances in ICD technology. Nonetheless, in selected circumstances, surgical ablation may lead to the best quality of life (e.g., spurious shocks with ICD). Patients with preserved left ventricular function have the lowest surgical risk but also good long-term survival, whatever the therapy. The surgical technique is a compromise between preservation of cardiac function and neutralization of the current or future arrhythmogenic substrates. It is based on two surgical concepts: exclusion and ablation. *Exclusion* is aimed at isolating the arrhythmogenic mechanism from the rest of heart. *Ablation* is aimed at neutralizing the arrhythmogenic foci. Surgical techniques include ventriculotomy, transmural resection, endocardial resection, cryoablation, and laser photocoagulation The latter two methods produce a well-demarcated mass of neutralized tissue that accomplishes the treatment goal without undue myocardial functional impairment. Cryosurgery is enhanced by cold cardioplegia, whereas laser photocoagulation can be accomplished on the normothermic, beating heart. Another surgical issue is the value of intraoperative mapping.

4. **Perioperative considerations.** Whether arrhythmia surgery is performed on or off pump and the requirement for cardioplegic circulatory arrest are dictated by the surgical procedure. Arrhythmia surgery can be accomplished safely with total intravenous anesthesia, obviating the need for volatile inhalation anesthetics that might modify arrhythmia substrates or the results of EP testing during the surgical procedure.

References

1. Atlee JL, Bosnjak ZJ. Mechanisms for cardiac dysrhythmias during anesthesia. *Anesthesiology* 1990;72:347–374.
2. **The Sicilian Gambit. A new approach to the classification of antiarrhythmic drugs based on arrhythmogenic mechanisms. Task Force of the Working Group on Arrhythmias of the European Society of Cardiology. *Circulation* 1991;84: 1831–1851.**
3. *The Sicilian Gambit. Antiarrhythmic therapy: a pathophysiologic approach.* Armonk, NY: Futura Publishing, 1994.
4. **Atlee JL, Bernstein AD. Cardiac rhythm management devices. Part I. Indications, device selection and function. *Anesthesiology* 2001;95:1265–1280.**
5. **Atlee JL, Bernstein AD. Cardiac rhythm management devices. Part II. Perioperative management. *Anesthesiology* 2001;95:1492–1506.**

6. **Gregoratos G, Cheitlin M, Conill A, et al. ACC/AHA guidelines for implantation of cardiac pacemakers and antiarrhythmia devices: a report of the ACC/AHA Task Force on Practice Guidelines (Committee on Pacemaker Implantation). *J Am Coll Cardiol* 1998;31:1175–1206.**
7. The American Heart Association in collaboration with the International Liaison Committee on Resuscitation (ILCOR). Guidelines 2000 for cardiopulmonary resuscitation and emergency cardiovascular Care. Part 6: advanced cardiovascular life support: section 2: defibrillation. *Circulation* 2000;102[Suppl 8]:I90–I94.
8. Morady F. Radio-frequency ablation as treatment for cardiac arrhythmia. *N Engl J Med* 1999;340:534–544.
9. Pappone C, Oreto G, Lamberti F, et al. Catheter ablation of paroxysmal atrial fibrillation using a 3D mapping system. *Circulation* 1999;100:1203–1208.
10. Falk RH. Atrial fibrillation. *N Engl J Med* 2001;344:1067–1078.
11. Page PL. Surgery for atrial fibrillation and other supraventricular tachyarrhythmias. In: Zipes DP, Jalife J, eds. *Cardiac electrophysiology,* 2nd ed. Philadelphia: WB Saunders, 2000:1065–1077.
12. Cox JL, Schussler RB, D'Agostino HJ Jr, et al. The surgical treatment of atrial fibrillation. III. Development of a definitive surgical procedure. *J Thorac Cardiovasc Surg* 1991; 101:569–583.
13. Guiraudon GM, Klein GJ, Guiraudon CM, et al. Surgical treatment of ventricular tachycardias. In: Zipes DP, Jalife J, eds. *Cardiac electrophysiology,* 2nd ed. Philadelphia: WB Saunders, 2000:1078–1086.

17. MANAGEMENT OF CARDIOTHORACIC SURGICAL EMERGENCIES

Stephen R. Longo and David B. Campbell

Emergency is a relative term. For the orthopedic or ophthalmologic surgeon, an emergency may require operative intervention within hours. In contrast, cardiothoracic emergencies may require surgical intervention within minutes or seconds. In general, cardiothoracic emergencies are precipitated by one of the following conditions: (i) intractable myocardial ischemia, (ii) obstruction of forward cardiac output, (iii) hemorrhage, or (iv) obstruction to airflow. Each can kill within minutes. This chapter reviews the emergencies in each of these categories, emphasizing throughout an appropriate sense of urgency and clinical priority.

I. The heart
A. Pericardial tamponade is associated with multiple medical and surgical illnesses. However, tamponade most often results from bleeding into the pericardial space after cardiac surgery.
1. **The pericardial space normally contains 25 to 50 mL of clear fluid.**
   a. Symptoms of cardiac tamponade usually are rapid in onset but depend on the rate at which pericardial fluid accumulates. A relatively small amount of fluid within the closed pericardial space is sufficient to interfere with cardiac filling. However, a chronic increase in pericardial fluid will produce cardiac tamponade only after a large volume has been added. This gradual accumulation of fluid stretches the pericardium; therefore, larger volumes are tolerated before symptoms occur. The **clinical features** of cardiac tamponade include dyspnea, orthopnea, tachycardia, pulses paradoxus, distant heart sounds, hepatic engorgement, and jugular venous distention.
   b. The **accumulation of fluid in the pericardial space** causes serious alteration in normal cardiac physiology by applying external pressure on the heart. The pressure causes a restriction of atrial and ventricular filling and a consequent drop in stroke volume. Cardiac output becomes rate dependent. Continuous monitoring of all cardiac pressures would demonstrate the following:
      (1) An increase and equalization of atrial and ventricular end-diastolic filling pressures. An absent or diminished y-descent in the central venous pressure (CVP) trace (Fig. 17.1).
      (2) Most authors have suggested that the decrease in cardiac output and stroke volume is caused by the decrease in ventricular filling [1]. **The primary problem is reduced ventricular preload,** not failure of myocardial contractility.

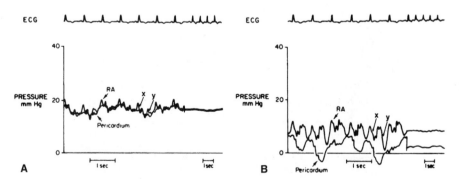

FIG. 17.1 Right atrial (*RA*) and pericardial pressures in cardiac tamponade. **A:** Note equal RA and pericardial pressure and the diminished y-descent of the RA waveform. **B:** After removal of 100 mL of fluid, the pericardial pressure is lower than RA pressure, and the normal large y-descent has returned. (From Lorell BH, Braunwald E. Pericardial disease. In: Braunwald E, ed. *Heart disease.* Philadelphia: WB Saunders, 1984:1481, with permission.)

2. Cardiac tamponade is most **commonly related to one of three causes:** (i) trauma, which may be penetrating or nonpenetrating; (ii) infection; or (iii) neoplastic disease. Other possible causes include the following:
   a. Acute myocardial infarction
   b. Postoperative bleeding (cardiac patients have a 3% to 6% incidence of tamponade). Common sources of bleeding are graft suture lines, arterial bleeding from the sternum, and generalized coagulopathy
   c. Aortic dissection with intracardiac leak or rupture
   d. Iatrogenic (central venous catheter placement, radiation, pacemaker, cardiac catheterization)
   e. Connective tissue disorders
   f. Uremia
3. The **diagnosis** of tamponade should be considered in any patient with hypotension and an elevated jugular venous pressure. Because immediate treatment may be life saving, prompt measures to establish the diagnosis should be undertaken. The following clinical findings may be helpful in making the diagnosis:
   a. Acute tamponade is well described by the **Beck triad: a small quiet heart, increased venous pressure, and hypotension**
   b. Equalization of the CVP, right ventricular end-diastolic pressure, pulmonary capillary wedge pressure, left atrial pressure, and left ventricular end-diastolic pressure
   c. **Pulsus paradoxus.** A decrease of more than 10 mm Hg in systolic arterial pressure occurs with inspiration (not a specific finding)
   d. Radiographically one sees an enlarged globular cardiac shadow with a convex or straight left heart border. The right costophrenic angle is reduced to less than 90 degrees and the lungs are clear.
   e. The electrocardiogram (ECG) is nonspecific but may show low-voltage, PR-segment depression and ST segment elevation. Occasionally **electrical alternans** may be seen (Fig. 17.2).

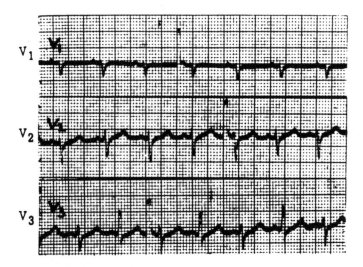

FIG. 17.2 Electrical alternans with cardiac tamponade. Lead V_3 demonstrates the variation in R-wave axis in alternate beats. Note that this phenomenon is not seen in all electrocardiographic leads. (From Goldman JM. *Principles of clinical electrocardiography,* 11th ed. Los Altos, CA: Lange Medical Publications, 1982:305, with permission.)

    f. Echocardiography permits diagnosis noninvasively. A characteristic echo-free space is seen between the epicardium and the pericardium. This is the most sensitive tool for making the diagnosis of pericardial effusion. Findings of tamponade may include diastolic collapse of the right ventricular free wall, right atrial inversion, left atrial collapse, and characteristic Doppler abnormalities. However, clotted blood in the pericardial space can complicate accurate echocardiographic diagnosis.

  4. Treatment. Definitive treatment of cardiac tamponade is drainage. It may be accomplished through pericardiocentesis (Figs. 17.3–17.4) or surgical decompression. Surgical approaches include the subxiphoid approach, which is easier to perform but offers a limited exposure. A left thoracotomy incision provides excellent exposure and is indicated if a larger field is required.

  5. Anesthetic management. The sequence of anesthesia and surgery depends on the hemodynamic state of the patient. In severely compromised patients, pericardiocentesis or subxiphoid exploration can be performed with the patient under local anesthesia. This is the preferred anesthetic when hypotension is severe. If a general anesthetic is planned, consider the following guidelines:

    a. Administer intravenous fluids before induction to optimize preload. Avoid or minimize manipulations that decrease venous return.

    b. Avoid drugs that cause myocardial depression. Ketamine is an option for induction.

    c. Heart rate must remain high to preserve cardiac output.

    d. Controlled ventilation significantly decreases preload and cardiac output. **If a general anesthetic is required, it is suggested that the patient be allowed to breathe spontaneously until the pericardial sac is opened. If spontaneous ventilation is not possible, ventilation with high rates and low tidal volumes** (to minimize mean airway pressure) **should be considered.**

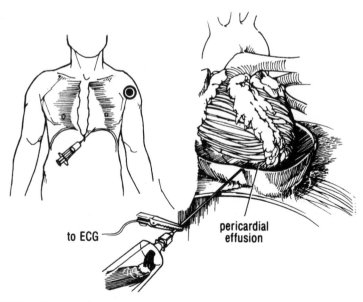

to ECG

pericardial effusion

FIG. 17.3 Technique of subxiphoid pericardiocentesis. The needle is directed toward the left shoulder. Needle electrogram permits identification of contact between needle tip and epicardium (causes ST elevation). (From Polomano RC, Miller SE. *Understanding and managing oncologic emergencies.* Columbus: Adria Laboratories, 1987:22, with permission.)

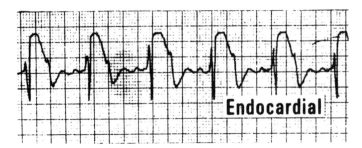

FIG. 17.4 QRS complex showing the "current of injury" or ST-segment elevation character-istic of contact of the needle electrode with the epicardium. (From Mansour KA, Dorney ER, Kisig SB. Techniques for insertion of perivenous and epicardial pacemakers. In: Hurst JW, Logue RB, Rachley CE, et al., eds. *The heart, arteries and veins.* 5th ed. New York: McGraw-Hill, 1982:1759, with permission.)

       e. Acute pulmonary edema has been reported after relief of pericardial tam-ponade and diuretics should be considered.

  B. Massive pulmonary embolism is a major cause of morbidity and mortality in the general patient population. More than 95% of pulmonary emboli arise from the lower extremity deep venous system [2]. Thrombi occurring in the right cardiac chambers or in other veins account for the remainder of pulmonary emboli. In 1856, **Virchow suggested three possible causes of venous thrombosis:** (i) stasis of blood, (ii) venous wall abnormalities, and (iii) abnormal states of coagulation. Patients that are predisposed to developing deep venous thrombosis include those immobilized for long periods of time, the elderly, the obese, and those with malignancies, conges-tive heart failure, and previous history of emboli [3].

     1. Major thromboemboli lead to a series of pathophysiologic events, which can be categorized as having a predominant respiratory or hemodynamic conse-quence. They may produce **symptoms** either by the direct effect of pulmonary arterial obstruction or by the secondary pulmonary bronchospasm and vaso-constriction. The most common symptoms are tachycardia, tachypnea, and rales. **The classic triad of dyspnea, pain, and hemoptysis is present in fewer than 25% of patients.**

     2. The **signs and symptoms** of acute pulmonary embolism vary widely and are nonspecific. Minor degrees of embolism probably occur frequently, but because they produce no circulatory or respiratory disturbance they go unnoticed [4]. However, massive pulmonary embolism produces a catastrophic picture that includes cyanosis, extreme dyspnea, chest pain, hemoptysis, and cardiovascu-lar collapse. The increase in pulmonary vascular resistance causes right ven-tricular failure. This hemodynamic compromise is worsened by concomitant hypoxemia and an acute change in matching of ventilation and perfusion.

       a. Pulmonary angiography is the definitive test. Angiography allows visualization of the pulmonary tree, outlining clearly which branches are occluded by clot. It is the most reliable diagnostic test for pulmonary embolism.

       b. A contrast spiral computed tomographic (CT) study provides direct imag-ing information that can demonstrate significant pulmonary embolism and altered segmental lung perfusion. CT is considered the initial exami-nation of choice because of its speed and availability.

       c. Echocardiography can play an important role in the diagnosis of pul-monary embolism. It is quick, easy to mobilize, and has minimal morbid-ity. Echocardiographic findings may include the following:

         1. Thromboemboli inside the right atrium or pulmonary artery

         2. Right ventricular dilation

3. Right ventricular hypokinesis
4. Reduced left ventricular volume
5. Pulmonary artery dilation
6. Tricuspid and pulmonary regurgitation

   d. A ventilation–perfusion scan is another noninvasive method of detecting pulmonary emboli. However, the scan's findings often are nonspecific and may demonstrate false-positive results.
   e. There are no specific findings on ECG to identify pulmonary embolism, but the ECG may show signs of right ventricular strain or bundle branch block.
3. Treatment
   a. Heparin anticoagulation is the standard treatment if the clinical evidence strongly supports the diagnosis of a pulmonary embolus.
   b. Thrombolytic therapy usually is contraindicated in postoperative patients because of the risk of hemorrhage. However, drugs such as tissue plasminogen activator (tPA), streptokinase and urokinase speed the resolution of both venous thrombi and pulmonary emboli.
   c. Surgical embolectomy for a massive embolus carries an operative mortality of 50% to 60% [5]. Even massive emboli may resolve spontaneously. Pulmonary embolectomy is an emergent procedure that may be performed without the use of cardiopulmonary bypass (CPB).
   d. Portable bypass via femoral cannulation can be life saving. Unfortunately, the diagnosis is seldom made promptly enough to alter the mortality of a massive pulmonary embolism.
   e. Inferior vena cava interruption or placement of an inferior vena cava filter is required in patients who have a contraindication to anticoagulation or who have recurrent emboli despite anticoagulation.
4. **Anesthetic considerations**
   a. The gradient between arterial and end-tidal PCO_2 reflects the amount of pulmonary dead space. When followed over time, at a constant minute ventilation, PCO_2 provides a relative index of ventilation–perfusion mismatch during surgery and recovery.
   b. In most cases, management consists primarily of resuscitation with use of tracheal intubation, hyperventilation with oxygen, muscle relaxants, hypnotic drugs, and inotropic support
   c. The goal should be to maximize cardiac output to preserve vital organ function until establishment of CPB. All anesthetic agents should be titrated to optimize cardiac function, preferably through cardiac output measurements.
   d. In the haste to establish bypass, it is vital to remember to administer heparin into a central vein. During surgical suctioning of clot from the pulmonary vessels, manual massage and ventilation of the lungs may enhance clot retrieval. The pleural space should be emptied and drained at the end of the operation. If tolerated, positive end-expiratory pressure often is useful to minimize reperfusion abnormalities and alveolar edema.
C. **Postoperative bleeding and reoperation**
   1. **Pathophysiology**
      a. Etiology. Coagulation problems in the cardiac surgical patient differ from those of other surgical patients. Coagulopathies may exist from preoperative and intraoperative drug therapy, such as high-dose heparin, warfarin (Coumadin) and IIb/IIIa platelet receptor antagonists (abciximab, eptifibatide, and tirofiban). In addition, the use of the artificial surface of the CPB circuit stimulates anticoagulants and fibrinolysis and causes qualitative and quantitative changes in platelets [6]. The surgical procedure itself may cause significant bleeding. There may be inadequate hemostasis at suture lines with bleeding from venous and arterial grafts or even the chest wall. Finally, elevated blood pressure can initiate bleeding that may be difficult to control.

    b. Complications. Continued bleeding may lead to significant morbidity and mortality. Knowledge of the normal hemostatic process is essential to understanding the etiology of the problem.

        1. Continued bleeding may lead to multiple transfusions and risks of hepatitis, human immunodeficiency virus, and pulmonary dysfunction.

        2. Hypothermia can result from multiple transfusions; therefore, blood products must be warmed to prevent coagulopathy. An active patient warming device may be indicated.

        3. Hypovolemia must be treated aggressively or it may lead to hypotension and shock.

        4. Calcium should be checked and supplemented as necessary during massive transfusion.

2. Clinical setting. Fluid replacement is dictated by the patient's hemodynamics, urine output, laboratory studies, and ongoing blood loss. When bleeding continues at rates of more than 300 mL/hour, returning to the operating room (OR) is prudent if results of coagulation studies are close to normal. If chest tube drainage suddenly ceases, the chest tubes should be examined for clots, with concern for impending tamponade.

3. Management

    a. Prevention

        Surgical hemostasis at the end of CPB remains the best prophylactic measure against postoperative bleeding. Adequate heparin reversal with confirmation by an activated clotting time is mandatory. Strict control of the systemic blood pressure should be emphasized. If hemostasis is clinically abnormal, laboratory tests should include prothrombin time, partial thromboplastin time, fibrinogen level, and platelet count. If bleeding continues despite normal coagulation studies, either platelet function is inadequate or a more complex coagulopathy exists. In this case, blood component therapy is indicated. Other adjunctive measures include the use of topical hemostatic agents such as "fibrin glue" and collagen preparations. The use of 1-deamino-8-arginine vasopressin (DDAVP) or ε-aminocaproic acid is controversial. These compounds may be effective in certain types of coagulopathies. The serine protease inhibitor aprotinin, an antifibrinolytic agent and kallikrein inhibitor, has established value in decreasing blood loss and transfusions. It must be administered before, during, and after the surgery for optimal effect. Aprotinin should be considered for reoperations and for complex and prolonged cardiac operations for which excessive bleeding is anticipated.

    b. Postoperative bleeding. Bleeding in excess of 300 to 400 mL/hour initially or in excess of 100 mL/hour within the first few postoperative hours should prompt return of the patient to the OR, particularly if the results of coagulation studies are reasonably normal. If signs of cardiac tamponade are present, urgent reoperation is required. If transport to the OR cannot occur immediately, the inferior aspect of the sternotomy wound can be opened to allow temporary drainage of the pericardium.

    c. Anesthetic considerations. Anesthetizing the hypovolemic patient presents particular challenges, especially if the bleeding is so rapid that transfusions cannot restore normovolemia. In this situation, it is critically important to achieve surgical control as rapidly as possible. A combination of amnestics (scopolamine or midazolam), muscle relaxants with or without narcotics, or ketamine may be the only anesthetics tolerated by a patient in shock. Knowledge of the prior filling pressures and other hemodynamic variables is important in guiding fluid resuscitation. All intravenous fluids should be warmed to avoid hypothermia. CPB rarely is required for surgical management of postoperative bleeding.

D. Emergency coronary artery bypass surgery

    1. Pathophysiology

        a. Surgical revascularization often is indicated for life-threatening clinical situations, such as cardiogenic shock, severe mitral valve regurgitation, repair of postinfarction ventricular septal defects, and unstable angina that does not respond to medical therapy. Myocardial ischemia may result in myocardial necrosis if not rapidly treated (less than 4 to 6 hours). The need for primary surgical revascularization has decreased with improvements in catheter-based interventions such as angioplasty and stenting.

   b. Emergency coronary artery bypass grafting (CABG) may be needed after a failed percutaneous coronary intervention such as angioplasty or coronary stent. The rate of emergency CABG surgery after percutaneous coronary intervention decreased to about 1% to 2% in recent years. When an operation is required, it is complicated further by delays, heparin, and platelet receptor antagonists.

2. Clinical setting

   a. Patients with unstable angina, non–Q-wave myocardial infarction, or recent percutaneous coronary intervention often are taking drugs that inhibit platelet aggregation. These drugs, abciximab (ReoPro), eptifibatide (Integrilin), and tirofiban (Aggrastat), function by preventing the binding of fibrinogen to the platelet glycoprotein IIb/IIIa receptor. Bleeding is the most common adverse reaction that occurs. Surgical interventions appear to be safe 2 to 4 hours after stopping eptifibatide or tirofiban. Both drugs have a shorter duration of action than abciximab and their effects on platelet activity rapidly diminish when the infusion is discontinued. This is advantageous for patients who experience serious bleeding or require emergency bypass surgery. Patients treated with IIb/IIIa receptor antagonists, who require emergent or urgent surgery, may need platelet transfusions. The high-affinity binding of the drug to existing platelets usually leaves little drug to interact with platelets subsequently given.

   b. Myocardial revascularization performed during an acute myocardial infarction has a higher mortality rate. Surgery during an acute myocardial infarction with necrosis results in ventricular arrhythmias, greater postoperative use of inotropic drugs, and an increased need for an intraaortic balloon pump.

3. Surgical management

   a. The goal of the operation is to provide satisfactory and complete myocardial revascularization in an expeditious manner. Most patients are unstable and cannot tolerate off-pump bypass techniques. Spending the extra time required for takedown of the internal mammary arteries may not be prudent; therefore, grafting is performed swiftly using the most appropriate conduits. The most critical lesions are bypassed first, with cardioplegia given down the grafts as they are completed.

   b. The technical aspects of the surgical procedure differ little from those used in elective CABG. However, several adjunctive measures may be of particular importance to myocardial preservation in such an emergency setting, including the following:

      (1) Intensified efforts to achieve (local) myocardial hypothermia, including cooling pads, electrolyte slush or irrigation solutions, bicaval cannulation with snares, and venting. The latter two techniques reduce the rewarming of the arrested heart that occurs when the warmer systemic venous blood returns to the heart.

      (2) Retrograde coronary sinus cardioplegia in an attempt to achieve better cardioplegic distribution and hypothermia.

      (3) "Warm induction protocols," which have been designed to achieve some measure of ischemic reversal and intracellular metabolic stabilization. Ventricular venting and anterograde–retrograde coronary perfusion before hypothermic cardioplegia may optimize myocardial preservation and maximize muscle salvage.

      (4) Period of controlled reperfusion of the heart after completion of the revascularization.

      (5) Reducing myocardial workload both before and after CPB by using an intraaortic balloon pump.

4. Anesthetic management

a. Time factor. The sooner the patient can be placed on CPB, the fewer myocytes will die. Steps to hasten the surgery are most beneficial in these patients.

b. History. Usually these patients arrive directly from the cardiac catheterization laboratory. It is important to ascertain the coronary anatomy, the interventions performed (angioplasty, transluminal perfusion catheter), and medications administered. Platelet transfusions may be needed if patients recently received aspirin or IIb/IIIa inhibitors. Intraaortic balloon support should be maintained until CPB is established. Patients may still be partially heparinized.

c. Monitoring. The cardiologist may have inserted femoral arterial and venous lines during catheterization. The lines should remain in place for intraoperative monitoring and to prevent bleeding. For unstable, severely ischemic patients, it may be prudent to delay preinduction insertion of a pulmonary artery catheter or a neck CVP line. The femoral artery can be used for blood pressure monitoring; the femoral vein line becomes the volume infusion line. The surgeon can provide transthoracic left atrial and right atrial monitoring lines before termination of CPB. At the conclusion of the surgery, a conventional jugular or subclavian pulmonary artery catheter can be inserted. Transesophageal echocardiography is an extremely valuable monitoring tool in these patients.

d. Technique. As in any patient with myocardial ischemia, the anesthetic technique must address maintenance of favorable myocardial oxygen supply–demand balance. It may be necessary temporarily to accept lower cardiac output values to reduce myocardial work until CPB can be established.

II. The lung and thorax

A. Pneumothorax

1. Pathophysiology

a. Pneumothorax is the accumulation of air within the pleural (potential) space. Pneumothorax often is categorized as small (less than 20% of pleural space volume), moderate (20% to 50%), or major (greater than 50% of pleural space occupied by air). Tension pneumothorax refers to progressive accumulation of air under positive pressure. This process is potentially lethal as the mechanical effects of mediastinal shift progressively impede cardiac venous return. Wheezing may occur as a result of extrinsic airway compression.

b. Etiology. The most common cause of pneumothorax is an iatrogenic puncture of the lung during attempts to place subclavian or internal jugular vein catheters. Vigorous positive-pressure ventilation causes barotrauma and may result in alveolar rupture, particularly if underlying disease (blebs or emphysema) is present. Chest trauma is an important cause of pneumothorax. Additionally, spontaneous rupture of congenital blebs or emphysematous bullae may occur.

c. During spontaneous ventilation, the leakage of air from the lung into the pleural space tends to be progressive because of normally negative intrathoracic pressure. A one-way valve mechanism can exist at the site of the leak, allowing a simple pneumothorax to progress to a tension pneumothorax. Positive-pressure ventilation will predictably exacerbate an ongoing leak and augment the risk of tension pneumothorax.

2. Clinical setting

a. Diagnosis of pneumothorax can be difficult in the OR setting but depends in part on adequate monitoring and attention to detail. The classic triad of hypoxemia, hypotension, and wheezing should be remembered. Decreasing oxygen saturation should always lead to suspicion of pneumothorax during anesthesia.

b. Access to the chest to listen to breath sounds often is limited during cardiothoracic operations. The esophageal stethoscope provides limited information because of its location adjacent to central rather than peripheral airways.

      c. A progressive increase in ventilator pressures (with a fixed volume) signals decreased lung compliance, which can be due to increasing size of a pneumothorax. Often, however, progression to a tension pneumothorax occurs before impressive difficulties are encountered.

      d. Hypotension, hypoxia, high inflation pressures, and the clinical findings of right heart failure and shock indicate that tension pneumothorax is the most likely diagnosis.

3. Management

      a. Outside the OR, an occasional small pneumothorax can be followed by obtaining serial chest x-ray films. Because of the high nitrogen content, several days may be required for resolution of the pneumothorax.

      b. In most cases, elimination of intrapleural air is prudent. Any pneumothorax should be regarded as life threatening because of its potential for progression to a **tension pneumothorax.** Tube thoracostomy is the standard treatment. The chest tube should be placed before anesthesia or positive-pressure ventilation is initiated. The precise point of insertion or the position of the chest tube is of much less importance than its presence. (Fig. 17.5).

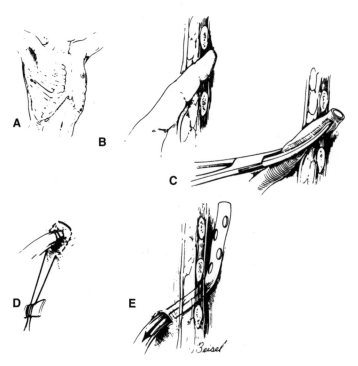

FIG. 17.5 Placement of tube thoracostomy. After applying local anesthesia, a skin incision is made with a knife **(A).** A finger or a clamp creates a tract **(B),** then a clamp is used to pass the tube into the pleural space **(C).** Note how the tube is tunneled to a different interspace from that of the skin incision (allowing the hole to seal spontaneously when the tube is removed). Care should be taken to pass the tube near the superior surface of the rib (to avoid the intercostals blood vessels) **(D).** The tube is held in place by a skin suture **(E).** The tube is connected to a water-seal and suction system to evacuate the pleural space and to prevent air from entering the chest cavity with negative-pressure inspiration. (From Waldhausen JA, Peirce WS. *Johnson's surgery of the chest.* 5th ed. Chicago: Year Book, 1985:15, with permission.)

Elimination of the air space permits apposition of the pleural surfaces and resolution of the air leak.

   c. There may be a need for emergency therapy of a tension pneumothorax. Placement of a needle (18-gauge or larger) through the appropriate chest wall will relieve the positive intrathoracic pressure and ameliorate the crisis. In the supine patient, insertion at the second or third intercostal space in the midclavicular line will avoid puncture of the heart or internal mammary artery. Needles and tubes should be placed just over the superior surface of the rib because the intercostal blood vessels lie next to the inferior surface.

   d. Operative treatment of pneumothorax is indicated for prolonged air leaks and for recurrent pneumothoraces. Video-assisted thoracic surgery with thorascopic instruments has replaced open thoracotomy for treatment. Visualization is adequate to identify congenital blebs and emphysematous bullae. Minimally invasive staplers are adequate for local resections. Pleurodesis can be induced by abrasion or with talc.

   e. **Anesthetic considerations.** Unless the pleural space is vented, spontaneous ventilation should be used whenever possible to decrease the risk of forcing additional air into the pleural space. Nitrous oxide should be avoided to prevent enlargement of gas in the closed pleural space. At the conclusion of a thoracic operation, the anesthesiologist should always inspect the chest tube water seal before spontaneous ventilation is resumed to prevent room air from being sucked into the pleural space with each breath.

B. **Hemorrhage within the airways**
  1. **Pathophysiology**
      a. **Etiology.** It is essential to determine that the blood is coming from the respiratory tract and not from the nasopharynx or gastrointestinal tract. Despite extensive evaluations, 5% to 15% of cases of gross hemoptysis remain undiagnosed [7].
         (1) Spontaneous parenchymal bleeding most frequently is infectious in etiology and often is due to tuberculosis, bronchiectasis, or, increasingly, aspergillosis.
         (2) Tumor, whether primary or metastatic, within the airway causes less severe hemoptysis, but highly vascular lesions (carcinoid, metastatic renal cell) may bleed profusely.
         (3) Iatrogenic hemoptysis may result from endoscopic biopsies of bronchial lesions and transbronchial biopsy techniques. Overinflation of a pulmonary artery catheter balloon, when the catheter tip is distally positioned, or allowing the catheter to remain in the "wedged" position for a prolonged period of time can lead to rupture of a pulmonary artery and massive hemoptysis.
         (4) Perhaps the most dreaded cause of massive hemoptysis is tracheo-innominate artery fistula, which most often is a complication of chronic tracheostomy or intubation.
      b. **Massive hemoptysis** (greater than 600 mL/24 hours) is an indication for immediate investigation and intervention because of the risk of asphyxiation and death. The choice of medical or surgical intervention relates to the anatomic basis for the hemoptysis. Urgent surgical intervention is considered in patients with definable lesions who have evidence of uncontrollable respiratory or hemodynamic compromise.
      c. **Hypoxemia.** The presence of a mass lesion, blood, or clots in the tracheobronchial tree leads to bronchial obstruction. The blood flow to the nonventilated segments represents right-to-left shunting that causes hypoxemia due to ventilation–perfusion mismatching. Serious underlying chronic lung disease and other medical problems often compound the problem.
  2. **Clinical setting.** Coughing up blood is a universally terrifying experience for patients. Physicians, too, should recognize that "conservative" treatment of massive hemoptysis is associated with 75% mortality. The incidence of rebleeding is high (80%), so decisions about definitive treatment should be made early.

3. Management

    a. First in priority is confirmation of true hemoptysis, followed by efforts to localize the site of bleeding. Details of the history usually will differentiate oropharyngeal or upper alimentary bleeding (with aspiration or regurgitation) from true bleeding within the airway. Simple lateralization of the source of bleeding to either the left or right lung is information of considerable value. The patient may volunteer information on which side feels abnormal or uncomfortable. A chest x-ray film often will reveal evidence of underlying disease, such as cancer or chronic inflammation. Infiltrates, particularly at the lung bases, are of limited help in localization because of aspiration and dependent drainage of airway blood. Bronchoscopy should be performed promptly in all patients to evaluate the source and nature of the bleeding. Fibrin casts and blood clots within the airway often are tenacious and difficult to remove with suction. It may be beneficial to perform all such bronchoscopies in the OR, where opportunities for intervention are available, including selective endobronchial intubation.

    b. Intermittent hemoptysis. The capacity to deal with airway bleeding using the flexible bronchoscope is limited by the small size of the working channel (approximately 2 mm) and the instruments available, but it is possible to use balloon occluders (i.e., Fogarty catheters) through or alongside the bronchoscope. For tumor bleeding in the large airways, the Nd-YAG laser can be extremely effective. Rarely, embolization of pulmonary artery branches may be performed, based on the history, bronchoscopic findings, and assessment of operative outcome. Selective bronchial artery embolization may be effective in patients with a bronchial (as opposed to an alveolar) source of bleeding.

    c. Massive or ongoing hemoptysis. The initial maneuvers should be designed to protect the patient from asphyxia. The flexible bronchoscope is of limited value, and the use of rigid bronchoscopy is preferred. High-frequency jet ventilation is favored by some centers because accumulation of blood within the instrument is minimized.

        (1) Isolation of the affected bronchus. If only limited resources are available, intubation of the nonbleeding side with a standard endotracheal tube can accomplish ventilation. A flexible bronchoscope may assist in optimal placement of the tube. Use of contrast material to inflate the cuff allows confirmation of the tube's position on the chest x-ray film. Ideal management involves swift insertion of a double-lumen endotracheal tube to provide isolation and selective ventilation of the "normal" lung and removal of blood and clots from the diseased lung. Active bleeding from the pathologic side can be quantified accurately if bleeding continues. The patient then can be transported either to the angiography suite or to the OR for further intervention. As soon as the tube is secured, the normal side should be cleared of blood and secretions that spilled over from the bleeding side.

        (2) Surgical management. Definitive resolution of hemoptysis generally involves pulmonary resection. Initial control of the bronchus (rather than the vascular structures) is achieved and conservative operations are preferred. As with all operations done with one-lung ventilation, hypoxia due to shunting can be minimized by temporarily occluding the pulmonary artery on the nonventilated side if necessary.

C. Immersion and hypothermia

  1. Pathophysiology

    a. Drowning is the second leading cause of accidental death among children next to motor vehicle accidents.

    b. The risk of fatal outcome increases steadily with length of submersion. There is a 10% risk of fatal outcome with submersion of 5 minutes or less and an 85% risk with submersions of 10 to 25 minutes [8].

    c. The common problem in drowning is aspiration. Fluid aspirated by the drowning victim frequently is a mixture of stomach contents and drowning medium.

    d. Loss of surfactant, alveolitis, pulmonary edema, and ventilation–perfusion mismatching are present. The lungs are at great risk for infection.

    e. Submersion victims frequently are hypothermic, offering some protection to the central nervous system. Declining mental status, ataxia, and hyperreflexia appear as temperatures fall to about 32°C. Below this temperature, stupor progresses and hyporeflexia appears along with muscle rigidity. Cardiac arrhythmias are common at any reduced temperature, with underlying bradycardias progressing to the fibrillation threshold at approximately 28°C.

    f. Ingestion of fresh water leads to rapid absorption and a transient increase in plasma volume. Large volumes can produce hypervolemia, hyponatremia, and red cell hemolysis.

    g. Ingestion of hypertonic solution (salt water) results in hemoconcentration, hypernatremia, and hyperchloremia.

2. Management

    a. Prehospital advanced cardiac life support is a critical part of the medical therapy.

    b. Core temperature measurements are made by means of rectal or esophageal probes. Survey and subsequent comprehensive examinations are made to detect other bodily injuries, including those of the cervical and thoracic spine.

    c. Monitoring should include blood pressure, blood gas analysis, oxygen saturation, pulse, ECG, neurologic status, and urine output.

    d. Intubation and airway suctioning or bronchoscopy is critical because aspiration of stomach contents is a common problem with drowning victims.

    e. The need for CPB should be immediately assessed. Passive rewarming with hyperthermia blankets, convection heaters, and insulation allows for rewarming at a rate of 0.5° to 1.0°C/hour. Temperatures below 30°C are best managed by active rewarming using CPB via femoral vessels, which offers the advantage of precise control of temperature, plasma volume, and systemic perfusion. Ventricular fibrillation is an absolute indication for immediate institution of CPB and defibrillation.

    f. As warming progresses, arterial blood gas values are monitored to assess the adequacy of ventilation and resolution of lactic acidosis.

    g. If necessary, cardioversion should be completed when the core temperature reaches 32°C.

    h. Toxicology screens for substance abuse and drug level assays may be important.

III. Chest trauma

Trauma is the leading cause of death in patients younger than 40 years. Cardiac injury has been reported in 6% to 7% of trauma victims [9]. The anesthesiologist should suspect cardiac injury in any patient with thoracoabdominal injuries. Thoracic emergencies can be life threatening because the intrathoracic organs are so well protected that, in general, severe trauma is necessary for injury to occur.

    A. Blunt trauma to the chest

        1. Pathophysiology. Because cardiac trauma is underdiagnosed, all patients with blunt trauma to the chest or abdomen should be suspected of having cardiac injuries. The forces responsible for organ damage in blunt trauma are direct (rib fractures), indirect (lung laceration from rib fractures), or shearing (pulmonary contusions, bronchial and vascular injuries). Cardiac injuries that result from blunt chest trauma include the following:

        A. Transection or dissection of the thoracic aorta

        B. Cardiac tamponade

        C. Myocardial contusion

        D. Laceration of a coronary artery

        E. Laceration of the pericardium, papillary muscles, valves or intraventricular septum

Noncardiac injuries that may result from blunt chest trauma include the following:

A. Tension pneumothorax/open pneumothorax
B. Rib fractures and flail chest
C. Pulmonary contusion
D. Diaphragmatic rupture
E. Tracheobronchial disruption
F. Esophageal disruption

Direct injury to the chest wall or diaphragm impairs respiratory mechanics, whereas injury to the lung parenchyma may compromise gas exchange [10]. Loss of integrity of the bony framework of the chest results in ineffective ventilation. "Flail chest" injuries are those in which a large segment of the chest wall is subject to paradoxical (inward) motion during spontaneous inspiration. The pneumothorax and pulmonary contusion that frequently coexist compound the inadequacy of spontaneous ventilation.

Serious tracheobronchial and vascular injuries frequently are not apparent on initial assessment. However, delayed diagnosis is potentially lethal. Unstable vital signs, worsening respiratory status, or subtle changes on chest radiographs should prompt further study with bronchoscopy and chest CT.

2. **Management**
   a. Supportive management of the patient after blunt chest trauma is the rule rather than operative management. Mechanical ventilation should be avoided, but severe injuries may mandate intubation to compensate for rib fractures, chest wall instability, or reduced minute ventilation secondary to shock. Associated brain or vascular injury may dictate early intubation for airway protection to minimize the risk of aspiration.
   b. Airway assessment and management are the primary, immediate, and ongoing goals. Supplemental oxygen should be administered while additional information is gathered from the patient and the transport team.
   c. Flail chest wall segments should be immobilized, and open wounds should be occluded until endotracheal intubation can be accomplished. Tube thoracostomy is necessary.
   d. Urgent intervention is required for manifestations of cardiac tamponade or tension pneumothorax (see Sections **I.A** and **II.A**). A pneumothorax should be treated with a tube thoracostomy (Fig. 17.5). Failure of the lung to reexpand or a significant air leak may require additional chest tubes or, rarely, surgical exploration. A large air leak that is not controlled with a chest tube suggests tracheal or bronchial rupture.
   e. The finding of mediastinal emphysema on physical examination or chest x-ray film should prompt endoscopic evaluation of the airway and esophagus.
   f. Tracheal and bronchial injuries are uncommon but often are unrecognized during the initial survey. Eighty percent of these injuries are within 2.5 cm of the carina. Injuries above the carina can be managed by advancement of an endotracheal tube past the injury. With bronchial injuries, an endotracheal tube can be advanced into the uninjured main stem bronchus. In the case of severe trauma to the lung, the surgeon's primary objective is to control the hilum of the involved lung.
   g. Direct esophageal injury is uncommon because of its location in the posterior mediastinum.

3. **Anesthetic considerations**
   a. In all cases, the anesthesiologist should be attentive to the signs of **pneumothorax or cardiac tamponade,** which may develop insidiously during nonthoracic surgery. Because of the potential for an undetected pneumothorax, nitrous oxide should be avoided. Note that a tension pneumothorax may develop in the nonoperative dependent lung during thoracotomy, causing impaired ventilation and circulatory compromise.

    b. Patients with blunt chest trauma may develop myocardial ischemia or contusion; therefore, continuous monitoring of ECG leads II and V_5 is prudent. Transesophageal echocardiography has increasingly become the instrument of choice for diagnosis.

    c. In severe lung or tracheobronchial trauma there is a risk of air embolism. Positive-pressure ventilation should be given at the lowest required pressures until the injury is explored and controlled.

    d. Regional anesthesia and patient-controlled analgesia are useful for controlling the pain of thoracic injury. Effective pain control with epidural and/or intercostal analgesia minimizes respiratory depression. Continuous epidural analgesia, through a catheter placed in the lumbar or thoracic epidural space, has proved to be extremely effective for postthoracotomy as well as posttraumatic thoracic pain relief.

B. Penetrating trauma to the chest

    1. Pathophysiology. The nature and extent of injury produced by penetrating trauma depends on the weapon or missile involved. The injuries produced by a knife are familiar to everyone who works in an OR [11]. Gunshot wounds, however, are considerably different. The "zone of injury" produced by high-velocity bullets extends far beyond the tract between entry and exit points. Explosive forces, shearing forces, and cavitation all combine to produce complex injuries.

    2. Clinical setting. Most penetrating chest trauma is the result of acts of violence. Penetrating chest trauma is much more likely to be an isolated injury than is blunt chest trauma.

    3. Management. As with blunt trauma, the immediate concerns are those of breathing and circulation. Effective management of the airway includes the ability to provide selective lung ventilation. Pneumothorax and pericardial tamponade are addressed as previously described.

        a. Adequate surgical exposure, while maintaining cardiopulmonary stability, is the key to effective operative treatment of all chest conditions. A variety of incisions, from "classic" posterolateral thoracotomy to sternotomy with extension of the incision into the neck, may prove invaluable to provide exposure and control.

        b. The care of patients with knife wounds to the chest first requires a decision about whether an operation is required. For purposes of decision making, these wounds can be separated into three groups by location:

            (1) *Median wounds,* even of apparently small dimension, may involve the heart.

            (2) *Cervicothoracic wounds* are always dangerous because of the vital structures in this area. Surgical exploration of these wounds should always be considered.

            (3) *Lateral wounds* to the lower thorax may have penetrated the diaphragm, with involvement of the spleen, colon, or liver.

            (4) In all cases, if a knife or impaling object is still in place, it should be left alone and removed only in the OR, where control of the lung and vasculature can be obtained if necessary.

        c. Patients with bullet injuries rarely require removal of the projectile [12]. The injuries caused in or around the path of the missile are the focus of attention, but the possibility of internal deflection and fragmentation of the bullet by bony structures must be recognized. A straight line between entry and exit or between entry and the x-ray location of the bullet is not necessarily the path taken.

        d. The wounding capacity of a bullet is a function of its kinetic energy, which is principally related to its velocity. Low-velocity bullet injuries generally are straightforward. Immediate but conservative repair is the surgeon's goal.

        e. High-velocity missiles travel at speeds greater than Mach 2 and may be responsible for massive tissue destruction. The bullet itself and the internal shock waves produced within the tissue cause primary injuries. Shattered bone and bullet fragments may act as multiple secondary projectiles and compound the severity of these injuries. All such patients require OR care. The threat to life is great, and the surgical team often is faced with no option but to perform an aggressive resection and debridement.

References

1. **Kahn RA. The patient with cardiac tamponade. In: Frost EAM, ed. *Preanesthetic Assessment 4*. New York: The McMahon Group, 1994:1–11.**
2. Chartier L, Bera J, Delomez M, et al. Free-floating thrombin in the right heart: diagnosis, management, and prognostic indexes in 38 consecutive patients. *Circulation* 1999;99: 2779–2783.
3. Ullmann W, Hemmer W, Hannekum A. The urgent pulmonary embolectomy: mechanical resuscitation in the operating theatre determines the outcome. *Thorac Cardiovasc Surg* 1999;47:5–8.
4. Pharo GH, Andonakakis A, Chandrasekaren K, et al. Survival from catastrophic intraoperative pulmonary embolism. *Anesth Analg* 1995;81:188–190.
5. Alpert JS, Dalen JE. Pulmonary embolism. In: Hurst JW, Logue RB, Schlant RC, et al., eds. *The heart—arteries and veins,* 4th ed. New York: McGraw-Hill, 1994:1875–1893.
6. Moreno-Cabral CE, Mitchell RS, Miller DC. Section three—postoperative problems. In: *Manual of postoperative management in adult cardiac surgery*. Baltimore: Williams & Wilkins, 1988:29–34.
7. Weinberger SE, Braunwald E. Cough and hemoptysis. In: Fauci AS, Braunwald EB, Isselbacher KJ, et al., eds. *Harrison's principles of internal medicine,* 14th ed. New York: McGraw-Hill, 1994:196–198.
8. **Mueller JB. The drowning/near drowning patient. In: Frost EAM, ed. *Preanesthetic assessment 3*. Boston: Birkhauser, 1991:111–123.**
9. **Kingsley CP. Perioperative anesthetic management of thoracic trauma. In: Grande CM, Smith CE, eds. *Anesthesiology clinics of North America—trauma*. Philadelphia: WB Saunders, 1999:183–195.**
10. Kelledy P, Abrams KJ. The heart in trauma surgery. In: Reich DL, ed. *Anesthesiology clinics of North America—anesthesia for the cardiac patient.* Philadelphia: WB Saunders, 1997:105–118.
11. **Sinfield A. The patient with cardiac trauma. In: Frost EAM, ed. *Preanesthetic assessment 4*. New York: The McMahon Group, 1994:168–183.**
12. Rossi NP, Lamberth WC Jr. Thoracic and pulmonary surgery. In: Liechty RD, Soper RT, eds. *Synopsis of surgery*. St. Louis: CV Mosby, 1985:337–338.

18. COAGULATION MANAGEMENT DURING AND AFTER CARDIOPULMONARY BYPASS

Linda Shore-Lesserson, Glenn P. Gravlee, and Jay C. Horrow

In essence, cardiopulmonary bypass (CPB) creates a blood "detour" to permit surgery on the heart. This detour must route the blood through an artificial heart and lung while maintaining its fluidity. Historically, fluidity represented the final frontier in the development of cardiac surgery, because effective mechanisms for blood gas exchange and for propelling the blood had been established more than a decade before surmounting the fluidity challenge. The challenge was to find a therapeutic approach that would inhibit blood's natural propensity to clot when it contacts foreign surfaces. Because the restoration of normal coagulation was desirable at the end of the surgical procedure, this clotting inhibition needed to be reversible, like turning a spigot on and off. The long-awaited solution was monumental: **anticoagulation with heparin followed by neutralization with protamine. This fundamental approach to establishing and reversing blood fluidity remains unchanged after almost 50 years,** although much fine-tuning has occurred. This chapter reviews anticoagulation and the restoration of coagulation in the patient undergoing CPB.

I. Physiology of blood clotting
A. Mechanisms of hemostasis
1. Plasma coagulation. Figure 18.1 depicts the plasma coagulation pathway. Blood contact with foreign surfaces classically was thought to activate the intrinsic pathway, whereas vascular injury or disruption was thought to activate the extrinsic pathway. These definitions seem counterintuitive, because vascular disruption should be intrinsic and foreign bodies extrinsic, but logic has held little sway in coagulation pathway nomenclature. Thankfully, distinctions between the intrinsic and extrinsic pathways have become less important, because both the activants and the pathways overlap (e.g., connection between VIIa and IXa). The coagulation factor numbering system was defined in order of discovery rather than use, which explains the illogical numerical progression through the pathways [1].
   a. Intrinsic pathway. Contact activation involves binding of factor XII to negatively charged surfaces, which leads to the common pathway through factors XI, IX, platelet factor 3, cofactor VIII, and calcium. Kallikrein also is formed in this reaction and serves as a positive feedback mechanism and as an initiator of fibrinolysis (a negative feedback mechanism) and inflammation.
   b. Extrinsic pathway. Tissue factor initiates the extrinsic pathway, which proceeds quickly to the common pathway with the aid of factor VII and calcium.
   c. Common pathway. Beginning with the assisted activation of factor X, this pathway proceeds to convert prothrombin (factor II) to thrombin and fibrinogen (factor I) to fibrin monomer, which initiates the actual substance of the clot. Fibrin monomer then cross-links to form a more stable clot with the aid of calcium and factor XIII.
   d. Thrombin is the most important enzyme in the pathway, because (in addition to activating fibrinogen) it
      (1) Provides positive feedback by activating cofactors V and VIII
      (2) Accelerates cross-linking of fibrinogen by activating factor XIII
      (3) Strongly stimulates platelet adhesion and aggregation
      (4) Facilitates clot resorption by releasing tissue plasminogen activator (tPA) from endothelial cells
      (5) Activates protein C, which provides negative feedback by inactivating factors Va and VIIIa
2. Platelet activation. As shown in Figure 18.1, a variety of stimuli initiate platelet activation, and thrombin is an especially potent one. This sets off a cascade of events that initiate platelet adhesion to endogenous or extracorporeal surfaces, followed by platelet aggregation and formation of a primary platelet plug. Fibrin clots and platelet plugs form simultaneously and mesh together, yielding a product more tenacious and difficult to dissolve than either alone.
   a. Von Willebrand factor (vWF) is essential to platelet adhesion, and fibrinogen is essential to platelet aggregation.
   b. Products released from platelet storage granules [adenosine diphosphate (ADP), epinephrine, calcium, thromboxane A_2, factor V, and vWF] serve to perpetuate platelet activation and the plasma coagulation cascade.

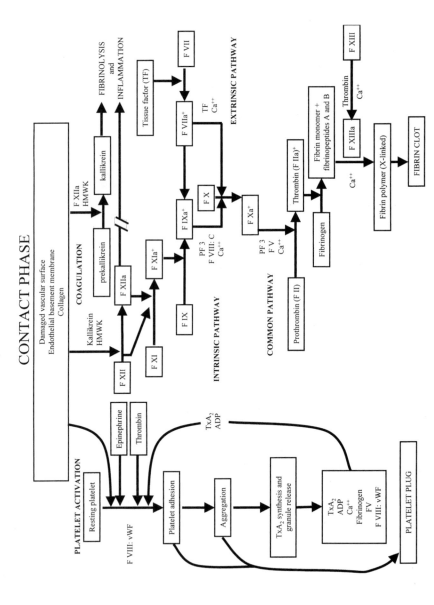

FIG. 18.1 Schematic representation of the hemostatic system depicting the vascular, platelet, and coagulation components.

3. Nature's system of checks and balances demands counterbalancing forces to discourage runaway clot formation and to dissolve clots. These counterbalances include the following:
   a. Proteins C and S, which inactivate factors Va and VIIIa
   b. Antithrombin III (ATIII), which inhibits thrombin as well as factors XIa, IXa, XIIa, and Xa
   c. Tissue factor inhibitor, which inhibits the initiation of the extrinsic pathway
   d. tPA, which is released from endothelium and converts plasminogen to plasmin, which in turn breaks down fibrin. Plasminogen activator inhibitor 1 in turn inhibits tPA to prevent uncontrolled fibrinolysis.

B. **Tests of hemostatic function**
   1. Table 18.1 lists commonly used tests of hemostatic function [1]. These tests may be used to detect hemostatic abnormalities preoperatively or after CPB. With the exception of the activated clotting time (ACT), typically they are not used during CPB except under extenuating circumstances, because most of them will be abnormal as a result of hemodilution, anticoagulation, and sometimes hypothermia.
      a. **Most studies suggest that routine preoperative hemostatic screening is not helpful in predicting patients who will bleed excessively during surgery.** If the patient's clinical history (e.g., nosebleeds; prolonged bleeding with small cuts, dental work, or surgery; easy bruising; strong family history of pathologic bleeding) suggests the need for hemostatic screening, selective use of these and other tests is appropriate. Similarly, when the patient is taking medications that alter hemostatic function, hemostatic function tests may be selectively indicated. Examples include the following:
         (1) Heparin: activated partial thromboplastin time (aPTT) or ACT
         (2) Low-molecular-weight heparin (LMWH): no test or anti-Xa heparin concentration
         (3) Warfarin: prothrombin time (PT) and/or international normalized ratio (INR)
         (4) Platelet inhibitors including aspirin: no testing, bleeding time, or platelet function tests

II. **Heparin anticoagulation**
A. **Heparin pharmacology [2]**
   1. Structure. As drugs go, heparin might be described as impure. Heparin resides physiologically in mast cells, and it is commercially derived most often from the lungs of cattle (bovine lung heparin) or the intestines of pigs (porcine mucosal heparin). Commercial preparations used for CPB typically include a range of molecular weights from 3,000 to 40,000 Da, with a mean molecular weight of approximately 15,000 Da. Each molecule is a heavily sulfated glycosaminoglycan polymer, so heparin is a strong biologic acid that is negatively charged at physiologic pH.
      a. Porcine mucosal and bovine lung heparin both are satisfactory for CPB and both have been widely used.
   2. Action. A specific pentasaccharide sequence that binds to ATIII is present on approximately 30% of heparin molecules. This binding potentiates the action of ATIII more than 1,000-fold, thereby allowing heparin to inhibit thrombin and factor Xa most importantly, but also factors IXa, XIa, and XIIa.
      a. **Inhibition of thrombin requires simultaneous binding of heparin to both ATIII and thrombin, whereas inhibition of factor Xa requires only that heparin bind to ATIII.** The former reaction limits thrombin inhibition to longer saccharide chains (18 or more saccharide units); hence, shorter chains can selectively inhibit Xa. This is the primary principle underlying therapy with LMWH.
         (1) Because thrombin inhibition is pivotal for CPB anticoagulation and because LMWH is poorly neutralized by protamine, LMWH is inadvisable as a CPB anticoagulant.

Table 18.1 Common clinical tests of hemostatic function

Test	Normal values	Comment
Platelets		
Platelet count	150,000–400,000/µL	Most widely accepted clinical test of platelet function;
Bleeding time (IVY)	<8 min	inconvenient; arms must be exposed
Coagulation system		
Whole blood clotting time (WBCT, Lee–White)	2.5–6 min	Prolonged by marked deficiencies in intrinsic system or final common pathway; formerly used to monitor heparin therapy
Activated clotting time (ACT)	Manual = 90–110 s Automated = 90–130 s^a = 100–140 s^b	Modified WBCT: commonly performed to monitor heparin in the operating room because of convenience
Prothrombin time (PT)	12–15 s; compare to control or INR 1.0–1.5	Tests extrinsic system and final common pathway; used to monitor warfarin anticoagulation
Activated partial thromboplastin time (aPTT)	35–45 s; compare to control	Tests intrinsic system and final common pathway; used to monitor heparin anticoagulation
Thrombin time	<14 s; compare to control	Tests final common pathway; prolonged by heparin, fibrinogen ≤100 mg/dL, abnormal fibrinogen and increased fibrin split products
Fibrinogen	250–500 mg/dL	Decreased in disseminated intravascular coagulation (DIC)
Fibrinolytic system		
Fibrin(ogen) split products	<10 µg/mL	Increased during fibrinolysis
d-Dimer	<0.5 µg/mL	Increased during fibrinolysis; specific assay of cross-linked fibrin degradation

^{a} Hemochron, International Technidyne, Edison, NJ, USA.
^{b} Medtronic, Hemo/Tec, Minneapolis, MN, USA.
^{c} INR, international normalized ratio.

    b. Heparin binds and activates cofactor II, a non–ATIII-dependent thrombin inhibitor. This may explain why heparin-induced anticoagulation can be effective even in the presence of marked ATIII deficiency, although the primary mechanism of action is ATIII inhibition.

3. Potency. Heparin potency is tested by measuring the anticoagulation effect in animal plasma. The United States Pharmacopoeia (USP) defines 1 unit of activity as the amount of heparin that maintains the fluidity of 1 mL of citrated sheep plasma for 1 hour after recalcification.

    a. Heparin dosing is best recorded in USP units, because commercial preparations vary in the number of USP units per milligram. The most common concentration is 100 units/mg (1,000 units/mL) [3].

4. Pharmacokinetics. **After central venous administration, heparin's effect peaks within 1 minute, and there is a small redistribution effect that most often is clinically insignificant** [4,5].

    a. Heparin's large molecular size and its polarity essentially limit its distribution to the intravascular space and endothelial cells.

    b. The onset of CPB increases circulating blood volume by approximately 1,500 mL; hence, plasma heparin concentration drops proportionately with the onset of CPB unless heparin is added to the CPB priming solution.

    c. Heparin can be eliminated by the kidneys or by metabolism in the reticuloendothelial system.

    d. Elimination half-life has been determined only by bioassay, i.e., by the time course of clotting time prolongation. By this standard, heparin's elimination time is dose dependent [6]. At lower doses, such as 100 to 150 USP units/kg, elimination half-time is approximately 1 hour. At CPB doses of 300 to 400 USP units/kg, elimination half-time is 2 or more hours; hence, clinically significant anticoagulation might persist for 4 to 6 hours in the absence of neutralization by protamine. Hypothermia and probably CPB itself prolong elimination.

5. Side effects. Heparin's actions on the hemostatic system extend beyond its primary anticoagulant mechanism to include activation of tPA, platelet activation, and enhancement of tissue factor pathway inhibitor.

    a. Lipoprotein lipase activation influences plasma lipid concentrations, which indirectly affects the plasma concentrations of lipid-soluble drugs.

    b. Heparin boluses decrease systemic vascular resistance. Typically this effect is small (10% to 20%), but rarely it can be more impressive and may merit treatment with a vasopressor or calcium chloride.

    c. Anaphylaxis rarely occurs.

    d. Heparin-induced thrombocytopenia (HIT) is covered elsewhere in this chapter.

B. Dosing and monitoring

  1. Dosing. The initial dose for CPB is 300 to 400 USP units/kg.

    a. Because heparin distributes primarily into the plasma compartment, increasing the dose with increasing body weight assumes that plasma volume increases in direct proportion to body weight. This is not the case, because fat does not require blood volume in proportion to weight. Consequently, there is seldom reason to exceed an initial dose of 35,000 to 40,000 units, even in patients weighing more than 100 kg, as lean body mass tends to peak at 90 kg for females and 110 kg for males.

    b. Heparin dosing for coronary revascularization procedures performed without CPB is controversial. Published doses range from 100 to 300 units/kg, but most centers use 100 to 150 units/kg and set minimum acceptable ACT values at 200 seconds.

    c. **The CPB priming solution should contain heparin at approximately the same concentration as that of the patient's bloodstream at the onset of CPB.** Because this most often would be 3 to 4 USP units/mL, a priming volume of 1,500 mL should contain at least 5,000 units of heparin. CPB priming solutions commonly contain 5,000 to 10,000 units of heparin.

    d. Supplemental heparin doses typically are guided by monitoring of anticoagulation.

2. **Monitoring.** Until the late 1970s, heparin dosing was guided by experiential practices and varied a great deal from hospital to hospital. Using ACT, a variation on the Lee–White clotting time, **Bull et al. [7] identified rather staggering variations in the approach to heparin dosing and in both the initial anticoagulant response and the time course of anticoagulation in response to a fixed dose of heparin.** This landmark work rapidly led to the realization that the anticoagulant response to heparin should be monitored, although a few centers continue to dose heparin empirically.

3. **Approaches to anticoagulation monitoring for CPB. The ACT is the most widely used test,** although some centers monitor blood heparin concentration as well.

   a. ACT uses an activant such as celite or kaolin to activate clotting, then measures the clotting time in a test tube. Heparin prolongs ACT with a roughly linear dose–response pattern (Fig. 18.2). Normal ACT depends upon the

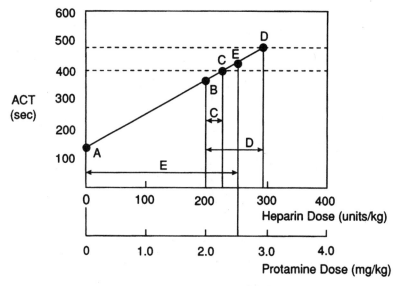

FIG. 18.2 Graph of a heparin (and protamine) dosing algorithm. In the graph, the control activated clotting time (*ACT*) is shown as *point A* and the ACT resulting from an initial heparin bolus of 200 units/kg is shown in *point B.* The line connecting *A* and *B* then is extrapolated and a desired ACT is selected. *Point C* represents the intersection between this line and a target ACT of 400 seconds, theoretically requiring an additional heparin dose represented by the difference between points *C* and *B* on the *horizontal axis* (*arrow C*). Similarly, to achieve an ACT of 480 seconds (*higher horizontal dotted line* intersecting the ACT versus heparin dose line at *point D*), one would administer the additional heparin dose represented by *arrow D.* To estimate heparin level and calculate protamine dose at the time of heparin neutralization, the most recently measured ACT value is plotted on the dose–response line (*point E* in the example). The heparin level present theoretically is represented by the difference between *point E* and *point A* on the *horizontal axis* (*arrow E*). The protamine dose required to neutralize the remaining heparin then may be calculated. Protamine 1.0 mg/kg is administered for every 100 units/kg of heparin present. (Modified from Bull BS, Huse WM, Brauer FS, et al. Heparin therapy during extracorporeal circulation: II. The use of a dose-response curve to individualize heparin and protamine dosage. *J Thorac Cardiovasc Surg* 1975;69:686; and Gravlee GP. Anticoagulation for cardiopulmonary bypass. In: Gravlee GP, Davis RF, Kurusz M, et al., eds. *Cardiopulmonary bypass: principles and practice,* 2nd ed. Philadelphia: Lippincott Williams & Wilkins, 2000:435–472, with permission.)

specific test and upon operator technique, but generally falls between 110 and 140 seconds.

b. Although originally described as a manual test, most centers now use one of two automated approaches to ACT (International Technidyne, Edison, NJ, U.S.A., or Medtronic HemoTec, Minneapolis, MN, U.S.A.). The two automated approaches yield slightly different values both at baseline and with anticoagulation because of different activators and endpoint detection techniques.

c. ACT is prolonged by hypothermia and hemodilution; hence, conditions often imposed by CPB alter the ACT-heparin dose–response relationship [8]. Some see this as risking underanticoagulation, whereas others see the hemodilution and hypothermia as legitimate anticoagulant aids.

d. The target ACT level for CPB is controversial. There is evidence supporting the safety of ACT values as low as 300 seconds, yet some centers accept only values exceeding 480 seconds.

    (1) As a clotting test, ACT is somewhat crude and may vary as much as 10% on repeated testing at heparin concentrations used for CPB [9], so it seems reasonable to build in a safety margin by accepting 400 seconds as a safe threshold for sustained CPB.

    (2) Aprotinin complicates the use of ACT, as indicated by marked prolongation of celite ACTs in the presence of heparin and aprotinin. This may represent enhanced anticoagulation to some degree, but in the presence of aprotinin it probably is wise to titrate heparin to a celite ACT level exceeding 750 seconds or to use a kaolin ACT instead. Kaolin ACT levels of 400 seconds appear safe, although higher levels probably are needed at deep levels of hypothermia (less than 25°C).

e. Whole blood heparin concentrations can be measured during CPB. The most commonly used technique is automated protamine titration (Medtronic HemoTec). Advocates of this monitoring technique argue that CPB-induced distortion of the ACT-heparin dose–response relationship mandates maintenance of the heparin concentration originally needed before CPB to achieve the target ACT level [10]. This approach substantially increases the amount of heparin given during CPB, which enhances suppression of thrombin formation. This benefit may accrue at the expense of more profound platelet activation that may aggravate and prolong platelet dysfunction after CPB.

    (1) Whole blood heparin concentrations of 3.0 to 4.0 units/mL most often are sufficient for CPB.

    (2) A drawback to monitoring heparin concentration is that patients vary in their sensitivity to heparin-induced anticoagulation; therefore, isolated use of heparin concentration could lead to dangerous underanticoagulation. If this technique is chosen, simultaneous use of ACT or another clotting time is strongly advised.

    (3) Heparin concentration monitoring may be a useful adjunct in the presence of aprotinin, especially when celite ACTs are being used.

    (4) Heparin concentration monitoring may be advantageous in selecting a protamine dose, because the dose will be chosen in relation to approximate actual blood heparin concentration. The weakness of this technique is its dependence on a calculated blood volume determination at a time when blood volume may vary substantially.

f. Other monitors of anticoagulation. Neither ACT nor heparin concentration is perfect, so other tests have been evaluated or are under investigation. aPTT and traditional thrombin time are so sensitive to heparin that those tests are not useful at the heparin concentrations needed for CPB. Detailed description of other tests are beyond the scope of this chapter. Tests under consideration include high-dose thrombin time (International Technidyne) and heparin management test (HMT; Cardiovascular Diagnostics, Raleigh, NC, U.S.A.).

C. Heparin resistance. Heparin resistance is loosely defined as the need for greater than expected heparin doses to achieve the target ACT for CPB. As noted earlier, ACT prolongation in response to heparin varies greatly. A number of factors that may decrease the ACT response to heparin are listed in Table 18.2 [2]. ATIII deficiency is blamed most often for heparin resistance and it does cause this phenomenon, but overall the correlation between ATIII concentrations and anticoagulant response to a bolus of heparin has been weak and inconsistent, perhaps because heparin resistance often is multifactorial.

   1. Clinical approach. **Most often heparin resistance can be managed by simply giving more heparin.** It is reasonable to consider administering supplemental ATIII if more than 600 USP units/kg has been required to reach the target ACT level. Similarly, if maintaining the target ACT during CPB requires administering more than 100 USP units/kg per 30 minutes of CPB, supplemental ATIII seems reasonable.

      a. ATIII can be provided in the form of fresh frozen plasma (FFP), liquid plasma, and ATIII concentrates.
         (1) FFP or liquid plasma dose typically is 2 to 4 units in adults.
         (2) For ATIII concentrates, an initial dose of 1,000 units often is sufficient.

D. Heparin-induced thrombocytopenia
   1. **HIT develops in 5% to 28% of patients receiving heparin and is marked by a fall in platelet count after exposure to heparin.** This results from heparin's proaggregatory effect on platelets. HIT is commonly categorized into two subtypes.
      a. HIT type I has a rapid onset (2 to 5 days) and is characterized by a mild decrease in platelet count without thrombosis or immune response.
      b. HIT type II is considerably more severe, most often occurs after more than 5 days of heparin administration (average onset time, 9 days), and is immune mediated. Antibody binding to the complex formed between heparin and platelet factor 4 (PF4) is responsible for the syndrome. Antibody binding to platelets and endothelial cells causes platelet activation, endothelial injury, and complement activation. The platelet clots formed are referred to in lay terms as "white clots." This syndrome is highly morbid and can be fatal.
         (1) **Among patients who develop HIT II, the incidence of thrombosis approximates 20%, the mortality of which can be as high as 40%.**
         (2) Diagnosis: demonstration of heparin-induced aggregation of platelets
            (a) Heparin-induced serotonin release assay: a functional test, often considered the "gold standard"

Table 18.2 Potential causes of heparin resistance

Hypercoagulable states	Drugs
1. Antithrombin III deficiency	1. Heparin
A. familial	2. Nitroglycerin[a]
B. acquired	**Protein binding**
2. Arteriosclerotic disease	1. Acid glycoprotein
A. unstable angina pectoris	2. Histidine-rich glycoprotein
3. Septicemia	3. Immunoglobulins
A. bacterial endocarditis	**Other**
4. Pregnancy	1. Neonates
5. Heparin-induced thrombocytopenia	2. Elderly patients
6. Thrombocytosis	

[a] Controversial cause. Probably not clinically significant.
Modified from Shore-Lesserson L, Gravlee GP. Anticoagulation for cardiopulmonary bypass. In: Gravlee GP, Davis RF, Kurusz M, et al., eds. *Cardiopulmonary bypass principles and practice.* Philadelphia: Lippincott, Williams & Wilkins, 2000: 456.

(b) Heparin-induced platelet activation assay: a functional test, may be nonspecific

(c) Enzyme-linked immunosorbent assay (ELISA) specific for the heparin/PF4 complex or for PF4 alone: patients with a positive antibody test do *not* always develop thrombosis. Antibodies associated with HIT often become undetectable 50 to 85 days after discontinuing heparin. The clinical syndrome does not always recur upon reexposure to the drug and sometimes resolves despite continued drug therapy. HIT can be associated with heparin resistance and thus should be in the differential diagnosis.

(3) Treatments for HIT and alternative anticoagulant sources

(a) Change tissue source, plasmapheresis, LMWH, heparinoids, heparin plus platelet inhibitors, hirudin, argatroban, and ancrod (see Section **E**).

(b) If heparin can be discontinued for a few weeks to months, often the antibody will disappear and allow a brief period of heparinization for CPB without complication.

E. Alternatives to unfractionated heparin

1. LMWH (shorter-chain heparin molecules). Intravenously administered LMWH has a half-life at least twice as long as that of unfractionated heparin and possibly several times as long for some LMWH compounds. Problems in CPB arise from the fact that protamine neutralization only reverses the factor IIa inhibition and leaves the predominant factor Xa inhibition intact. LMWH therapy also complicates heparin monitoring because aPTT (and presumably ACT) is much less sensitive to Xa inhibition and will not accurately measure the full anticoagulant effect. Factor Xa inhibition can be measured, but not with a simple bedside test. In HIT, LMWHs cross-react with heparin/PF4 complex antibodies. Reactivity of the particular LMWH with the patient's platelets should be confirmed *in vitro*.

2. Heparinoids. Two glycosaminoglycans with heparin-like properties are available for clinical use: dermatan sulfate and danaparoid (Org 10172). They are referred to as heparinoids because they represent a class of synthetic or naturally occurring heparin analogues. Danaparoid is a natural composite of heparan sulfate (80%), dermatan sulfate (20%), and chondroitin sulfates. They have been used successfully in CPB when heparin use was contraindicated.

3. Hirudin [11]
   a. Thrombin inhibitor isolated from the salivary glands of the medicinal leech (*Hirudo medicinalis*)
   b. Independent of ATIII and inhibits clot-bound thrombin
   c. Inhibits thrombin activation of protein C
   d. Hirudin is a small molecule (molecular weight 7 kDa) that is eliminated by the kidney and is easily filtered at the end of CPB.
   e. r-Hirudin dose: 0.25 mg/kg bolus and an infusion to maintain the hirudin concentration at 2.5 μg/mL as determined by ecarin clotting time
   f. Ecarin clotting time: a card for use in the TAS analyzer (Cardiovascular Diagnostics) analyzer has been used in large series of HIT patients [12].
   g. r-Hirudin–treated patients maintain platelet counts and hemoglobin levels and have few bleeding complications, if renal function is normal.

4. Bivalirudin (Hirulog)
   a. Shorter half-life and wider therapeutic window than hirudin
   b. Synthetic polypeptide that directly inhibits thrombin by binding simultaneously to its active catalytic site and its substrate recognition site
   c. Dose during interventional procedures: 1.0 mg/kg bolus followed by a 2.5 mg/kg/hour infusion, yielding a median ACT of 346 seconds
   d. Clearance through renal elimination and proteolysis
   e. Studies in interventional procedures suggest lower bleeding rates than unfractionated heparin (UFH) and similar efficacy.

   5. Argatroban. A direct thrombin inhibitor that is approved by the U.S. Food and Drug Administration (FDA) for anticoagulation in HIT patients but not yet approved for use in CPB. Clinical trials are in progress.
   6. Other direct thrombin inhibitors, such as melagatran, are investigational. They are not FDA approved for CPB or other use.
   7. Ancrod
      a. Derived from Malayan pit viper venom
      b. Lyses fibrinogen
      c. Stimulates release of tPA from the vascular endothelium
      d. Elimination half-life is 3 to 5 hours
      e. Goal of safe CPB anticoagulation (plasma fibrinogen concentration 0.4 to 0.8 g/L) takes at least 12 hours
      f. Restoration of plasma coagulation after CPB requires FFP and cryoprecipitate

III. Neutralization of heparin
   A. Protamine pharmacology. Protamine, commercially prepared from fish sperm, was first used clinically in combination with insulin to delay absorption and prolong its effect. When an attempt was made to combine protamine with heparin to achieve a similar delay, it was found to inactivate heparin instead. The combination of a strongly cationic substance (protamine) with a strongly anionic substance (heparin) produces a stable complex that is devoid of anticoagulant activity. **Heparin–protamine interaction occurs in proportion to weight. One milligram of protamine neutralizes 1 mg of heparin** [13].
   B. Protamine dose. Because protamine appears to distribute within the circulatory system as heparin does, the protamine dose required to neutralize a given dose of heparin equals the number of milligrams of heparin remaining in the patient's circulation at the time of neutralization. Clinical protocols for determining an initial dose of protamine are based on an estimation of blood heparin concentration and blood volume. Direct assay of heparin concentration is expensive and unnecessary. Indirect assay using protamine effect *in vitro* is more accurate than ratio-based estimates and is easily performed.
      1. Empiric ratio to heparin administered. Most clinicians choose a dose of protamine based on the number of units of heparin administered (milligrams of protamine to units of heparin, assuming that 1 mg of protamine will neutralize 100 units of heparin). **Clinical efficacy has been documented using a ratio as low as 0.6 mg protamine to 100 units of heparin administered.** Most centers choose a ratio of 1 mg of protamine to 100 units of heparin. Initial doses using this ratio or the dose–response method (see Section **III.B.2**) result in a mild-to-moderate protamine excess relative to heparin that ensures total neutralization and minimizes the likelihood of subsequent heparin rebound. Doses exceeding 1 mg/100 units tend to be excessive and may increase bleeding.
         a. For example, consider a patient who received 25,000 units of heparin before CPB, with no subsequent heparin required, and 5,000 units in the bypass pump prime. If the entire contents of the pump are returned after bypass to the patient, the ratio of 1:100 would result in 300 mg of protamine as the neutralizing dose. If the pump contents are not returned or if the cells only are returned after washing, the dose would be slightly more than 250 mg, as the cell washing virtually eliminates heparin. A ratio of 0.6 to 0.75 mg to 100 USP units would result in 180 mg of protamine as the neutralizing dose, and this would be reasonable as a starting point if CPB has lasted for more than 1 hour, as some heparin would be excreted or metabolized in that time frame.
      2. Estimated from heparin dose response. Another method for calculating protamine dose is to extrapolate the dose from a heparin dose–response curve previously constructed (Fig. 18.2). This method estimates the existing heparin concentration in terms of its activity at the time of reversal in units of heparin per kilogram. Using an arbitrary ratio of protamine to heparin (e.g., 1 mg of protamine to 100 units of heparin) then determines the protamine dose. Note that both the assumption of a linear relationship between heparin dose and

ACT prolongation, and extrapolation of the line beyond the measured endpoints degrade the predictive ability of this technique.

3. Calculated from *in vitro* protamine effect. The Hemochron protamine dose assay (PDA) measures the effect of a predetermined quantity of protamine on circulating heparin using the Hemochron celite ACT. Shortly before protamine is to be given, a standard ACT (ACTs) is measured simultaneously with a special ACT, the PDA (ACTp). When filled with 2 mL of blood, the ACTp tube adds 20 μg/mL of protamine so that the resultant clotting time is at least partially neutralized. The protamine dose then can be easily calculated.

  a. Note that this technique assumes linearity and may extrapolate.

C. **Protamine administration.** Always administer protamine slowly. The rate of administration is more important than the route of administration in preventing adverse hemodynamic effects (see Section **III.E.1**). One can either use a syringe or dilute the drug in a small volume of intravenous fluid and infuse by gravity or calibrated pump. Because the syringe technique results in multiple boluses, restricting its use to doses less than 1 mg/kg, or 20 mg in any 60-second period, appears advisable.

  1. The injected dose of protamine cannot neutralize heparin bound to plasma proteins or within endothelial cells. Release of heparin from these stored areas after initial protamine administration may result in reappearance of heparin anticoagulant effect (heparin rebound). Small additional doses of protamine will provide neutralization when repeat testing shows a heparin effect in a bleeding patient.

D. **Monitoring heparin neutralization**

  1. ACT. After protamine administration, the ACT test should return a value no more than 10% above the value before heparin administration. If more prolonged, residual heparin activity is likely. An ACT value that remains prolonged despite additional protamine suggests a technical error or, less commonly, some other hemostatic abnormality.

  2. Protamine titration. Protamine titration yields a qualitative or semiquantitative value for the circulating concentration of residual heparin. Because protamine has anticoagulant properties *in vitro,* it prolongs the coagulation time of normal blood in test tubes.

  3. Automated protamine titration. This test can be performed manually or by using an automated ACT device (Medtronic HemoTec).

E. **Adverse Effects [14].**

  1. **Hypotension from rapid administration. Administration of a neutralizing dose of protamine (about 3 mg/kg) over 3 minutes or more quickly decreases both systemic and pulmonary pressures as well as venous return.** This predictable response may be blunted, but not predictably avoided, by volume loading. Release of vasoactive compounds from mast cells or other sites may be responsible for this adverse response.

  2. Anaphylactoid reactions. Although protamine is a foreign protein, immune responses occur infrequently following exposure so that true allergy to protamine is uncommon. Table 18.3 lists those patients at potential risk.

Table 18.3 Patients at potential risk for true allergy to protamine

Condition	Risk increase
Prior reaction to protamine	189-fold
Allergy to true (vertebrate) fish	24.5-fold
Exposure to NPH insulin	8.2-fold
Allergy to any drug	3.0-fold
Prior exposure to protamine	No increase!

Adapted from Kimmel SE, et al. *J Am Coll Card* 1998;32:1916.

      3. Pulmonary vasoconstriction. Occasionally, protamine increases pulmonary arterial pressure, resulting in right ventricular failure, decreased cardiac output, and systemic hypotension. Formation of large heparin–protamine complexes may stimulate production of thromboxane by pulmonary macrophages, causing vasoconstriction.

      4. Antihemostatic effects. Protamine activates thrombin receptors on platelets, causing partial activation and subsequent impairment of platelet aggregation. Transient thrombocytopenia also occurs in the first hour after a full neutralizing dose of protamine.

  F. Treatment of adverse protamine reactions. Systemic hypotension within 10 minutes of protamine administration suggests protamine as the cause. Specific treatment depends on other hemodynamic events.

      1. Normal or low pulmonary pressures suggest either rapid administration or an anaphylactoid reaction. Rapid fluid administration alone often suffices to treat the former, whereas the latter cause usually requires aggressive volume resuscitation, large doses of epinephrine, and possibly other vasoactive compounds and inhaled bronchodilators. Refer to other sources for the treatment of acute anaphylaxis, including use of systemic steroids.

      2. High pulmonary pressures suggest a pulmonary vasoconstriction reaction. Inotropes with pulmonary dilating properties, such as isoproterenol or milrinone, will support the failing heart while facilitating movement of blood across the pulmonary circulation. With extreme hemodynamic deterioration, reinstitution of CPB may be necessary. In this case, give a full heparin dose (at least 300 units/kg). Occasionally, heparin alone will correct the pulmonary hypertension (presumably by breaking up large heparin–protamine complexes, the putative stimulant to thromboxane production) so that CPB no longer becomes necessary.

  G. Prevention of adverse responses

      1. Rate of administration. Always administer fully neutralizing doses of protamine slowly (minimum duration 3 minutes). Rather than depend on volume loading to prevent hypotension, just dilute the drug and give it slowly. Place the calculated dose in 50 mL or more of clear fluid and connect a small-drop (approximately 60 drops/mL) administration set to limit the infusion rate.

      2. Route of administration. The preponderance of evidence suggests that peripheral vein infusion offers no benefit over central venous infusion as long as the infusion is dilute and not rapid. Injection directly into the aorta provides no reliable protection and risks introduction of embolic material, such as small bubbles, pieces of rubber stopper, or glass.

      3. High-risk subgroups. Patients without previous exposure to protamine, including those with diabetes or prior vasectomy, require no special measures before initial exposure. **Even patients who have received protamine-containing insulin preparations rarely develop an adverse response.** Only patients with a prior history of an adverse response to protamine warrant special treatment. See Table 18.3 for the relative risks of protamine administration to these subgroups.

      4. Prior protamine reaction. Prepare a special, dilute protamine solution of about 1 mg in 100 mL and administer over 10 minutes. If no adverse response occurs, administer the fully neutralizing dose as described earlier. Skin tests taken before giving protamine provide little predictive value and frequently are falsely positive. Special immunologic tests for protamine allergy [radioallergosorbent test (RAST), ELISA] also demonstrate many false-positive results.

  H. Alternatives to protamine

      1. Allow heparin's effect to dissipate. This approach results in continued hemorrhage with massive transfusion requirements and bouts of hypovolemia and consumptive coagulopathy. Although this may be the only option available, ideally it should be avoided.

      2. Platelet concentrates. PF4 is released from activated platelets. It combines with and neutralizes heparin. However, platelet concentrates do not effectively restore coagulation following CPB, so this approach is not recommended.

3. Hexadimethrine. This synthetic polycation, no longer readily available in the United States because of renal toxicity, can avoid true allergic reactions to protamine. However, like protamine, it forms complexes with heparin that can incite pulmonary vasoconstriction if administered quickly.
4. Methylene blue. Even large doses do not effectively restore the ACT. However, inhibition of nitric oxide synthetase can incite pulmonary hypertension, so this approach is not recommended.
5. Investigational substances. Recombinant PF4 showed initial promise, but its development was abandoned. "Designer" polycation molecules, which retain neutralizing ability while adverse responses have been "engineered" out, show some promise for the future. Lactoferrin, a large human protein produced in copious amounts in cow's milk by transgenic means, displays only a modest neutralizing ability. Heparinase I, an enzyme produced by harmless soil bacteria, shows initial promise and at the time of this writing remains in late-stage clinical trials.

IV. **Hemostatic abnormalities in the cardiac surgical patient** [1,15]
   A. **Management of the patient taking preoperative antithrombotic drugs.** Table 18.4 lists commonly used antithrombotic drugs and their mechanisms of action.
      1. Anticoagulant therapy. Patients receiving warfarin anticoagulant medications should be advised to discontinue the medication 3 to 4 days before the anticipated cardiac surgery. Generally an INR value less than 2 is considered an acceptable recovery of vitamin K-dependent clotting factors. In fact, some residual

Table 18.4 Common antithrombotic drugs

Drug	Mechanism	Clinical uses
Heparin	Antithrombin III agonist, anti-Xa and anti-IIa	Deep vein thrombosis, atrial fibrillation, unstable angina, surgical, extracorporeal circulation, heart valve, shunts
Low-molecular-weight heparin	Antithrombin III agonist, anti-Xa	Deep vein thrombosis, unstable angina
Warfarin	Inhibit production of vitamin K-dependent coagulation factors	Deep vein thrombosis, atrial fibrillation, heart valve
Acetylsalicylic acid (aspirin)	Inhibit cyclooxygenase, inhibit thromboxane, prevent platelet activation	Atherosclerotic cardiovascular disease, cerebrovascular disease, percutaneous coronary intervention
Dipyridamole	Adenosine enhancing, inhibit thromboxane	Peripheral vascular disease
Abciximab	Glycoprotein IIb IIIa receptor antagonist (monoclonal antibody)	Percutaneous coronary intervention, stent
Eptifibatide	Glycoprotein IIb IIIa receptor antagonist (small peptide)	Percutaneous coronary intervention, stent
Tirofiban	Glycoprotein IIb IIIa receptor antagonist (nonpeptide)	Percutaneous coronary intervention, stent
Ticlopidine	Thienopyridine, ADP receptor antagonist	Percutaneous coronary intervention, stent, cerebrovascular disease
Clopidogrel	Thienopyridine, ADP receptor antagonist	Percutaneous coronary intervention, stent

ADP, adenosine diphosphate.

inhibition of the extrinsic coagulation pathway advantageously accentuates anti-coagulation for CPB. If anticoagulation is so vitally important that it must be maintained until the time of surgery, an intravenous infusion of heparin may be started preoperatively. Heparin may be discontinued a few hours before surgery or continued into the operative period.

2. Antiplatelet therapy

   a. Aspirin. Many studies support the use of aspirin in the prevention of thrombosis in coronary and cerebral vascular disease. Patients taking aspirin therapy who are undergoing cardiac surgery have a propensity for increased bleeding postoperatively; however, the benefits of aspirin therapy, weighed against a potential for bleeding, often leads to preoperative continuation of aspirin therapy. Most patients do not bleed excessively with this approach. An increase in bleeding, if it exists, is not accompanied by an increase in transfusion requirements due to blood conservation strategies in use.

   b. Glycoprotein IIb/IIIa (GPIIb-IIIa) inhibitors. The GPIIb-IIIa receptor is the platelet fibrinogen receptor, which causes fibrinogen bridging and subsequent platelet aggregation. GPIIb-IIIa inhibitors inhibit platelet aggregation and have been increasingly used during interventional cardiology procedures. Their beneficial effects include reductions in mortality and cardiac events after angioplasty and stent procedures. However, there is strong potential for hemorrhagic complications if the patients present for emergent cardiac surgery. Currently the three intravenous GPIIb-IIIa inhibitors in clinical use are abciximab, tirofiban, and eptifibatide. Abciximab (ReoPro; Centocor, Malvern, PA, U.S.A.) is a monoclonal antibody to the GPIIb-IIIa receptor that stoichiometrically inhibits fibrinogen binding. Tirofiban and eptifibatide are receptor blockers whose effects are reversible after discontinuation of therapy. Their short duration of action may mitigate some perioperative bleeding complications [16].

   c. ADP receptor inhibitors. The thienopyridine derivatives ticlopidine (Ticlid; Sanofi, New York, NY, U.S.A.) and clopidogrel (Plavix; Sanofi) noncompetitively antagonize at a platelet ADP receptor known as the P2T receptor. Blockade of this receptor by ticlopidine or clopidogrel elevates cyclic adenosine monophosphate levels to induce profound and rapid platelet disaggregation. Ticlopidine has generally been replaced by clopidogrel because of fewer side effects with the latter [17]. Antiplatelet activity endures for the life span of the platelet because the P2T receptor is permanently altered. Clopidogrel and aspirin are synergistic; hence, this therapeutic combination may lead to excessive postoperative bleeding.

B. **Abnormalities acquired during cardiac surgery**

   1. Endothelial dysfunction. Contact of blood with extracorporeal surfaces initiates a "total body inflammatory response" characterized by activation of coagulation, fibrinolysis, and inflammation. This leads to an abnormal cellular–endothelial interaction.

   2. Persistent heparin effect. This is uncommon, because most clinicians fully neutralize the administered heparin.

   3. Platelet abnormalities (Table 18.5)

      a. Thrombocytopenia occurs frequently after CPB due to dilution of the blood volume with extracorporeal circuit volume and to platelet consumption or sequestration. This thrombocytopenia can be severe (less than 50,000/μL) but, in the absence of other hemostasis abnormalities, often does not lead to excessive bleeding. With modern techniques, platelet counts after CPB most often exceed 100,000/μL.

      b. Platelet dysfunction. **The most prevalent yet elusive cause of hemostatic abnormalities after CPB is platelet dysfunction.** Platelets are rendered inactive by contact activation from the extracorporeal surfaces, hypothermia, receptor down-regulation, and by heparin and protamine. Heparin activates platelets to render them less functional after CPB, and protamine depresses platelet function.

Table 18.5 Causes of platelet dysfunction in cardiac surgery

CPB-related causes
Hypothermia
Materials-induced activation
Trauma-induced activation (cardiotomy suction)
Fibrinolysis
Glycoprotein Ib receptor down-regulation
Glycoprotein IIb/IIIa receptor down-regulation/destruction
Thrombin receptor down-regulation/destruction
Drug-related causes
Heparin
Nitrates
Phosphodiesterase inhibitors
Protamine

4. Coagulopathy. Hemodilution and consumption of coagulation factors by microvascular coagulation combine to cause the deficiencies of coagulation seen after CPB. Despite the use of large doses of heparin, contact activation causes microvascular activation of factor XII and initiates the intrinsic pathway of coagulation.

5. Fibrinolysis. Fibrinolysis can be primary or secondary during CPB (Fig. 18.3). Primary fibrinolysis occurs from release of endothelial plasminogen activators. Secondary fibrinolysis describes activation of plasmin as a result of a feedback response to fibrin formation. Circulating plasmin degradation products adversely affect platelet function.

6. Pharmacology. As noted earlier, heparin and protamine impair platelet function. Other drugs commonly used during CPB (milrinone, nitroglycerin, nitroprusside) adversely affect platelet function *in vitro,* but their clinical implications remain unknown.

7. Hypothermia. Hypothermia impairs the enzymatic cascades of the coagulation pathway. Platelets are activated during mild hypothermia and are depressed during moderate-to-severe hypothermia.

C. **Pharmacologic prophylaxis**

1. Platelet protection

   a. Antifibrinolytic agents. See **IV.C.2.**

   b. Coated surfaces. Heparin-bonded circuits attenuate the inflammatory response to CPB and may confer some platelet protective properties.

2. Antifibrinolytic agents [18]

   a. Synthetic antifibrinolytic agents: ε-aminocaproic acid (EACA) and tranexamic acid (TA). EACA and TA act as lysine analogues that bind to the lysine-binding sites of plasmin and plasminogen (Fig. 18.3). TA is a more potent analogue of EACA that has a higher affinity for plasminogen than does EACA. Fibrin degradation products inhibit platelet function. Thus, plasmin inhibition may protect platelets. **The benefits of EACA and TA have been demonstrated, especially in high-risk cardiac surgery, and are most obvious when these agents are used prophylactically (i.e., initiated before CPB and maintained throughout CPB).** *Dosing:* EACA 100 to 150 mg/kg bolus, 10 to 15 mg/kg/hour, *or* 4 to 6 g bolus, 1 g/hour. Recent reports suggest constant plasma activity may be best achieved with smaller initial boluses (approximately 50 mg/kg) followed by higher maintenance doses (20 to 25 mg/kg/hour). *Dosing range:* TA 10 to 20 mg/kg bolus, 1 to 2 mg/kg/hr, *or* 5-g bolus, repeat bolus to total 15 g. The latter dosing scheme probably is much higher than necessary, but it is preferred in some centers.

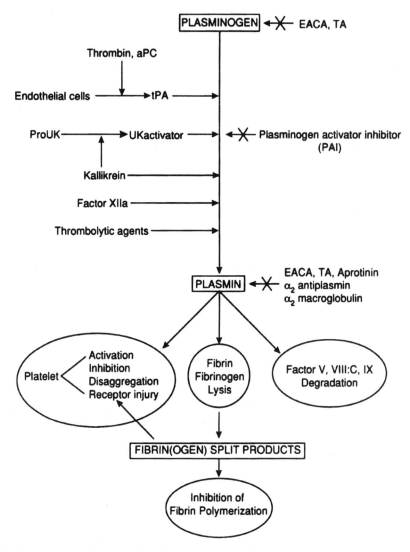

FIG. 18.3 Schematic diagram of the fibrinolytic system displaying endogenous and exogenous activators and inhibitors of fibrinolysis. The antihemostatic actions of plasmin and fibrin(ogen) split products (FSPs) are illustrated. *aPC,* activated protein C; *EACA,* ε-aminocaproic acid; *TA,* tranexamic acid; *tPA,* tissue plasminogen activator; *UK,* urokinase.

   b. Aprotinin is a high-molecular-weight proteinase inhibitor of bovine origin
      that inhibits plasmin, kallikrein, and other serine proteases. Aprotinin is
      effective in minimizing activation of the hematologic system during CPB
      and in preventing fibrinolysis. **Like EACA and TA, it reduces peri-
      operative blood loss and transfusion. Under most circumstances,
      its use does not appear to be superior in this context to the use of
      EACA or TA.**

Full Hammersmith dose regimen: 2 million kallikrein-inhibiting units (KIU) as a bolus, 2 million KIU added to the pump prime, and 500,000 KIU/hour as an infusion. It is effective in primary and repeat cardiac surgery. Beneficial effects have been documented using half Hammersmith doses; however, these beneficial effects may be less consistent and have been less frequently documented. In the future, it seems likely that aprotinin dosing may be based on patient weight instead of the more traditional empiric Hammersmith and half-Hammersmith protocols.

3. Accurate heparin and protamine dosing. Attempts to individualize heparin and protamine doses in order to minimize bleeding rely on patient-specific doses of each drug based on patient sensitivity. A number of different heparin and protamine management strategies have been reported to result in reduced perioperative bleeding.

   a. Higher heparin concentrations have been associated with increased mediastinal tube bleeding postoperatively, possibly due to heparin rebound or platelet dysfunction. This leads to the practice of giving just enough heparin to maintain a "threshold" minimum acceptable ACT.

   b. Some investigators postulate that higher heparin levels allow for reduced activation of the coagulation cascade and may blunt the consumptive coagulopathy that occurs with microvascular coagulation. This leads to the practice of maintaining heparin at a specific concentration in the blood, which leads to large doses of heparin and high ACTs. Heparin management strategies are still being investigated.

   c. Lower protamine doses have been used successfully to neutralize heparin after CPB and have been associated with reduced bleeding and transfusion requirements. This relationship between higher heparin and lower protamine doses has been suggested to result in less postoperative bleeding.

4. Inhibition of inflammation

   a. Coated surfaces. Heparin-bonded CPB circuits make the extracorporeal circuit more biocompatible and thus effectively attenuate the inflammatory response to CPB. Despite this benefit, use of these circuits has not uniformly reduced morbidity. Use of a reduced heparin dose in conjunction with heparin-bonded circuits has shown reductions in postoperative chest tube drainage and transfusion requirements, but probably increases the risk of clot formation in the CPB circuit, particularly if circuit flows should be low or nil.

   b. Steroids. Methylprednisolone 500 to 1,000 mg has proved helpful in some studies.

   c. Aprotinin acts by kallikrein inhibition, but this can only be achieved in the high-dose range (e.g., full Hammersmith protocol).

   d. Modified ultrafiltration has the most effect in pediatrics.

   e. Complement inhibitors are mostly experimental agents. They act to prevent activation of complement by kallikrein inhibition or direct complement antagonism. Reduction of the inflammatory response theoretically would reduce morbidity.

V. **Management of postbypass bleeding [1]**

   A. **Evaluation of hemostasis**

      1. Achieve surgical hemostasis
      2. Confirm adequate heparin neutralization
      3. Point-of-care testing to diagnose and treat bleeding. Point-of-care tests should be used appropriately in order to accurately and rapidly pinpoint the cause of a hemostasis defect. Etiologies of post-CPB bleeding should be prioritized by the clinician and should be tested in logical order. These tests should include heparin neutralization, platelet function, platelet number, coagulation, and fibrinolysis (Table 18.6)

         a. Tests of heparin neutralization: heparinase ACT, protamine titration test, heparinase thromboelastography (TEG). *Note:* The standard ACT is not a specific test of heparin neutralization. **Treatment of this abnormality includes protamine administration.**

Table 18.6 Point-of-care tests of platelet function

Test/monitor	Mechanism
Bleeding time	Collagen-activated in vivo adhesion
Thromboelastography/Sonoclot	Viscoelastic clot strength
Hemostatus	Platelet-activated clotting time
Ultegra	Activated fibrinogen bead agglutination
Platelet Works	Platelet count ratio
Platelet Function Analyzer (PFA-100)	In vitro activated bleeding time
Clot Signature Analyzer	High shear and collagen activation
Hemodyne	Platelet-mediated force transduction
Standard aggregometry	Optical density
Whole blood aggregometry	Electrical impedance

   b. Tests of platelet function: TEG maximal amplitude, Hemostatus [19], Ultegra, Platelet Works, Platelet Function Analyzer-100, whole blood aggregometry. *Note:* Bleeding time is too sensitive to measure platelet dysfunction after CPB. **Treatment of this abnormality includes administration of desmopressin acetate (DDAVP) 0.3 μg/kg and possibly a transfusion of platelet concentrates.**
   c. Coagulation tests: PT, aPTT, thrombin time, ACT. **Treatment of this abnormality includes transfusion of FFP.**
   d. Tests of fibrinolysis: euglobulin lysis time, TEG lysis index. **Treatment of this abnormality includes administration of an antifibrinolytic agent. Secondary fibrinolysis should be treated by replacement of consumed coagulation factors (FFP).**
      Note: **Treatment of any abnormal laboratory value should not take place unless warranted by the clinical situation. Treat the patient, not the number!**
B. *Treatment of postbypass hemostatic disorders*
C. **Transfusion medicine and the use of algorithms.** Allogeneic transfusions after CPB are common because of the wide range of hemostatic insults incurred. The lack of adequate testing of hemostasis and the subjectivity of a diagnosis of microvascular bleeding lead to indiscriminate transfusion practices.
   1. Transfusion of red blood cells, platelets, and plasma is fraught with adverse effects, not least of which include infectious disease transmission, acute lung injury, and immunomodulation. The rational use of transfusion algorithms should create an approach to transfusion medicine that is stepwise, logical, and based upon the hemostatic defects that are most common and easily treated.
   2. One of the most critical tests that should be measured "early" in a transfusion algorithm is an accurate point-of-care test of platelet function. This will minimize the occurrence of indiscriminate transfusion practices because subjective assessment of microvascular bleeding often leads to empiric transfusion practices. Rapid and accurate diagnosis of a hemostasis abnormality after CPB is critical. TEG predicts abnormal bleeding after CPB and has been used successfully in a number of algorithms to reduce the incidence of transfusion [20,21]. Other point-of-care monitors used in rational algorithms have proved effective in reducing transfusions.

References
 1. **Horrow JC, Fitch JCK. Management of coagulopathy associated with cardiopulmonary bypass. In: Gravlee GP, Davis RF, Kurusz M, et al., eds.** *Cardiopulmonary bypass: principles and practice,* **2nd ed. Philadelphia: Lippincott Williams & Wilkins, 2000:506–533.**
 2. Shore-Lesserson L, Gravlee GP. Anticoagulation for cardiopulmonary bypass. In: Gravlee GP, Davis RF, Kurusz M, et al., eds. *Cardiopulmonary bypass: principles and practice,* 2nd ed. Philadelphia: Lippincott Williams & Wilkins, 2000: 435–472.

3. Merton RE, Curtis AD, Thomas DP. A comparison of heparin potency estimates obtained by activated partial thromboplastin time and British pharmacopoeial assays. *Thromb Haemost* 1985;53:116–117.
4. Gravlee GP, Angert KC, Tucker WY, et al. Early anticoagulation peak and rapid distribution after intravenous heparin. *Anesthesiology* 1988;68:126–129.
5. Heres EK, Speight K, Benckart D, et al. The clinical onset of heparin is rapid. *Anesth Analg* 2001;92:1391–1395.
6. Olsson P, Lagergren H, Ek S. The elimination from plasma of intravenous heparin. An experimental study on dogs and humans. *Acta Med Scand* 1963;173:619–630.
7. **Bull BS, Korpman RA, Huse WM, et al. Heparin therapy during extracorporeal circulation. I. Problems inherent in existing heparin protocols. *J Thorac Cardiovasc Surg* 1975;69:674–684.**
8. Cohen EJ, Camerlengo LJ, Dearing JP. Activated clotting times and cardiopulmonary bypass I: the effect of hemodilution and hypothermia upon activated clotting time. *J Extracorp Technol* 1980;12:139–141.
9. Gravlee GP, Case LD, Angert KC, et al. Variability of the activated coagulation time. *Anesth Analg* 1988;67:469–472.
10. Despotis GJ, Summerfield AL, Joist JH. Comparison of activated coagulation time and whole blood heparin measurements with laboratory plasma anti-Xa heparin concentration in patients having cardiac operations. *J Thorac Cardiovasc Surg* 1994;108:1076–1082.
11. Greinacher A, Volpel H, Janssens U, et al. Recombinant hirudin (lepirudin) provides safe and effective anticoagulation in patients with heparin-induced thrombocytopenia. A prospective study. *Circulation* 1999;99:73–80.
12. **Koster A, Hansen R, Grauhan O, et al. Hirudin monitoring using the TAS ecarin clotting time in patients with heparin-induced thrombocytopenia type II. *J Cardiothorac Vasc Anesth* 2000;14:249–252.**
13. Metz S, Horrow JC. Pharmacologic manipulation of coagulation: protamine and other heparin antagonists. In: Lake CL, Moore RA, eds. *Blood: hemostasis, transfusion, and alternatives in the perioperative period.* New York: Raven Press, 1995:119–130.
14. **Horrow JC. Protamine: a review of its toxicity. *Anesth Analg* 1985;64:348–361.**
15. Horrow JC. Transfusion medicine and coagulation disorders. In: Kaplan JA, ed. *Cardiac anesthesia,* 4th ed. Philadelphia: WB Saunders, 1999:1111–1154.
16. Brown DL, Fann CS, Chang CJ. Meta-analysis of effectiveness and safety of abciximab versus eptifibatide or tirofiban in percutaneous coronary intervention. *Am J Cardiol* 2001;87:537–541.
17. Bertrand ME, Rupprecht HJ, Urban P, et al. Double-blind study of the safety of clopidogrel with and without a loading dose in combination with aspirin compared with ticlopidine in combination with aspirin after coronary stenting: the Clopidogrel Aspirin Stent International Cooperative Study (CLASSICS). *Circulation* 2000;102:624–629.
18. **Levi M, Cromheecke ME, de Jonge E, et al. Pharmacologic strategies to decrease excessive blood loss in cardiac surgery: a meta-analysis of clinically relevant endpoints. *Lancet* 1999;354:1940–1947.**
19. Despotis GJ, Levine V, Saleem R, et al. Use of point-of-care test in identification of patients who can benefit from desmopressin during cardiac surgery: a randomised controlled trial. *Lancet* 1999;354:106–110.
20. **Shore-Lesserson L, Manspeizer HE, DePerio M, et al. Thromboelastography-guided transfusion algorithm reduces transfusions in complex cardiac surgery. *Anesth Analg* 1999;88:312–319.**
21. **Nuttall GA, Oliver WC, Santrach PJ, et al. Efficacy of a simple intraoperative transfusion algorithm for nonerythrocyte component utilization after cardiopulmonary bypass. *Anesthesiology* 2001;94:773–781.**

III. CIRCULATORY SUPPORT AND ORGAN PRESERVATION

19. CARDIOPULMONARY BYPASS CIRCUITS: DESIGN AND USE

Mark Kurusz, Kane M. High, Alfred H. Stammers, and John M. Toomasian

This chapter describes the cardiopulmonary bypass (CPB) circuit; how it is configured, used, and monitored; and safety devices and necessary communications to prevent malfunctions and decrease risk of errors. Medical management of the patient on CPB is discussed in Chapter 7 and specific CPB pathophysiologic effects are discussed in Chapter 20.

I. **Goals of cardiopulmonary bypass.** The essential goals of CPB are to provide a still, bloodless heart with blood flow temporarily diverted to an extracorporeal circuit that functionally replaces the heart and lungs. The components of CPB may be classified as follows:

A. **Respiration**

1. **Ventilation. Provide adequate and controllable CO_2 elimination to maintain P_aCO_2 within the desired range.** As temperature decreases, CO_2 production decreases. This requires less "ventilation" through the oxygenator, which is accomplished by decreasing the "inspired" gas flow into the oxygenator. The choice of the desired P_aCO_2 depends on the particular management scheme (α-stat vs. pH-stat) and is discussed in Chapter 20.

2. **Oxygenation. Provide adequate O_2 transport to blood.** The large surface area of the membrane oxygenator provides adequate oxygen transport under most conditions. Under normal operating conditions, higher P_aO_2 values are maintained ($P_aO_2 = 150$ to 300 mm Hg) than are generally maintained during mechanical ventilation. It is possible to maintain the P_aO_2 in a more physiologic range with use of inline blood gas monitoring. However, because membrane oxygenators have little reserve capacity and moderate hyperoxia has not been associated with any clinically apparent ill effects, there is a small margin of safety if the P_aO_2 during CPB is maintained slightly elevated.

B. **Circulation. Maintain a desired perfusion pressure and flow while minimizing trauma to the formed elements of the blood.** Owing to abnormal pressures and shear stresses during extracorporeal blood flow, some hemolysis during CPB is inevitable. Elevations in free plasma hemoglobin are slight and transient, except after prolonged CPB or with excessive use of cardiotomy suction.

C. **Temperature regulation**

1. **Decreased body metabolism with hypothermia**

   a. **Hypothermia permits the use of lower systemic blood flows,** thereby decreasing blood trauma and probably enhancing central nervous system protection during CPB. Also, the return of less blood to the heart at a lower flow rate may provide a drier operative field. Typical blood temperature ranges for hypothermia and a suggested classification scheme are given in Table 19.1 [1].

   b. Reducing body temperature to profound hypothermic levels makes it possible to reduce metabolism to the point where the body tolerates **total circulatory arrest** for an extended period. Usually nasopharyngeal or tympanic temperatures in the range from 16° to 20°C are used. With this degree of hypothermia, it is generally agreed that circulatory arrest periods of up to 45 minutes can be safely undertaken [2].

2. **Providing hypothermic myocardial preservation.** Intravascular (anterograde and retrograde) and topical cooling are excellent adjuncts to flaccid hyperkalemic myocardial arrest used for myocardial preservation [3]. The heart can be actively chilled by cold cardioplegic solution (blood based or crystalloid

Table 19.1 Typical temperature ranges for hypothermia

Classification	Temperature (°C)
Tepid	34–35
Mild	30–34
Moderate	25–30
Deep	20–25
Profound	<20

alone), by ice slush or cold topical saline applied to the surface of the heart by the surgeon, or by a cooling jacket wrapped around the heart. To minimize warming of the myocardium by surrounding tissue (and to avoid cold injury to the phrenic nerve), an insulating pad is applied to the posterior surface of the heart in the pericardial well to prevent direct heat transfer between warmer tissues and the heart. **Cardioplegia typically decreases the myocardial temperature to approximately 8° to 12°C.** When a single right atrial–inferior vena cava (RA–IVC) cannula is used to provide venous return, myocardial temperatures need to be monitored carefully because venous blood returning to the RA is at patient body temperature. Two cannulas, one in the IVC and another in the superior vena cava (SVC), can be used to keep venous blood from entering and warming the heart. This is termed **bicaval cannulation.**

II. The cardiopulmonary bypass circuit

A. Circuit design.
The essential elements of the CPB system remain the same despite different manufacturers and different component designs. These components can be assembled in myriad configurations depending on institutional or surgical preference. Figure 19.1 shows a detailed schematic of a CPB circuit when using a membrane oxygenator with hard-shell venous reservoir and a blood cardioplegia delivery system. Tracing the path of blood flow in this diagram, desaturated blood exits the patient's vena cava through an RA–IVC cannula and is **drained by gravity siphon** through large-bore polyvinyl chloride (PVC) tubing into a venous reservoir that is an integral part of the membrane oxygenator. Blood then is drawn from the reservoir by the systemic flow pump (roller or centrifugal) and pumped through a heat exchanger (also integral to the membrane oxygenator) and a membrane bundle (usually hollow fiber), through an arterial filter and bubble trap, and back through the arterial cannula inserted into the ascending aorta. A recirculation line from the oxygenator outlet is used when priming the system and can be used as a blood source for blood cardioplegia; it is kept clamped during CPB. A purge line from the inflow side of the arterial filter transmits any accumulated air from the arterial filter to the venous reservoir.

Other roller pumps on the CPB console are used to vent the heart, suction blood, or deliver blood cardioplegia. Ancillary components of the CPB system include various safety devices (discussed later), a cooler/heater water source for the heat exchangers, gas blender and flow meter, anesthetic vaporizer, and sensors for monitoring arterial and venous blood parameters.

B. Pumps.
There currently are two types of blood pumps used in the CPB circuit: roller pumps and the centrifugal (kinetic) pumps. Use in clinical practice in the United States is approximately evenly divided between the two types of pumps.

1. Roller pump
a. Principles of operation.
The roller pump causes blood to flow by compressing plastic tubing between the roller and the horseshoe-shaped backing plate as the roller turns in the raceway (Fig. 19.2). Each pump has **two roller heads** placed 180 degrees apart to maintain continuous roller head contact with the tubing. The revolutions per minute (rpm) for roller pumps used for systemic flow typically range from 50 to 150 rpm, depending on the pump head tubing internal diameter (ID). **Flow from a systemic roller pump is linear with rpm.** With larger ID tubing (e.g., ½-inch ID), lower rpm are required to achieve the same output compared to smaller ID tubing. The **stroke volume,** or output in milliliters per rpm, of a roller pump can vary slightly depending on tubing material, elasticity, or temperature but generally ranges from 12.7 (¼-inch ID tubing) to 41.9 mL (½-inch) when using a 6-inch dual roller pump. The **total pump output** is displayed in milliliters or liters per minute on the pump control panel. Roller pumps also are used to deliver cardioplegic solution, remove blood or air from heart chambers or great vessels, or suction shed blood from the operative field.

b. Adjustment of occlusion
(1) To minimize hemolysis, the occlusion, or separation between the rollers and the backing plate (or raceway), must be properly set. In

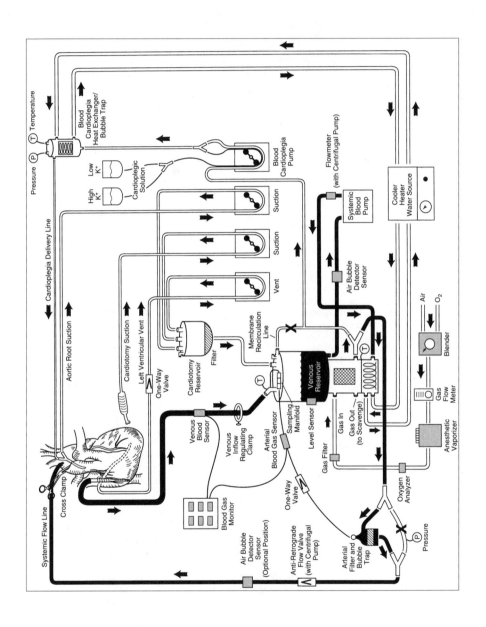

essence, this provides a mechanism for setting the resistance to back-flow past the roller head. The occlusion is set by adjusting the distance between the raceway and each of the roller heads, which control the cross-sectional area inside the tubing at the point of compression by the roller.

Total occlusion is not used because increased hemolysis and excessive tubing wear will result. However, a problem with hemolysis can develop if too large an area is left between the pump head and the backing plate. In this case, a rapid regurgitant backflow causing large-velocity gradients and excessive red blood cell (RBC) shear stresses can occur, in turn causing hemolysis. Too little occlusion also can lead to decreased forward flow to the patient.

The conventional **method for setting occlusion** involves holding the distal systemic flow line, which is primed with clear fluid, vertically so that the top of the fluid column is 30 to 40 inches above the pump. The occlusion is adjusted until the fluid level falls at a rate of 1 inch/min. Two alternative methods are (i) clamping the outlet tubing from the roller pump and slowly advancing the rollers to pressurize fluid within the line, stopping the pump, and then adjusting the occlusion until a slow decline in pressure monitored distal to the pump head is observed; and (ii) clamping the distal tubing and adjusting the occlusion while slowly rotating the pump head so as to maintain pressure in the tubing greater than that anticipated during CPB (e.g., 300 to 400 mm Hg); this method requires a valved shunt between the outlet and inlet tubing of the pump [4]. For suction or vent pumps, the occlusion is set by clamping the tubing on the inlet side of the roller pump and gradually occluding the rotating rollers until tubing within the pump head just collapses.

(2) Although not totally occlusive, roller pump output is not significantly affected by the patient's systemic blood pressure. **When occlusion is properly set, the pump flow rate does not significantly decrease as the afterload (arterial pressure) increases.** Because of this, high pressures can quickly develop in the CPB systemic flow line if the arterial cannula is blocked as a result of either tube kinking or a tubing clamp. Pressures high enough to cause line separation or

---

FIG. 19.1 Schematic of typical cardiopulmonary bypass circuit. The systemic circuit (*bolded in the diagram*) includes the venous line, membrane oxygenator with integral hard-shell venous reservoir (**lower center**), systemic blood pump, arterial filter, and return to the patient via the arterial cannula. Venous cannulation is by a right atrial–inferior vena cava, "two-stage" cannula and arterial cannulation is in the ascending aorta. The systemic blood pump may be either a roller or centrifugal type. The cardioplegia delivery system (**right**) is a one-pass, combination blood/crystalloid type that draws arterialized blood from the membrane recirculation line. The cooler/heater water source may be operated to supply water to both the oxygenator heat exchanger and cardioplegia delivery system. The air bubble detector sensor may be placed on the tubing between the venous reservoir and systemic pump, between the pump and membrane oxygenator inlet or between the oxygenator outlet and arterial filter (neither shown), or on the tubing after the arterial filter (optional position on drawing). One-way valves prevent retrograde flow (some circuits with a centrifugal pump also incorporate a one-way valve after the pump and within the systemic flow arterial tubing). Other safety devices include an oxygen analyzer placed between the anesthetic vaporizer (if used) and the oxygenator gas inlet; and a reservoir level sensor attached to the housing of the hard-shell venous reservoir (**left**). *Arrows,* directions of flow; *P* and *T,* pressure and temperature sensors, respectively; *X,* placement of tubing clamps. A hemoconcentrator (described in text) is not shown. (Modified from Hessel EA II, Hill AG. Circuitry and cannulation techniques. In: Gravlee GP, Davis RF, Kurusz M, et al., eds. *Cardiopulmonary bypass: principles and practice,* 2nd ed. Philadelphia: Lippincott Williams & Wilkins, 2000:70, with permission.)

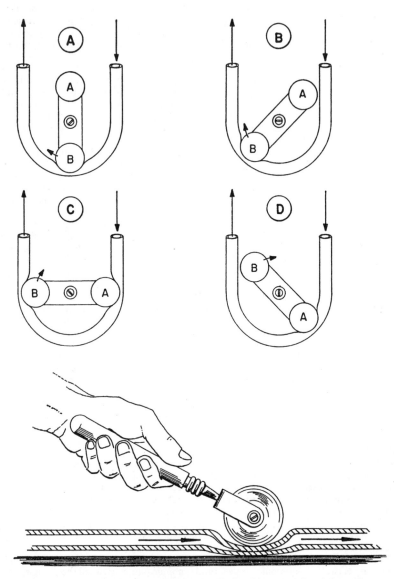

FIG. 19.2 Drawing of a dual roller pump and tubing. The principle of the roller pump is demonstrated by the hand roller in the **lower drawing** moving along a section of tubing pushing fluid ahead of it and suctioning fluid behind it. The **upper four drawings** in sequence (**A–D**) show how roller pump B first moves fluid ahead of it and suctions fluid behind it (**A**). As the pump rotates clockwise, the second roller A begins to engage the tubing (**B**). As the rotation continues there is a very brief period with volume trapped between the two rollers (**C**) and no forward flow, which imparts some pulsatility. In position **D,** roller B leaves the tubing while the second roller A continues to move fluid in the same direction. Not shown are the roller pump backing plate, tubing holders, and tube guides for maintaining the tubing within the raceway. Fluid flows in direction of the *arrows*. (From Stofer RC. *A technic for extracorporeal circulation.* Springfield, IL: Charles C. Thomas, 1968:22, with permission.)

rupture can occur, but most CPB consoles today are equipped with high-pressure cutoff mechanisms to prevent this complication. If the inlet tubing to the roller pump is restricted, it is possible for a roller pump to quickly create extreme negative pressures, which physically pulls gas out of solution (**cavitation**). However, this usually does not occur because the tubing that enters the roller pump is short and is connected directly to a reservoir that contains enough blood to preclude development of significant negative pressure.

2. **Centrifugal/kinetic pump**

   a. There are several models of centrifugal pumps used for CPB (Fig. 19.3). A common type consists of three vaneless rotor cones, capable of spinning at high velocity (e.g., 2,000 to 3,000 rpm), mounted in a clear plastic housing, causing circular motion (sometimes referred to as a **constrained vortex**)

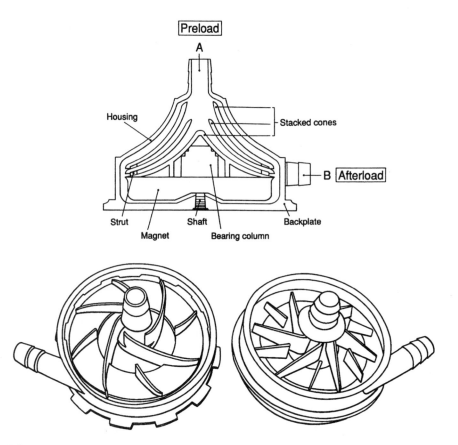

FIG. 19.3 Drawings of centrifugal pump heads. A cross-sectional view of a smooth, cone-type pump is shown on the **top.** Blood enters at (*A*) and is expelled on the right (*B*) due to kinetic forces created by the three rapidly spinning cones. Impeller-type pumps with vanes are shown in the **bottom** drawings. (Modified from Trocchio CR, Sketel JO. Mechanical pumps for extracorporeal circulation. In: Mora CT, ed. *Cardiopulmonary bypass: principles and techniques of extracorporeal circulation.* New York: Springer-Verlag, 1995:222, 223, with permission.)

of the blood and generating flow and pressure by centrifugal force. The cones spin by means of an indirect magnetic connection to a drive shaft on the centrifugal pump console. The two outer cones are attached at a few points to each other and to the innermost cone. Blood enters through an integral molded connector at the top along the axis of the pump and exits peripherally through another integral connector on the base of the pump housing. Other commercially available centrifugal pumps contain single vaned rotators or impellers that increase pump efficiency, thus allowing slightly lower rpm.

   b. **The centrifugal pump is nonocclusive** and flow is dependent on the pressure change created by the spinning cone(s) within the pump. The flow rate is affected by the size of the cannula, length of the tubing, diameter of the tubing, restrictions in the tubing, and changes in the patient's systemic vascular resistance (SVR). That is, as the pressure distal to the pump increases, the flow decreases if there is no change in rpm. Such decreases in flow can be partially compensated for by increasing the rpm. An electromagnetic or ultrasonic flow meter placed in the systemic flow line is required when a centrifugal pump is used and most often is located between the pump and patient to accurately determine the flow rate. To prevent retrograde flow when a centrifugal pump is not operating or if the rpm are insufficiently high to overcome afterload, a large-bore one-way valve may be inserted into the tubing distal to the pump [5].

   Centrifugal pumps will not pump blood if they become filled with air (rendering them unusable for suction or vent pumps) because they rely on centrifugal force to generate pressure. However, they can easily transmit small bubbles into the systemic circulation if they are present in the blood. A summary of the advantages and disadvantages of centrifugal and roller pumps is given in Table 19.2.

C. Oxygenators. "Oxygenators" provide an environment for CO_2 and O_2 exchange similar to that in the pulmonary alveolar capillary unit. In designing an oxygenator, it is desirable that ventilation (i.e., CO_2 elimination) be independent from oxygenation so that each can be controlled without affecting the other. This is possible with membrane oxygenators, which today are used nearly universally for CPB.

   1. **General principles of design and operation must be followed in the use of oxygenators.**
      a. **Optimize gas transport** by minimizing the gas transport distance (diffusion distance) in the blood, maximizing the effective area for gas diffusion, and increasing the blood transit time in the oxygenator.
      b. **Minimize formed element trauma** by minimizing shear stresses and providing smooth blood-contacting surfaces.
      c. **The priming volume should be as small as possible** to minimize hemodilutional effects.
   2. **Membrane oxygenators.** The artificial membrane lung more closely imitates the natural pulmonary anatomy by interposing a thin membrane between the blood and gas. This creates a distinct blood space and gas space within the oxygenator (Fig. 19.4).

Table 19.2 Comparison of roller and centrifugal pumps

	Advantages	Disadvantages
Roller	Predictable pump flow based on pump speed	Can pump **large** quantities of air
	Capable of pulsatile flow	Can overpressurize lines, causing them to burst
Centrifugal	Cannot pump **large** quantities of air	Output not necessarily indicated by pump speed
	Cannot overpressurize lines	Not capable of pulsatile flow

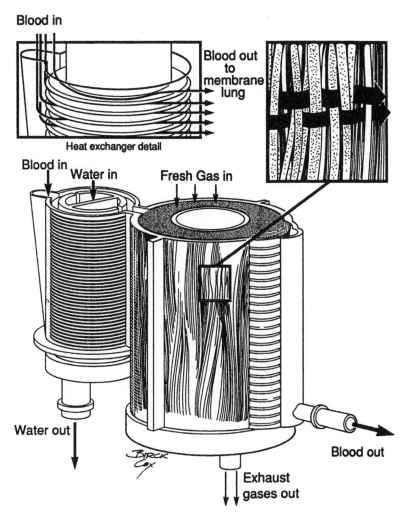

FIG. 19.4 Drawing of a microporous hollow-fiber membrane oxygenator. In this example, the stainless steel heat exchanger (**top left**) incorporates fins that channel blood into thin layers to increase heat exchanger efficiency. After passing through the heat exchanger, blood permeates through the membrane bundle and around individual hollow fibers (**top right**) for gas exchange; gas flows through the hollow fibers. The **center** drawings show the membrane transected for illustration purposes. Both the heat exchanger and gas exchanger portions of the membrane lung contain manifolds that distribute blood flow evenly to minimize the blood pressure drop at clinical flow rates. (From High KM, Bashein G, Kurusz M. Principles of oxygenator function: gas exchange, heat transfer, and operation. In Gravlee GP, Davis RF, Kurusz M, et al., eds. *Cardiopulmonary bypass: principles and practice,* 2nd ed. Philadelphia: Lippincott Williams & Wilkins, 2000:57, Used with permission.)

Current adult membrane oxygenators have a large surface area, approximately 1.8 to 4.5 m^2, which is either fan folded, coiled, or configured as capillary tubes. Blood passes through the oxygenator as a thin film, minimizing the diffusion distance for gases in the blood and thereby maximizing gas exchange.

a. Types of membrane oxygenators. The majority of membrane oxygenator materials are hollow-fiber capillaries of microporous polypropylene, microporous polypropylene sheets, or thin sheets of silicone rubber. Membranes constructed of sheets of silicone rubber are nonporous and rely entirely on gas diffusion through the silicone rubber for gas exchange. In contrast, the polypropylene sheets and fibers have small pores that potentially allow physical connections between the gas and blood spaces.

(1) Hollow-fiber membranes. The microporous fibers are wound together into a bundle to promote blood mixing. Whereas earlier designs relied on blood flowing through the hollow fibers surrounded by ventilating gas, most designs used today rely on gas flow through the capillaries with blood around them. This configuration reduces blood pressure drop across the oxygenator.

As mentioned earlier, at the onset of bypass there is a direct blood–gas interface present at these pores until a thin protein layer covers the hollow fibers to form a molecular membrane. Because of these porous channels, it is extremely important that gas phase pressure not exceed blood phase pressure (e.g., due to a blocked oxygenator gas exhaust port) when using any microporous membrane oxygenator. This is necessary in order to prevent possible systemic air embolism (see Section **V**).

(2) Microporous sheets. These devices originally were introduced in the mid-1970s. They generally have a larger surface area than hollow-fiber types and require larger priming volumes, but they are more effective in trapping and expelling air that may inadvertently enter the membrane oxygenator.

(3) Nonporous membrane oxygenators. "True" membrane oxygenators are manufactured by coiling silicone rubber sheets in a cylindrical fashion. Blood is kept on one side of the membrane and gas on the other. Gas transfer through the membrane is dependent on the permeability of the membrane, the diffusion distance of the gas in blood, and the driving pressure of gas on either side of the membrane. Membranes must be 20 to 30 times more permeable to CO_2 than to O_2 because of the lower driving pressure for CO_2 exchange. These oxygenators are infrequently used for standard CPB because of relatively larger priming volumes than microporous types and the need to correctly "size" the oxygenator to patient weight. They are used for long-term extracorporeal life support because of their ability to function for days or weeks.

b. Characteristics of operation. Because of the relatively high resistance to blood flow through most membrane oxygenators, blood must be drawn from the venous reservoir and actively pumped through the oxygenator by the roller or centrifugal pump. Excessive pressure through the membrane can cause rupture, creating either a blood leak or air embolism, depending on flow conditions.

A major advantage of membrane oxygenators over bubble oxygenators is their capability for exerting independent control of CO_2 and O_2 gas exchange. Because all gas present in the blood phase is in solution, an air–oxygen blender is used to control the P_aO_2. The gas flow ("sweep rate") can be controlled independently to remove carbon dioxide, allowing better control of blood gases on CPB. This lack of a blood–gas interface allows gentler handling of blood with a lower rate of hemolysis during longer duration CPB.

The major disadvantage of microporous membrane oxygenators is a usable life of approximately 6 hours, after which time plasma infiltration into the micropores limits gas exchange. The nonporous membrane oxygenators generally are more expensive, more complex to set up, and require larger priming volumes.

D. Reservoirs. Venous reservoirs may be either a **rigid hard-shell** or **collapsible soft-bag** type. Because it is open to atmosphere, the advantage of a hard-shell reservoir is its ability to automatically dissipate any entrained venous line air. Most current hard-shell venous reservoirs also function as a cardiotomy reservoir for debubbling and filtration of suction or vent blood. Determination of volume status is more precise with a hard-shell reservoir than with a soft-bag reservoir. Soft-bag venous reservoirs require that a separate hard-shell cardiotomy reservoir be used. The advantage of a soft-bag venous reservoir is absence of an air–blood interface and the inability to pump large volumes of air if it is depleted. Whatever type is used, **the venous reservoir should be of large capacity** and permit easy viewing of the blood level at all times.

E. Venous and arterial cannulas

    1. Venous cannulas. Venous blood returning to the right heart is drained by gravity to the venous reservoir through either two venous cannulas separately inserted into the IVC and SVC or, more commonly, a single cannula inserted directly into the RA–IVC. Occasionally a single large-bore cannula is inserted into the RA.

        If both the IVC and SVC are cannulated and secured with heavy ligatures (commonly referred to as caval tapes) around the cavae and cannulas, all blood returning through the venae cavae is diverted to the CPB venous reservoir. This precludes ejection of blood from the left ventricle and is called **total bypass.** This type of cannulation is used to create a bloodless operative field and to prevent rewarming of the heart by venous blood. If a single atrial cannula is used, it most often is a **single** "two-stage" cannula in which blood is drained from the RA–IVC by this single tube with concentric flow channels.

        When using a two-stage cannula or bicaval cannulation without caval tapes, some blood may pass into the RA, go through the right heart, and into the pulmonary circulation. Restricting venous return to the CPB circuit can control the amount of blood passing into the RA. Assuming the heart is not arrested by cardioplegia, restriction of blood return to the CPB circuit then causes blood to pass through the pulmonary circulation, and some arterial pulsation can occur. This condition is called **partial bypass.** Representative venous cannulas are shown in Figure 19.5.

        With the recent trend toward minimally invasive cardiac surgery, smaller-bore venous cannulas have been used through small chest wall incisions or peripherally from the femoral or jugular veins. Because of their smaller diameter and longer length than centrally placed venous cannulas, adequate venous drainage sometimes is augmented by applying regulated wall vacuum to the hard-shell venous reservoir [6]. This technique is referred to as **vacuum-assisted venous drainage (VAVD)** and requires a pressure-relief valve in the hard-shell reservoir to prevent pressurization of the reservoir that is connected to suction and vent roller pumps. The pressure within the venous reservoir can be measured, as a backup, to ensure that pressure within the system is not too negative or positive. Use of VAVD permits shortening of the venous line by decreasing the necessary height difference between the patient's RA and venous reservoir and because the conventional siphoning effect is not necessary when using VAVD. VAVD also can be used to remove venous line priming fluid before starting CPB in an effort to decrease CPB hemodilution [7].

        A centrifugal pump can be used in the venous line as another form of assisted venous drainage [8]. **Kinetic-assisted venous drainage (KAVD)** isolates suction to the venous drainage line, which augments venous drainage in a fashion similar to VAVD; however, the negative pressure can be controlled more precisely by the speed of the centrifugal pump. However, with both VAVD and KAVD, optimal venous drainage depends on precise position of the cannula tip within the RA–SVC junction.

        Several factors affect venous return to the pump circuit. The driving pressure for blood flow in the venous cannulas is the hydrostatic pressure head

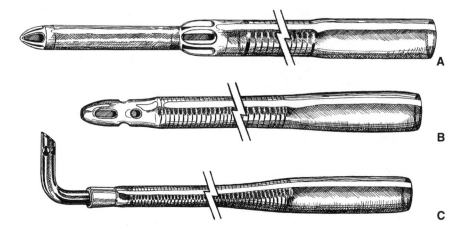

FIG. 19.5 Drawings of commonly used venous cannulas. **A:** Tapered, "two-stage" right atrial–inferior vena cava (RA–IVC) cannula. **B:** Straight, wire-wound "lighthouse" tipped cannula for RA or separate cannulation of the superior vena cava (SVC) or IVC. **C:** Right-angled, metal-tipped cannula for cannulation of the SVC or IVC. (From Hessel EA II, Hill AG. Circuitry and cannulation techniques. In: Gravlee GP, Davis RF, Kurusz M, et al., eds. *Cardiopulmonary bypass: principles and practice,* 2nd ed. Philadelphia: Lippincott Williams & Wilkins, 2000:72, with permission.)

from the RA to the venous reservoir less any pressure drop incurred in the venous system of the CPB circuit. **Remedies to consider when venous return is less than desired include the following:**

   a. **Relieving inflow obstruction** caused by caval wall obstruction of the inlet of the cannula(s) or too deep insertion of the IVC cannula (e.g., into the portal vein)

   b. **Undoing kinking** of the cannula(s), particularly as it passes over the sternal retractor

   c. **Increasing or decreasing the height difference** (elevating the operating room table or lowering the venous reservoir or vice versa) between the cavae and the venous reservoir, i.e., increase or decrease (if the height differential is so great that the venous return cannula is tending to collapse the cavae) the hydrostatic pressure head

   d. **Removing all clamps** from the venous line at the pump or operative field

   e. **Using larger venous cannula(s)** because they have less flow resistance and allow greater flows at the same pressure drop. Single venous cannulas for individual cannulation of the IVC and SVC range in size from 10 to 46 Fr. Selection is based on the patient's weight and anticipated CPB flow requirements. The **single** "two-stage" cannulas range from small [40 × 32 Fr (outside cannula by inside cannula)] to large (51 × 36 Fr) and are chosen by the patient's weight and flow requirements.

2. **Arterial cannulas.** Arterialized blood is returned to the patient from the CPB circuit through an arterial cannula placed either in the ascending aorta or, less commonly, the femoral artery. Size of the cannula is chosen to minimize the pressure drop across the cannula at the patient's calculated CPB flow rate. A standard cardiac index of 2.2 to 2.4 L/min/m² for adults and 2.6 to 3.0 L/min/m² for pediatric patients is used to determine the **calculated flow rate** required at normothermia. Representative arterial cannulas are shown in Figure 19.6.

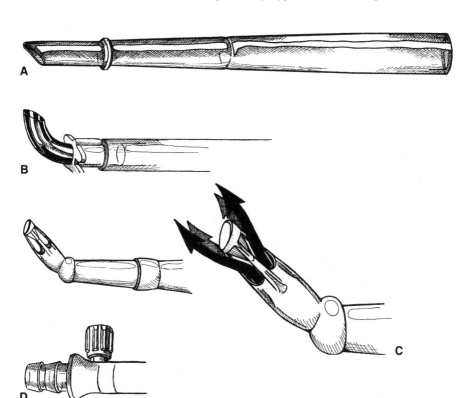

FIG. 19.6 Drawings of commonly used arterial cannulas. **A:** Tapered, bevel-tipped cannula with molded flange near tip. **B:** Angled, thin-walled, metal-tipped cannula with molded flange for securing cannula to aorta. **C:** Angled, diffusion-tipped cannula designed to direct systemic flow in four directions (**right**) to avoid a "jetting effect" that may occur with conventional single-lumen arterial cannulas. **D:** Integral cannula/tubing connector and luer port (for de-airing) incorporated onto some newer arterial cannulas. (Modified from Hessel EA II, Hill AG. Circuitry and cannulation techniques. In: Gravlee GP, Davis RF, Kurusz M, et al., eds. *Cardiopulmonary bypass: principles and practice,* 2nd ed. Philadelphia: Lippincott Williams & Wilkins, 2000:77, with permission.)

Pump flow must be high enough to prevent the occurrence of metabolic acidosis, which usually requires maintaining a mixed venous Po_2 greater than 30 mmHg (measured at blood temperature) or mixed venous O_2 saturation greater than 65%. Generally accepted CPB systemic flows are shown in Table 19.3.

As a general rule, the pressure drop across the cannula should not exceed 100 mm Hg. Size then is determined by the smallest cannula that can provide calculated flow with a gradient less than 100 mm Hg. Pressure gradients are determined by manufacturers, and pressure drop flow charts come with cannula packages. Gradients also can be determined by allowing fluid to flow through the pump circuit and the cannula and by measuring the pressure from a port located just before the cannula. "High-flow" cannulas are thin walled and allow a greater flow with a smaller outside diameter. Newer diffusion-flow arterial cannulas minimize jetting at the cannula tip [9].

Table 19.3 Typical adult cardiopulmonary bypass flow indices with hypothermia

Temperature (°C)	Cardiac index (L/min/m²)
34–37	2.4
30–34	2.0
25–30	1.8
20–18	1.5
<18	1.0

F. Cardioplegia delivery. Hyperkalemic crystalloid or mixed blood/crystalloid (usually 4:1 ratio) solution is intermittently delivered from the CPB console to the aortic root or coronary ostia (**anterograde**) or coronary sinus (**retrograde**) when the aorta is cross-clamped to quickly arrest and cool the heart. Dosages of cardioplegic solution often are based on patient weight (10 mL/kg) or body surface area (450 mL/m²) and are guided by the achieved myocardial temperature (approximately 10°C). When blood cardioplegia is used, the initial dose typically contains a higher potassium concentration (approximately 20 to 30 mEq/L) than subsequent maintenance doses (approximately 5 to 10 mEq/L) to avoid systemic hyperkalemia. The cardioplegia delivery system contains a small heat exchanger/bubble trap and temperature monitoring port. The water source for this heat exchanger is independently regulated from the one used for the oxygenator that controls body temperature (Fig. 19.1)

Cardioplegic solution often is administered every 15 to 30 minutes during the period of aortic cross-clamp to maintain the heart arrested and hypothermic. Cardioplegic solution also may be administered to de-air vein grafts before the surgeon secures distal anastomoses. **Retrograde cardioplegia** often is used to perfuse and cool areas of myocardium beyond coronary blockages and during aortic valve replacement to avoid direct coronary ostial delivery routes. Most of the volume of cardioplegic solution becomes part of the circulating blood volume after perfusion of the coronary vasculature.

Some newer cardioplegia delivery systems rely on a separate console with a piston-type pump and built-in heat exchanger to deliver precise doses of potassium-containing perfusate that can be adjusted over a wide range of delivery hematocrits and temperatures [10].

G. Ancillary equipment

1. Blood filters

   a. Filter types. There are two primary types of filters used for blood filtration during CPB: depth filters and screen filters. A **depth filter** is composed of packed fibers of Dacron. They filter by absorption on their large wetted surface areas. With depth filters, particulate removal depends on the following:

   1. Amount of wetted surface area
   2. Chemical structure of the particles and filter material
   3. Diameter of blood flow pathways

   Screen filters are made of a woven mesh of polyester fibers with specific pore sizes in the mesh; the screen has accordion pleats to increase the surface area and permit acceptable blood pressure drop at clinical flow rates. Particulate material is trapped in this filter because the particles are larger than the pores; gaseous microemboli also are trapped due to surface tension effects from the wetted pores. The pore size must be larger than 20 μm to permit adequate blood flow without excessive blood pressure drop. Both types of filters make effective gross bubble traps.

   b. Filter location. Virtually all filters used in the arterial line are screen type. A **bypass line** (Fig. 19.1) around the arterial line filter is recommended should the filter become obstructed. The pressure drop across the filter can be measured to monitor potential obstruction of the filter, which is rare today because of better control of anticoagulation. The bypass line around the arterial filter normally is occluded by a tubing clamp that can be readily released in the event of filter obstruction.

Because the cardiotomy reservoir receives blood that contains a significantly larger quantity of debris [11] along with room air, it contains an integral filter that relies on a combination of both depth and screen-type filters. Other filters used for CPB can be placed in a number of locations, including the ventilating gas line (0.2 μm) and the cardioplegia delivery circuit, or for removal of leukocytes (systemic flow line or cardioplegia delivery line).

2. **Blood and vent suctioning.** Suction often is used during CPB to remove blood and cardioplegic solution from the operative field, to drain cardiac chambers or great vessels, or to remove air. When the fluid drained is primarily cardioplegic solution, the operating room (OR) wall suction system can be used. This fluid does not enter the CPB circuit. When the fluid is primarily blood, the pump suction lines are used to return the fluid to the circuit and the patient.

The pump suction lines are powered by a roller pump to draw a vacuum (Fig. 19.1). Generally, two pump heads on the CPB console are dedicated to this purpose; a separate suction pump is used for venting. Blood from the pump suction or vent lines is pumped into the cardiotomy or venous reservoir and returned to the patient. Usually these roller pumps are activated only when needed by the surgeon. **Operating these roller pumps at a high rate or continuously is a major source of hemolysis and should be avoided.** Indiscriminate use of suction or vent pumps causes aspiration of room air, which is less easily removed by the cardiotomy filters and defoamers and can increase the risk of transmission of gaseous microemboli.

3. **Arterial line pressure monitor.** Electronic transducers are used to monitor the pressure in the arterial line. These transducers can be used in conjunction with aneroid-type gauges that display phasic pulsations with aortic cannulation. Both types of pressure displays usually are connected to the circuit at a luer-port on the CPB systemic flow line after the oxygenator or from a luer-port on the arterial line filter. This monitor is extremely **important for detecting restrictions to flow in the arterial line** caused by the presence of an inadvertent clamp or kink in the line.

4. **Heat exchangers.** Heat exchangers are an integral part of the CPB oxygenator. A mixture of hot and cold water is circulated through the heat exchanger and provides a **temperature gradient** to cool or warm the blood. Generally, perfusate temperature should not be less than 12° to 15°C when cooling nor greater than 38°C when warming. Management of rewarming during CPB is discussed in detail in Chapter 7.

5. **Temperature sensors.** The temperature of the blood in the venous and systemic flow lines is continuously monitored during CPB to determine the temperature gradient during cooling and rewarming, which is kept at less than 10°C between arterial and venous blood. The temperature is measured by either thermocouple or thermistor and is displayed on the CPB console.

6. **Anesthesia vaporizer.** An anesthesia vaporizer can be placed in the ventilating gas line to the oxygenator. This vaporizer typically is the same as those found on anesthesia machines. Isoflurane is the agent usually used because of its low blood solubility and its prominent **vasodilating effect.** The vaporizer should not be located directly above the oxygenator or other plastic components because anesthetic liquid that spills onto these devices while the vaporizer is being filled can cause damage or cracking [12].

7. **Ultrafiltration.** Occasionally during CPB it is necessary to remove excess water (with electrolytes) to increase the patient's hematocrit. This process is easily accomplished on CPB by the use of ultrafiltration. In comparison with diuretics, ultrafilters (or, as they are more commonly called, **hemoconcentrators**) are readily controllable and do not cause excessive losses of potassium.

Hemoconcentrators consist of hollow-fiber membranes that allow the separation of water and electrolytes from formed elements and larger molecules (i.e., proteins) in the blood. Blood is either shunted from the arterial line filter purge line or pumped from a reservoir or the oxygenator's recirculation line through the hemoconcentrator by an auxiliary roller pump. Pressure is created by the resistance to flow within the hemoconcentrator and occasionally by a downstream clamp that partially occludes the return line. This hydrostatic pressure forces water out of the blood and across the membrane, which concentrates the remaining blood. Effluent removal rates vary but, depending on the hematocrit, rates up to 75 mL/min can be achieved [13].

H. Heparin or other surface-modifying treatments for blood-contacting surfaces of circuit components now are available. These circuits may allow CPB to be performed with **lower than normal systemic heparin anticoagulation** of the patient, although this seldom is recommended [14]. This capability is particularly useful in patients with massive bleeding after trauma but who require operation on the heart or great vessels. Use of these circuits is restricted by their questionable efficacy, cost, and somewhat limited experience. It must be realized that *every* component in the circuit (tubing, connectors, oxygenator, filters) must be surface treated if lower than normal levels of heparin-induced anticoagulation are used.

III. Priming and disposition of perfusate. Owing to advances in understanding concepts of hemodilution and hypothermia and ongoing concerns about transmission of blood-borne diseases, the use of a total nonblood prime now is standard CPB procedure in adults and large children. For smaller patients or those with low preoperative hematocrits, **retrograde autologous priming** may be used to lessen hemodilution associated with CPB [15]. Hypothermia increases the viscosity of the blood, thereby increasing flow resistance. Hemodilution decreases the blood viscosity and enhances tissue perfusion at lower flow rates. Hemodilution therefore decreases RBC trauma, and lessens the need for banked blood. Hemodilution to a hematocrit level of 20-25% is commonly employed during CPB.

A. Priming solutions. Four major factors must be considered when priming the bypass circuit.

1. Osmolality. The fluid should be isotonic or slightly hypertonic to preserve the interstitial–intravascular fluid balance.

2. Electrolytes. Normal electrolyte balance must be maintained to avoid electrolyte depletion after bypass.

3. Volume. An adequate volume of priming solution must be used to fill the circuit to a safe level and to allow adequate systemic CPB flow rates. The tubing size and length for the circuit determine the total volume of fluid needed to prime the CPB system, along with the volume required to prime components such as the venous reservoir, oxygenator, arterial line filter, and cardioplegia delivery system. The total volume used must be enough to allow initiation of CPB with adequate blood flow rates but not so much as to cause excessive hemodilution.

4. Hemodilution. It is undesirable to reduce the hematocrit to less than 18% with the initiation of bypass. Recent, retrospective, multiinstitutional data suggest that the hematocrit should be maintained at 20% or more during CPB [16]. The **initial bypass hematocrit** can be estimated using the following equation:

$$Hct_{int} = \frac{(Hct \times EBV)}{(EBV + \text{volume of prime} + \text{prebypass IV fluids})}$$

where EBV = estimated blood volume of patient, Hct_{int} = initial hematocrit on CPB, Hct = preoperative hematocrit, and IV = intravenous.

Solutions used for priming vary from institution to institution. The routine adult priming protocols for Stanford University Medical Center, Pennsylvania State University, the University of Texas at Galveston, and Geisinger Medical Center are compared in Table 19.4. Generally, an isotonic, balanced electrolyte solution such as Plasma-Lyte A is used. Sodium bicarbonate typically is used as a buffer. Osmotic agents such as mannitol often are added to improve renal function, and a colloid solution such as 6% hetastarch or albumin can be included

Table 19.4 Standard adult cardiopulmonary bypass primes

Stanford University Medical Center		Pennsylvania State University	
Normosol R	1,500 mL	Plasma-Lyte A	1,500 mL
Mannitol (25%)	25 g	Mannitol (25%)	25 g
Heparin (1,000 USP units/mL)	10,000 units	Heparin (1,000 USP units/mL)	5,000 units
Sodium bicarbonate (8.4%)	35 mEq	Sodium bicarbonate (8.4%)	45 mEq
Amicar (ϵ aminocaproic acid)	5–10 g	**Geisinger Medical Center**	
		Plasma-Lyte A	1,400 mL
		Mannitol (25%)	12.5 g
University of Texas at Galveston		Heparin (1,000 USP units/mL)	5,000 units
Plasma-Lyte A	900 mL	Sodium bicarbonate (8.4%)	25 mEq
D5W with 0.45% sodium chloride	400 mL	Amicar (ϵ aminocaproic acid)	5–10 g
Hespan (6% hetastarch)	500 mL		
Salt-poor albumin (25%)	5 g		
Heparin (1,000 USP units/mL)	5,000 units		
Sodium bicarbonate (8.4%)	20 mEq		

in the priming solution to maintain oncotic pressure and coat the artificial blood surfaces. The prime should be heparinized to prevent dilution of the heparin dose given before bypass. Aminocaproic acid or aprotinin may be added to the solution when those agents are being used prophylactically to enhance postoperative hemostasis.

B. **Methods of priming.** The goal of priming is to wet and debubble the bypass circuit completely. The actual methods used to accomplish this vary among perfusionists. Generally, a 100% CO_2 flush of the arterial line filter, membrane oxygenator, and tubing for several minutes is used to remove all room air from the circuit [17]. Carbon dioxide is used because of its high water solubility, which is 30 times greater than that of air. This is followed by addition and recirculation of priming solution through the circuit (with the venous and systemic flow lines connected). All circuit elements and stopcocks must be primed. Any CO_2 bubbles that are not washed from the circuit are quickly absorbed into the prime. A **prebypass filter** often is used during priming to remove particulates contained in circuit components from manufacturing or assembly.

The prime is recirculated at the maximum calculated flow rate to test the circuit, monitor for excessive CPB line pressure, and verify the integrity of connections. Recirculation with gas flow (FIO_2 set at 0.21 to avoid hyperoxia of prime) allows removal of excessive CO_2 from the circuit before commencing bypass. An attempt should be made to approach a physiologic acid–base status before initiating CPB.

C. **Disposition of perfusate.** After bypass is stopped, residual perfusate in the CPB circuit can be salvaged by transfer into a completely de-aired sterile IV bag for transfusion. Bags containing residual perfusate should be labeled. Most often this blood is administered in the immediate postbypass period. Alternatively, a cell salvage system that has been used during the case can concentrate and wash residual perfusate before transfusion. A hemoconcentrator can be used to process residual perfusate. **Depending upon the initial protamine dose, supplemental protamine sulfate should be considered after transfusion of any unwashed residual perfusate to counteract heparin contained in the salvaged perfusate.** Washed cell salvage products do not contain clinically significant amounts of residual heparin.

IV. Equipment monitoring and communication. Safe CPB depends on close coordination of activities by all team members [18]. Essential and effective communication facilitates such coordination. Instructions or announcements are necessary during CPB as the surgical procedure progresses, and all such **notifications should be acknowledged.**

   A. **Oxygenator function.** The immediate, life-sustaining function of the artificial lung is oxygenation of the blood; ventilation follows. Therefore, the single best monitor of oxygenator function is oxygenation. **Adequacy of oxygenation must be determined early and throughout CPB.** Blood gas values (arterial and venous) should be determined at regular intervals throughout CPB or whenever changes are made in oxygenator gas flow or composition or CPB systemic blood flow rate.

   B. **Cardioplegia delivery.** When cardioplegic solution is delivered from the CPB console, the flow, pressure, and temperature should be monitored to avoid overpressurization of the aortic root or, particularly, of the coronary sinus if retrograde cardioplegia is being used. The aortic root pressure should not exceed 75 to 100 mm Hg and the coronary sinus pressure should not exceed 35 to 40 mm Hg. Monitoring cardioplegic solution and myocardial temperature can reasonably ensure adequate cardioplegia and guide intervals for reinfusion.

   C. **Placement of vents. All vents should be tested before use** by briefly immersing the tip in a basin of saline or pool of blood in the pericardial cavity to verify its suctioning effect. It is important to avoid excessive negative pressures, which can cause hemolysis. Some teams use a one-way valved, vacuum-relief connector incorporated into the vent line before the roller pump. Alternatively, a small-gauge needle can be inserted into the vent line to relieve pressure in the event of vent occlusion. **The perfusionist should be notified when vents are placed, discontinued, or removed** because a significant portion of blood return to the CPB reservoir may occur through a vent.

   D. **Physiologic variables.** Circuit performance must be monitored and managed continuously during CPB to maintain adequate perfusion and organ system viability. Some physiologic variables are under **direct external control** (e.g., total systemic blood flow; input pressure waveform; systemic venous pressure; hematocrit and composition of priming fluid; arterial blood oxygen, carbon dioxide, and nitrogen levels; and temperature of the perfusate and patient) [19]. **The patient determines other variables,** some of which are still, in part, determined by external control (e.g., SVR; total body oxygen consumption; mixed venous blood oxygen levels; lactic acidemia and pH; regional and organ blood flow; and organ function) [19]. Monitoring physiologic function during CPB differs little in principle from normal intraoperative monitoring practices for surgical procedures of similar magnitude without CPB.

   From a practical standpoint, in addition to monitoring patient blood pressures [including central venous (CVP), pulmonary artery (PA), and/or left atrial (LA) pressures] and temperatures, the electrocardiogram and the electroencephalogram (if used) should be monitored. All can warn of abnormal or unexpected conditions. Urinary output should be monitored periodically as a relative indication of adequate perfusion. Blood coagulation status also is monitored throughout CPB. A less specific assessment should be made of the patient's neuromuscular blockade or anesthetic depth. Decreasing mixed venous blood O_2 levels or overt patient movement may indicate light anesthesia.

   E. **Circuit variables.** Parameters that should be continuously monitored by the perfusionist include the following:

      1. **Blood flow** on the arterial side of the circuit by calibrated and properly occluded roller pump or electronic flowmeter display when using a centrifugal pump. Venous blood drainage to the CPB circuit is assessed indirectly by monitoring the blood volume in the venous reservoir. The venous reservoir **blood volume** should be maintained to provide a safe "reaction time," that is, to allow enough time for the systemic blood flow rate to be reduced before dangerously low volumes or depletion of the reservoir volume occurs (Fig. 19.7).

      2. **Arterial tubing "line" pressure** is monitored to warn of possible arterial cannula malpositioning or kinks in the arterial line.

      3. **Gas flow and composition** of the oxygenator ventilating gas are adjusted in response to changing patient temperature and blood gas values. The **inhala-**

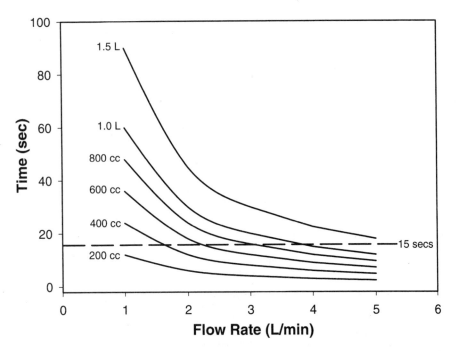

FIG. 19.7 Graph of reaction times with various cardiopulmonary bypass (CPB) reservoir volumes. Each curve depicts decreasing reservoir volume plotted as a function of flow rate and time (in seconds) in the event there is a cessation in venous drainage. As the flow rate is increased, the perfusionist's time to make an appropriate reduction in CPB systemic flow is reduced. The *dashed horizontal line* shows the flow rate that should not be exceeded for a given reservoir volume to maintain 15 seconds' reaction time. (From Kurusz M, Davis RF, Conti VR. Conduct of cardiopulmonary bypass. In: Gravlee GP, Davis RF, Kurusz M, et al., eds. *Cardiopulmonary bypass: principles and practice,* 2nd ed. Philadelphia: Lippincott Williams & Wilkins, 2000:556, with permission.)

          tional anesthetic is adjusted in conjunction with the anesthesiologist to provide anesthesia and manipulation of SVR.
     4. Temperatures include arterial and venous blood and heat exchanger water sources for the oxygenator and cardioplegia delivery system. In addition, it is advisable to monitor at least **two patient temperatures** in the event there is a probe malfunction or malposition.
     5. Suction and vent pump speed should be regulated to avoid excessive speed and occlusion at the suction or vent tip.
  F. Communication. The perfusionist should communicate to the surgeon or anesthesiologist activities that are performed according to protocol or in response to instruction. Any **significant abnormal conditions** should be communicated, including the following:

1. Abruptly increased CPB systemic flow line pressure
2. Sustained decreased venous drainage
3. Nonfunctioning vent or suction
4. Sustained elevated or low patient arterial blood pressure
5. Elevated CVP, LA, or PA pressure
6. Elevated cardioplegia delivery pressure and/or lower than expected flow
7. Any life-threatening equipment malfunction or failure

Other abnormal situations can occur during CPB that are less acute but potentially damaging, including the following:

1. Elevated serum potassium or lower than expected hematocrit
2. Higher than expected CPB fluid volume requirements
3. Higher than expected use of vasopressors or need for increased systemic blood flow for decreased SVR
4. Lower than expected mixed venous O_2 saturation
5. Resumption of cardiac electrical or mechanical activity when the aorta is cross-clamped
6. Air entrainment in the venous line
7. Variation of patient temperature(s) from desired parameters

If deep hypothermia and low flow or circulatory arrest are required, the duration of cooling, patient temperature(s), and elapsed time of low flow or circulatory arrest should be communicated periodically. Similarly, the perfusionist should communicate all changes in CPB systemic blood flow, whether in response to direct instruction or protocol.

V. Prevention of malfunctions and errors. Mechanical malfunction of equipment and components can occur during CPB. Although the incidence is extremely low [20], these problems require quick thinking on the part of the perfusionist and members of the OR team. Each problem must be determined rapidly and evaluated, and corrective measures instituted. Specific protocols to deal with problems can save valuable time when dealing with emergencies during CPB.

  A. Malfunctions of the systemic pump

    1. **Electrical failure** of the pump due to a power interruption in the OR can occur. In this instance, perfusion is maintained by using the manual crank or battery backup to maintain systemic perfusion. The hand crank should always be available and should be stored on the CPB console. When needed, it is applied to the axle of the roller pump head and turned in the proper direction. Newer hand cranks are ratcheted so that they will operate in one direction only to prevent accidental reversal of flow. Hand cranks for centrifugal pumps are geared to permit adequate rpm. A battery-operated light source must be readily available so that the perfusionist can observe the level in the oxygenator reservoir. With manual operation it is possible for the venous reservoir to be emptied, with possible systemic air embolism.

    2. The **pump motor controller can fail** and the arterial roller pump will accelerate to its maximum speed, a condition referred to as **runaway arterial pump head.** In this instance, the pump's electrical plug must be pulled out immediately and the arterial and venous lines clamped. The roller pump tubing then is changed to another pump head. A centrifugal pump may **decouple** when the magnetic attachment to the motor is lost. This condition is manifested by a high-pitched whining sound and can be corrected by turning the speed control knob to zero, clamping the arterial and venous lines to prevent exsanguination of the patient, and then removing and repositioning the pump head on the console before restarting the pump.

    3. **"Pump creep"** is a phenomenon in which the systemic roller pump continues to rotate very slowly after pump rotation has been stopped with the speed control knob. The danger in pump creep lies in the possibility that air will be inadvertently pumped into the arterial CPB flow tubing or that the arterial tubing ("line") will be overpressurized. For these reasons, it is a safe practice to activate the pump's off switch and **clamp the arterial line when no pumping is desired.**

    4. **Occlusion malfunction.** There have been some instances of occlusion malfunction of the arterial pump head. This malfunction may cause the roller head to become totally occlusive to the point where it cannot move. Total occlusion of a roller pump may cause the circuit breaker for that pump head to trip and the rollers to stop. If it cannot be easily corrected, the tubing must be changed to another roller pump. The opposite problem in occlusion malfunction can occur if the rollers become totally nonocclusive. This will result in in-

adequate flows to the patient and may cause hemolysis. If that happens, the pump must be stopped and the occlusion properly reset.

B. **Oxygenator failure.** Hypoxemia of blood leaving the oxygenator may result from either O_2 **supply failure** or **failure of the oxygenator** itself. Failure to oxygenate the blood can be detected either by observing the color of the arterial blood or by an inline blood gas sensor. If oxygenation failure is noted at the onset of bypass and is due to the oxygenator itself, it may be possible to take the patient off bypass while the heart is still ejecting and change the oxygenator. If the problem becomes apparent later during bypass after the aorta has been cross-clamped and the heart arrested, the oxygenator must be changed during a period of circulatory arrest, preferably after inducing hypothermia.

Loss of oxygen supply can occur due to loss of wall O_2 pressure or leaks in the O_2 supply line in the room and can be detected by use of an oxygen analyzer in the oxygenator gas delivery line, preferably placed close to the oxygenator on the gas inlet side (Fig. 19.1). The availability of a backup O_2 supply near the pump console is advisable. The tubing and connectors that supply O_2 to the oxygenator may develop leaks or cracks, leading to an oxygenator failure.

C. **Inadequate anticoagulation.** The causes and management of inadequate anticoagulation are discussed in Chapter 18. If clots appear in the oxygenator, a dose of heparin equal to that initially administered before CPB should be given again immediately and preferably drawn from a different bottle of heparin. If the arterial line filter becomes totally obstructed, the filter bypass line must be opened to maintain CPB systemic blood flow.

D. **Drug or transfusion errors.** Bolus drugs should be administered into the CPB circuit while the patient is on bypass to ensure adequate delivery. All syringes used by the perfusionist should be labeled, dosages verified before administration, and confirmed after administration. **All blood bank and pharmacy products should be double checked** before administration to ensure the blood unit or pharmacy product matches the patient for whom it is designated.

E. **Switching of arterial and venous lines.** There have been some cases of inadvertent switching of the arterial and venous lines, resulting in blood draining from the aorta and pumping into the venous circulation, leading to excessive venous pressure, possible damage to the vena cava, or air entrainment into the aorta as a result of negative pressure around the cannula insertion site. This can be immediately noted by a **widening of the pulse pressure** observed on the aneroid manometer that is connected to the CPB circuits' arterial line (rather than the usual decrease in pulse pressure) and distention of the vena cava when starting CPB. This phenomenon can be prevented by verification of the arterial line pressure, which should closely mimic the systemic arterial pressure.

The CPB systemic inflow line usually is smaller (⅜-inch ID) than the venous line (½-inch ID), so this mistake should not occur. If the same-sized tubing is used for both lines, they should be color coded or otherwise designated from one another to permit easy identification. If reversal of the CPB systemic flow and venous lines occurs, it should be readily appreciated. **Patency of the arterial cannula and systemic tubing should be verified before starting CPB** by the presence of a pulsatile aortic pressure in the CPB systemic flow tubing correlating with the systemic blood pressure. If switching of the lines occurs, CPB must be stopped immediately and the connections corrected after proper de-airing before restarting CPB.

F. **Inadvertent air infusion [21].** As previously mentioned, both roller and centrifugal pumps can deliver air to the arterial circulation. One of the primary functions of the perfusionist is to ensure during the course of CPB that the reservoir from which the pump draws blood does not become dangerously low or empty and allow air to enter the systemic flow line or arterial cannula. Even if the reservoir has not become completely empty, air can be entrained into the arterial line in the form of bubbles that have been mixed into the blood (**vortexing**). If VAVD is being used, a pressure-relief valve must be incorporated into the venous reservoir to avoid buildup of positive pressure from suction or vent pumps that, if not relieved, can cause rapid **retrograde venous line air transmission.** As mentioned earlier, vents should always be tested before use. If air is observed entering the heart or aorta, CPB should be immediately stopped and treatment begun according to the protocol outlined in Table 19.5.

G. **Safety devices**

1. **Devices to detect and prevent air embolism.** Besides the most important safety device—a vigilant perfusionist—many available mechanical and electronic safety devices are designed to detect and prevent air embolism.

    a. **Low-level alarm.** An ultrasonic or capacitance sensor is attached to the side of the hard-shell reservoir at a user-determined level. When the blood level is above the sensor, no alarm sounds, but if the blood level drops below the sensor, an alarm sounds and a light flashes. Low-level alarms can be engaged to automatically shut off the arterial pump or to simply warn of a low-level condition.

    b. **Air bubble detector.** The air bubble detector has been used for many years and has a good track record in prevention of massive systemic air embolism. A sensor head clamps onto the arterial tubing and an ultrasonic signal detects bubbles greater than 0.5 to 1.0 mL in size. Pump shutoff is automatic unless the air bubble detector is turned off or overridden. Discrete bubbles are necessary to trip the detector, and **the detector can fail to detect foam** (microbubbles) passing through the arterial line.

    c. **Arterial line filter.** This device is placed in the systemic CPB flow line between the oxygenator and the patient. It captures gross air emboli physically. Arterial screen filters are effective in retaining gaseous microemboli.

Table 19.5 Intraoperative and postoperative management strategies for treatment of air embolism

---

1. Perfusionist: Stop CPB immediately, clamp arterial and venous lines, and notify surgeon and anesthesiologist.
2. Locate and confirm source of air; if due to pressurized CPB component, isolate component from patient before relieving pressure.
3. Perfusionist: Purge air from CPB systemic flow line and refill with fluid.
4. Surgeon: Aspirate air (if present) from arterial cannula; if possible, initiate cardiac massage until CPB restarted.
5. Anesthesiologist: Place patient in steep head-down position; be prepared to temporarily occlude carotid arteries.
6. Confirm sufficient volume in CPB reservoir and resume CPB with active aortic root venting.
7. Administer vasopressors to raise perfusion pressure.
8. If suspected cerebral air embolism, cool patient on CPB and consider instituting retrograde cerebral perfusion; consider packing patient's head in ice.
9. Anesthesiologist: Ventilate lungs vigorously with 100% oxygen; administer corticosteroids (2–4 g methylprednisolone and/or 20 mg dexamethasone, and continue for 3–4 days postoperatively).
10. Administer 25 g mannitol and maintain for 48 hours postoperatively.
11. Aim for early patient arousal and assess for return of normal mentation.
12. Consult a neurologist if CNS damage is suspected.
13. Consider CT scan or MRI if patient fails to awaken or develops delayed mental deterioration.
14. Consider hyperbaric oxygen treatment (6 ATA using recommended U.S. Navy diving tables) and make necessary ground transportation arrangements; repeat hyperbaric oxygen therapy as necessary.
15. Do not give up resuscitative efforts unless patient dies or is diagnosed as brain dead.

ATA, atmospheres of absolute pressure; CNS, central nervous system; CPB, cardiopulmonary bypass; CT, computed tomography; MRI, magnetic resonance imaging.
(From Kurusz M, Mills NL. Management of unusual problems encountered in initiating and maintaining cardiopulmonary bypass. In: Gravlee GP, Davis RF, Kurusz M, et al., eds. *Cardiopulmonary bypass: principles and practice,* 2nd ed. Philadelphia: Lippincott Williams & Wilkins, 2000:596, with permission.)

To maximize its effectiveness, it should be operated with an **open purge line** to allow any entrained air to escape.

   d. **Purge line.** The one-way purge line is an important safety device. It originates from the top of the arterial line filter and connects to a venous reservoir port or manifold for blood sampling. By allowing a continuous flow of approximately 200 mL/min to drain from the top of the arterial filter to the reservoir, it serves as an air purge from the arterial filter. This one-way purge line prevents the accidental injection of air into the systemic side of the circuit that might otherwise occur during blood sampling or drug injection.

   e. **Other one-way valves.** These valves can be used to prevent air from being pumped through a suction or vent line in the wrong direction if either the pump is operated in reverse or the tubing is loaded into the pump head incorrectly at the time of assembly. Large-bore, one-way valves are available for use with centrifugal pumps to prevent retrograde flow.

 2. **Devices to monitor blood oxygenation, ventilation, electrolytes, and acid–base status.** Reliable and accurate continuous inline monitoring of blood gas parameters and electrolytes has become more routinely used. These indicators assess the adequacy of perfusion and measure the oxygen content in arterial and venous blood, acid–base balance with hydrogen ion concentration, and metabolite levels. The advantage of these systems is rapid detection of changes in patient and CPB perfusion status rather than reliance on intermittent blood sampling. **These devices must be calibrated to conventional laboratory sample values and are used primarily for trending purposes.**

 3. **Devices to monitor coagulation status.** Because patient response to heparin varies greatly depending on factors including levels of antithrombin III, previous doses of heparin, and potency of the heparin administered, **it is imperative to monitor the degree of anticoagulation.** The standard for measurement of coagulation is currently the activated clotting time (ACT). Quantitative measurements of heparin concentration by the automated protamine titration method also are used in some centers. Measurement of the ACT and other coagulation tests are discussed in greater detail in Chapter 18.

 H. **Checklists and protocols.** Checklists and protocols are no substitute for common sense and experience. However, they have been found useful in promoting safe conduct of CPB. Protocols can describe selection of circuit components and required priming volumes referenced to patient size or diagnosis. Protocols can be created for specific surgeon preferences (e.g., cannulas) or pediatric applications. Detailed protocols may list in outline form specific steps for circuit assembly, priming, and management during certain less frequently performed and specialized procedures, such as cardiac transplantation, left heart bypass for repair of the descending aorta, or deep hypothermia and circulatory arrest with retrograde or select anterograde cerebral, or retrograde cerebral perfusion for inadvertent air embolism. **Protocols should be developed with input from all OR team members** and periodically reviewed and updated to remain contemporary with current clinical practice.

   Prebypass checklists are useful for verifying proper CPB circuit assembly and function. Checklists can be abbreviated or be all inclusive. They are most effective if they contain only those items that, if omitted, would have a direct and adverse effect on the safe conduct of perfusion [22]. The sections of a checklist might include items related to patient and procedure; sterility of CPB components; proper pump assembly and function; adequacy of electrical connections; adequacy of oxygenator gas supply; arrangement and integrity of CPB lines; composition of cardioplegic solution; testing and activation of alarms; calibration and placement of monitors and probes; operational capacity of water supply system; verification of anticoagulation; and availability of backup supplies and equipment.

VII. Summary. CPB has evolved into a routine, safe, and reliable system that requires intensive specialized training to operate [23,24]. It is the function of the perfusionist to maintain and operate this equipment during CPB. However, anesthesiologists and surgeons caring for patients undergoing CPB bear the responsibility of understanding this equipment and its function in order to manage cardiovascular surgery patients properly [25].

References
1. Engelman RM, Pleet AB, Rousou JA, et al. Influence of cardiopulmonary bypass perfusion temperature on neurologic and hematologic function after coronary artery bypass grafting. *Ann Thorac Surg* 1999;67:1547–1555.
2. Kirklin JW, Barratt-Boyes BG. Hypothermia, circulatory arrest, and cardiopulmonary bypass. In: *Cardiac surgery,* 2nd ed. New York: Churchill Livingstone, 1993:97.
3. Buckberg GD. Myocardial protection: an overview. *Semin Thorac Cardiovasc Surg* 1993; 5:98–106.
4. Lee-Sensiba K, Azzaretto N, Carolina C, et al. New roller pump disposable provides safety and simplifies occlusion setting. *J Extracorpor Technol* 1997;29:19–24.
5. Springer MA, Korth DC, Guiterrez PJ, et al. An in vitro analysis of a one-way arterial check valve. *J Extracorpor Technol* 1995;27:29–33.
6. Munster K, Andersen U, Mikkelsen J, et al. Vacuum assisted venous drainage (VAVD). *Perfusion* 1999;14:419–423.
7. Rousou JA, Engelman RM, Flack JE 3rd, et al. The "primeless pump": a novel technique for intraoperative blood conservation. *Cardiovasc Surg* 1999;7:228–235.
8. Toomasian JM, McCarthy JP. Total extrathoracic cardiopulmonary support with kinetic assisted venous drainage: experience in 50 patients. *Perfusion* 1998;13:137–43.
9. Groom RC, Hill AG, Kuban B, et al. Aortic cannula velocimetry. *Perfusion* 1995;10:183–188.
10. Stammers AH. Advances in myocardial protection: the role of mechanical devices in providing cardioprotective strategies. *Int Anesthesiol Clin* 1996;34:61–84.
11. Solis RT, Noon GP, Beall AC, et al. Particulate microembolism during cardiac operation. *Ann Thorac Surg* 1974;17:332–344.
12. Jones L, Knight PG, Alley R, et al. Adverse effects of Forane, Ethrane, and halothane on the William Harvey H-1700 bubble oxygenator. *Proc Am Acad Cardiovasc Perfusion* 1987;8:178–181.
13. Faulkner SC, Kurusz M, Manning JV Jr, et al. Clinical experience with the Amicon Diafilter during cardiopulmonary bypass. *Proc Am Acad Cardiovasc Perfusion* 1987;8: 66–69.
14. Aldea GS, O'Gara P, Shapira OM, et al. Effects of anticoagulation protocol on outcome in patients undergoing CABG with heparin-bonded cardiopulmonary bypass circuits. *Ann Thorac Surg* 1998;65:425–433.
15. Rosengart TR, DeBois WJ, O'Hara M, et al. Retrograde autologous priming for cardiopulmonary bypass: a safe and effective means of decreasing hemodilution and transfusion requirements. *J Thorac Cardiovasc Surg* 1998;115:426–439.
16. DeFoe GR, Ross CS, Olmstead EM, et al. Lowest hematocrit on bypass and adverse outcomes associated with coronary artery bypass grafting. Northern New England Cardiovascular Disease Study Group. *Ann Thorac Surg* 2001;71:769–776.
17. Hargrove M, McCarthy AP, Fitzpatrick GJ. Carbon dioxide flushing prior to priming the bypass circuit, an experimental derivation of the optimal flow rate and duration of the flushing process. *Perfusion* 1987;2:177–180.
18. Kurusz M, Wheeldon DR. Risk containment during cardiopulmonary bypass. *Semin Thorac Cardiovasc Surg* 1990;2:400–409.
19. Kirklin JW, Barratt-Boyes BG. Hypothermia, circulatory arrest, and cardiopulmonary bypass. In: *Cardiac surgery,* 2nd ed. New York: Churchill Livingstone, 1993, p 75.
20. Mejak BL, Stammers A, Rauch E, et al. A retrospective study on perfusion accidents and safety devices. *Perfusion* 2000;15:51–61.
21. Kurusz M, Butler BD, Katz J, Conti VR. Air embolism during cardiopulmonary bypass. *Perfusion* 1995;10:361–391.
22. Kurusz M, Harshaw RC. The contribution of checklists to perfusion safety: lessons from aviation. In: Steenbrink J, Wijers-Hille MJ, deJong DS, eds. *Fourth European Congress on Extracorporeal Circulation Technology,* June 12–15, 1991. Utrecht: Foundation European Congress on Extracorporeal Circulation, 1995:177–185.
23. **Stammers AH. Extracorporeal devices and related technologies. In: Kaplan JA, ed. *Cardiac anesthesia,* 4th ed. Philadelphia: WB Saunders, 1999:1017–1060.**
24. **Stammers AH, ed. Cardiopulmonary bypass: emerging trends and continued practices. *Intl Anesthesiol Clin* 1996;34.**
25. **Gravlee GP, Davis RF, Kurusz M, et al., eds. *Cardiopulmonary bypass: principles and practice,* 2nd ed. Philadelphia: Lippincott Williams & Wilkins, 2000.**

20. PATHOPHYSIOLOGY OF CARDIOPULMONARY BYPASS

Eugene A. Hessel II and Peter G. Hild

Cardiopulmonary bypass (CPB), often regarded by lay persons and medical personnel alike as a routine procedure, frequently is taken for granted. This attitude may be attributable to the large number of cases performed and the relatively low incidence of morbidity and mortality associated with CPB.

It should be remembered that CPB technology is relatively new. Improvements in oxygenator design, addition of various filters and defoaming devices, improved monitoring of anticoagulation, and greater understanding of blood damage by high flow rates and shear stresses have contributed to the relative safety of modern CPB. However, the low frequency of complications associated with CPB is due more to the human organism's ability to adapt to physiologic insults than to any inherent safety of CPB techniques.

The three major physiologic aberrations introduced by CPB are (i) alterations of pulsatility and blood flow patterns; (ii) exposure of blood to nonphysiologic surfaces and shear stresses; and (iii) exaggerated stress responses. In addition, modern CPB usually involves varying degrees of hypothermia and hypotension and their attendant physiologic changes. Improving the safety of CPB will depend on greater understanding of these aberrations [1].

I. Cardiopulmonary bypass as a perfusion system

   A. Normal circulatory homeostasis. Normally, maintenance of adequate cardiac output, O_2 delivery, and metabolic waste elimination are governed by metabolic needs of the body. Heart rate, ventricular filling pressures, myocardial contractility, and systemic vascular resistance (SVR) are modulated by autonomic nervous system tone and circulating catecholamine levels.

   Autonomic nervous system activity is modulated by the various baroreceptors and chemoreceptors in the central nervous system (CNS) and periphery in response to changes in blood pressure, pH, P_aO_2, and P_aCO_2. These changes are in turn directly related to tissue metabolism. As metabolic requirements increase, sympathetic tone is increased. Consequently, cardiac output and O_2 delivery are increased.

   B. Circulatory control during cardiopulmonary bypass. "Cardiac output" on CPB is the pump flow rate, which can be set at any level desired. Systemic and venous blood pressures are partially dependent on the patient's autonomic tone but are easily manipulated by increasing or decreasing venous drainage and by administering vasopressors or vasodilators. Thus, the circulation during CPB is controlled in large part by the perfusionist and the anesthesiologist.

   1. **Systemic blood flow.** Systemic blood flow is determined by pump flow of the heart lung machine, which is set by the perfusionist. This should be guided by the patient's age, temperature, depth of anesthesia, and hematocrit. At mild hypothermia (about 35°C) and with a hematocrit of about 24% in an adult, flow typically is set at about 2.4 L/min/M², which meets the oxygen needs of an anesthetized patient. Whether this remains true during the lighter levels of anesthesia used with "fast-track" protocols remains to be defined. Recall that the normal adaptation to a reduced hematocrit is a rise in the cardiac output, which should be taken into account when selecting flow rates, especially at normothermia or lower hematocrits [2]. However, the maximal flow during CPB is limited by venous return from the patient, which is influenced by the height of the operating table above the heart-lung machine; placement and resistance in venous cannulas and lines; blood volume; and venous tone. Maximal flow also is limited by the capacity of the heart-lung machine and size of the arterial cannula. High flows through the arterial cannula produce high-pressure gradients and turbulence, which damage the blood and produce adverse jet effects (e.g., dislodgment of atheroemboli). If there is significant aortic regurgitation or bronchial collateral flow, this shunts pump flow away from the body, and pump flow must be increased appropriately.

   2. **Arterial pressure.** As in the normal state, arterial pressure is the product of cardiac output (i.e., pump flow during CPB; see Section **1** above) and SVR. The latter is determined by blood viscosity and by smooth muscle tone in the arterioles. Viscosity is principally influenced by hematocrit and temperature, both of which often change considerably during CPB. Viscosity remains reasonably constant if hematocrit (expressed as a percentage) and temperatures (expressed in degrees Celsius) are the same (i.e., viscosity at 35°C with a hematocrit of

35% is about the same as when temperatures and hematocrit are 27°C and 27%, or 20°C and 20%, respectively). It follows that at normothermia, if hematocrit falls from 40% to 20%, viscosity (and hence SVR) will fall about 50% and at a constant pump flow (cardiac output), the mean arterial pressure (MAP) will fall about 50%.

SVR also is determined by vascular tone, which is influenced by pulsatility (SVR lower with pulsatile flow), sympathetic nervous system activity, depth of anesthesia, catecholamines, angiotensin and arginine vasopressin (AVP), acid–base and electrolyte status, various mediators of the systemic inflammatory response (SIR; see Section **V.H.1**), and administration of vasoactive drugs.

Controversy exists regarding the importance of and optimal arterial pressure during CPB (see below). If pressure is too low, perfusion of critical vascular beds may be compromised, especially if vascular disease is present. Conversely, excessive arterial pressure increases noncoronary collateral flow to the heart during aortic cross-clamping (hence "washing out" myocardial protection with cardioplegia) and bronchial flow to the lungs (increases blood return to left heart) and places strain on arterial clamps and suture lines. Likewise there is controversy as to the best means of raising MAP when it is deemed to be too low (e.g., increasing pump flow vs. raising hematocrit or administering a vasoconstrictor).

3. **Venous pressure.** Venous pressure is determined by blood volume, venous tone (sympathetic nervous system, depth of anesthesia, vasoactive drugs), resistance to flow out the venous cannula (placement, size, kinks, distortion of heart), height of operating table, and total flow. Venous return normally is by gravity (siphon) but sometimes is augmented by applying vacuum or suction to the venous lines.

Elevated venous pressure can seriously compromise organ perfusion and can lead to peripheral edema.

4. **Distribution of blood flow.** In addition to total blood flow, one must be concerned about flow in each organ [3]. Recent studies have noted a hierarchy of distribution of blood flow during normothermia and hypothermia as total flow is reduced [4,5]. Even at "normal flow" (i.e., 2.4 L/m/M²) muscle flow is significantly reduced during CPB. As flow is progressively reduced, first splanchnic, then renal, and then (only at extremely low flows) cerebral flows are reduced.

C. **Circulatory changes during cardiopulmonary bypass**
   1. **Changes at onset of CPB.** At commencement of CPB, there usually is a fall in systemic blood pressure due to several factors.
      a. Usual pump flow rates are comparable to cardiac output before initiating CPB. Decreases in blood pressure from decreased "cardiac output" are unusual.
      b. The major cause of decreased blood pressure at the initiation of CPB is a dramatic decrease in SVR. This phenomenon results from
         (1) Decreased blood viscosity secondary to hemodilution by the pump priming fluid
         (2) **Decreased vascular tone secondary to**
            (a) Dilution of circulating catecholamines
            (b) Temporary hypoxemia. Hypoxemia from initial circulation of pump asanguineous priming fluid may lead to decreased vascular tone.
            (c) Low pH and low calcium and magnesium levels in the priming fluid
   2. **Circulatory status during hypothermic CPB**
      a. **Increased SVR.** There may be considerable patient-to-patient variations in SVR during CPB. However, as CPB progresses, there will generally be a steady increase in systemic pressure due to increasing SVR if flow rates are kept constant, but SVR rarely exceeds values present before CPB initiation. The observed increase in SVR during the course of CPB probably is caused by several factors:
         (1) Decreased vascular cross-sectional area from closure of portions of the microvasculature

       (2) Vasoconstriction brought on by
         (a) Hypothermia
         (b) Increasing levels of circulating catecholamines, arginine vaso-
              pressin (AVP), and angiotensin II
       (3) Increase in blood viscosity secondary to hypothermia, and rising
          hematocrit (due to urine output or translocation of fluid into the in-
          terstitial compartment)
  b. Decreased SVR. Transient decreases in SVR and systemic pressure may
     be observed shortly after infusion of cardioplegic solutions, especially if the
     solutions contain nitroglycerin.
  c. Flow rate. Pump flow rates are completely under external control and can
     be manipulated at will within the limits of venous return to the pump.
     Pump flow rates usually are expressed as mL/kg/min or, more frequently,
     L/min/m². In awake patients, it is generally accepted that a cardiac index
     less than 2.0 to 2.2 L/min/m² is not sufficient to provide tissues with an ad-
     equate oxygen supply. This also appears to be the lower limit of sufficient
     cardiac output during **normothermic** CPB. With increasing degrees of
     hypothermia, the patient's oxygen demand decreases, and consequently
     pump flow rates may be reduced significantly. Kirklin and Barratt-
     Boyes [6] calculated curves relating oxygen consumption to pump flow
     rates at different temperatures (Fig. 20.1). These hyperbolic curves are
     mathematically expressed by the equation:

$$V_{O_2} = 0.4437 \, (Q - 62.7) + 71.6$$

and describe "best-fit" lines for measured V_{O_2} at varying nonpulsatile flow
rates from several animal studies. The small x's on each curve represent
clinically used flow rates at each temperature at the University of Alabama.

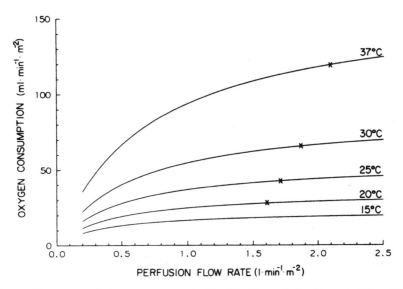

FIG. 20.1 Nomogram relating oxygen consumption (V_{O_2}) to perfusion flow rate (Q) and temperature (T). (From Kirklin JW, Barratt-Boyes BG. Hypothermia, circulatory arrest, and cardiopulmonary bypass. In: Kirklin JW, Barratt-Boyes BG, eds. *Cardiac surgery,* 2nd ed. New York:
Churchill Livingstone, 1993:91, with permission.)

Pump flow rates greater than 2.2 L/min/m² at normothermia do not result in greater tissue oxygen consumption and expose blood to greater damage from higher shear rates. The significance of O_2 consumption will be discussed later.

   d. **Arterial blood pressure.** Although acceptable flow rates are fairly well established, there is considerable controversy about acceptable arterial pressures during CPB. At any given flow rate, there is marked variability in arterial pressure from patient to patient. The overriding concern with low arterial pressures is adequacy of organ perfusion. The brain and kidney are the organs at greatest risk. Short periods of hypotension with MAP less than 30 mm Hg are well tolerated. Fox et al. [7] demonstrated that cerebral autoregulation is well preserved during moderately hypothermic CPB. Govier et al. [8] demonstrated that cerebral blood flow was relatively constant down to MAP of about 30 mm Hg in patients who were normotensive preoperatively and in whom α-stat blood gas management was used during hypothermic CPB. In this study, flow rates were held constant and low arterial pressure represented low SVR. More recent studies support the premise that cerebral autoregulation remains essentially intact. When pH-stat arterial blood gas management is used (see Section **IV.C.4**), cerebral blood flow may become more pressure dependent [9–11]. Despite these findings, many anesthesiologists use vasopressors and vasodilators to keep MAP between arbitrarily set limits of 50 and 100 mm Hg during CPB. Some centers report lower perfusion pressures than those described earlier, with no greater reported incidence of mortality [12].

3. **Circulatory changes during the rewarming phase of CPB**
   a. As the perfusate temperature is increased to rewarm the patient, variable circulatory responses are observed depending on the anesthetics used, patient hematocrit, underlying disease, and other factors. Frequently SVR and MAP increase during rewarming from 25°C to 32°C. Occasionally, as temperature increases above 32°C, SVR and MAP will decrease.
   b. A more consistent decrease in SVR and MAP usually occurs with release of the aortic cross-clamp and reperfusion of the heart. Despite cardioplegia and hypothermia, there is some degree of ongoing metabolic activity and utilization of myocardial energy stores during the ischemic period. When the heart is reperfused, accumulated metabolites are washed out of the heart into the general circulation. Some of these metabolites, most notably **adenosine,** are potent vasodilators that induce a marked decrease in SVR.

4. **Warm CPB.** Recently there has been a trend to conduct CPB at near normothermic levels [13]. The putative advantages include avoiding adverse effects of hypothermia, shortening duration of bypass required for cooling and rewarming, avoiding hazards of overheating (especially of the brain) during rewarming, less bleeding, and perhaps earlier extubation. Normothermic bypass narrows the ratio of oxygen demand (Vo_2) to oxygen delivery (Do_2). This suggests the need to maintain hematocrit and pump flow rates higher than accepted during hypothermic CPB. SVR and MAP also tend to be lower, leading to the practice of administering more fluids and vasoconstrictors and using higher pump flow rates. Deeper levels of anesthesia likely are necessary. Obviously the safe durations of low flow or circulatory arrest are shortened should these strategies be needed. Cerebral outcome has been a concern. This partially explains the popularity of using mild degrees of hypothermia (about 35°C), so called "tepid" bypass, which may offer substantial cerebral protection without the disadvantages of deeper levels of hypothermia. Cognitive outcome has been found to be comparable among patients maintained at 35°C versus 30°C [14].

5. **Changes in the microcirculation and adequacy of tissue perfusion during CPB**
   a. During CPB, cardiac output and arterial pressure can be easily maintained at "normal" values. However, several observations suggest that tissue

perfusion and O_2 delivery can be impaired to varying degrees during CPB, including

   (1) Postoperative organ dysfunction, both temporary and permanent
   (2) Variable decreases in O_2 consumption during normothermic CPB at flows and pressures that are comparable to pre-CPB values
   (3) Variable increases in serum lactate levels

b. The microcirculation lies between the precapillary arterioles and the postcapillary venules and includes the capillary bed, interstitial fluid space, and microcirculatory lymphatics. Normal microcirculatory physiology is poorly understood and requires further clarification. However, it is clear that microcirculatory function during CPB may be impaired by

   (1) Constriction of precapillary arteriolar sphincters (caused by catecholamines, angiotensin, vasopressin, thromboxane, and decreased release of nitric oxide) with or without formation of arteriolar-venular shunts
   (2) Increased interstitial fluid volume (edema)
   (3) Decreased lymphatic drainage
   (4) Loss of pulsatile flow
   (5) "Sludging" in the capillaries due to hypothermia
   (6) Altered deformability of red blood cells (RBCs)
   (7) Microaggregation and adhesion of white cells, platelets, and fibrin onto the endothelium related to the systemic inflammatory reaction and contact activation described below
   (8) Microemboli (gas, lipids, aggregates of white blood cells, platelets, and fibrin, and foreign materials), a major source of which is the cardiotomy suction.

   Attempts to optimize microcirculatory function during CPB may include use of vasodilators to inhibit arteriolar constriction, addition of mannitol to the pump priming fluid to inhibit interstitial fluid accumulation, use of pulsatile perfusion techniques, and hemodilution to a hematocrit between 20% and 30% to optimize capillary flow, use of microfiltration, minimizing return to unprocessed cardiotomy suction blood directly into the heart-lung machine, and antiinflammatory strategies (see below).

6. **Pulsatile versus nonpulsatile flow during CPB.** One of the major physiologic derangements introduced by CPB is loss of pulsatility of flow. Intuitively, it seems desirable to reproduce normal flow patterns as closely as possible during CPB. However, there is considerable controversy about the merits of pulsatile perfusion compared with conventional nonpulsatile perfusion.

   a. **How to produce pulsatile flow.** Several methods are commonly used to maintain arterial pulsations during CPB.
      (1) If partial CPB is being used, venous drainage can be reduced to permit some cardiac ejection.
      (2) If an intraaortic balloon is in place, it can be used to impart pulsatility to the flow.
      (3) Pulsations can be produced by roller pumps designed to rotate at varying speeds.
      (4) Use of ventricular pumps

   b. **Damping effects of the aortic cannula.** The first two methods of producing pulsations are more effective because they generate the pulse in the aorta itself. Although many pumps produce effective pulsations in the pump outflow, the amount of pulsatile energy transmitted into the aorta is limited by the damping effects caused by the narrow aortic cannula, membrane oxygenators, and arterial microfilters. This makes it unlikely that much pulsatile power can be transferred into the patient by roller pumps [15].

   c. **Nature of the pulse waveform.** The energy and dynamics of the normal arterial pressure waveform are complex. It is becoming increasingly evident that the more closely the pulse contour resembles the normal arterial pulse, the less the physiologic disruption from extracorporeal perfusion. Many early studies that found no significant differences between the two techniques used pulse contours that were nearly sine wave in nature, in contrast to pulsations with the rapid systolic upstroke and slower diastolic runoff of a normal arterial pulse.

   d. Benefits

      (1) Transmission of more energy to the microcirculation

         (a) Reduces critical capillary closing pressure

         (b) Improves lymphatic flow

         (c) Improves tissue perfusion; enhances diffusion of oxygen and other substrates and hence cellular metabolism

      (2) Reduction of adverse neuroendocrine responses (mainly vasoconstrictive) to nonpulsatile flow that emanate from baroreceptors, the kidneys, and the endothelium (regulation of nitric oxide release)

      (3) The above two effects may result in increased oxygen consumption; reduced acidosis; reduced edema formation; improved perfusion of brain, heart, and kidney; and potentially reduced morbidity and mortality.

   e. Liabilities

      (1) Increased cost and complexities

      (2) Requires use of larger arterial cannulas

      (3) Is associated with higher nozzle velocities out of the arterial cannula (risking cellular and endovascular injury and thromboembolism)

      (4) Risk of generating gaseous microemboli and damage to oxygenator circuit

   f. Clinical outcome. Clinical outcome data have been conflicting [16,17]. In the absence of clear-cut benefit, use of pulsatile flow has not gained much popularity for clinical CPB.

II. Cardiopulmonary bypass as an O_2 delivery system

  A. Oxygenator function. The details of oxygenator design and the efficiency of those designs are discussed in detail in Chapter 19. The oxygenator serves the function of the lungs, namely, oxygenation of and elimination of CO_2 from venous blood. During CPB, the intricacies of pulmonary physiology are eliminated, and gas exchange occurs merely by bringing blood and gas into direct contact (bubble oxygenator) or close proximity (membrane oxygenator). The resulting P_aO_2 and P_aCO_2 are determined by the F_IO_2 of the gas mixture and the rate at which the gas mixture flows through the oxygenator. Varying amounts of CO_2 may be added to the gas mixture flowing through the oxygenator.

  B. Blood gas monitoring during cardiopulmonary bypass. Modern oxygenators are efficient gas exchangers, and the perfusionist easily and precisely controls arterial blood gas tensions. Frequent blood gas determinations are becoming less necessary with the advent of inline blood gas monitors in the CPB circuit. During normothermic CPB, arterial blood gases are maintained near conventional values: pH 7.40, P_aCO_2 35 to 45 mm Hg, and P_aO_2 more than 100 mm Hg.

III. Adequacy of perfusion

  A. How to define

    1. A pragmatic answer is that if the patient survives without evidence of organ dysfunction, then bypass has been adequate. In addition to being retrospective, this evaluation depends highly on the sensitivity of the test used to evaluate postoperative organ function. However, studies of this nature have provided much useful information to guide improvements in conducting CPB.

    2. Maintain adequate oxygen delivery to all organs

    3. Avoid activation of undesirable reactions, e.g., neuroendocrine stress response and SIR

    4. Maintaining adequate systemic blood flow, arterial and venous pressures, arterial pulsatility, arterial and venous blood gases, and arterial oxygen content and delivery. The definition of "adequate" is influenced by the patient's age and temperature, and by the type and depth of anesthesia.

  B. Monitoring

    1. Global

a. Oxygen consumption (V_{O_2}) measurement, although not commonly used clinically, experimentally has provided much insight into the proper conduct of CPB. It can be easily calculated from simultaneously measured arterial and venous oxygen contents and knowledge of pump flow:

$$V_{O_2} = \text{Pump flow} \times (C_aO_2 - C_vO_2)$$

Kirlin and Barratt-Boyes [6] suggested that maintaining V_{O_2} at 85% of the predicted maximum for a given temperature will provide adequate O_2 delivery (Fig. 20.1).

b. Oxygen delivery (D_{O_2}) can be easily calculated during CPB ($D_{O_2} = C_aO_2 \times$ pump flow) but this is not commonly done.

c. Mixed venous oxygen saturation (S_vO_2), content (C_vO_2), or oxygen extraction ratio (OER) provide clues to the adequacy of the balance of oxygen delivery (O_2D) to oxygen demand (V_{O_2}). OER is the ratio of V_{O_2}/O_2D. Normally S_vO_2 is about 75% and OER about 25%. When these two values approach 50%, critically compromised oxygen delivery is suggested. Inline monitoring of venous saturation is commonly used during CPB. Unfortunately this can fail to detect regional ischemia if the vascular bed is small or if there is too little desaturated blood returning from a poorly perfused bed to influence mixed venous oxygen. Thus, although a low venous oxygen saturation should always be remedied, a normal or high venous saturation is not always reassuring [18].

2. **Monitoring specific organ function during CPB as a means of ensuring adequate tissue perfusion**
   a. Cerebral function. Electroencephalography, cerebral evoked responses, cerebral blood flow (transcranial Doppler), and cerebral oximetry can be used to monitor cerebral perfusion, but the effects of anesthetic medication and hypothermia may limit their usefulness. Jugular venous saturation, pressure, and temperature may give insight into how well the brain is being supported.
   b. Renal function. Urine output is the simplest measure of renal function. However, different blood flow patterns, varying perfusion pressures, effects of hypothermia, and the presence or absence of diuretics in the pump priming fluid may affect urine output and render it an inaccurate indicator of overall tissue perfusion.
   c. Splanchnic. No monitoring usually is used clinically at this time, but use of gastric tonometry (saline or air, pH, or P_{CO_2}), Doppler assessments of mucosal blood flow, hepatic blood flow measurement, and hepatic venous O_2 saturation monitoring have been used in clinical investigations.

IV. **Hypothermia and cardiopulmonary bypass**
   A. **Effects of hypothermia on biochemical reactions.** The Q_{10} for chemical reactions is a measure of changes in rate of reaction for 10°C rise in temperature. For human tissues, Q_{10} is approximately 2. That is, for each 10°C decrease in body temperature, the rate of reaction (i.e., metabolic rate or oxygen consumption) is roughly halved.
   B. **Effects of hypothermia on blood viscosity.** Hypothermia increases blood viscosity. In the early history of CPB, hemodilution was not performed, and the high morbidity and mortality (e.g., stroke, organ infarcts) probably were secondary to this hyperviscous state. Today patients are hemodiluted to hematocrits of 20% to 30% during CPB. Although O_2-carrying capacity is decreased from hemodilution, O_2 delivery is improved because the decreased viscosity provides improved microcirculatory flow.
   C. **Changes in blood gases associated with hypothermia**
      1. **Changes in oxygen–hemoglobin dissociation curve.** As the temperature decreases, the affinity or strength of binding between O_2 and hemoglobin increases. A lower partial pressure of O_2 is required to force a given amount of O_2 into the hemoglobin molecule. The oxygen–hemoglobin dissociation curve is shifted to the left. Release of O_2 from hemoglobin at the tissue level is less efficient.

2. **Changes in solubility of O$_2$ and CO$_2$.** As temperature decreases, gases become more soluble in liquid. For a given amount of O$_2$ or CO$_2$, more gas will be dissolved in the plasma and the partial pressure of the gas will decrease. This is much more significant for CO$_2$ because it is more soluble in plasma at any given temperature.

3. **Neutrality of water.** Neutral water is water in which the [H$^+$] is equal to the [OH$^-$]. At 37°C, the pH of neutral water is 6.8. At 25°C the pH of neutral water is 7.0. As temperature decreases, the pH at which water is "neutral" changes in a linear fashion. The neutral pH increases 0.017 units for each degree Celsius decrease in temperature (Fig. 20.2).

4. **Differing strategies for measuring and managing blood gases during CPB**

   Blood gases are measured at 37°C in blood gas analyzing machines. If the patient's body temperature is lower than this value, the pH and P$_a$CO$_2$ would have to be (and can be) corrected to determine their actual values at the patient's temperature. If the patient's temperature is 27°C and the pH and Pco$_2$ as measured at 37°C are 7.40 and 40, respectively, then the pH and P$_a$CO$_2$ corrected to a body temperature of 27°C would be about 7.55 and 25. Conversely, if the pH and P$_a$CO$_2$ as measured at 37°C are 7.25 and 55, then the corrected values at 27°C would be about 7.40 and 40.

   At issue are the appropriate temperature-corrected pH and P$_a$CO$_2$ values during hypothermia. One method (*pH-stat*) attempts to keep the *temperature-corrected* pH and P$_a$CO$_2$ at 7.40 and 40, respectively. The other method (*alpha-stat*) attempts to keep the ratio of OH$^-$/H$^+$ ions constant so that enzyme systems function appropriately. This will be accomplished if the *uncorrected* pH and P$_a$CO$_2$ as measured at 37°C are 7.40 and 40!

   The rationale and the pros and cons of these two regimens are discussed in Chapter 23.

V. Systemic effects of the bypass environment

CPB is a highly unphysiologic experience that triggers an "explosion" of adverse events (Fig. 20.3), some of which have already been described.

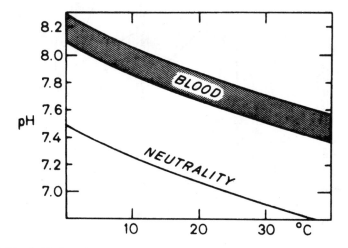

FIG. 20.2 Blood pH of exotherms and homeotherms, and pH of neutral water as a function of body temperature. (From Ream AF, Reitz BA, Silverberg G. Temperature correction of Pco$_2$ and pH in estimating acid–base status: an example of the Emperor's new clothes? *Anesthesiology* 1982;56:42, with permission.)

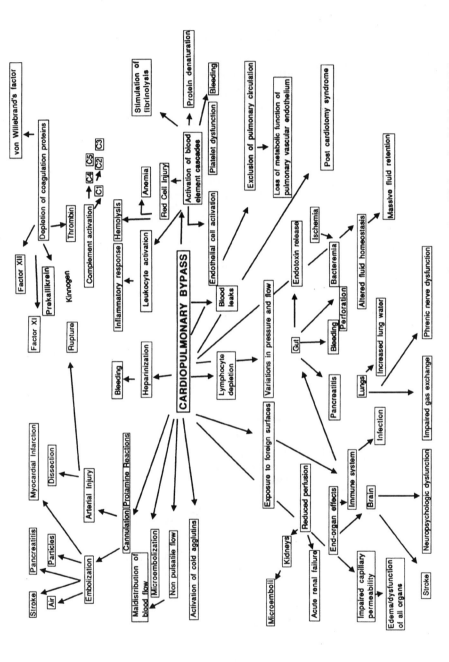

FIG. 20.3 The "explosion" of adverse events triggered by cardiopulmonary bypass. (From Elefteriades JA. Mini-CABG: a step forward or backward? The "pro" point of view. *J Cardiothorac Vasc Anesth* 1997;11:663, with permission.)

A. Hematology

1. **Coagulation.** Changes in the coagulation cascade, platelets, and fibrinolytic cascade are discussed in Chapter 18.
2. **Changes in formed elements**
   a. **Red blood cells**
      (1) During CPB, red cells become stiffer and less distensible. This change may interfere with microcirculatory blood flow. Stiffer RBCs are more susceptible to hemolysis.
      (2) During CPB, RBCs are exposed to nonphysiologic surfaces and shear stresses. The degree of **hemolysis** is increased by both higher flow rates and the accompanying increase in rate of shear and by a greater gas–fluid interface in the CPB apparatus. Oxygen-derived free radicals may contribute to hemolysis during CPB. As red cells are lysed, the **free hemoglobin** produced is bound to haptoglobin. When the amount of free hemoglobin generated exceeds the binding capacity of haptoglobin, serum hemoglobin concentrations increase and hemoglobin begins to be filtered by the kidney, resulting in hemoglobinuria.
   b. **Leukocytes.** CPB affects primarily neutrophils [polymorphonuclear leukocytes (PMNs)] and, to a lesser degree, monocytes. Shortly after the onset of CPB there is a marked decrease in circulating PMNs. Neutrophil counts decrease to a greater extent and remain decreased longer when a membrane oxygenator is used. The reason for this difference is unknown. The neutrophils are sequestered primarily in the pulmonary circulation. However, margination, diapedesis, and both intravascular and extravascular accumulation of PMNs have been demonstrated in the microcirculation of heart and skeletal muscle. Blockage of vessels by PMNs or microcirculatory derangements induced by substances released from PMNs may contribute to organ dysfunction after CPB.

      As CPB progresses, a rebound neutrophilia becomes evident and is more pronounced in patients treated with corticosteroids. The neutrophilia is less dramatic during hypothermia, but circulating PMN levels increase dramatically with rewarming. Both neutrophils released from the pulmonary circulation and younger cells released from the bone marrow contribute to the observed neutrophilia.

      Effects of CPB on host defense functions of PMNs are controversial. Studies demonstrating decreased responsiveness of PMNs to chemotactic and aggregating stimuli indicate impaired defense mechanisms. However, other studies show that the bacteriocidal activity of PMNs is increased for up to 3 days after CPB.

      Other effects on leukocytes are discussed in the Section **H** on inflammatory response.
3. **Changes in plasma proteins.** Proteins are globular molecules with highly specific structures. Generally polar, hydrophilic groups are oriented toward the outside of the molecule, and nonpolar hydrophobic groups are located internally. When proteins approach a gas–liquid interface, strong electrostatic forces at that interface produce varying degrees of molecular unfolding by disrupting the internal sulfhydryl and hydrogen bonds.
   a. **Consequences of protein denaturation**
      (1) **Altered enzymatic function.** Denatured proteins lose some or all of their function. This may be one mechanism by which coagulation becomes impaired during and after CPB.
      (2) **Aggregation of proteins.** Denatured proteins have a tendency to aggregate and may produce precipitates. Immunoglobulin M aggregates are strong activators of the complement cascade.
      (3) **Altered solubility characteristics.** Denatured proteins are less soluble in plasma and cause increased blood viscosity.
      (4) **Release of lipids.** Denaturation of lipoproteins and the protein fractions of chylomicrons result in chylomicron aggregates and free lipid globules in the circulation. These lipid emboli may become large enough to occlude small vessels.

(5) Absorption of denatured proteins onto cell membranes. RBCs may become "sticky." Resulting RBC aggregates promote capillary sludging and may contribute to microcirculatory dysfunction.

   b. Membrane oxygenators may induce less protein denaturation by virtue of the absence of a direct gas–fluid interface.

   c. **Colloid osmotic pressure.** Because of the hemodilution associated with use of asanguineous solutions to prime the heart-lung machine, plasma protein concentration and hence colloid osmotic pressure (COP) fall with onset of CPB if no colloids are added to the prime. The impact of a fall in COP on fluid balance during CPB is discussed in Section **B** below. There is controversy about the need and benefits of avoiding the fall in COP by use of albumin or artificial colloids (e.g., dextrans, starches) in the prime.

   4. **Activation of humoral cascade systems**

   a. **Coagulation and fibrinolytic cascade systems.** See Chapter 18.

   b. **Complement system.** See Section **H** below.

   c. **Kallikrein–kinin cascade** See Section **H** below.

B. **Fluid balance and interstitial fluid accumulation during cardiopulmonary bypass.** The following equation, based upon Starling's hypothesis, is thought to describe the fluid fluxes at the microcirculatory level:

$$\text{Tissue fluid accumulation} = K[(P_c - P_{IS}) - \sigma(\pi_c - \pi_{IS})] - Q_{lymph}$$

where K = filtration coefficient ("permeability") of capillary membrane, P_c = mean intracapillary hydrostatic pressure, P_{IS} = mean interstitial hydrostatic pressure, σ = reflection coefficient to macromolecules, π_c = intracapillary oncotic pressure, π_{IS} = interstitial oncotic pressure, and Q_{lymp} = lymph flow.

CPB tends to shift this balance toward accumulation of interstitial fluid by affecting several of these factors. Membrane permeability is increased [19] by activation of many of the components of the SIR and intermittent ischemia (hypoperfusion or microemboli)/reperfusion (see Section **V.H**), whereas plasma oncotic pressure regularly falls due to the use of largely colloid free asanguineous priming fluids. Intermittent (e.g., lifting the heart) or continuous inadequate venous drainage may increase mean capillary hydrostatic pressure, whereas immobility, lack of pulsatile flow, and loss of negative intrathoracic pressure impede lymphatic flow.

C. **Heart.** Frank myocardial infarction associated with modern cardiac surgery is relatively uncommon, but a lesser degree of myocardial injury and cell necrosis that may produce myocardial stunning, dysfunction, and morbidity in vulnerable patients (e.g. those with limited baseline function) may be more common.

Factors that contribute to myocardial injury include those that affect microcapillary perfusion in general (see Section **I.C.5**), but also ventricular distention, prolonged ventricular fibrillation, coronary air embolization, hypotension, catecholamines, endotoxemia, and ischemia/reperfusion associated with aortic cross-clamping or temporary individual coronary occlusion. It is thought that higher perfusion pressures and perhaps pulsatile flow (e.g., intraaortic balloon pump) are desirable to maintain adequate myocardial perfusion in patients with cardiac hypertrophy (e.g., chronic hypertension or valvular heart disease) and severe coronary artery disease during those periods of CPB when the ascending aorta is unclamped.

Myocardial injury and its prevention are discussed further in Chapter 22.

D. **Central nervous system.** Cerebral dysfunction (ranging from neuropsychiatric and cognitive deficits to frank stroke or coma) not infrequently follows CPB and is a major concern. Its etiology is multifactorial and includes hypoperfusion, macroemboli, microemboli, and the inflammatory response to CPB.

Cerebral perfusion and oxygen delivery receive highest priority by the host during CPB [4,5,20–22] but are influenced by MAP (rather than pump flow *per se*), jugular venous pressure, temperature, hematocrit, pH/P_aCO_2 management, and the presence of preexisting cerebrovascular disease.

The causes of cerebral dysfunction and strategies to minimize adverse cerebral outcomes are discussed further in Chapter 23.

E. **Renal function**
  1. **Significance of urine output during CPB.** Urine output is a crude indicator of renal function. There is no correlation between the amount of urine output during CPB and the incidence of postoperative renal failure. Urine output is greater when MAP is higher, when pulsatile perfusion is used, and when mannitol is added to pump priming fluids.
  2. **Decreased tubular function.** Tubular function is depressed by hypothermia alone. During CPB, tubular function is further depressed, resulting in reductions in urine output.
  3. **Renal blood flow.** Global renal blood flow usually decreases during CPB as a result of diminished flow rates and pressures or loss of pulsatility. As in other low-flow or shock-like states, there is a redistribution of renal blood flow from the cortex to the outer medulla. This redistribution of blood flow appears to be less severe during pulsatile perfusion.
  4. **Hemoglobinuria.** Intravascular hemolysis resulting in hemoglobinuria can cause acute tubular necrosis. It is not clear whether the mechanism is precipitation of pigment in the renal tubules with subsequent blockage of tubular flow or glomerular-tubular injuries caused by red cell stroma and other substances liberated from lysed RBCs.
  5. **Renal failure.** Renal failure after CPB is a persistent cause of morbidity and mortality in cardiac surgical patients. Its incidence is reported to be less than 1% in adult patients but may be as high as 2% to 10% in infants undergoing open intracardiac operations. Development of renal failure depends more on the preoperative and postoperative hemodynamic states than on various manipulations used to maintain urine output during CPB.
F. **Splanchnic, visceral, and hepatic effects.** The incidence of clinically recognized major gastrointestinal complications (e.g., bleeding, ulcers, pseudo-obstruction, mesenteric ischemia, infarction or perforation, acalculous cholecystitis, and pancreatitis) postoperatively is low (1% to 2%), but when they occur they are associated with high mortality (36% to 65%). Risk factors include advanced age, open ventricle operations, emergency procedures, prolonged bypass, use of vasopressors, and postbypass low cardiac output syndrome.

  Although global splanchnic blood flow (and hepatic venous oxygen saturation) appears to be mostly well preserved during CPB, recall that the hierarchy of regional blood flow indicates that splanchnic flow will be compromised early whenever systemic flow is reduced during CPB, and is likely to be reduced with administration of predominant vasoconstrictors such as phenylephrine, norepinephrine, and arginine vasopressin. Furthermore, despite apparently adequate global perfusion, many subjects exhibit increased intestinal permeability with development of edema, decreased gastric or intestinal mucosal pH and increased mucosal PCO_2 (by tonometry), decreased mucosal blood flow (by Doppler flowmetry), and endotoxemia, all of which suggest that mucosal ischemia occurs frequently in the gastrointestinal tract during CPB. The cause of this ischemia awaits further clarification, but its occurrence may play a role in the development of SIR syndrome and other gastrointestinal complications.

  Jaundice may occur in up to 23% of patients after surgery in which CPB was used, but severe jaundice (bilirubin levels at least 6 mg/dL) occurs in only 6% of patients. As with renal failure, hepatic dysfunction is more dependent on hemodynamic status before and after CPB than on any direct effect of CPB. The probability of postoperative jaundice is high when right atrial pressures are elevated, when there is significant hypoxia during operation, when there is persistent hypotension after CPB, or when large amounts of blood are transfused. If postoperative hemodynamics and nutritional status are kept normal, hepatic function will improve gradually.
G. **Pulmonary function**
  1. **Complete versus partial CPB.** Complete CPB implies that all systemic venous blood is drained into the oxygenator; hence, there is no blood flow to the right heart or pulmonary circulation. Complete CPB uses two venous cannulas

with "tapes" (analogous to tourniquets) around them to prevent blood from entering the right atrium. Partial CPB uses a single venous cannula or two venous cannulas without tapes. During partial CPB, variable amounts of blood can flow into the right atrium and ventricle, through the lungs, and eventually reach the left heart. During partial CPB, some anesthesiologists maintain minimal ventilation of the lungs to avoid delivery of hypoxic blood to the left heart.

2. **Pulmonary dead space and ventilation–perfusion mismatching after CPB.** Variable degrees of pulmonary dysfunction are seen after CPB. There is an almost inevitable increase in extravascular lung water during CPB. Development of intrapulmonary shunts and increased dead space ventilation result in less efficient matching of ventilation to perfusion. Increased dead space is reflected in greater end tidal-arterial CO_2 gradients after CPB in the majority of patients. Ventilation–perfusion (V/Q) mismatching results in increased alveolar-arterial O_2 gradients and decreased P_aO_2. These are the most consistent abnormalities noted after CPB.

3. **Pulmonary sequestration of neutrophils and release of vasoactive compounds.** PMNs sequestered in the lung during CPB may undergo release reactions causing localized, intense vasoconstriction or membrane damage with subsequent edema formation, resulting in increased dead space ventilation and V/Q mismatching.

4. **Metabolic functions of the lung**
   a. **Inactivation of catecholamines.** Under normal circumstances, the lung is a major site of inactivation of norepinephrine. During CPB the lungs are bypassed, and lack of pulmonary catecholamine degradation may contribute to the increasing levels of catecholamines seen during CPB. After CPB and reinstitution of pulmonary blood flow, inactivation of catecholamines resumes. However, decreasing catecholamine levels during this time result primarily from decreased production.
   b. The lung also plays a role in the renin-angiotensin system and in the metabolism of prostaglandins and serotonin. The physiologic impact of CPB on these functions is not well understood and merits further investigation.

5. **Sequestration of narcotics in the lungs.** This phenomenon has been reported to occur with fentanyl, which is widely used in cardiac anesthesia. The lungs have a high affinity for fentanyl. During CPB, plasma levels of fentanyl slowly decrease. On reperfusion of the lungs there is an increase in the plasma fentanyl concentration from release of sequestered fentanyl.

6. **Changes in pulmonary vascular resistance and hypoxic pulmonary vasoconstriction**
   a. **Pulmonary vascular resistance.** Numerous factors influence pulmonary vascular tone after CPB. Many congenital cardiac lesions are associated with increased pulmonary resistance. Efforts to limit increases in pulmonary vascular resistance (PVR) and maintain pulmonary blood flow include hyperventilation and administration of sodium bicarbonate to maintain an alkaline pH, and maintenance of adequate oxygenation. Increased catecholamine levels during and after CPB may contribute to increased PVR. Likewise, catecholamine infusions can induce pulmonary vasoconstriction. Notable exceptions are isoproterenol and dobutamine. Effects of CPB on increased PVR associated with underlying disease are unclear.
   b. **Hypoxic pulmonary vasoconstriction.** Direct effects of CPB and hypothermia on hypoxic pulmonary vasoconstriction are poorly understood. However, use of volatile anesthetics and vasodilators after CPB may interfere with hypoxic pulmonary vasoconstriction, leading to V/Q mismatching and decreasing P_aO_2.

7. **Postpump pulmonary dysfunction** [23]. Pulmonary dysfunction after CPB may range from mild decreases in P_aO_2, probably related to the nearly ubiquitous postoperative atelectasis, to full-blown respiratory failure resembling the adult respiratory distress syndrome. Most patients exhibit some immediate

decrease in P_aO_2 postoperatively, and it is difficult to predict which patients will develop more serious pulmonary insufficiency. Controversy exists about lung management during CPB.

Although full-blown respiratory failure after CPB now is relatively rare, its incidence is directly related to preoperative pulmonary dysfunction, duration of CPB, and postoperative hemodynamic status. Events during CPB that may contribute to development of pulmonary dysfunction include the following:

a. Decreased pulmonary blood flow resulting from

   (1) Emboli of various composition leading to localized areas of V/Q mismatching and edema formation

   (2) Localized vasoconstriction due to elevated endogenous catecholamines, exogenous catecholamine infusions, or substances released from PMNs trapped in the pulmonary capillaries

b. Edema formation enhanced by membrane damage from

   (1) Complement activation. Activated complement components increase capillary permeability.

   (2) Vasoactive compounds released from PMNs. These enhance capillary permeability and may lead to localized areas of interstitial edema.

   (3) Oxygen free radicals. Direct cellular toxins can lead to altered permeability at the capillary level.

c. Edema formation from increased pulmonary hydrostatic pressure, which is caused by

   (1) Inadequate left ventricular venting

   (2) Increased bronchial blood flow

H. Inflammatory and immunologic effects

   1. Systemic inflammatory response. CPB is associated with an unphysiologic activation of the *innate immune system* resulting in a whole-body SIR resembling that associated with sepsis and trauma [24–27a]. It represents a spectrum of responses ranging from the near-universal evidence of some inflammation (fever, leukocytosis), to more severe signs (tachycardia, diaphoresis increased cardiac output, increased oxygen consumption, decreased SVR, increased capillary permeability with increased extracellular fluid), to organ dysfunction (cardiac, renal, pulmonary, gastrointestinal, hepatic, CNS along with coagulopathies, disseminated intravascular coagulation, or intravascular thrombosis), and finally to the relatively rare multiple organ dysfunction syndrome and death. The explanation for why different patients exhibit differing degrees of this syndrome is largely unknown, but the baseline condition of the patient, extremes of age, and the extent and duration of the surgery are factors. Although all major surgeries can stimulate SIR, CPB appears to significantly exacerbate it.

   Some important stimuli that have been suggested include contact activation (exposure of blood to foreign surfaces in the CPB circuit and in the cardiotomy suction), nonphysiologic flow (e.g., nonpulsatile, high shear rates), tissue injury (ischemia and reperfusion, in particular), and endotoxemia. Contact activation is responsible for activation of complement via the alternate pathway with production of anaphylatoxins (C3a and C5a), which cause release of mediators from mast cells and basophils, result in increased capillary permeability, stimulate macrophages to release tumor necrosis factor (TNF), and stimulate expression of the leukocyte adhesion molecule P-selectin on the endothelium. The end product of complement activation (C5b–9 complex) is the membrane attack complex (also called the terminal attack complex), which causes cell lysis. The rise in concentration of complement proteins in plasma associated with CPB was one of the first recognized manifestations of SIR, which appeared to correlate with adverse outcomes [28] (Fig. 20.4), although the importance of this relationship is less clear now. Contact activation also activates the coagulation, fibrinolytic, and kallikrein–bradykinin cascades. Kallikrein plays a seminal role in activation and amplification of the inflammatory response (accelerates XII activation; activates complement; promotes fibrinolysis, the formation of renin, and the release of bradykinin). Bradykinin increases vascular permeability and release of tissue plasminogen activator.

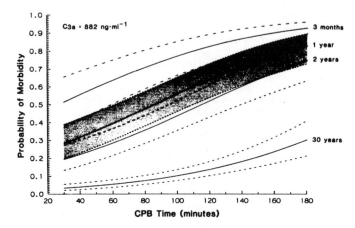

FIG. 20.4 Probability of morbidity related to duration of cardiopulmonary bypass in pediatric patients of different ages. Mean C3a level of 882 mg/mL at conclusion of cardiopulmonary bypass. (From Kirklin JK, Westaby S, Blackstone EH, et al. Complement and the damaging effects of cardiopulmonary bypass. *J Thorac Cardiovasc Surg* 1983;86:853, with permission.)

Ischemia and reperfusion, especially of the heart and lungs, also is thought to activate SIR. Endotoxemia frequently is detected during CPB and has been attributed to its translocation from the bowel due to splanchnic hypoperfusion and ischemia (which occurs commonly during CPB). Endotoxin (also known as lipopolysaccharide) then binds with lipopolysaccharide-binding protein, and this complex potently stimulates macrophages to release TNF.

The development of SIR syndrome involves both humoral mediators and activated cells. In addition to complement proteins and kallikrein–bradykinin, mediators include cytokines [TNF, interleukins 1, 6, and 8 (IL-1, IL-6, IL-8), and interferon-γ], leukotrienes, thromboxane, prostaglandins, platelet-activating factor, and tissue factor, which are produced variously by macrophages, endothelial cells, lymphocytes, and platelets. Activation of endothelial cells, neutrophils, macrophages, lymphocytes, and platelets contributes importantly to SIR. Expression of adhesion molecules (e.g., P-selectin, intercellular adhesion molecule, and CD11a/CD18) on endothelial cells and neutrophils leads to adhesion of the latter to the endothelium with subsequent migration and degranulation. This leads to microvascular obstruction and tissue injury from release of oxygen free radicals, elastase, and other toxic substances. Systemic endothelial cell activation occurs in response to cytokines (TNF, IL-1), endotoxin, C5a, hypoxia, and oxygen free radicals. In addition to expression of adhesion molecules, this causes release of more cytokines and increased production of nitric oxide (causing vasodilation).

These humoral mediators and activated cells lead to injury of various organs (e.g., heart, lung, kidney, CNS) by a number of mechanisms, including microvascular occlusion, thrombosis, fibrinolysis, capillary leak and edema, and direct trauma due to oxygen free radicals, neutrophil elastase, and membrane attack complex. Oxygen free radicals (superoxide, hydrogen peroxide, and hydroxyl radicals) have been implicated in cell and membrane damage during ischemic–hypoxic conditions. Oxygen free radicals are produced by activated PMNs and by the action of xanthine oxidase in hypoxic tissues.

In most patients the early SIR resolves without significant injury as a result of discontinuation of the stimulus, dissipation of mediators, or the action of naturally occurring antagonists [e.g., TNF-α receptor, IL-1 receptor antagonists, antiinflammatory cytokines (e.g., IL-10, transforming growth factor B), and antiendotoxin antibodies]. Excessive antiinflammatory response may overwhelm defensive inflammatory mechanisms and contribute to infection. This competing syndrome is called counter or compensatory antiinflammatory response syndrome (CARS).

Various strategies have been promoted to minimize the SIR syndrome, including use of heparin-coated circuits, centrifugal pumps, pulsatile flow, membrane oxygenators, hypothermia, priming with colloids, ultrafiltration, leukodepletion or leukofiltration, administration of corticosteroids or aprotinin, anticytokine therapy, antiendotoxin therapy, digestive decontamination, and administration of antibodies to block adhesion molecules or their activation. To date few have been proven to be clinically effective.

2. **Suppression of the adaptive immune system.** CPB is associated with suppression of the *adaptive system*, which renders the patient immune insufficient and at risk for infection. The severity of this suppression is related to the magnitude and duration of the surgery and the volume of transfused blood. This is partly related to the CARS discussed earlier. Other factors contributing to immune suppression include reduced levels of immunoglobulins and complement from dilution, protein denaturation, and consumption. Leukocytes suffer from degranulation and exhibit reduced chemotactic and metabolic function. Natural killer cells, T cells, B cells, and the reticuloendothelial system display reduced function. Immune cells display decreased antibody production and reduced response to phytohemagglutinin and IL-2. There are reduced numbers of CD3+, CD4+, and CD8+ T cells.

I. **Endocrine, metabolic, and electrolyte effects, and stress response.** CPB is associated with a marked exaggeration of the stress response associated with all types of surgery. This is manifested by large increases in epinephrine, norepinephrine, AVP (or antidiuretic hormone), adrenocorticotropic hormone, cortisol (mainly after bypass), growth hormone, and glucagon. Elevated catecholamines may have adverse effects on regional and organ blood flow patterns. Catecholamines also increase myocardial oxygen consumption, which may adversely affect the balance of myocardial oxygen supply and demand at the critical time of reperfusion. Other stress hormones also increase catabolic reactions, leading to increased energy consumption, tissue breakdown, and possible impairment of wound healing.

Hyperglycemia is encountered frequently during CPB, especially in patients with diabetes mellitus, and may contribute to neurologic dysfunction and wound infection. It is difficult to control with insulin and is a reason to avoid administration of glucose-containing solutions during cardiac surgery. Contributors to hyperglycemia include decreased insulin production, insulin resistance (possibly related to stress hormones), decreased consumption (related to insulin resistance and hypothermia), increased glycogenolysis and gluconeogenesis (related to stress hormones), and increased reabsorption of glucose by the kidney.

Renin, angiotensin II, and aldosterone levels all tend to rise during CPB, whereas the level of atrial natriuretic peptide typically falls at the start of CPB but rises during rewarming and after bypass. Many patients display the so-called sick euthyroid syndrome with reduced triiodothyronine (T_3), thyroxine (T_4), and free thyroxin levels but normal thyroid-stimulating hormone levels. The etiology of this is unclear, but it provides the rationale for administration of thyroid hormone in some patients with low cardiac output syndrome. Thromboxane and prostacyclin levels also rise with CPB.

Both ionized calcium and total and unfiltratable fractions of magnesium commonly fall whereas potassium levels may fluctuate widely during CPB. The latter may be related to diuretics, catecholamines, preoperative spironolactone (Aldactone) and β-blockers, potassium-containing cardioplegia, and renal dysfunction. The importance of maintaining normal levels of these ions to maintain normal muscle and cardiac function and prevent dysrhythmias is apparent.

J. **Effects of cardiopulmonary bypass on pharmacology.** CPB can have profound effects on plasma concentrations of drugs, on pharmacokinetics, and on pharmacodynamics. Some factors contributing to this include sudden hemodilution, changes in protein binding [effects of heparin (released free fatty acids which bind to proteins and may displace bound drugs)], hypothermia, altered distribution of blood flow, exclusion of the lungs from circulation, and absorption into the CPB circuit.

The observed changes in drug concentrations are influenced by phase of operation, mode of administration (bolus vs. infusion), and site of administration (peripheral, central line, or into the pump). If bicaval cannulation is used for venous drainage, it has been shown that systemic appearance may be delayed for up to 5 minutes when a drug is administered into a central line. Therefore, drugs should be administered directly into the heart-lung machine. The uptake of volatile anesthetics by extracorporeal oxygenators, which may be different for each agent and model of oxygenator, has not been fully elucidated.

Because of all these permutations, it is difficult to generalize about the pharmacology of individual drugs during CPB. With onset of CPB, plasma drug levels usually fall due to hemodilution (but protein-free fraction may rise), whereas volumes of distribution and rates of clearance are reduced during CPB and rates of elimination often are reduced after bypass. However, the interested reader is referred to extensive chapters by Hall [29] and Mets [30] for data on specific drugs.

VI. Pediatric versus adult cardiopulmonary bypass. The many differences between infants and small children and adults tend to exacerbate the pathophysiologic responses to CPB [31]. These include less mature organ systems; impaired thermoregulation; reactive pulmonary vasculature; the frequent presence of a patent ductus arteriosus, patent foramen ovale, and persistent left superior vena cava; and the presence of aortopulmonary collaterals and increased bronchial collateral flow (the presence of the latter two increase return of blood to left heart and may steal blood from the brain). In marked contrast to adults, the prime volume of the extracorporeal circuit may equal or exceed the blood volume of the patient by several fold, resulting in extreme dilution of all blood components. Arterial and venous cannulas are large in comparison to patient structures. The conduct of bypass often includes more extreme degrees of hypothermia, low flow, and even circulatory arrest.

On the other hand, children are less likely to have the various acquired and degenerative diseases that characterize the elderly population (e.g., atherosclerosis, chronic hypertension, diabetes, chronic obstructive pulmonary disease) and their CNS is more "plastic" and probably more tolerant to oxygen deprivation.

VII. Summary. This chapter focused primarily on the aberrations of normal physiology imposed by the bypass environment, with secondary emphasis on specific organ dysfunction. Certainly not all of the pathophysiology described is seen in every patient undergoing CPB. Many patients appear to suffer no ill effects at all. The absence of significant organ dysfunction probably is the best indicator of successful CPB. Post-CPB organ dysfunction constitutes a spectrum ranging from mild dysfunction in one or more organ systems to death resulting from multiorgan failure. The probability of significant morbidity increases with duration of CPB and decreasing age of the patient within the pediatric age group (Fig. 20.4).

The impact of preexisting organ dysfunction on post-CPB morbidity is not well defined, but it seems likely that poor overall condition before CPB results in greater morbidity after CPB. For unexplained reasons, women seem to have greater morbidity and mortality after cardiac surgery [32].

Finally, it should be emphasized that placing a patient on CPB is a physiologic trespass against that patient (Fig. 20.3). Absence of significant damage caused by CPB depends primarily on a particular patient's ability to compensate for the derangements introduced by that trespass.

References

1. **Gravlee GP, Davis RF, Kurusz M, et al. eds. *Cardiopulmonary bypass: principles and practice*, 2nd ed. Philadelphia: Lippincott Williams & Wilkins, 2000.**
2. Cook DJ. Optimal management of flow, pressure, temperature and hematocrit during cardiopulmonary bypass. *Semin Cardiothorac Vasc Anesth* 2001;5:265–272.
3. Rudy LW, Heymann MA, Edmunds LH. Distribution of systemic blood flow during cardiopulmonary bypass. *J Appl Physiol* 1973;34:194–200.
4. Slater JM, Orszulak TA, Cook DJ. Distribution and hierarchy of regional blood flow during hypothermic cardiopulmonary bypass. *Ann Thorac Surg* 2001;72:542–547.

5. Boston US, Slater JM, Orszulak TA, et al. Hierarchy of regional oxygen delivery during cardiopulmonary bypass. *Ann Thorac Surg* 2001;71:260–264.
6. Kirklin JW, Barratt-Boyes BG. Hypothermia, circulatory arrest, and cardiopulmonary bypass. In: Kirklin JW, Barratt-Boyes BG, eds. *Cardiac surgery, 2nd ed.* New York: Churchill Livingstone, 1993:61–127.
7. Fox LS, Blackstone EH, Kirklin JW, et al. Relationship of whole body oxygen consumption to perfusion flow rate during hypothermic cardiopulmonary bypass. *J Thorac Cardiovasc Surg* 1982;83:239–248.
8. Govier AV, Reves JG, McKay RD, et al. Factors and their influence on regional cerebral blood flow during nonpulsatile cardiopulmonary bypass. *Ann Thorac Surg* 1984;38: 592–600.
9. Johnsson P, Messeter K, Ryding E, et al. Cerebral blood flow and autoregulation during hypothermic cardiopulmonary bypass. *Ann Thorac Surg* 1987;43:386–390.
10. Murkin JM, Farrar JK, Tweed WA, et al. Cerebral autoregulation and flow/metabolism coupling during cardiopulmonary bypass: the influence of $PaCO_2$. *Anesth Analg* 1987;66: 825–832.
11. Soma Y, Hirotani T, Yozu R, et al. A clinical study of cerebral circulation during extracorporeal circulation. *J Thorac Cardiovasc Surg* 1989;97:187–193.
12. Kolkka R, Hilberman M. Neurologic dysfunction following cardiac operation with low-flow, low-pressure cardiopulmonary bypass. *Thorac Cardiovasc Surg* 1980;79:432–473.
13. Cook DJ. Changing temperature management for cardiopulmonary bypass. *Anesth Analg* 1999;88:1254–1271.
14. Grigore AM, Mathew J, Grocott HP, et al. Prospective randomized trial of normothermic versus hypothermic cardiopulmonary bypass on cognitive function after coronary artery bypass graft surgery. *Anesthesiology* 2001;95:1110–1119.
15. Wright G. Mechanical simulation of cardiac function by means of pulsatile blood pumps. *J Cardiothorac Vasc Anesth* 1997;11:299–309.
16. Louagie YA, Gonzalez M, Colland E, et al. Does flow character of cardiopulmonary bypass make a difference? *J Thorac Cardiovasc Surg* 1992;104:1628–1638.
17. Murkin JM, Martzke JS, Buchan AM, et al. A randomized study of the influence of perfusion technique and pH management in 316 patients undergoing coronary artery bypass surgery: I. Mortality and cardiovascular morbidity. *J Thorac Cardiovasc Surg* 1995; 110:340–348.
18. McDaniel LB, Zwischenberger JM, Vertrees RA, et al. Mixed venous oxygen saturation during cardiopulmonary bypass poorly predicts regional venous desaturation. *Anesth Analg* 1994;8:466–472.
19. Smith EEJ, Naftel DC, Blackstone EH, et al. Microvascular permeability after cardiopulmonary bypass. *J Thorac Cardiovasc Surg* 1987;94:225–233.
20. Cook DJ, Orszulak TA, Daly RC, et al. Minimum hematocrit for normothermic cardiopulmonary bypass in dog. *Circulation* 1997;96[Suppl II]:II200–II204.
21. **Prough DS, Rogers AT. What are the normal levels of cerebral blood flow and cerebral oxygen consumption during cardiopulmonary bypass in humans? *Anesth Analg* 1993;76:690–693.**
22. **Schell RM, Kern FH, Greeley WJ, et al. Cerebral blood flow and metabolism during cardiopulmonary bypass. *Anesth Analg* 1993;76:849–865.**
23. Weissman C. Pulmonary function after cardiac and thoracic surgery. *Anesth Analg* 1999; 88:1272–1279.
24. Boyle EM Jr, Pohlman TH, Johnson MC, et al. Endothelial cell injury in cardiovascular surgery. The systemic inflammatory response. *Ann Thorac Surg* 1997;63:277–284.
25. Hall RI, Smith MS, Rocker G. The systemic inflammatory response to cardiopulmonary bypass: pathophysiologic, therapeutic and pharmacologic considerations. *Anesth Analg* 1997;85:766–782.
26. Asimakopoulos G. Systemic inflammation and cardiac surgery: an update. *Perfusion* 2001;16:353–360.
27. Hennein HA. Inflammation after cardiopulmonary bypass: therapy for the postpump syndrome. *Semin Cardiothorac Vasc Anesth* 2001;5:236–255.
27a. Laffey JG, Boylan JF, Cheng DCH. The systemic inflammatory response to cardiac surgery. Implications for the anesthesiologist. *Anesthesiology* 2002;97:215–252.

28. Kirkland JB, Westaby S, Blackstone EH, et al. Compliment and the damaging effects of cardiopulmonary bypass. *J Thorac Cardiovasc Surg* 1983;86:845–857.
29. Hall RI. Changes in the pharmacokinetics and pharmacodynamics of drugs administered during cardiopulmonary bypass. In: Gravlee GP, David RF, Kurusz M, et al., eds. *Cardiopulmonary bypass: principles and practice,* 2nd ed. Philadelphia: Lippincott Williams and Wilkins, 2000:265–302.
30. Mets B. Cardiac pharmacology. In: Thys D, Hillel Z, Schwartz J, eds. *Textbook of cardiothoracic anesthesiology.* New York: McGraw-Hill, 2001:421–432.
31. **Jonas RA, Elliot MF, eds. *Cardiopulmonary bypass in neonates, infants, and young children.* Oxford: Butterworth-Heinemann, 1994.**
32. Hogue CW, Sundt T, III, Barzilai B, et al. Cardiac and neurologic complications identify risks for mortality for both men and women undergoing coronary artery bypass graft surgery. *Anesthesiology* 2001;95:1074–1078.

21. CIRCULATORY ASSIST DEVICES

Ronald L. Harter and Robert E. Michler

The perioperative use of circulatory assist devices has become more common as the spectrum of available devices has enlarged. Although still far from routine, the use of various types of circulatory assist devices has expanded from serving primarily as a "last ditch" exercise in futility to an intervention that, while fraught with potentially devastating complications, can provide an opportunity for patient survival when all less aggressive means have been exhausted.

This chapter overviews issues surrounding the perioperative management of patients requiring circulatory assist devices, whether the device is a "simple" intraaortic balloon pump (IABP) or a univentricular or biventricular assist device. We explore the current state of totally artificial hearts and examine potential future directions for these devices.

I. Intraaortic balloon pump

A. Indications for placement

Thought by some to be reserved for placement after one or more failed attempts at separation from cardiopulmonary bypass (CPB), the numbers of IABPs placed in the cardiac catheterization laboratory approaches or exceeds the number placed intraoperatively. Invasive cardiologists often place IABPs when high-grade lesions of proximal coronary vessels supplying large regions of myocardium are diagnosed, or when myocardial ischemia persists or myocardial infarction (MI) occurs after an intervention such as coronary stent placement. Recent retrospective outcome studies for preoperative versus intraoperative placement of IABP for coronary artery bypass graft (CABG) patients suggest that preoperative IABP placement improves outcome and shortens hospital stay, especially for patients with low ejection fractions or those undergoing urgent or emergent CABG [1].

Indications for intraoperative IABP placement vary widely among centers and even among surgical teams. Left ventricular (LV) failure despite maximal inotropic support and/or evidence of ongoing regional myocardial ischemia that is not amenable to surgical revascularization constitute the primary intraoperative indications. The definitions of "LV failure," "maximal inotropic support," and "ongoing regional myocardial ischemia" may vary widely among institutions. Independent predictors of death among patients with intraoperative IABP insertion include New York Heart Association class III or IV symptom level, mitral valve replacement or repair, prolonged CPB, urgent or emergent operation, emergent reinstitution of CPB, preoperative renal dysfunction, diabetes mellitus, right ventricular (RV) failure, complex ventricular ectopy, pacer dependence, and IABP placement via the ascending aorta [1].

B. Contraindications to placement

1. **Aortic insufficiency.** Use of the IABP is relatively contraindicated in patients with aortic valve insufficiency. Because the IABP inflates in the descending aorta during diastole to promote retrograde flow into the ascending aorta, this potentially increases aortic valvular regurgitation, further distending the LV at the expense of coronary perfusion.

2. **Sepsis.** As with any prosthetic intravascular device, bacteremic infections are difficult to treat if the prosthetic surfaces become seeded with bacteria.

3. **Severe vascular disease.** Placement of an IABP may be technically difficult in patients with atherosclerosis or other vascular pathologies. Such patients are more prone to arterial thrombosis during use of an IABP. Patients with abdominal aortic aneurysms are at increased risk for aortic rupture, although balloons have been successfully passed and used in such patients. For patients with severe aortoiliac or femoral arterial disease, another option is to place the balloon directly into the descending thoracic aorta. This option obviously requires a subsequent trip to the operating room to remove the device when such support becomes unnecessary.

C. Functional design.

The IABP consists of an inflatable balloon at the end of a catheter that typically is advanced into the descending thoracic aorta percutaneously from the groin (Fig. 21.1). The balloon inflates during diastole, displacing blood from the thoracic aorta and increasing aortic diastolic pressure. Balloon inflation improves coronary perfusion pressure, increasing coronary blood flow to both the LV and the RV. During early systole, rapid balloon deflation reduces LV afterload and wall tension. IABP can improve myocardial energy balance at most by 15%.

Systole   **Diastole**

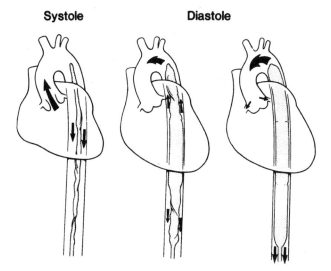

FIG. 21.1 Placement of the intraaortic balloon pump (IABP) in the aorta. The IABP is shown in the descending aorta, with the tip at the distal aortic arch. During systole the balloon is deflated to enhance ventricular ejection. During diastole the balloon inflates, forcing blood from the proximal aorta into the coronary and peripheral vessels.

The IABP drive console consists of a pressurized gas reservoir that is connected to the balloon supply line through an electronically controlled solenoid valve. The gas used to inflate the balloon is either CO_2 or helium. The advantage of CO_2 is its increased blood solubility, which reduces the consequences of balloon rupture with potential gas embolization. The advantage of helium is its decreased density, which thereby decreases the Reynolds number and allows the same flow through a smaller drive line. A tube with a smaller diameter decreases the potential for injury to the artery.

D. Intraaortic balloon pump placement

1. Insertion of the IABP usually is accomplished either percutaneously or by surgical cutdown into the femoral artery using the Seldinger technique for placement of a large-diameter introducer.

2. The balloon is passed through the introducer.

3. The balloon is ideally positioned so that its tip is at the junction of the descending aorta and the aortic arch, just distal to the origin of the subclavian artery, as shown in Figure 21.1. This positioning minimizes the risk of subclavian or renal artery injury or occlusion. Radiographically, the tip should lie between the anterior portion of the second intercostal space and the first lumbar vertebra.

4. When the IABP is placed intraoperatively, transesophageal echocardiography can confirm proper tip location before initiation of balloon assistance. Fluoroscopy, if available, can facilitate positioning.

E. Intraaortic balloon pump control. Several parameters are important during the setup and operation of an IABP.

1. **Synchronization of the IABP.** Synchronization of the IABP with the cardiac rhythm is accomplished by using either the largest electrical deflection of the electrocardiographic signal (usually the QRS complex) or the arterial pressure waveform. If there is a natural pulse pressure greater than 40 mm Hg, use of the arterial waveform for synchronization is generally preferred in the

operating room because the electrical artifact produced by the electrocautery inhibits most electrocardiography-triggered IABP control units. Recent monitoring systems have advanced suppression circuitry designed to reduce electrical noise from electrocautery. Most current consoles can differentiate pacer spikes from a QRS complex, allowing proper timing of IABP inflation even when atrial or atrioventricular pacing is in use.

2. **Timing of balloon inflation and deflation.** When setting the timing of IABP inflation (Fig. 21.2), it is important to time the onset of the pressure rise caused

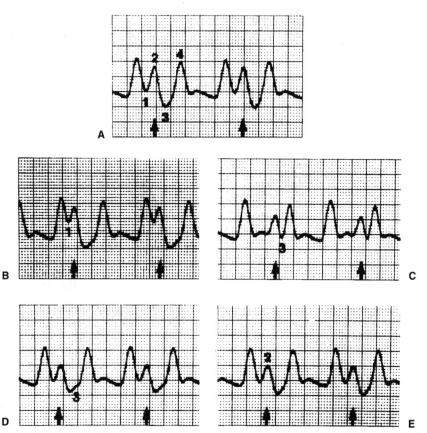

FIG. 21.2 Manipulation of the timing of inflation and deflation of intraaortic balloon pump. Tracings illustrate 1:2 support for the sake of clarity. **A:** Normal tracing. Augmentation commences after the dicrotic notch (*1*) augments diastolic pressure (*2*) and reaches its nadir just before the next contraction (*3*). Peak systolic pressure in the next (nonaugmented) beat is decreased (*4*). **B:** Early inflation. Augmentation commences before aortic valve closure (*1*), thereby increasing afterload and possibly inducing aortic regurgitation. **C:** Late inflation. Diastolic augmentation is inadequate, and end-diastolic pressure is no different from that in the unassisted cycle (*3*). **D:** Early deflation. Diastolic augmentation and afterload reduction are impaired. **E:** Inadequate filling time. Timing is satisfactory, but diastolic augmentation is impaired. (From Sladen RN. Management of the adult cardiac patient in the intensive care unit. In: Ream AK, Fogdall RP, eds. *Acute cardiovascular management in anesthesia and intensive care.* Philadelphia: Lippincott, 1982:509, with permission.)

by balloon inflation with the dicrotic notch of the arterial waveform, which signifies aortic valve closure and the start of diastole. If inflation begins sooner, the IABP will impede ventricular ejection. If it begins later, the effectiveness of the balloon in augmenting coronary perfusion and reducing afterload will be limited.

Deflation should be timed so that the arterial pressure just reaches its minimum level at the onset of the next ventricular pulse. If it deflates too soon, the aorta will not be maximally evacuated before ventricular contraction, and coronary perfusion will not be optimized. If the balloon deflates too late, it will impede LV ejection.

3. **Ratio of native ventricle pulsations to IABP pulsation.** Pumping frequently is initiated at a ratio of 1:2 (one IABP beat for every two cardiac beats), so the natural ventricular beats and augmented beats can be compared to determine IABP timing and efficacy. Depending on the patient's condition, the ratio often will be increased to 1:1 to obtain maximal benefit.

4. **Stroke volume of the balloon.** The volume of gas used to inflate the balloon is determined by the balloon used and the patient's size. Exceeding the volume for which the balloon was designed risks rupture with arterial gas embolization. Typically, balloon volume is set to 50% to 60% of the patient's ideal stroke volume [2].

5. **Balloon filling.** The time required for the balloon to fill and empty is determined by the density of the gas used, gas pressure, the length and diameter of the gas line, and balloon volume. These values usually are constant for any particular balloon. At high heart rates, the time required for balloon filling may limit balloon stroke volume.

F. **Intraaortic balloon pump weaning.** Weaning the patient from the IABP should be considered when inotropic support has been reduced substantially, allowing "room" to increase inotropic support as IABP support is reduced. Weaning is done primarily by gradually (over 6 to 12 hours) decreasing the ratio of augmented to native heartbeats (from 1:1 to 1:2 to 1:4 or less) and/or decreasing balloon volume while maintaining acceptable hemodynamics, which often necessitates a concomitant increase in inotropic support. The balloon is never turned off while it remains in the aorta except when the patient is anticoagulated, as during CPB, because of the risk of thrombus formation on the balloon.

Comparison of intraarterial pressure tracings of augmented ventricular pulsations to native pulsations can serve as an indicator of ventricular performance. As ventricular performance improves, the amplitude of the native pressure tracing will increase relative to the augmented pressure tracing. By comparing the magnitude of these two pulses over time, one can obtain a qualitative assessment of ventricular performance. Once the IABP is removed, it is important to continue close examination of the distal ipsilateral leg because partial or total femoral arterial occlusion may occur.

G. **Management of anticoagulation during intraaortic balloon pumping.** During extended IABP use, anticoagulation is generally indicated. In the immediate post-CPB period, anticoagulants may not be required for the first few hours or until drainage from the chest tubes is acceptable (less than 100 to 150 mL/hour). Low-molecular-weight dextran sometimes is chosen to prevent thrombosis in patients with IABP because its antithrombotic effects are fairly mild, although no reversal agent exists. Heparin can prevent IABP-related thrombosis and its ready reversibility offers appeal, but many surgeons are reluctant to initiate heparin therapy within the first 6 hours after CPB. If heparin is used, adequate anticoagulation should be confirmed every 4 to 6 hours with activated clotting time (ACT) or activated partial thromboplastin time (aPTT) maintained at 1.5 to 2 times normal values.

H. **Complications.** The incidence of IABP complications has decreased significantly from its early use, but significant morbidities persist. The most frequent complications are vascular in nature, with a reported incidence of 6% to 33% [1]. These complications include events such as limb ischemia, compartment syndrome, mesenteric infarction, aortic perforation, and aortic dissection. Risk factors for these complications include a history of peripheral vascular disease, female gender, tobacco smoking, diabetes mellitus, and postoperative IABP placement.

Other complications include infection, primarily at the groin site of a transcutaneous introducer, and coagulopathies (especially thrombocytopenia). Neurologic complications include paresthesia, ischemic neuritis, neuralgia, foot drop, and rarely paraplegia [3]. Balloon rupture with gas embolus has become increasingly common, presumably as a result of severity of aortic atherosclerotic calcifications among an increasingly elderly patient population. When this occurs, blood usually is seen in the gas drive line and the arterial pressure deflection caused by the IABP is lost. Most pumps have an alarm that indicates low balloon pressure. Air embolism from the pressure monitoring line to the brain is a larger risk from the IABP than from a radial artery catheter, because the monitoring port is located at the tip of the balloon catheter, which is close to the origin of the carotid arteries. Blood gases should be drawn through the IABP pressure monitoring line only if no other locations are available, paying meticulous attention to ensure that no air bubbles or other debris are flushed through the tubing.

I. **Limitations.** The ability of the IABP to augment cardiac output and unload the LV is limited, because the IABP does not directly affect LV function. With severe LV failure, an IABP will not provide sufficient flow to sustain the circulation. When the LV cannot eject blood into the aorta, the IABP will simply cause pulsations in the arterial waveform without increasing blood flow. In this situation, a ventricular assist device (VAD) must be considered, although readily correctable technical problems with the IABP, such as malpositioning, kinking of the gas line, or improper inflation-deflation timing, should be considered.

Early IABPs were not effective during rapid cardiac rhythms. Improvements in the pneumatic circuitry and compressor response time now permit some IABP models to provide hemodynamic improvement at rates up to 190 beats/min. Irregular heart rhythms persist as a limitation to IABP efficacy, because optimal timing of inflation and deflation cannot be achieved with large variations in the R-R interval.

J. **Pediatric intraaortic balloon pump.** Enthusiasm regarding IABP use in children was scarce after early reports of high mortality associated with IABP use in the early 1980s. Improved balloon and control panel circuitry design now make IABP an option even in neonates. A variety of balloon sizes and lengths are available for pediatric use. Choosing the correct balloon is critical for success and to minimize complications. Vascular access in small neonates may be best achieved via direct cannulation of the descending aorta; the femoral or external iliac artery can be used successfully in larger (more than 4 kg) infants and children.

Many children with congenital heart disease are not expected to derive substantial benefit from IABP, because the RV is frequently the chamber most in need of support. However, children with certain types of congenital cardiac defects may benefit from IABP perioperative support.

II. **Ventricular assist devices.** Since DeBakey first used a pneumatic device in 1966 for a patient with LV failure, profound technologic advances have produced a number of devices for mechanical support of the failing LV.

A. **Types of ventricular assist devices.** The two primary types of VADs are rotary and displacement. Displacement pumps are used most frequently in adults. Rotary pumps can be used in adults or children.

1. **Rotary.** Rotary pumps are small in size and weight, operate quietly, and have relatively low power consumption. However, current designs are prone to thrombus formation and bearing failure, which limit their longevity to several weeks.

a. **Axial flow.** Axial flow pumps represent a relatively recent advance in rotary VADs, so information on their efficacy is limited. Their small size, easy implantability, and high efficiency may increase their popularity in coming years. Examples of these devices include the Sun Waseda (Sun Medical Company, Waseda University, Tokyo, Japan), Jarvik 2000 (Texas Heart Institute, Houston, TX, U.S.A.), NASA/DeBakey (MicroMed Technology Inc., Houston, TX, U.S.A.), TCI HeartMate II (Axipump; TCI/Nimbus Inc.,

Pittsburgh PA, U.S.A.), Hemopump (Medtronic Inc., Minneapolis MN, U.S.A.), and Impella (Cardiotechnik AG, Aachen, Germany). These devices presently are used infrequently [4].

   b. Centrifugal. Centrifugal pumps (Fig. 21.3) have been used clinically in humans for several years, with pumps such as those produced by Biomedicus (Medtronic Biomedicus Inc., Minneapolis MN, U.S.A.) and Sarns (Sarns, Inc./3M, Ann Arbor MI, U.S.A.). A report of the Baylor University experience from 1986 to 1994 noted that 56.3% of patients on Biomedicus support were weaned successfully.

      Other centrifugal models include the Gyro Pump (Baylor College of Medicine, Houston TX, U.S.A.), the magnetically suspended centrifugal pump (Terumo Corporation, Tokyo, Japan), and the Rotodynamic pump (Cleveland Clinic Foundation, Cleveland OH, U.S.A.) [4].

2. Displacement. Displacement pumps are classified as **intracorporeal or extracorporeal.** Sometimes the term "paracorporeal" is used interchangeably with "extracorporeal"; both terms refer to the location of the pumping chamber being outside the body. They provide pulsatile flow but are more bulky than rotary models.

   a. Intracorporeal. The two most commonly used intracorporeal displacement-type VADs are manufactured by TCI (Thermocardiosystems, Woburn MA, U.S.A.) HeartMate (Fig. 21.4) and Novacor (Baxter Healthcare Corp., Deerfield IL, U.S.A.) (Fig. 21.5). Human use of TCI pumps has been limited

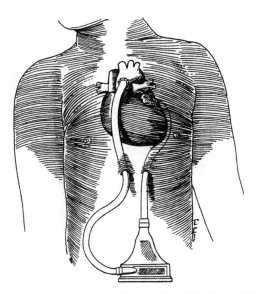

FIG. 21.3 Centrifugal pump. (From Arabia FA, Copeland JG, Larson DF, et al. Circulatory assist devices: applications for ventricular recovery or bridge to transplant. In: Gravlee GP, Davis RF, Kurusz M, et al., eds. *Cardiopulmonary bypass: principles and practice,* 2nd ed. Philadelphia: Lippincott Williams & Wilkins, 2000:131–145, with permission.)

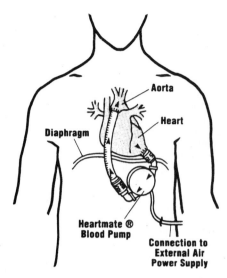

FIG. 21.4 TCI HeartMate. (From Arabia FA, Copeland JG, Larson DF, et al. Circulatory assist devices: applications for ventricular recovery or bridge to transplant. In: Gravlee GP, Davis RF, Kurusz M, et al., eds. *Cardiopulmonary bypass: principles and practice,* 2nd ed. Philadelphia: Lippincott Williams & Wilkins, 2000:131–145, with permission.)

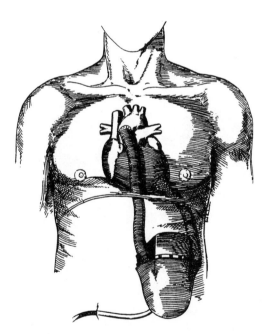

FIG. 21.5 Novacor left ventricular assist device (electromechanical). (From Arabia FA, Copeland JG, Larson DF, et al. Circulatory assist devices: applications for ventricular recovery or bridge to transplant. In: Gravlee GP, Davis RF, Kurusz M, et al., eds. *Cardiopulmonary bypass: principles and practice,* 2nd ed. Philadelphia: Lippincott Williams & Wilkins, 2000: 131–145, with permission.)

mostly to two models. The vented electric (VE) TCI requires a percutaneous vent tube to equalize pressure in the motor chamber. Incorporation of porcine bioprosthetic valves and textured surfaces greatly reduces the need for anticoagulation with this device. The implantable pneumatic (IP) TCI induces fewer bleeding complications but more infections than the VE TCI. As of July 1998, 1,387 HeartMate devices had been implanted worldwide. Sixty-five percent of HeartMate recipients were transplanted. Although device explantation can be technically challenging, successful weaning and explantation with good long-term survival have been reported. Requirement of right ventricular assist device (RVAD) support following placement of a TCI left ventricular assist device (LVAD) is a poor prognostic sign, with 100% mortality reported in one study of TCI LVAD recipients. A comparison of TCI recipients to heart transplant candidates who did not receive VAD placement demonstrated improved survival to transplant and better survival after transplantation among TCI LVAD recipients. At present, the HeartMate pumps can be used only in patients with body surface area greater than 1.5 m^2.

As of mid-1999, the Novacor device had been used in nearly 1,000 patients. Battery packs permit patients with the Novacor device to walk alone for periods up to 4 hours. Although the noise level of the Novacor had been problematic, the newer N100 PC system achieved significant noise reduction. Gram-positive infection incidence has been reduced by irrigation of the exit site with vancomycin [4].

    b. Extracorporeal. The Abiomed BVS 5000 (Abiomed Inc., Danvers, MA, U.S.A.) (Fig. 21.6) is a pulsatile, dual-chamber extracorporeal VAD. Filling is adjusted by changing the height of the device on the bedside intravenous pole. It is a safe system because there is no vacuum, and it is inexpensive and simple to operate. This pump generally provides effective support for periods of 30 days or less. Bleeding frequently complicates use of this device, with a reported reoperation rate as high as 50%. When used as a bridge to transplantation, one report showed 50% survival to transplantation with the Abiomed device compared to 85.5% with the Thoratec VAD (Thoratec Laboratories Corp., Pleasanton, CA, U.S.A.) [4]. Among patients with organ failure at the time of VAD placement, Abiomed output (4.0 to 4.5 L/min) often is insufficient to restore organ function. As of December 1998, 790 patients bridged to transplantation with the Abiomed VAD had a survival rate of 52% [4].

The Thoratec VAD (Fig. 21.7) is commonly used. As of December 1998, 570 patients had bridged to transplantation with this device, with overall survival of 53% in patients ranging from 17 to 144 kg. Better survival has been reported among patients with early rather than late cardiogenic shock. Implantation of this device requires full CPB support. Postoperative bleeding occurs less frequently than it does with the Abiomed or Biomedicus devices. The Thoratec TLC-11 portable VAD driver, which weighs 9.1 kg, has improved patient mobility. Several other paracorporeal displacement VADs are commercially available [4].

B. Indications for ventricular assist device placement

    1. Post-CPB. Patients with ventricular failure post-CPB that persists despite maximal pharmacologic support, often in combination with IABP support, require placement of a pneumatic VAD if they are to survive the immediate postoperative period. It is essential to implement circulatory support quickly, and devices such as the Thoratec or the Abiomed can be placed rapidly with limited additional surgical dissection [4].

    In a report of Abiomed VAD use for postcardiotomy heart failure, 62% of patients receiving an Abiomed VAD after CPB were weaned successfully and 54% were discharged from the hospital. Those requiring Abiomed support after admission to the intensive care unit postcardiotomy were weaned in 64% of cases, with 36% ultimately being discharged from the hospital. Multiple organ system failure and sepsis were the most common causes of death [5].

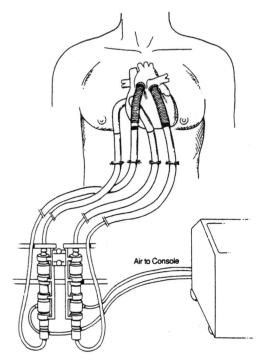

FIG. 21.6 Abiomed circulatory support system with inflow and outflow cannulas, prosthetic ventricles, and console. (From Arabia FA, Copeland JG, Larson DF, et al. Circulatory assist device: applications for ventricular recovery or bridge to transplant. In: Gravlee GP, Davis RF, Kurusz M, et al., eds. *Cardiopulmonary bypass: principles and practice,* 2nd ed. Philadelphia: Lippincott Williams & Wilkins, 2000:131–145, with permission.)

2. **Post-MI.** Initial experience with VAD placement for severe LV failure early after MI suggested little benefit and was associated with mortality rates as high as 75%. More recent studies, however, have demonstrated more encouraging outcomes when VAD placement is initiated early after acute MI. Patients in cardiogenic shock receiving a TCI HeartMate 1000 IP LVAD 9 days or less after an acute MI had a 13% mortality rate [6]. These results seem encouraging in light of the high mortality rate typically reported for this patient population.
3. **Bridge to cardiac transplantation.** Technologic advancements have created VADs that are largely implantable, with increasingly smaller portions of the device remaining outside the body. The potentially acceptable duration of circulatory assistance offered by these devices continues to increase, as side effect profiles continually improve. Consequently, VAD support for several months is becoming more common.

Although the costs associated with placement of a VAD are sizable, they may be comparable to those of prolonged hospitalization with maximal medical support. A retrospective study of patients receiving either inotropic therapy or HeartMate LVAD support as a bridge to transplantation demonstrated that LVAD patients had better clinical and metabolic function at the time of transplant and better 6-month posttransplantation survival rates than did patients who received only intravenous inotropic support [7]. A prospective comparison of the Novacor N100 and the TCI HeartMate assist systems as bridges to trans-

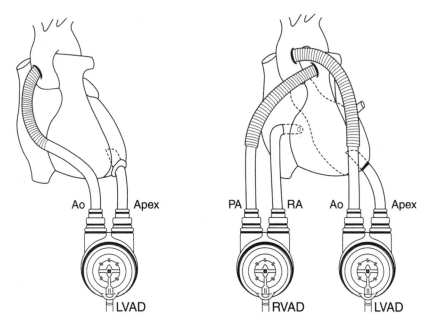

FIG. 21.7 Thoratec ventricular assist device. (From Mahmood AK, Courtney JM, Westaby S, et al. Critical review of current left ventricular assist devices. *Perfusion* 2000;15:399–420, with permission.)

plantation demonstrated no difference in survival to transplant. However, the Novacor group exhibited a significantly greater incidence of thromboembolic neurologic complications, whereas the HeartMate group had more infectious and technical complications [8].

    4. Permanent use. Improved VAD portability and reduced morbidity have enabled increasing numbers of patients to survive many months with an intracorporeal VAD. As a result of VAD improvements and the limited supply of human hearts available for transplantation, VAD placement now is being considered as an alternative to cardiac transplantation. Recent design advances have permitted development of a totally implantable artificial heart. The first of these devices, the AbioCor (Abiomed), was implanted by a University of Louisville surgical team on July 2, 2001. The device is attached to the native atria; weighs about 2 pounds; and consists of two artificial ventricles, each with valves, and a motor-driven hydraulic pump. An external lithium battery pack and coil provide the power, transmitting an electrical charge transcutaneously to an internal coil and lithium battery. The external batteries are rechargeable, maintain a charge for 4 hours, and signal when the power is becoming low. Three such devices have been implanted to date [9].

  C. Ventricular assist device placement. The TCI HeartMate VAD inflow cannula inserts into the LV apex, whereas the outflow cannula attaches to the ascending aorta. Percutaneous drive lines for power connection and venting or pneumatic activation can be tunneled from the pump in the left hemithorax to an exit site on the right midabdominal wall. This pump position permits outflow into the descending thoracic aorta [9,10]. The device also can be positioned intraabdominally with the cannulas traversing the diaphragm. More commonly, however, the pump is placed in a pocket behind either the rectus abdominus muscle or the posterior rectus fascia. Although intraperitoneal positioning probably reduces the risk of infection, it increases the risk of bowel perforation or obstruction. Although placement options for the Novacor VAD are the same as those for the HeartMate VAD, the preperitoneal position has been used almost exclusively for that device. Either the HeartMate or the Novacor VAD can be used for RVAD support, which would use right atrial inflow and pulmonary artery outflow.

Abiomed BVS-5000 VADs are easier to place than HeartMate or Novacor devices, because the pump is extracorporeal and CPB support is not required. The inflow cannula attaches to either the left atrium or the LV apex. The outflow cannula is a preclotted woven Dacron (Ethibond; US Surgical, Norwalk, CT, U.S.A.) graft that tends to minimize bleeding at the graft interstices. The LVAD outflow cannula is placed into the ascending aorta. Should this VAD need to be replaced, the procedure can be performed in the operating room or at the bedside in approximately 1 minute. The Thoratec LVAD inflow cannula is placed in the LV apex or the left atrium, with outflow to the ascending aorta.

When used as an RVAD, these devices permit inflow via the right atrium or RV, and outflow into the main pulmonary artery. The outflow cannula should be placed on the proximal pulmonary artery, taking care not to injure or distort the pulmonic valve [11].

D. Control and operation of ventricular assist devices. In the Biomedicus pump, the ventricle is not completely unloaded, resulting in some ventricular ejection and reduction in device filling. When rotational speed is increased, pump flow does not always increase, depending on cannula size and position as well as on preload and afterload. Anticoagulation is not required if VAD flow remains greater than 2 L/min. Minimizing the interval between separation from CPB and initiation of VAD support appears to be critical for providing successful support [4].

HeartMate and Novacor VAD patients typically do not tolerate ventricular fibrillation or asystole well, although ventricular tachyarrhythmias are common, particularly in post-MI patients requiring VAD support. In general, ventricular tachycardia is poorly tolerated early after VAD placement. Implantable pacers and/or defibrillators and aggressive antiarrhythmic pharmacotherapy may be necessary. V-E HeartMate and Novacor devices have two external batteries that provide tether-free support for 4 to 6 hours. It is essential to provide the necessary teaching for the patient, the patient's family, and other home caregivers before hospital discharge [10].

The Abiomed BVS-5000 pump is a dual-chamber device. The upper ("atrial") chamber is a passive gravity-filled reservoir, and the lower ("ventricular") chamber performs the pumping action. The atrial chamber fills continuously throughout systole and diastole, and filling occurs by gravity. Thus, adjusting the height of the device relative to the patient will affect filling and output. The drive console timing is independent of native cardiac rhythm. The duration of pump systole and diastole are automatically altered in response to changes in preload and afterload, maintaining a relatively constant stroke volume of 88 mL. Operator input is not required during normal operation of this device. Consequently, a reduced rate of pump cycles per minute may serve as a clinical indicator of inadequate preload or of excessive afterload. During weaning, separate controls are available that allow the operator to manually convert to a fixed rate.

The Thoratec VAD system is a pneumatic assist device. The amount of drive pressure required to produce systole and the amount of vacuum required to produce diastole can each be adjusted as needed. The stroke volume of the device is 65 mL with a maximal flow of 6.5 L/min. Typically drive line pressures 75 to 100 mm Hg above the patient's systolic blood pressure, a vacuum of −30 to −40 mm Hg, and systolic ejection time greater than 300 msec will produce a desirable adult LVAD output. There are three modes of support with the Thoratec VAD: volume or fill mode; R-wave synchronous mode; and asynchronous mode. The asynchronous mode is most commonly used at the time of implantation during air removal maneuvers and can be set to low rates during intervals of echocardiographic assessment of LV recovery. The fill or volume mode is most commonly used after initial implantation, when weaning is not being considered. Support is optimal in this mode, providing more complete washing of the blood sac, to theoretically reduce the risk of thrombus formation. The R-wave synchronous mode allows VAD systole to occur during native LV diastole. It can be programmed to eject with every other or every third diastole, analogous to 1:2 or 1:3 modes with IABP [11]. This mode is most useful for VAD weaning.

E. **Beneficial effects of ventricular assist devices.** In patients with severe LV failure, the myocardium can dramatically improve during VAD support in a process commonly referred to as remodeling. LV echocardiography before and during LVAD support has demonstrated marked reductions in LV mass; thus, the pathologic hypertrophy exhibited in end-stage cardiomyopathy can improve dramatically [12]. Furthermore, myocardial gene expression in LVAD-supported hearts changes in a way that is compatible with decreased susceptibility to apoptotic cardiomyocyte death [13]. These changes are not necessarily permanent. Recurrence of end-stage cardiomyopathy has been reported in patients whose LVAD support was discontinued for several months; these patients required a second LVAD placement [14]. Once a VAD has been functioning for a period of time, left atrial, pulmonary arterial, and central venous pressures all drop to normal levels, and systemic arterial pressure increases to normal levels [10].

It has been demonstrated that patients receiving more than 30 days of VAD support with the HeartMate device had better posttransplantation perioperative survival than patients who are transplanted less than 30 days after VAD placement. It is generally believed that the longer duration of VAD support provides for greater improvement of overall physiologic status with subsequent improved outcome [15]. Patients who do not demonstrate normalization of blood urea nitrogen and creatinine levels [16] and/or bilirubin levels [16,17] after initiation of a VAD are significantly less likely to survive to cardiac transplantation than are patients who exhibit improvement in these laboratory values.

F. **Anticoagulation and antiplatelet drugs with ventricular assist devices.** With placement of HeartMate and Novacor devices, perioperative bleeding is a common complication. This is not surprising, considering that many of these patients have undergone prior sternotomy and anticoagulant and/or antiplatelet medication regimens chronically. Congestive hepatic dysfunction may be present. The U.S. Food and Drug Administration (FDA) reports a 40% to 44% reexploration rate for bleeding among Novacor and HeartMate patients. Striking a balance between the bleeding propensities induced by preexisting coagulopathies and prevention of thrombosis on the foreign surfaces of a VAD creates an imposing therapeutic challenge. The Cleveland Clinic protocol includes routine vitamin K, fresh frozen plasma, and aprotinin administration perioperatively for VAD patients. In some cases, coagulopathy may be best managed by packing the surgical wound for 24 hours, then returning to the operating room to close the wound when coagulopathy becomes less pronounced. After the acute phase, once bleeding has diminished to acceptable levels, HeartMate recipients frequently are placed solely on aspirin therapy. Novacor recipients traditionally had been placed on coumadin and various antiplatelet regimens, but recent reduction in the thrombogenicity of Novacor cannulas may allow those patients to have a less stringent anticoagulant regimen [10].

The St. Louis University group [18] suggests the following anticoagulation regimen for Thoratec devices. The device is inserted during CPB with full heparinization and a half-Hammersmith aprotinin regimen. Upon separation from CPB, heparin is fully reversed with protamine sulfate and anticoagulation is held for 24 hours, after which heparin is infused at 10 USP units/kg/hour to produce an aPTT of 1.5 times control. Once oral intake resumes, warfarin is initiated and titrated to produce an international normalized ratio (INR) of 2.5 to 3.0. Heparin is stopped when the INR is greater than 2.5, but resumed at 10 units/kg/hour if INR drops below 2.5. If the patient remains stable, aspirin 81 mg/day is added on postoperative days 10 to 14. Using this protocol, the overall bleeding complication rate was 31%, with device-related thromboembolic events occurring in 8.1% of patients.

G. **Weaning from ventricular assist devices.** Although the majority of VADs are not removed until transplantation, VAD weaning and explantation can occur if myocardial function returns to a level that permits separation with minimal pharmacologic assistance. Serial echocardiographic studies allow quantitative assessment of ventricular size and function. Once weaning is considered, echocardiographic evaluation of ventricular function during periods of minimal VAD support should be performed. The patient should be fully heparinized, and the pump essentially turned off with a single stoke every 20 seconds or so to avoid thrombus formation in the device. If LV function appears adequate over a period of at least 10 minutes, the device may be placed in a fixed rate mode in order to create some afterload for the LV. If LV function remains adequate over the ensuing days, elective explantation may be a consideration. Hetzer et al. [19] report a technique whereby the intrathoracic portions of the cannulas are left in place, which allows the device to be explanted without reentry into the thorax. This technique is associated with good long-term results.

Decreasing the pump speed and observing the function of the native ventricle permits weaning from centrifugal pumps. However, pump flows less than 2 L/min risk thrombus formation on the pump rotor, so care must be taken to ensure adequate anticoagulation. With pneumatic assist pumps, the first weaning step is to reduce the diastolic vacuum, which reduces blood flow into the pump. Atrial pressure then increases to permit the native heart to fill and eject, hence providing an opportunity to observe the native ventricle's performance.

H. Complications and limitations

1. **Thromboembolic events.** Early experience with Novacor VADs was complicated by thromboembolic events in as many as 41.6% of patients [10]. In 1998 the inflow and outflow conduits of the Novacor VAD were changed to a less thrombogenic material, which reduced the incidence of central nervous system embolic events by 50% [4]. Embolic complications are less common with the Abiomed device, although Korfer et al. [5] noted a 19% incidence of cerebral infarction. Slater et al. [20] reported an 8% incidence of thromboembolic complications with the Thoratec VAD and just a 2.7% incidence of thromboemboli in more than 200 patients on TCI HeartMate IP support. What is particularly impressive about the HeartMate results is that most of those patients either received no anticoagulation or were treated only with aspirin or with aspirin and dipyridamole [20].

2. **Infections.** Septicemia can occur either as a complication of VAD placement or as a result of catheter (i.e., "line") sepsis, because patients frequently require long-term invasive monitoring. Infections also can occur in the VAD device, including its drive lines and cannulas. Infection rates of 10% to 66% have been reported [4,10,18]. Infection of the device, its pump pocket, or endocarditis of the device's valves often requires explantation, although in some cases local debridement and povidone iodine (Betadine) irrigation will control the infection sufficiently to permit continued VAD support until transplantation.

3. **RV failure.** RV failure occurs in up to 25% of patients receiving LVAD support. In some cases, RV failure is not evident until LV assistance has been provided, as the improved aortic flow then may cause the concomitant increased venous return to the right heart to outstrip the flow capacity of an impaired RV. Either acute or chronic pulmonary hypertension may contribute to poor RV performance. Optimizing RV performance with "inodilators," such as milrinone, and pulmonary arterial dilators, such as nitric oxide, may prevent the need for RV mechanical support, although biventricular support is unavoidable in many cases.

4. **Vacuum-related events.** Probe patent foramen ovale occurs in approximately 25% of the general population and can cause severe intracardiac shunting if left atrial pressure is reduced below right atrial pressure (with the aid of a diastolic vacuum). Accordingly, the foramen should **always** be checked (by visual inspection or transesophageal echocardiography) and surgically closed at the time of insertion of the LV assist cannulas. In patients with an open chest, diastolic vacuum may draw air into the circulation before the chest is closed. Similarly, the negative inflow pressure generated by centrifugal pumps potentially can draw air into the circulation at suture lines or central venous catheters at their insertion sites.

5. **Mechanical events.** Thrombus formation inside the cannula or extrinsic compression of the cannula or atrium by clot or tissue can prevent adequate flow of blood into the pump. This can rapidly progress to profound hypoperfusion. Fortunately, primary pump failure is rare with currently used VADs despite months of continuous use.

6. **Economic considerations.** A retrospective study of patients receiving either inotropic therapy or HeartMate LVAD support as a bridge to transplantation demonstrated that patients with LVAD implantation before transplant had similar average daily costs compared to patients receiving intravenous inotropic support [7]. A multicenter study currently under way is comparing the cost-effectiveness of long-term VAD support with medical management [21].

7. **Psychosocial concerns.** Shapiro et al. [22] noted that 25 of 30 LVAD recipients required one or more psychiatric interventions. Adjustment disorder was seen most commonly, followed by organic mental syndrome, family distress, and major depression.

I. **Contraindications.** Although there are no absolute contraindications to VAD placement, VAD support would likely be detrimental in patients with active sepsis or significant bleeding diatheses. In addition, there must be some anticipated improvement in ventricular performance or the prospect of cardiac transplantation, although those decisions are difficult to make in the acute clinical setting.

J. **Pediatric ventricular assist devices.** Although experience with VAD use among the pediatric population is not nearly as extensive as for adults, early results appear promising. Assist devices have been used in infants less than 10 kg and have been used successfully as a bridge to transplantation with successful support for more than 1 year. Helman et al. [23] report greater than 60% survival to the time of transplant. Compared to pediatric patients receiving extracorporeal membrane oxygenation support, children receiving VAD support had a lower incidence of moderate-to-severe neurologic impairment, with no differences in other long-term outcome [24].

III. **Anesthetic management of patients with ventricular assist devices**

A. **Ventricular assist device placement.** Management of these patients depends to some degree on the clinical setting. Scheduled elective placement of a VAD in a patient with end-stage cardiac function permits ample time for anesthetic preparation and planning. As with any patient with severe cardiac dysfunction, myocardial depressants should be avoided and meticulous attention to fluid management is essential to optimize preload. In patients with a pulsatile VAD, vacuum should be avoided while the chest is open to reduce the risk of air entrainment. One must maintain adequate blood volume to permit the VAD to fill while avoiding intravascular volume overload that could precipitate failure of the unassisted ventricle.

Inotropic support likely will be necessary before initiation of VAD support and also may be needed after VAD placement to support an unassisted ventricle. Vasodilators may enhance output from the unassisted ventricle. VAD placement in the setting of failed separation from CPB gives less opportunity to prepare an anesthetic plan, but the same principles apply. Standard monitors are appropriate in these patients, as well as an arterial catheter and a central venous pressure catheter or Swan-Ganz catheter (if an RVAD is not used). A left atrial catheter may be useful for monitoring left heart filling pressures. Transesophageal echocardiography is helpful for determining adequate positioning of the inflow cannula and to assess changes in ventricular function resulting from initiation of VAD therapy. It is important to maintain good communication with the individual controlling the assist device in order to optimize its function.

B. **Ventricular assist device removal.** As with VAD placement, anesthetic management for VAD removal depends upon the setting in which the VAD is being removed. Elective removal from a patient in whom significant improvement in ventricular function has occurred is a far different scenario from VAD removal for infectious or hemorrhagic complications in a patient with persistent severe ventricular dysfunction. In the former setting, a requirement for significant inotropic support during intervals of diminished VAD support suggests that the patient may not be able to tolerate explantation. In the latter case, one expects maximal inotropic support in conjunction with pulmonary vasodilators such as nitric oxide.

C. Management of the ventricular assist device patient for noncardiac surgery.

Electromechanical interference (EMI) has the potential to temporarily or, in some cases, permanently disrupt electronic circuitry within certain VADs. The electronics for timing and driving Novacor, Thoratec, and Abiomed VADs are shielded from EMI because they are housed within the external controller. Some of the timing circuitry of TCI VADs is located within the device and, therefore, is not completely shielded from EMI. TCI IP-LVAD models should be put in the fixed-rate mode with the timing circuit disconnected if electrocautery interferes with the device or if a need for defibrillation is likely.

Electrocautery interferes with the ability of the TCI VE-LVAD to sustain cardiac output. If electrocautery is necessary in such patients, it can be applied in 1-second bursts with 10 seconds or more between bursts to allow cardiac output to recover. Alternatively, if the surgeon can attain adequate exposure using an ultrasonically activated scalpel, such as the Harmonic scalpel (Ultracision Inc., Smithfield, RI, U.S.A.), VAD function should not be affected. If defibrillation is needed, the drive line should be disconnected from the external controller, which will require the pump to be driven pneumatically or manually for the interval of defibrillation [25].

Should magnetic resonance imaging studies be necessary in the patient on VAD support, the Abiomed is the only current VAD device that is not adversely affected by the intense magnetic field. TCI, Thoratec, and Abiomed VADs all will experience a drop in output that may be permanent in some VAD models. Thus, magnetic resonance imaging is not recommended for VAD patients unless they have an Abiomed device [25].

Emergent surgery in patients on a VAD produces an obvious risk for hemorrhagic complications. In such settings, multiple transfusions of blood components frequently are required. The benefit of antifibrinolytic agents, such as aprotinin, in this setting has yet to be determined. In less emergent operative settings, there may be an opportunity to discontinue oral antiplatelet and anticoagulant medications for a sufficient interval to allow coagulation status to be near normal. To minimize thromboembolic risk, intravenous heparin should be administered during that interval [26].

References

1. Melhorn U, Kroner A, deVivie ER. 30 years clinical intra-aortic balloon pumping: facts and figures. *Thorac Cardiovasc Surg* 1999;47[Suppl 2]:298–303.
2. Booker PD. Intra-aortic balloon pumping in young children. *Paediatr Anaesth* 1997;7: 501–507.
3. Hurle A, Llamas P, Meseguer J, et al. Paraplegia complicating intraaortic balloon pumping. *Ann Thorac Surg* 1997;63:1217–1218.
4. **Mahmood AK, Courtney JM, Westaby S, et al. Critical review of current left ventricular assist devices. *Perfusion* 2000;15:399–420.**
5. Korfer R, El-Banayosy A, Arusoglu L, et al. Temporary pulsatile ventricular assist devices and biventricular assist devices. *Ann Thorac Surg* 1999;68:678–683.
6. Park SJ, Nguyen DQ, Bank AJ, et al. Left ventricular assist device bridge therapy for acute myocardial infarction. *Ann Thorac Surg* 2000;69:1146–1151.
7. Bank AJ, Mir SH, Nguyen DQ, et al. Effects of left ventricular assist devices on outcomes in patients undergoing heart transplantation. *Ann Thorac Surg* 2000;69:1369–1375.
8. El-Banayosy A, Arusoglu L, Kizner L, et al. Novacor left ventricular assist system versus HeartMate vented electric left ventricular assist system as a long-term mechanical circulatory support device in bridging patients: a prospective study. *J Thorac Cardiovasc Surg* 2000;119:581–587.
9. SoRelle R. Third AbioCor artificial heart implanted in Houston. *Circulation* 2001;104: e9033.
10. **McCarthy PM, Hoercher K. Clinically available intracorporeal ventricular assist devices. *Prog Cardiovasc Dis* 2000;43:37–46.**
11. **Dowling RD, Etoch SW. Clinically available extracorporeal assist devices. *Prog Cardiovasc Dis* 2000;43:27–36.**
12. Altemose GT, Gritsus V, Jeevanadam V, et al. Altered myocardial phenotype after mechanical support in human beings with advanced cardiomyopathy. *J Heart Lung Transplant* 1997;16:765–773.

13. Bartling B, Milting H, Schumann H, et al. Myocardial gene expression of regulators of myocyte apoptosis and myocyte calcium homeostasis during hemodynamic unloading by ventricular assist devices in patients with end-stage heart failure. *Circulation* 1999; 100[Suppl II]:II-216–II-223.

14. Helman DN, Maybaum SW, Morales DLS, et al. Recurrent remodeling after ventricular assistance: is long-term myocardial recovery attainable? *Ann Thorac Surg* 2000; 70:1255–1258.

15. Ashton RC, Goldstein DJ, Rose EA, et al. Duration of left ventricular assist device support affects transplant survival. *J Heart Lung Transplant* 1996;15:1151–1157.

16. Farrar DJ, Hill JD et al. Recovery of major organ function in patients awaiting heart transplantation with Thoratec ventricular assist devices. *J Heart Lung Transplant* 1994; 13:1125–1132.

17. Reinhartz O, Farrar DJ, Hershon JH, et al. Importance of preoperative liver function as a predictor of survival in patients supported with Thoratec ventricular assist devices as a bridge to transplantation. *J Thorac Cardiovasc Surg* 1998;116:633–640.

18. McBride LR, Naunheim KS, Fiore AC, et al. Clinical experience with 111 Thoratec ventricular assist devices. *Ann Thorac Surg* 1999;67:1233–1239.

19. Hetzer R, Muller J, Weng Y, et al. Cardiac recovery in dilated cardiomyopathy by unloading with a left ventricular assist device. *Ann Thorac Surg* 1999;68:742–749.

20. Slater JP, Rose EA, Levin HR, et al. Low thromboembolic risk without anticoagulation using advanced-design left ventricular assist devices. *Ann Thorac Surg* 1996;62:1321–1328.

21. Rose EA, Moskowitz AJ, Packer M, et al. The REMATCH trial: rationale, design, and end points. *Ann Thorac Surg* 1999;67:723–730.

22. Shapiro PA, Levin HR, Oz MC. Left ventricular assist devices. Psychosocial burden and implications for heart transplant programs. *Gen Hosp Psychiatry* 1996;18:30S–35S.

23. Helman DN, Addonizio LJ, Morales DLS, et al. Implantable left ventricular assist devices can successfully bridge adolescent patients to transplant. *J Heart Lung Transplant* 2000;19:121–126.

24. Ibrahim AE, Duncan BW, Blume ED, et al. Long-term follow-up of pediatric cardiac patients requiring mechanical circulatory support. *Ann Thorac Surg* 2000;69:186–192.

25. **Madigan JD, Choudhri AF, Chen J, et al. Surgical management of the patient with an implanted cardiac device. *Ann Surg* 1999;230:639–647.**

26. Schmid C, Wilhelm M, Dietl K, et al. Noncardiac surgery in patients with left ventricular assist devices. *Surgery* 2001;129:440–444.

22. INTRAOPERATIVE MYOCARDIAL PROTECTION

John W. C. Entwistle III and Andrew S. Wechsler

I. Introduction

Cardiac surgery is performed to preserve or restore cardiac function in a diseased heart. However, the performance of the procedure is, by necessity, accompanied by myocardial injury. Protection of the myocardium is required to minimize the detrimental effects on the heart. A proper strategy of myocardial protection encompasses events before, during, and after the initiation of myocardial ischemia, including treatment of the patient both pre-operatively and postoperatively. As such, all medical personnel involved in the perioperative care of the cardiac patient should be cognizant of implications toward myocardial preservation. A strategy of myocardial preservation may be made infinitely complex, but most patients will be adequately served through the use of a limited number of techniques and agents designed to minimize the difference between oxygen delivery and utilization during ischemia. The new popularity of beating heart surgery has required the development of different strategies for myocardial protection, but they remain based on the balance between supply and demand of oxygen. In addition, the use of minimally invasive techniques, such as port access, has increased the role of the anesthesiologist in the perioperative aspects of myocardial protection.

II. History of myocardial protection

A. Before the introduction of the cardiopulmonary bypass machine, the earliest cardiac procedures were performed without myocardial protection. Topical myocardial cooling and **systemic hypothermia** were used to facilitate the conduct of the operation.

B. In 1955, Melrose advocated the use of hyperkalemic cardioplegia to provide cardiac quiescence during the operation. This approach was abandoned because of the permanent myocardial injury (**"stone heart"**) produced by the high potassium concentrations used.

C. In 1956, Lillehei introduced the technique of administration of cardioplegia through the right atrium or coronary sinus (**"retrograde cardioplegia"**) for use in operations on the aortic valve.

D. Procedures used to provide myocardial standstill, such as intermittent aortic cross-clamping, were primarily performed to facilitate the conduct of the operation, with less regard to the ischemic consequences to the myocardium. Interest and research in chemical cardioplegia persisted but was not used clinically.

E. **Topical myocardial cooling** with iced saline or slush was used as an early form of myocardial protection.

F. A correlation was made between poor myocardial protection and the onset of **myocardial necrosis** in patients who succumbed to postoperative cardiogenic shock. Clinical confirmation was obtained when a high rate of perioperative myocardial infarction was demonstrated in patients undergoing either coronary artery bypass grafting or valvular procedures.

G. In 1973, Gay and Ebert reintroduced **hyperkalemic cardiac arrest** but with potassium concentrations of less than 20 mmol, thus preventing the occurrence of stone heart syndrome seen with the earlier use of potassium cardioplegia. This marked the beginning of the use of a technique that provided a combination of effective myocardial protection and cardiac quiescence.

H. In the late 1970s, Follette et al. [1] and Buckberg popularized the use of **blood cardioplegia,** citing the advantages gained by using the intrinsic advantages of potassium-enriched blood, such as its natural buffers and oxygen delivery capabilities.

III. Cardiac physiology

A. The myocardium has a high rate of energy consumption under normal circumstances. This requires a constant supply of oxygen to the myocardium. **Myocardial ischemia** occurs when the supply of oxygen is exceeded by the demand, and infarction occurs when this occurs for a prolonged period of time.

B. **Oxygen delivery** to the myocardium is dependent upon the concentration of hemoglobin in the blood, the arterial oxygen saturation, and the flow of oxygenated blood to the myocardium. Under normal conditions, the blood flow to the myocardium is controlled by **autoregulation,** in which blood flow is matched to myocardial requirements. Autoregulation is not active when the blood pressure is above or below the autoregulatory range.

C. The **subendocardium** receives its nutritive flow primarily during diastole and is vulnerable to variations in blood flow.
   1. Flow is dependent upon the transmural gradient, which is the difference between the aortic diastolic pressure and the intraventricular end-diastolic pressure.
   2. Oxygen delivery may be insufficient because of either a decrease in perfusion pressure (systemic hypotension or coronary artery disease) or an increase in ventricular end-diastolic pressure (aortic stenosis, ventricular fibrillation, or ventricular distension).
D. The heart depends upon a continuous supply of oxygen to maintain full function
   1. Adenosine triphosphate (ATP) is made at a rate of 36 moles per mole of glucose in the presence of oxygen.
   2. Under anaerobic conditions, ATP production falls to 2 moles of ATP per mole of glucose. Lactate and hydrogen accumulate in the tissues, which further inhibits glycolysis and other cellular functions.
E. Myocardial **oxygen consumption** is dependent upon the work performed by the heart (Fig. 22.1) [2,3].
   1. Normal working ventricular myocardium consumes 8 mL of O_2 per 100 g of myocardium per minute.
   2. This decreases to 5.6 of O_2 per 100 g of myocardium in the empty beating heart and to 1.1 mL of O_2 per 100 g of myocardium per minute in the potassium-arrested heart.
   3. Myocardial cooling provides an additional decrease to 0.3 mL of O_2 per 100 g of myocardium.

IV. Mechanisms of myocardial ischemic injury. The mechanisms by which ischemia and reperfusion injure the heart are complex, and the contributions of the individual components of this process are hotly debated. It is possible that the process of reperfusion may be as equally harmful to the myocardium as is the ischemic insult itself. Thus, in the field of myocardial protection, it is important to have an understanding of the components thought to contribute to the damage, because amelioration of these factors that lead to injury may lessen the injury, whereas ignoring important aspects of ischemia and reperfusion injury may make all other protective interventions ineffective.

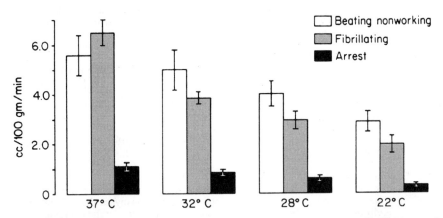

FIG. 22.1 Left ventricular myocardial oxygen uptake of the beating empty, fibrillating, and arrested perfused hearts at varying myocardial temperatures. The greatest decrease in myocardial oxygen uptake at a given temperature occurs with mechanical arrest. The addition of hypothermia decreases the oxygen consumption to a lesser degree. (From Buckberg GD, Brazier JR, Nelson RL, et al. Studies of the effects of hypothermia on regional myocardial blood flow and metabolism during cardiopulmonary bypass. I. The adequately perfused beating, fibrillating, and arrested heart. *J Thorac Cardiovasc Surg* 1977;73:87–94, with permission.)

A. Depletion of high-energy phosphates occurs during ischemia. Breakdown products may be washed away with reperfusion, prohibiting the rapid conversion back to ATP.

B. Intracellular acidosis develops during anaerobic metabolism, and the accumulation of hydrogen ions interferes with the function of many intracellular enzymes.

C. Calcium is important in numerous cellular functions. The intracellular fluxes in calcium concentration are responsible, in part, for contraction and relaxation of the myocardium. Alterations in intracellular **calcium homeostasis** have been documented after ischemia and reperfusion. Changes in the rate of calcium uptake or release within the cell can have profound functional consequences.

D. Direct myocellular injury from ischemia may cause myocardial dysfunction

E. In addition to the alterations in calcium homeostasis that have been documented, intracellular **calcium overload** can occur at the time of reperfusion as calcium is released from the sarcoplasmic reticulum or enters the cell through calcium channels, such as the sodium–calcium exchanger or the L-type calcium channel. Alterations in intracellular calcium levels may activate enzymes, trigger second messenger cascades, or alter excitation–contraction coupling. Calcium concentrations may be so high that contracture develops.

F. Generation of **oxygen-derived free radicals** occurs upon reperfusion. These are highly unstable compounds that are capable of damaging proteins, nucleic acids, phospholipids, and other cellular components. Natural free radical scavengers prevent damage under normal circumstances, but these endogenous systems are depleted during a significant period of ischemia and are quickly overwhelmed.

G. Complement activation may occur as part of the generalized inflammatory process that occurs with injury.

H. Adverse **endothelial cell–leukocyte interactions** occur after ischemia and reperfusion. Under normal conditions, the endothelium and neutrophils are the producers of, and responsive to, numerous signaling compounds. There is a delicate balance between vasoconstriction and vasodilation, as well as between the promotion and prevention of thrombosis. Adenosine, nitric oxide, endothelin, and thromboxane are a few of the potent substances whose production and effects are altered after ischemia and reperfusion. This may produce a state of altered endothelial cell–leukocyte interaction, leading to areas of myocardial malperfusion and damage from increased endothelial adherence [4].

I. Myocellular **edema** may result from ischemia and reperfusion injury. Edema may occur in response to numerous injurious events and can alter the function of all of the cells within the myocardium. Edema has been implicated in contractile dysfunction, decreased ventricular compliance, and capillary plugging that inhibits reperfusion of the coronary microcirculation.

J. Damage to **nonmyocyte components** of the heart may cause systolic and diastolic dysfunction. This includes injury to the endothelium of the coronary circulation, as well as to fibroblasts and other structural components of the heart.

V. Consequences of ischemia and reperfusion injury. The severity of myocardial injury after a period of ischemia and reperfusion depends on numerous factors, including the length of ischemia (Fig. 22.2) [5]; the temperature of the myocardium; the conditions of the myocardium before, during, and after the ischemia; and the method in which the myocardium is reperfused. The resulting myocardial injury can be described according to established criteria.

A. Brief periods of ischemia may produce no readily identifiable functional deficit.

B. Myocardial stunning represents ischemia and reperfusion injury in its mildest form. Although stunning may be severe, it represents viable myocardium that has systolic and/or diastolic dysfunction in the presence of normal myocardial perfusion. By definition, there is no necrosis in stunned myocardium. Given sufficient time, this stunned myocardium will manifest complete functional recovery in the absence of additional injury. Stunned myocardium is distinct from hibernating myocardium, which is viable myocardium that is chronically underperfused and subsequently has down-regulated its contractile elements. Upon revascularization, this myocardium begins to return to its normal phenotype and subsequently returns to normal function.

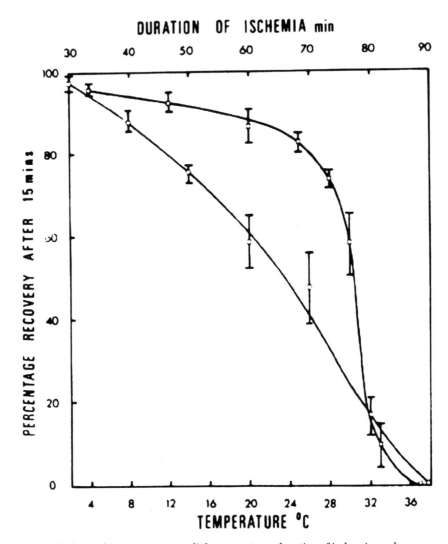

FIG. 22.2 Relationship among myocardial temperature, duration of ischemia, and recovery of aortic blood flow. Two sets of experiments are shown. In the duration of ischemia studies *(top horizontal axis, open circles)*, the heart was made ischemic for varying times at 30°C and then reperfused. The percentage myocardial recovery is shown on the *vertical axis*, and it declines steadily with time. In the temperature studies *(lower horizontal axis, open squares)*, hearts were subjected to 60 minutes of ischemia at varying myocardial temperatures and then reperfused. As the temperature of the myocardium is decreased below 28°C, myocardial recovery increases. (From Hearse DJ, Stewart DA, Braimbridge MV. Cellular protection during myocardial ischemia. The development and characterization of a procedure for the induction of reversible ischemic arrest. *Circulation* 1976;54:193–202, with permission.)

C. **Myocardial necrosis** occurs when myocytes are irreversibly injured. Necrosis may not be readily identifiable by functional or histologic means early after injury and thus may not be distinguishable from stunned myocardium. However, these cells eventually die, despite reperfusion, and are replaced by noncontractile scar.

VI. **Purpose of cardioplegia.** Historically, most cardiac operations performed over the past few decades have been done under conditions of cardiac arrest. Despite the recent popularity of beating heart surgery, cardiac arrest still is predominantly used during valve repair/replacement, cardiac transplantation, and procedures on the aortic root. Cardioplegia serves separate, but often interrelated, purposes.

A. The first is to provide **cardiac quiescence.** Most cardiac procedures are more easily performed on the flaccid, noncontracting heart than on the beating heart. Additionally, this lessens the possibility of air embolism occurring during open procedures performed on the left-sided chambers of the heart. Although cardiac standstill originally was produced via cooling of the heart, potassium-based cardioplegia can provide rapid and reversible arrest.

B. Second, interruption of myocardial blood flow facilitates the operation by providing a **bloodless field** and enhancing visibility. During most cardiac procedures, a crossclamp is applied across the ascending aorta, which eliminates continuous coronary flow. Through the use of cardioplegia, the energy requirements of the myocardium can be significantly reduced, thus increasing the safety and allowable duration of this interruption of blood flow.

C. Through the reduction in myocardial energy consumption, there is preservation of myocardial function, despite significant periods of myocardial ischemia.

D. Current methods of cardioplegic myocardial arrest allow for the rapid resumption of contractile activity at the end of the procedure. The period of contractile arrest can be lengthened by the administration of additional doses of cardioplegia, and it can be shortened by the restoration of myocardial blood flow, with washout of the cardioplegia. This control allows the surgeon to minimize the time of cardiopulmonary bypass awaiting the return of cardiac function while providing maximal myocardial protection during the performance of the procedure.

VII. **Intervention before the onset of ischemia.** Optimal myocardial protection requires a complete, well-conceived strategy that takes into consideration the unique characteristics of the individual patient. Aortic insufficiency, ventricular hypertrophy, and severe obstructive coronary disease are a few of the factors that may alter the intraoperative management in order to obtain maximal cardiac protection. In addition to planning ahead, there are several interventions before the onset of ischemia that influence the effectiveness of myocardial protection. Almost all aspects of myocardial protection involve maintaining balance between myocardial oxygen supply and demand.

A. **Minimization of on-going ischemia** may require the use of nitrates, anticoagulants, antiplatelet agents, or insertion of an intraaortic balloon pump in the preoperative period. Hypertension, tachycardia, and patient anxiety should be controlled. Oxygen should be used liberally.

B. **Rapid revascularization.** Any sign of ischemia should warrant aggressive diagnosis and management. If ischemia cannot be readily controlled and infarction is imminent, then emergent operation to alleviate ischemia is required unless otherwise contraindicated. In this setting, rapid reversal of ischemia may require the use of saphenous vein grafts as opposed to arterial conduit, if the harvesting of the internal mammary artery would unduly delay resolution of the ischemia. Similarly, the choice between on-pump and beating heart revascularization may depend upon the urgency of the operation.

C. **Nutritional repletion** may be possible in the setting of elective cardiac surgery. The depleted heart has little reserve and may not tolerate ischemia as well. Depressed glycogen levels have been correlated with poor postoperative outcomes, and repletion with the preoperative administration of **GIK solution** (glucose, insulin, potassium) has been demonstrated to reduce complications.

D. **Avoidance of ischemia.** Although regional myocardial ischemia is required during any bypass operation, the intraoperative global cardiac ischemia that accompanies aortic cross-clamping may be avoided through one of several mechanisms.

1. Coronary artery bypass grafting may be performed using beating heart techniques. This strategy allows continuous perfusion of the coronary vasculature, with the exception of the territory being bypassed, while the anastomosis is being performed. With the use of an **intraluminal flow-through device,** some blood flow can be maintained to the distal vessel during the creation of the anastomosis, except for brief periods of time. However, perfusion pressure must be maintained within the physiologic range to avoid cardiac and peripheral ischemia. Insertion of an intraaortic balloon pump may be useful in this setting if hemodynamic instability results from cardiac manipulation.

2. Bypass grafting may be performed with minimal cardiac ischemia through the use of cardiopulmonary bypass without aortic cross-clamping. In the setting of the empty beating heart, perfusion to both the body and coronary arteries is supported by the bypass machine, eliminating the hemodynamic instability and subsequent hypoperfusion that may be associated with cardiac manipulation in some off-pump patients. Although this technique does not avoid the systemic effects of extracorporeal perfusion, it eliminates the effects of systemic hypothermia and avoids the myocardial effects of cardioplegia. By eliminating the work performed by the heart, myocardial energy requirements may drop to 20% of those in the working heart.

3. Intracardiac procedures may be performed without significant cardiac ischemia with the patient on bypass, without aortic cross-clamping. Although visibility may be limited, procedures such as tricuspid or mitral valve repair or replacement, or atrial or ventricular septal defect repair may be performed with continuous coronary perfusion. On procedures of the left heart, the left ventricle must remain decompressed to avoid the ejection of air through the aortic valve and subsequent air embolization. This technique is likely to increase in frequency with the adoption of newer ventricular remodeling procedures.

E. **Fibrillatory arrest** creates a nearly motionless heart to allow the performance of many cardiac procedures. It may be produced through either electrical stimulation or myocardial cooling.

   1. Normothermic fibrillatory arrest is produced by placing an alternating current generator in contact with the ventricular myocardium. As long as contact is maintained, the ventricle will remain in fibrillation, allowing procedures to be performed upon the heart with little ventricular motion. In this state, the left side of the heart can be opened to allow procedures such as closure of an atrial septal defect, without the fear of ejecting air in to the arterial circulation.

      a. Because the myocardium remains warm, energy consumption remains high.

      b. The fibrillating myocardium has increased wall tension.

      c. Perfusion to the endocardium is compromised, thus allowing possible subendocardial infarction.

      d. Therefore, this technique is not recommended.

   2. **Hypothermic fibrillatory arrest** [6] occurs as the myocardial temperature falls when the body is cooled. Energy consumption of the myocardium is less than during warm ventricular fibrillation, but not as low as during complete arrest. Procedures such as coronary artery bypass grafting or mitral valve replacement may be performed without interruption of myocardial perfusion. Fibrillation should be avoided in the setting of ventricular hypertrophy (Fig. 22.3) [7].

   3. Intermittent aortic cross-clamping may be combined with hypothermic myocardial ventricular fibrillation during performance of the distal anastomoses of a bypass operation to improve visibility while minimizing the time of myocardial ischemia.

F. **Prevention of ventricular distention** is important because increases in wall tension dramatically increase oxygen consumption while at the same time decreasing delivery.

   1. After the patient is on bypass and the heart is no longer ejecting blood into the aorta, a vent is inserted into the left ventricle through the right superior pulmonary vein.

   2. The vent is actively drained into the cardiotomy reservoir of the cardiopulmonary bypass machine at a rate of 100 to 300 mL/min to keep the left ventricle decompressed.

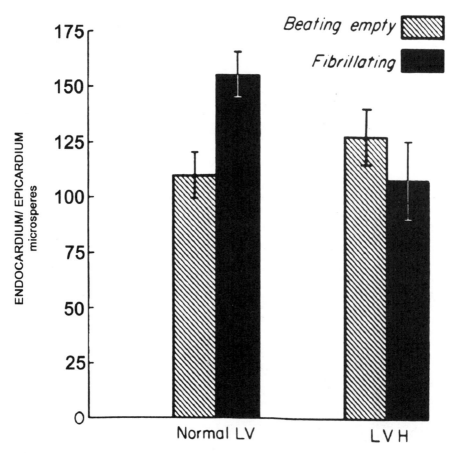

FIG. 22.3 Left ventricular myocardial flow distribution in the normal and hypertrophied heart. In left ventricular hypertrophy, endocardial blood flow is compromised during fibrillation, as the ratio of endocardial to epicardial flow decreases. This does not occur in the normal ventricle. (From Hottenrott CE, Towers B, Kurkji HJ, et al. The hazard of ventricular fibrillation in hypertrophied ventricles during cardiopulmonary bypass. *J Thorac Cardiovasc Surg* 1973;66:742–753, with permission.)

G. **Myocardial preconditioning** refers to the concept that myocardium that has undergone a brief limited period of ischemia may be better able to tolerate a subsequent, longer period of ischemia [8].
   1. Experimentally, hearts exposed to a brief ischemic stimulus sustain a smaller area of necrosis following a second longer period of ischemia. Numerous stimuli may induce the preconditioning response, including ischemia, hyperthermia, or the use of drugs (bradykinin, nitric oxide, phenylephrine, endotoxin, adenosine).
   2. Clinically, the effect of preconditioning is controversial. However, it is more likely to be relevant in the absence of myocardial protection, making it potentially more applicable in the setting of beating heart surgery or when myocardial protection is suboptimal, as with severe ventricular hypertrophy or occlusive coronary artery disease.

H. The use of warm, oxygenated cardioplegic solution to induce myocardial arrest (**warm induction**) minimizes energy consumption by arresting the ventricle, and it provides oxygen and substrates to the myocardium. Distribution of the cardioplegia to the subendocardium is maximized because the heart is arrested in diastole. This preischemic administration of cardioplegia has been shown to be beneficial in myocardial protection [9].

I. Diastolic arrest is the most common method of myocardial protection when aortic cross-clamping is used. Potassium-rich solutions are used to produce and maintain arrest until reperfusion. The electrical potential across the cellular membrane is determined by the concentrations of the ions on either side of the membrane at any given time. The resting potential across the cellular membrane is about -90 mV. During activation, the membrane depolarizes (becomes less negative), which allows the influx of sodium through voltage- and time-dependent sodium channels. Intracellular calcium concentrations rise, producing contraction. Relaxation occurs when calcium is sequestered into its intracellular sites. With the addition of cardioplegia, with a potassium concentration of 8 to 10 mEq/L, depolarization occurs. Sodium influx occurs, but the channels close in a time-dependent manner. However, because the concentration of potassium remains elevated in the extracellular space, the membrane remains depolarized, and the sodium channels remain closed and inactivated. Thus, the cell is unexcitable in a state of diastolic arrest. As the cardioplegia washes out of the extracellular space, the cell will repolarize and become excitable again. This is one reason why cardioplegia may require multiple doses over the course of the procedure.

VIII. Intervention during ischemia. The period of myocardial ischemia is when the myocardium is most vulnerable to injury. Numerous interventions are possible in order to minimize the injury, but not all are required in every circumstance. The overall strategy of myocardial protection must be individualized to the situation at hand.

A. Determination of the desired **myocardial temperature** is central to planning the protective strategy [10–12]. Although procedures can be performed on either the warm or hypothermic heart, the other components of the protective strategy must be chosen with the myocardial temperature in mind.

  1. Hypothermia is useful because the myocardial oxygen consumption decreases by 50% for every 10°C decrease in myocardial temperature ($\mathbf{Q_{10}}$ **effect**). Thus, the greatest absolute decrease in myocardial energy consumption occurs as the myocardial temperature decreases to 25°C, with relatively lesser gains with a progression to profound hypothermia. The major advantage of hypothermia is that it allows the interruption of myocardial blood flow for short periods of time, enabling the conduct of the operation to occur with minimal myocardial ischemic damage [2]. However, hypothermia itself is associated with injury to the myocardium, including alterations in cellular fluidity and transmembrane gradients, with the production of myocardial edema and a resultant decrease in ventricular performance. When desired, myocardial cooling can be produced through several mechanisms.

  a. Myocardial cooling most frequently is produced through the **administration of cardioplegia.** Cardioplegia usually is given at a temperature of 4° to 10°C and will produce myocardial cooling to 15° to 16°C. Cardioplegia may be administered through either the anterograde route via the native coronary arteries or the retrograde route through a special cannula placed in the coronary sinus.

  b. Profound systemic hypothermia as a method of routine myocardial protection is impractical because it takes a long time to cool and rewarm. However, myocardial cooling in the absence of systemic hypothermia can allow the unintentional rewarming of the myocardium through contact of the heart with the body and the return of warm blood to the heart through the cavae and noncoronary collaterals.

  c. Topical cooling can be achieved through the use of chilled saline or slush or through the use of a cooling jacket. Ice may produce uneven myocardial cooling. Slush may produce injury to the phrenic nerve through prolonged contact and increase atelectasis and pleural effusions. In addition, topical methods of cooling do not provide cooling to deep myocardium and thus are better suited for cooling the right ventricle than the left ventricle. In the setting of ventricular hypertrophy, topical methods clearly are inadequate. Topical cooling may be a useful adjunct to cooling with cardioplegia, especially with retrograde cardioplegia to improve cooling of the right ventricle.

2. Warm cardioplegia may be used before the initiation of ischemia as warm induction (see above). However, the entire operation may be conducted with **warm cardioplegia.** Because the myocardium is maintained at a warm temperature, metabolic activity continues, albeit at a lesser degree because mechanical activity of the heart is abolished. This constant oxygen requirement prohibits the use of significant periods of ischemia during the conduct of the operation [13,14].

    a. Warm cardioplegia must be supplied continuously to avoid ischemic injury.

    b. Its use is associated with less postoperative myocardial infarction and a lower incidence of low-output state.

    c. It requires the use of blood cardioplegia because crystalloid-based cardioplegia cannot carry enough oxygen to meet the demands of warm myocardium.

    d. Warm cardioplegia may not provide adequate protection in the presence of severe coronary artery disease, where uneven distribution may lead to poor protection.

3. **Tepid cardioplegia,** administered at 29°C, may provide some of the benefits of warm cardioplegia while minimizing the effects of hypothermia upon the myocardium.

B. The ideal **composition of cardioplegia** is hotly debated. Cardioplegia comes in two basic varieties, namely, crystalloid and blood. Blood cardioplegia is the most commonly used solution in adult cardiac surgery today, although the "recipe" varies significantly between surgeons. Cardioplegia can be made infinitely complex in nature by the use of additives and variations in administration. Most of these additives are chosen to combat the presumed causes of ischemia-reperfusion outlined in Section **IV.** The available evidence is controversial concerning the superiority of one cardioplegic regimen over the other [15]. Although benefits to blood cardioplegia may include improved systolic functional recovery, decreased ischemic injury, and decreased myocardial anaerobic metabolism, there appears that there is no long-term advantage with regard to ventricular function.

1. **Crystalloid cardioplegia** is uncommonly used in adult patients in the United States. A notable exception is in the preservation of the donor heart during cardiac transplantation.

    a. Crystalloid solutions do not contain hemoglobin and thus deliver dissolved oxygen only. At cold temperatures, oxygen delivery is adequate to sustain the myocardium. Therefore, crystalloid cardioplegia can be used only with a strategy of myocardial hypothermia.

    b. All components may be rigorously controlled. However, each additive increases the complexity of the cardioplegia. In addition, most additives serve to replace substances already present in blood cardioplegia.

2. **Blood cardioplegia** is produced by mixing blood to crystalloid in a defined ratio, with a final hematocrit usually of 16 to 20 vol%.

    a. Blood contains hemoglobin and thus has a high oxygen-carrying capacity. However, at low temperatures, the oxygen–hemoglobin dissociation curve is shifted to the left, diminishing the amount of oxygen available to the myocardium. However, due to the hemoglobin, blood cardioplegia may be administered either warm or cold. The frequency of administration varies with the temperature.

    b. Blood contains buffers, free radical scavengers, colloids, and numerous other substances that may have important benefits in myocardial protection. Because of these components, fewer additives may be required with blood cardioplegia.

    c. Blood has increased viscosity compared to crystalloid, and this is compounded with the addition of hypothermia. However, blood cardioplegia produces good myocardial protection, suggesting that the concerns over viscosity and capillary sludging are overstated.

  d. The ideal hematocrit for blood cardioplegia is unknown, but it may depend on the temperature of the myocardium and the frequency of administration. **Microplegia** refers to the use of blood that is minimally diluted with crystalloid containing only the elements necessary for achieving cardiac arrest. Theoretically, the avoidance of hemodilution lessens myocardial edema and thus improves postoperative left ventricular function.
- **C. Route of cardioplegia delivery.** Cardioplegia may be administered in either an anterograde or a retrograde direction.
  - **1. Anterograde cardioplegia** is delivered to the myocardium through the coronary arteries.
    - **a.** Usually, it is delivered through a cannula placed into the aortic root, after the aortic cross-clamp is applied. Flow often is started at a rate of 150 mL/(min·m^2) and adjusted to maintain a minimum aortic root pressure. Rapid infusion leads to uneven distribution and poor protection. A typical initial dose is 10 to 15 mL/kg, up to 1,000 mL. A low perfusion pressure results in uneven distribution of cardioplegia, and high perfusion pressure may cause damage to the endothelium. Perfusion pressure is typically between 70 and 100 mm Hg.
    - **b.** Anterograde cardioplegia through the aortic root cannot be used in the presence of significant aortic valve insufficiency. First, it is difficult to obtain adequate aortic root pressure when the aortic valve is incompetent. Second, cardioplegia enters the left ventricle, causing increased intraventricular pressure and wall tension and impeding delivery of the cardioplegia to the subendocardium. In this setting, anterograde cardioplegia may be administered directly down the left and right coronary arteries by using special cannulas that are placed into the coronary ostia after the aortic root is opened.
    - **c.** In the presence of severe occlusive coronary artery disease, especially in the absence of collateral vessels, uneven distribution of cardioplegia may occur through the anterograde route. Topical cooling with iced saline or slush may improve cooling in this setting.
    - **d.** During coronary artery bypass grafting, additional doses of cardioplegia can be given down each graft as it is completed. Not only does this allow the surgeon to check the flow of the graft, but it allows cardioplegia to be given distal to a flow-limiting lesion where the initial dose of cardioplegia may not have been adequate.
  - **2. Retrograde delivery** of cardioplegia may be used as either an adjunct to anterograde delivery or as the primary route of myocardial protection [16]. Cardioplegia is administered to the myocardium through the coronary veins by way of the coronary sinus.
    - **a.** A special cannula is directed into the coronary sinus through a small hole in the right atrium. Cardioplegia is delivered at a pressure of less than 40 mm Hg. Higher pressures may cause damage.
    - **b.** Improper placement of the catheter can cause injury to the coronary sinus.
    - **c.** Because the coronary veins draining the right ventricle enter the coronary sinus near the right atrium, or enter the right atrium directly, retrograde cardioplegia may not adequately protect the right ventricle because the tip of the cardioplegia catheter is positioned further into the coronary sinus.
    - **d.** Retrograde delivery has been associated with a larger leak of cardiac enzymes in the postoperative period, but there have not been associated clinical consequences of this leak.
    - **e.** The primary advantage of retrograde cardioplegia is in the performance of valvular procedures. In aortic valve replacement, multiple doses of cardioplegia can be administered without stopping the procedure and cannulating the coronary ostia individually. In mitral procedures, retraction on the heart limits effective distribution of anterograde cardioplegia, so repeat doses require release of the retractors. However, in retrograde cardioplegia, multiple doses can be given without changing the retractors, thus simplifying the procedure.

    f. During all-arterial grafting with *in situ* (internal mammary and gastro-epiploic) arteries, additional doses of cardioplegia can be administered through the retrograde route because they cannot be given down the completed grafts.

    g. During acute coronary artery occlusion, where collateral vessels have not developed, retrograde cardioplegia may provide some protection to the ischemic myocardium before the bypass can be completed.

3. **Anterograde and retrograde cardioplegia often are used together,** in a variety of different combinations. Studies have demonstrated that the combined use provides better myocardial protection than with either method alone (Fig. 22.4) [17].

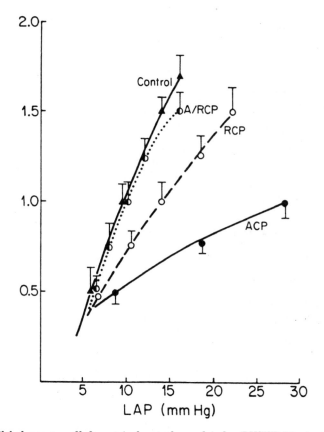

FIG. 22.4 Global recovery of left ventricular stroke work index (LVSWI) 30 minutes after discontinuation of extracorporeal circulation. As left atrial pressure (LAP) increases, LVSWI increases in control hearts. Hearts protected with anterograde perfusion only (ACP, ●) recover less function compared to hearts protected with retrograde perfusion (RCP, ○). Hearts with combined anterograde and retrograde perfusion (A/RCP, ◑) exhibit recovery of LVSWI similar to control values (▲) in this model. (From Partington MT, Acar C, Buckberg GD, et al. Studies of retrograde cardioplegia. II. Advantages of antegrade/retrograde cardioplegia to optimize distribution in jeopardized myocardium. *J Thorac Cardiovasc Surg* 1989;97:613–622, with permission.)

      a. Anterograde cardioplegia can be used to arrest the myocardium, with additional doses given retrograde with venting of the aortic root. This maximizes the distribution of cardioplegia.

      b. Anterograde and retrograde cardioplegia can be administered throughout the procedure in either an alternating or a simultaneous manner [18]. With the alternating technique, retrograde cardioplegia is administered frequently and interrupted for anterograde cardioplegia down each completed graft or through the aortic root. With the simultaneous method, retrograde cardioplegia is continued while anterograde cardioplegia is given down each graft, minimizing the time spent administering cardioplegia. Venovenous collaterals prevent venous hypertension in the coronary sinus. Clinical outcomes are similar between the two methods.

   4. The **frequency of cardioplegia administration** is determined by several factors, most importantly the temperature of the myocardium.

      a. Warm myocardium requires a constant supply of oxygen and thus constant administration of cardioplegia. The cardioplegia may be interrupted for brief periods to allow improved visualization. Significant hemodilution is possible when cardioplegia with a high crystalloid content is used continuously because of the high volume of cardioplegia required. In addition, large doses of potassium are required to maintain electromechanical quiescence in the warm perfused myocardium.

      b. With cold myocardium, visualization can be maximized with intermittent administration of cardioplegia. Each administration is essentially a period of reperfusion, so the initial pressure of cardioplegia should be controlled as it is during reperfusion.

      c. **Single-dose cardioplegia** can be used with cold myocardium if the duration of the operation will be limited and if there is no significant coronary artery disease to limit the distribution of cardioplegia.

      d. **Multidose regimens** are preferable in most circumstances. The initial dose produces cardiac arrest. Subsequent doses, through the aortic root, down a completed graft, or retrograde, serve to wash out metabolic byproducts and replenish substrates. These advantages may not hold in the immature myocardium.

  D. The list of **potential additives to cardioplegia** is tremendous, and a comprehensive listing and discussion would be overwhelming. Table 1 gives a partial list of common additives. The vast majority of additives available serve to combat one or more of the putative causes of ischemia-reperfusion injury. In addition, most additives have functions similar to substances already found in the blood. The cardioplegic solution must balance the goals of simplicity, cost, and effectiveness.

   1. The **electrolyte composition** of cardioplegia is important for producing and maintaining rapid myocardial arrest and limiting myocardial edema.

      a. **"Intracellular" cardioplegia** has an electrolyte composition that mimics that of the intracellular space. It produces myocardial arrest by eliminating

Table 22.1 Common additives to cardioplegia

Component	Purpose
KCl	Produce/maintain diastolic arrest
THAM/histidine	Buffer
Mannitol	Osmolarity, free radical scavenger
Aspartate/glutamate	Metabolic substrate
$MgCl_2$	Mitigates against effects of calcium
CPD	Lowers free calcium concentration
Glucose	Metabolic substrate
Blood	Oxygen-carrying capacity

CPD, citrate-phosphate-dextrose, THAM, tromethamine.

the sodium gradient across the cellular membrane and thereby eliminating phase 0 of the action potential.

(1) Intracellular solutions are crystalloid. Bretschneider solution is a popular example.

(2) The osmolar gap produced by the low sodium concentration allows the use of several additives without producing a hyperosmolar solution.

(3) These solutions are primarily used today for organ preservation in cardiac transplantation.

b. **"Extracellular" solutions** have an electrolyte concentration similar to serum. Diastolic arrest is produced by depolarization of the cellular membrane by high potassium concentrations.

(1) Potassium concentrations of 8 to 30 mM are used to produce arrest. Cardioplegia administration must continue until there is electrical silence, because persistent electrical activity utilizes ATP stores. Especially when hypothermia is used, subsequent doses of cardioplegia can use lower concentrations of potassium as long as electrical arrest persists.

(2) Other methods of producing cardiac arrest include the use of magnesium or local anesthetics. However, due to the simplicity of potassium-induced arrest, these methods are not commonly used.

c. **Calcium** is critical to cardiac function. However, high calcium concentrations are detrimental to the myocardium. Limiting the calcium in the cardioplegia helps to maintain arrest.

(1) Calcium-free cardioplegia produces arrest due to lack of calcium influx across the plasma membrane. However, this may lead to the **"calcium paradox"** in which calcium is depleted from the cell. Upon reperfusion, calcium reenters the cell and can cause severe damage. Therefore, solutions devoid of calcium are not used.

(2) Instead of limiting calcium concentration, the effects of calcium can be limited with nifedipine or diltiazem, which are calcium channel blockers. These drugs may improve myocardial metabolism, but the negative inotropic properties limit their clinical use.

d. The addition of **magnesium** to cardioplegia may counter the effects of calcium, eliminating the need to reduce calcium levels in blood cardioplegia [19]. The benefits of magnesium addition depend on the relative concentrations of the two ions, and there is no benefit to the addition of magnesium to calcium-free cardioplegia.

2. The **pH** of the myocardium is critical to the function of the heart. During ischemia, there is a fall in intracellular pH as lactate accumulates within the cell. Buffers in the cardioplegia are important to limit the change in pH associated with the period of ischemia.

a. Blood contains many naturally occurring buffers, including the histidine and imidazole groups on proteins.

b. Buffers commonly added to cardioplegia include tromethamine (THAM), Tris, and histidine. These buffers can buffer large amounts of hydrogen ion and have a pK_a in the vicinity of 7.40, which makes them good choices. The addition of buffers probably is more important when using crystalloid cardioplegia than with blood.

c. The method used to monitor pH during hypothermia is important because of the normal rise in pH associated with a fall in temperature.

(1) With the **α-stat protocol,** the pH of the blood sample is corrected to 37°C, to provide a pH value that is independent of patient temperature.

(2) Under the **pH-stat** protocol, the pH value is measured at the temperature of the patient and is corrected to 7.40 by the addition of CO_2 into the perfusion circuit. Although this protocol may lead to improved cerebral protection, it results in impaired ventricular function compared to the other method.

3. The **osmolality** of cardioplegia is important in limiting the myocardial edema, which may be detrimental to ventricular recovery. Because blood is iso-osmolar,

additives serve to make it hyperosmolar with respect to unmodified blood, unless the blood is diluted with hypotonic crystalloid. With crystalloid cardioplegia, on the other hand, the final solution may range from hypotonic to hypertonic, depending on the type and amount of additives used. Mannitol, glucose, and albumen are commonly used to increase the osmolality of the cardioplegia. Mannitol has been shown to lessen myocellular edema and improve postoperative ventricular function when used to produce a mildly hypertonic solution.

4. **Glutamate and aspartate** are intermediates in the Krebs cycle and serve to restore high-energy phosphate levels. The addition of these amino acids has been demonstrated to be beneficial in preserving myocardial function, both experimentally and clinically, although the benefit may be limited to substrate-depleted myocardium [20].

IX. **Interventions during reperfusion.** The period of reperfusion is critical to preserving myocardial function. Several potential mechanisms of ischemia-reperfusion injury are active in the reperfusion period, and any chance of minimizing these sources of injury requires action at, or slightly before, the time of reperfusion. If the conditions of reperfusion are not optimized, then potentially viable myocardium may be irreversibly injured. There are many components of the reperfusion period that are important in determining the amount of myocardium that is salvaged.

A. Improved functional recovery occurs if replacement of substrates can begin before the onset of mechanical function. This may be accomplished by one of two means.

1. In cold myocardium, removal of potassium from blood cardioplegia allows continued arrest with washout of metabolic byproducts. As the heart rewarms, function returns slowly. If the heart fibrillates, prompt electrical cardioversion minimizes the period of increased wall tension.

2. Warm hyperkalemic blood cardioplegia administered at the end of the procedure is termed a "hot shot" or **terminal warm blood cardioplegia** [21,22]. This allows the maintenance of electromechanical arrest with replenishment of metabolic substrates. It has been shown to preserve intracellular ATP and amino acid levels and to produce improved metabolic recovery.

B. **Controlled reperfusion.** The pressure of reperfusion is important in limiting the damage to the myocardium [23]. The endothelium is injured during ischemia, and its vasoregulatory properties are limited. This damage can be worsened through unregulated reperfusion.

1. After cross-clamp removal, the perfusion pressure should be limited to 40 mm Hg for the first 1 to 2 minutes of reperfusion by decreasing pump flows. The pressure during this period should not be increased abruptly with phenylephrine, or other agents, until after 1 or 2 minutes.

2. Pump flows are increased to maintain a mean pressure of 70 mm Hg subsequently. Pressors may be required to achieve this. Hypertension should be avoided.

C. The contractile state of the ventricle is critical to recovery, particularly in the early postischemic period. **Ventricular distention** is detrimental to the myocardium, especially during this period.

1. The ventricle should remain empty during the early period of reperfusion, while contractile function is recovering. This can occur by maintaining full bypass with right heart decompression.

2. In the presence of aortic insufficiency, venting of the left ventricle through a vent placed via the superior pulmonary vein can maintain decompression.

3. Ventricular fibrillation is likewise harmful in the warm myocardium, especially as the ventricle begins to fill with blood. Rapid electrical **cardioversion** is required to prevent the rapid depletion of substrates. Prophylactic lidocaine is given near the completion of bypass to lessen the frequency of arrhythmia.

D. **De-airing of the heart** is important to prevent the embolization of air, either down the coronary arteries or into the cerebral or peripheral vessels. The right coronary artery is particularly vulnerable, due to its anterior location on the aortic root. Air down this coronary can lead to malperfusion in its distribution and subsequent right ventricular dysfunction in the early postoperative period. Techniques for removal can include the following:

1. Placement of a vent through the right superior pulmonary vein into the left ventricle, particularly in the case of mitral valve procedures.
2. Venting of the aortic root with a small cannula placed to suction controlled by the perfusionist.
3. Aspiration of the left ventricle by piercing the apex of the heart with an intravenous catheter.
4. Restoring some blood flow through the heart. The perfusionist fills the right atrium with blood by temporarily impeding venous return, then the anesthesiologist fills the lungs with air. This produces increased blood flow through the pulmonary vasculature and into the left side of the heart to displace air that can then be removed with a vent.

Adequacy of air removal from the left cardiac chambers can be assessed with the use of intraoperative transesophageal echocardiography. It is important that air removal from the left chambers precede the onset of left ventricular ejection, to minimize the incidence of air embolization.

E. **Oxygen-derived free radicals** normally are produced in living cells, but the rate of production increases significantly at the moment of reperfusion. At the same time, the natural defense mechanisms are weakened.

1. To be effective, scavengers must be present and active at the initial moment of reperfusion.
2. Because each dose of cardioplegia in a multidose protocol is a period of reperfusion, scavengers may be important in the cardioplegia.
3. Free radical injury involves a cascade of radicals. Different scavengers are active at different points along the cascade. The physical properties of scavengers dictate their distribution within the myocardium, potentially limiting access to areas of free radical production. Therefore, the optimal use of free radical scavengers likely involves the use of several agents with activity at different points along the cascade.
4. Blood cardioplegia contains many natural free radical scavengers. Addition of extra scavengers may not be critical [24].

F. **Calcium management.** Intracellular hypercalcemia at the time of reperfusion can have detrimental effects. Although calcium is necessary at the time of reperfusion, the calcium concentration in the initial reperfusate may be effectively decreased with citrate or calcium channel blockers (diltiazem).

X. **Special circumstances**

A. **Beating heart surgery** is relatively new, especially compared to the traditional on-pump techniques of revascularization. The anesthetic management in beating heart surgery is discussed elsewhere in this text. There are a few caveats of myocardial protection that deserve mention.

1. Coronary perfusion pressure must remain adequate, especially because there are already flow-limiting lesions in the vessels. Similarly, hypertension increases the afterload and ventricular wall tension, decreasing myocardial perfusion.
2. The order in which bypasses are performed is critical. If required, the internal mammary artery to the left anterior descending artery often is a good choice for the first bypass, because an open graft can provide perfusion and stability to the myocardium during manipulations of the heart for subsequent bypasses.
3. Proximal anastomoses may be performed early, such that flow may be delivered down each graft after the distal is completed.
4. The use of flow-through shunts may permit adequate perfusion of the distal vessel while the anastomosis is completed.
5. Bypasses to totally occluded vessels often are well tolerated by the heart because occlusion during the anastomosis often is without significant ischemia. This is especially true when collateral vessels are well established.
6. Off-pump surgery probably represents a hypercoagulable state compared to its on-pump counterpart. The coagulopathy from extracorporeal circulation and the establishment of hypothermia are avoided. Many surgeons do not fully

reverse the heparinization with protamine, instead aiming for an activated clotting time (ACT) of approximately 180 seconds at the conclusion of the procedure. In addition, many surgeons use the newer antiplatelet agents, such as clopidogrel (Plavix), to inhibit graft thrombosis in the early postoperative period.

B. Redo operations often present with unique problems in relation to myocardial preservation.

1. Patent bypass grafts are a potential source of atheroemboli and subsequent myocardial infarction. The rate of postoperative infarction is higher in redo operations than for primary grafting procedures. Avoidance of graft manipulation can minimize the embolization of loose debris.

2. Dense adhesions from the prior operation may limit the safe dissection required to perform the standard maneuvers required for myocardial protection. Therefore, the risk of obtaining exposure to permit topical cooling of the right ventricle, placement of a left ventricular vent, or temporary occlusion of a patent internal mammary graft may outweigh the potential benefits of these maneuvers. Therefore, the surgeon must be well versed in alternative exposures or methods of myocardial protection.

   a. For a patent internal mammary artery that cannot be safely occluded, hypothermic fibrillatory arrest may represent the best alternative.

   b. A right thoracotomy approach to the mitral valve provides excellent exposure, especially in a reoperation. Dissection of the aorta through the right chest is possible for placement of a cross-clamp, but many procedures can be done with femoral cannulation and a beating or fibrillating heart on bypass.

C. Port-access surgery. Popularized by Heartport, Inc., port-access surgery allows common cardiac procedures to be performed through smaller incisions. The operative procedure should be similar to that for standard cardiac surgery, but the limited exposure requires alternative methods of cardioplegia administration, ventricular venting, and aortic occlusion. The technology, which is still evolving, provides the surgeon with the ability to use the limited exposure, but the entire operative team must embrace the new technology for it to be successful. Transesophageal echocardiography is important for the preparation and conduct of the operation. Myocardial protection requires vigilance of the surgeon, anesthesiologist, and perfusionist. Because very little of the heart is exposed, the monitors play an increased role in the assessment of the electromechanical state of the heart and provide vital information with regard to the pressures within the unseen cardiac chambers.

D. Acutely ischemic myocardium requires that energy demands on the myocardium be diminished as soon as possible and that delivery of oxygen to the ischemic territory is prompt.

1. The patient should be prepared for surgery promptly. Delays should be minimized to those necessary for patient safety. The patient should be well oxygenated, and perfusion pressure is critical. A preoperative intraaortic balloon pump may be useful.

2. Once on bypass, normothermic induction of cardioplegia can provide substrate to the stressed myocardium that is still perfused.

3. The acutely ischemic area should be revascularized first, with cardioplegia administered down the graft to the occluded vessel. There may be advantages to warm reperfusion to this segment of myocardium, and perfusion can be continued at a controlled pressure while other grafts are placed.

4. Special attention is directed to the period of time at which cardiopulmonary bypass is terminated, as the ischemic myocardium is likely to exhibit contractile dysfunction. It may be necessary to place the patient back on bypass temporarily to adjust inotropes or volume status and to give the myocardium additional time to recover contractile function before permanent separation from bypass is possible. Improper weaning may result in myocardial infarction in regions that are potentially recoverable.

E. The **pediatric heart** is unique in its physiology and thus requires special attention. Some of the differences are due to the disease states seen in the pediatric population, whereas others are inherent differences in the immature myocardium. Many of these are due to differences in myocardial gene expression seen in the fetal and neonatal heart, and result in differences in myocardial metabolism and energy consumption compared to the adult heart. For a complete discussion of the management of the pediatric myocardium, see the review by Allen et al. [25].

1. The normal immature myocardium is more resistant to ischemic injury than adult myocardium. However, cyanosis, pressure overload, or volume overload, which are all common in hearts with congenital defects, make these hearts more susceptible to ischemic injury.

2. In contrast to the cardiac surgery in the adult heart, crystalloid cardioplegia frequently is used in pediatric cardiac surgery. Although most studies have not demonstrated a difference in outcome, blood cardioplegia may be beneficial in the neonatal heart that has been subjected to hypoxic stress.

3. The immature myocardium is more susceptible to damage from high calcium concentrations due to its diminished capacity for calcium sequestration. Calcium levels may be reduced with citrate. In addition, magnesium supplementation of the cardioplegia provides increased protection from transient increases in intracellular calcium concentration.

4. The hypoxic immature heart is sensitive to the delivery pressure of cardioplegia. This must be controlled to both provide adequate distribution yet prevent myocardial edema and damage from high pressure delivery.

References

1. Follette DM, Mulder DG, Maloney JV, et al. Advantages of blood cardioplegia over continuous coronary perfusion or intermittent ischemia. Experimental and clinical study. *J Thorac Cardiovasc Surg* 1978;76:604–619.

2. **Buckberg GD, Brazier JR, Nelson RL, et al. Studies of the effects of hypothermia on regional myocardial blood flow and metabolism during cardiopulmonary bypass. I. The adequately perfused beating, fibrillating, and arrested heart. *J Thorac Cardiovasc Surg* 1977;73:87–94.**

3. Sink JD, Hill RC, Attarian DE, et al. Myocardial blood flow and oxygen consumption in the empty-beating, fibrillating, and potassium-arrested hypertrophied canine heart. *Ann Thorac Surg* 1983;35:372–379.

4. Nakanishi K, Zhao Z-Q, Vinten-Johansen J, et al. Coronary artery endothelial dysfunction after ischemia, blood cardioplegia, and reperfusion. *Ann Thorac Surg* 1994;58:191–199.

5. Hearse DJ, Stewart DA, Braimbridge MV. Cellular protection during myocardial ischemia. The development and characterization of a procedure for the induction of reversible ischemic arrest. *Circulation* 1976;54:193–202.

6. Akins CW, Carroll DL. Event-free survival following nonemergency myocardial revascularization during hypothermic fibrillatory arrest. *Ann Thorac Surg* 1987;43:628–633.

7. **Hottenrott CE, Towers B, Kurkji HJ, et al. The hazard of ventricular fibrillation in hypertrophied ventricles during cardiopulmonary bypass. *J Thorac Cardiovasc Surg* 1973;66:742–753.**

8. Perrault LP, Menasche P. Preconditioning: Can nature's shield be raised against surgical ischemic-reperfusion injury? *Ann Thorac Surg* 1999;68:1988–1994.

9. **Rosenkranz ER, Vinten-Johansen J, Buckberg GD, et al. Benefits of normothermic induction of blood cardioplegia in energy-depleted hearts with maintenance of arrest by multidose cold blood cardioplegic infusions. *J Thorac Cardiovasc Surg* 1982;84:667–677.**

10. Bufkin BL, Mellitt RJ, Gott JP, et al. Aerobic blood cardioplegia for revascularization of acute infarct: Effects of delivery temperature. *Ann Thorac Surg* 1994;58:953–960.

11. Hayashida N, Ikonomidis JS, Weisel RD, et al. The optimal cardioplegic temperature. *Ann Thorac Surg* 1994;58:961–971.

12. Yau TM, Weisel RD, Mickle DAG, et al. Optimal delivery of blood cardioplegia. *Circ.* 1991;84[Suppl III]:III-380–III-388.

13. Naylor CD, Lichtenstein SV, Fremes SE, Warm Heart Investigators. Randomised trial of normothermic versus hypothermic coronary bypass surgery. *Lancet* 1994;343:559–563.

14. Yau TM, Ikonomidis JS, Weisel RD, et al. Ventricular function after normothermic versus hypothermic cardioplegia. *J Thorac Cardiovasc Surg* 1993;105:833–843.

15. Fremes SE, Christakis GT, Weisel RD, et al. A clinical trial of blood and crystalloid cardioplegia. *J Thorac Cardiovasc Surg* 1984;88:726–741.
16. Schaper J, Walter P, Scheld H, et al. The effects of retrograde perfusion of cardioplegic solution in cardiac operations. *J Thorac Cardiovasc Surg* 1985;90:882–887.
17. **Partington MT, Acar C, Buckberg GD, et al. Studies of retrograde cardioplegia. II. Advantages of antegrade/retrograde cardioplegia to optimize distribution in jeopardized myocardium. *J Thorac Cardiovasc Surg* 1989;97:613–622.**
18. Shirai T, Rao V, Weisel RD, et al. Antegrade and retrograde cardioplegia: Alternate or simultaneous? *J Thorac Cardiovasc Surg* 1996;112:787–796.
19. Hearse DJ, Stewart DA, Braimbridge MV. Myocardial protection during ischemic cardiac arrest. The importance of magnesium in cardioplegic infusates. *J Thorac Cardiovasc Surg* 1978;75:877–885.
20. Rosenkranz ER, Okamoto F, Buckberg GD, et al. Safety of prolonged aortic clamping with blood cardioplegia. III. Aspartate enrichment of glutamate-blood cardioplegia in energy-depleted hearts after ischemic and reperfusion injury. *J Thorac Cardiovasc Surg* 1986;91:428–435.
21. **Caputo M, Dihmis WC, Bryan AJ, et al. Warm blood hyperkalemic reperfusion ("hot shot") prevents myocardial substrate derangement in patients undergoing coronary artery bypass surgery. *Eur J Cardiothorac Surg* 1998;13:559–564.**
22. Teoh KH, Christakis GT, Weisel RD, et al. Accelerated myocardial metabolic recovery with terminal warm cardioplegia. *J Thorac Cardiovasc Surg* 1986;91:888–895.
23. **Okamoto F, Allen BS, Buckberg GD, et al. Studies of controlled reperfusion after ischemia. XIV. Reperfusion conditions: Importance of ensuring gentle versus sudden reperfusion during relief of coronary occlusion. *J Thorac Cardiovasc Surg* 1986;92:613–620.**
24. Julia PL, Buckberg GD, Acar C, et al. Studies of controlled reperfusion after ischemia. XXI. Reperfusate composition: Superiority of blood cardioplegia over crystalloid cardioplegia in limiting reperfusion damage—Importance of endogenous oxygen free radical scavengers in red blood cells. *J Thorac Cardiovasc Surg* 1991;101:303–313.
25. **Allen BS, Barth MJ, Ilbawi MN. Pediatric myocardial protection: An overview. *Semin Thorac Cardiovasc Surg* 2001;13:56–72.**

23. PROTECTION OF THE BRAIN DURING CARDIAC SURGERY

Ivan Iglesias and John M. Murkin

I. **Central nervous system dysfunction associated with cardiac surgery**
   A. **Neurologic morbidity.** In most series reported to date, the incidence of clinically apparent neurologic injury or frank stroke is 2% to 6% for closed chamber cardiac procedures [e.g., coronary artery bypass graft (CABG) surgery]. Up to 25% to 65% of strokes after CABG surgeries are bilateral or multiple [1]. For open chamber procedures (e.g., valve surgery), the reported incidence historically has been 4.2% to 13% [2]. However, more subtle neurologic changes, such as development of primitive reflexes (e.g., snouting, palmomental reflex, visual field defects, and subtle motor-sensory limitation) [3,4], can be demonstrated in the early postoperative period in up to 61% of all patients undergoing cardiopulmonary bypass (CPB). This incidence apparently is independent of the nature of the surgical procedure (valve surgery versus coronary bypass) and likely represents central nervous system (CNS) injury secondary to exposure to CPB [4]. By 2 months postoperatively, the prevalence of such new subtle neurologic dysfunction decreases to about 20% and persists for at least 1 year.
   B. **Cognitive dysfunction.** It has been demonstrated that within the first postoperative week, up to 83% of all patients undergoing coronary artery bypass surgery using CPB demonstrate a degree of cognitive dysfunction. Of these patients, 38% have symptoms of intellectual impairment and 10% are considered to be overtly disabled. Concentration, retention and processing of new information, and visuospatial organization are the most frequently affected domains. At 1 and even 5 years of follow-up, more than 35% of patients still show some degree of neuropsychologic dysfunction [3].
   C. **Comparison groups.** The incidence of new postoperative CNS dysfunction in CABG patients has been compared with that of patients undergoing major abdominal vascular or thoracic surgical procedures. Most of these patients usually have concomitant disease including hypertension, diabetes mellitus, diffuse atherosclerosis, and chronic lung disease. After adjusting for identified risk factors, patients undergoing any surgical procedure have been found more likely to suffer a cerebrovascular accident (CVA) than nonoperated controls, with an odds ratio of 3.9. Even after excluding high-risk surgery (cardiac, vascular, and neurologic), the odds ratio is 2.9, which suggests the perioperative period itself predisposes patients to stroke [5]. The comparison indicates in all these patients a high incidence of subtle postoperative CNS morbidity that is not entirely related to CPB.
      1. **Nonspecific stresses associated with anesthesia, major surgery, and convalescence** in CABG patients may account for up to 50% of subtle neurologic and cognitive dysfunction detected in the early postoperative period.
      2. **Undergoing CPB exerts a direct and independent adverse effect** producing further subtle CNS dysfunction, which is resolved in about 70% of cases within 2 months.
      3. **Patients undergoing CPB have a 2% to 6% incidence of overt neurologic injury and CVA** specifically related to cardiac surgery and CPB.
   D. **Risk factors.** Table 23.1 lists the risk factors for CNS injury during cardiac surgery. Specific factors are discussed in more detail in subsequent sections.
II. **Cerebral physiology**
   A. **Cerebral autoregulation.** In normal subjects, cerebral blood flow (CBF) remains constant at $50 \text{ mL}/(100 \text{ g} \cdot \text{min})$ over a wide range of mean arterial pressure (MAP) from 50 to 150 mm Hg. This *autoregulatory plateau* reflects the tight matching between cerebral metabolic rate for O_2 ($CMRo_2$) and CBF, mediated in part by endothelial-derived relaxing factor (EDRF-nitric oxide). With decreased metabolic activity resulting from certain anesthetics or hypothermia, lowered $CMRo_2$ produces a resultant reduction in CBF and establishment of a lower autoregulatory plateau. It is apparent and should be considered that rather than a single cerebral autoregulatory curve, there are instead a series of autoregulatory curves. Each autoregulatory curve represents a differing set of metabolic conditions of the brain (e.g., normal metabolic activity) at 37°C versus lowered metabolic activity at 28°C. The autoregulatory plateau is a manifestation of intact cerebral flow and metabolism coupling, and it varies with metabolic rate.

Table 23.1 Risk factors for central nervous system

Patient related
  Age >70 years
  Overt cerebrovascular disease
  Extensive aortic atherosclerosis
  Diabetes mellitus
Produce related
  Open chamber procedures
  Duration of cardiopulmonary bypass >90 minutes
  Perioperative hemodynamic instability
  Multiple aortic instrumentations (repeated clampings, cannulations)
Equipment related
  Use of bubble rather than membrane oxygenators
  Lack of arterial inflow line filters
  Use of nitrous oxide

    With intact autoregulation, adequate substrate (blood flow) can be delivered at a lower perfusion pressure during conditions of lowered metabolic rate (e.g., anesthesia, hypothermia) in the absence of cerebral vasodilators (Fig. 23.1). Cerebral autoregulation is lacking in patients with diabetes mellitus and appears to be lost during deep hypothermia (e.g., <20°C) and for several hours after deep hypothermic circulatory arrest (DHCA). This results in pressure-passive CBF; in these instances, hypotension may entail increased risk for cerebral hypoperfusion.

B. pH Management. There is an inverse relationship between solubility of respiratory gases and blood temperature. With cooling of blood, CO_2 partial pressure (P_aCO_2) decreases and arterial pH (pH_a) increases, producing an apparent respiratory alkalosis *in vivo*. To compensate for this condition during hypothermic CPB, total

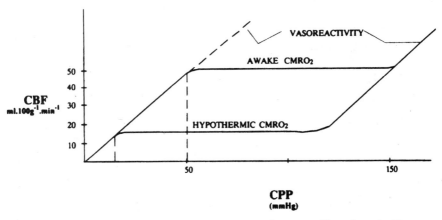

FIG. 23.1 Cerebral autoregulatory curves during normothermia and hypothermia. The *upper curve* demonstrates a higher cerebral blood flow (*CBF*) autoregulatory plateau that is appropriate for the higher cerebral metabolic rate for O_2(*CMRo$_2$*) in the awake state, versus a lower CBF plateau during hypothermia. With maximal cerebral vasodilation, lower cerebral perfusion pressure (*CPP*) results in lower CBF that is appropriate at a lower CMRo$_2$ (hypothermia), but not at higher CMRo$_2$. (From Murkin JM. The pathophysiology of cardiopulmonary bypass. *Can J Anesth* 1989;36:S41–S44, with permission.)

CO_2 must be increased by addition of exogenous CO_2 to the oxygenator, known as *pH-stat pH management.*

1. **α-Stat maintains pH_a 7.4 and P_aCO_2 40 mm Hg at 37°C without addition of exogenous CO_2.** Intracellular pH is primarily determined by the neutral pH (pH_N) of water. Because pH_N becomes progressively more alkaline with decreasing temperature, intracellular pH becomes correspondingly more alkaline during hypothermia. Because this intracellular alkalosis occurs in parallel with the hypothermia-induced increased solubility of CO_2 and increased blood pH, the normal transmembrane pH gradient of approximately 0.6 units remains unchanged, thus preserving optimal function of various intracellular enzyme systems. *This preservation of normal transmembrane pH gradient is the crux of α-stat pH theory,* and, in fact, we function *in vivo* according to α-stat principles. Because different tissues have differing temperatures (e.g., exercising muscle at 41°C vs skin at 25°C), they also will have correspondingly different pH_a values (e.g., 7.34 vs 7.6, respectively), although the net pH_a at 37°C will be 7.4. *α-Stat management acknowledges the temperature-dependence of normal pH_a* and strives to maintain a constant transmembrane pH gradient by maintaining P_aCO_2 at 40°C and pH_a at 7.4 as measured *in vitro* at 37°C. For this strategy during CPB, total CO_2 is kept constant by not adding exogenous CO_2 and thus not compensating for increased solubility of CO_2. Blood samples measured at 37°C will show pH_a 7.4 and P_aCO_2 40 mm Hg, but those same samples measured at 28°C would have pH_a 7.56 and P_aCO_2 26 mm Hg (Fig. 23.2).

2. **pH-stat management involves addition of exogenous CO_2 to maintain P_aCO_2 40 mm Hg and pH_a 7.4 when corrected for the patient's body temperature *in vivo*.** Until the mid-1980s, pH-stat management was generally the most common mode of pH management during moderate hypothermic CPB. Because it is a potent cerebral vasodilator, such increases in total P_aCO_2 associated with pH-stat have been shown to produce cerebral vasodilation, im-

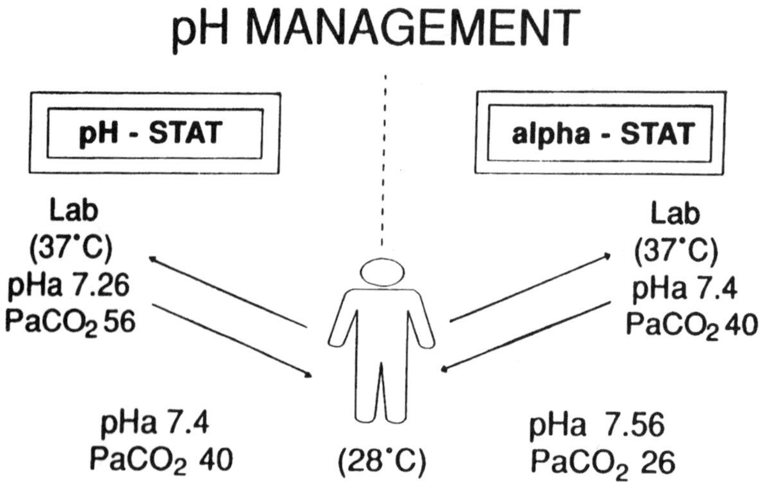

pH MANAGEMENT

FIG. 23.2 Contrasting arterial blood gas values as seen *in vitro* at 37°C or *in vivo* at 28°C when using α-stat or pH-stat management. Using pH-stat, laboratory values *in vitro* would be pH_a 7.26 and P_aCO_2 56 mm Hg, whereas temperature-corrected values *in vivo* would be pH_a 7.4 and P_aCO_2 40 mm Hg. If α-stat were used, laboratory values *in vitro* would be pH_a 7.4 and P_aCO_2 40 mm Hg, whereas temperature-corrected values *in vivo* would be pH_a 7.56 and P_aCO_2 26 mm Hg.

pairing cerebral flow and metabolism coupling and producing loss of cerebral autoregulation (Fig. 23.3) [6]. There now is evidence that pH-stat management can increase the incidence of postoperative cognitive dysfunction when CPB duration exceeds 90 minutes [4]. This likely reflects increased delivery of micro-emboli into the brain resulting from CO_2-induced vasodilation.

III. Etiology of central nervous system damage

  A. **Focal ischemia.** In the context of CPB, focal ischemia most often is a consequence of isolated cerebral arteriolar obstruction by a particulate or gaseous embolus. Emboli vary in size, nature (particular vs gaseous), and origin (patient vs equipment). Open chamber procedures entail greater risk of embolic debris than do closed chamber procedures.

  Areas of brain localized at the boundary limits of major cerebral arteries (e.g., anterior and middle, or middle and posterior cerebral arteries, or superior and posteroinferior cerebellar arteries) are known as *arterial boundary zones or watershed zones* (Fig. 23.4), and these can manifest as isolated lesions as a consequence of transient global ischemia (see following sections). Although formerly believed to be pathognomic of profound hypoperfusion, it now is recognized that watershed zone infarction may be caused by cerebral emboli.

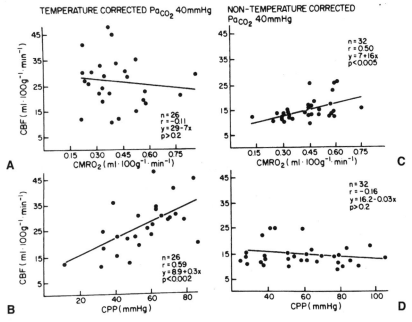

FIG. 23.3 Linear regression analysis of cerebral blood flow (*CBF*) and cerebral metabolic rate for oxygen (*CMRO$_2$*), or cerebral perfusion pressure (*CPP*), for patients managed using α-stat (nontemperature-corrected) or pH-stat (temperature-corrected) management during moderate hypothermia (28°C). With pH-stat (**A**), there is no correlation between CBF and CMRO$_2$, demonstrating loss of cerebral flow and metabolism coupling, whereas with α-stat (**C**) there is a highly significant ($p < 0.005$) correlation. CBF significantly ($p < 0.002$) correlates with CPP using pH-stat (**B**), reflecting pressure-passive CBF and loss of autoregulation, whereas with α-stat (**D**), CBF is independent of CPP. (From Murkin JM, et al. Cerebral autoregulation and flow/metabolism coupling during cardiopulmonary bypass: the influence of P_aCO_2. *Anesth Analg* 1987;66:825–832, with permission.)

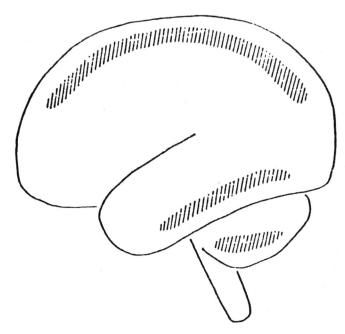

FIG. 23.4 *Hatched areas* showing the most frequent locations of boundary area, or watershed zone infarcts in the brain, situated between the territories of major cerebral or cerebellar arteries. (From Torvik A. The pathogenesis of watershed infarcts in the brain. *Stroke* 1984; 2:221–223, © 1984 American Heart Association, with permission.)

1. **Detection of emboli**
   a. **Brain histology.** Isolated areas of perivascular and focal subarachnoid hemorrhage, neuronal swelling, and axonal degeneration are seen with higher frequency in the brains of patients dying after cardiac surgery than after non-CPB major vascular surgery. After surgery using unfiltered CPB circuits, fibrin and platelet emboli and calcific and atheromatous debris were seen frequently in small arterioles and capillary beds. Small cerebral capillary and arterial dilatations (SCADS) have been demonstrated histologically, occurring in nonsurvivors after proximal aortic instrumentation after either CPB or coronary angiography. These SCADS are increasingly believed to be due in part to lipid microemboli from usage of unprocessed cardiotomy suction blood [7].
   b. **Intraoperative emboli detection.** Intraoperative fluorescein retinal angiography has demonstrated that extensive retinal microvascular embolization occurs during CPB. The incidence and extent of retinal obstruction are much greater with bubble than with membrane oxygenators, despite use of 40-μm arterial line filters. Use of transcranial Doppler (TCD) insonation enables assessment of blood flow perfusion characteristics through the middle cerebral artery (MCA). TCD insonation permits measurement of blood flow velocity and detection and quantification of emboli. Proximal aortic instrumentation and initiation of CPB have been identified as particularly emboligenic intraoperative events. After valve replacement surgery, cerebral emboli are detected as the heart fills and begins to eject, underscoring the importance of meticulous de-airing techniques (see following sections).

2. Sources of emboli

  a. Patient-related sources

    (1) **Aortic atheroma.** Atheromatous debris can be embolized during aortic clamping or cannulation. Intraoperative aortic ultrasonography using either transesophageal echocardiography (TEE; high sensitivity, low specificity) or epiaortic scanning (EAS) (high sensitivity, high specificity) enables visualization of aortic wall and can be used to guide cannulation sites. Ultrasonography has demonstrated that plaque may fracture or shear off and embolize during CPB as a consequence of trauma from aortic clamping and cannulation or from blood "jetting" from the aortic cannula. Proximal aortic atherosclerosis is thus a significant risk factor for neurologic injury.

    (2) **Intraventricular thrombi.** During closed chamber procedures in patients with recent mural thrombi, manipulation of the heart can dislodge thrombi that embolize once the heart begins to fill and eject.

    (3) **Valvular calcifications.** Valve surgery, particularly valve replacement surgery, is associated with increased risk of cerebrovascular accident resulting from embolization of intracavitary valve debris.

  b. Procedure-related sources.

    (1) Open chamber procedures (e.g., septal repair, ventricular aneurysmectomy, valve surgery) also expose the arterial circulation to air or particulate debris. Closed chamber procedures also can be associated with ventricular air. Use of a ventricular vent, particularly if active suction is applied and the heart is empty, produces localized subatmospheric pressure at the vent tip within the left ventricle (LV) and cause air to be entrained retrograde from the vent insertion site (usually through the superior pulmonary vein) into the LV. Use of TEE can assist in visualization and guide the removal of residual intracavitary air (see following discussion). Inadvertent opening of the left atrium (LA) or LV while the heart is beating also caused rapid air entrainment and increased potential for cerebral emboli.

    (2) Aortic cannulation and clamping are associated with cerebral embolization, particularly in the presence of extensive aortic atherosclerosis.

    (3) Duration of CPB is an independent risk for postoperative brain dysfunction. After 90 minutes of CPB, the incidence of cognitive dysfunction is increased compared to CPB of shorter duration. It is important to note that duration of CPB may be increased by factors that may themselves contribute to neurologic injury [3].

  c. Equipment-related sources.

    (1) Incorporation of a 25-μm filter into the aortic inflow line effectively reduces cerebral embolic load and has been shown to decrease the incidence of postoperative cognitive dysfunction.

    (2) Membrane oxygenators give rise to markedly fewer gaseous microemboli than do bubble oxygenators, but this does not entirely eliminate the risk of air emboli. Unless filtered out, air entrained into the venous side of a membrane oxygenator can transit the membrane and appear in the arterial inflow line.

    (3) Use of a 20- to 40-μm filters in the cardiotomy return line prevents particulate debris from the operative site from entering the CPB circuit. Use of cardiotomy blood washing techniques (cell saver) is associated with reduced amounts of cerebral lipid microemboli.

    (4) Use of nitrous oxide (N_2O) before commencement of CPB has been associated with increased evidence of ischemic damage, likely because residual N_2O increases the size of any microgaseous emboli in the cerebral circulation. This is especially true for several hours after CPB when high FIO_2 should be used to minimize the size of residual gaseous microemboli.

B. Global ischemia

 1. **Watershed areas.** Collateral perfusion of the brain can occur via extracerebral anastomoses (primarily through the circle of Willis) or by way of intracerebral anastomoses between major cerebral arteries, known as *arterial boundary zones* (watershed zones; Fig. 23.4). Rapid severe hypoperfusion can produce ischemic lesions within these boundary zones found at the territorial limits of the major cerebral arteries. The most frequently affected area is the parieto-occipital sulci located at the limits of the anterior, middle, and posterior cerebral arteries. Despite a global ischemic stress, these watershed lesions may be focal and asymmetrical. Placement of electroencephalographic (EEG) electrodes using a parasagittal montage (see following) may allow increased sensitivity for border zone ischemia detection.

 2. **Cerebral perfusion pressure.** During moderate hypothermia (28° to 30°C) using α-stat pH management, autoregulation is preserved in patients without overt cerebrovascular disease over the cerebral perfusion pressure (CPP) range from 20 to 100 mm Hg. There are several conditions in which autoregulation may be lost (Table 23.2). With profound hypothermia (15° to 20°C), there appears to be loss of autoregulation as a result of hypothermia-induced vasoparesis. There is evidence that diabetic patients have impaired cerebral autoregulation even at moderate hypothermia. During CPB, there may be dissociation between MAP and CPP as a result of unrecognized cerebral venous hypertension. Particularly with use of a single two-stage venous cannula, cerebral venous drainage may be impaired (Fig. 23.5). Consequently, jugular venous pressure should be measured proximally within the superior vena cava (SVC; e.g., via introducer port of pulmonary artery catheter) to detect this.

 3. **Circulatory arrest.** During circulatory arrest for surgical procedures, profound hypothermia (16° to 18°C) is used to minimize $CMRo_2$ and increase tolerance for ischemia (see following). During circulatory arrest under normothermic conditions, O_2 levels are depleted within a few seconds of onset of ischemia, EEG activity is lost (isoelectric EEG) within 30 seconds, high-energy phosphates are exhausted within 1 minute, and ischemic neuronal damage is found after periods of anoxia as brief as 5 minutes. For certain cardiac electrophysiologic procedures (e.g., diagnosis and treatment of certain refractory arrhythmias), transient ventricular fibrillation (VF) often is induced at normothermia and without circulatory support. Duration of VF must be limited to less than 1 minute, and prompt hemodynamic resuscitation with at least 4 minutes of reperfusion should be maintained between episodes of VF [8]. Monitoring and management of these patients should follow the principles outlined herein.

 4. **Neuronal ischemia markers.** Several potential markers of neuronal injury have been studied to detect and quantify the presence of neuronal damage. Adenylate kinase, neurospecific enolase, creatine phosphokinase (CPK) BB, and protein S100β have been studied among others. Although protein S100β has been demonstrated to increase after cardiac surgery correlated with age, aortic cross-clamp time, and CPB duration, it now is recognized to be nonspecific and released from sternotomy blood, thus confounding its utility as a perioperative marker. Although biochemical markers may provide an indication of the existence of cerebral damage, the lack of correlation with anatomic areas and controversies about methodology limit their present usefulness as clinical monitors of neuronal ischemia [3].

Table 23.2 Factors associated with loss of cerebral autoregulation

pH-stat management (Fig. 23.3)
Diabetes mellitus
Profound hypothermia (<20°C)
Deep hypothermic circulatory arrest
Previous cerebrovascular accident

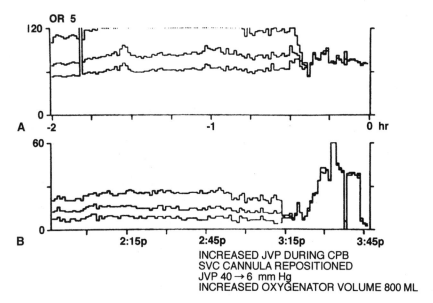

FIG. 23.5 A: Systolic, mean, and diastolic arterial blood pressures, with commencement of cardiopulmonary bypass (*CPB*) indicated at 3:15 p.m., after which mean arterial pressure (MAP) is shown. **B:** Pulmonary artery systolic, mean, and diastolic pressures with proximal jugular venous pressure (*JVP*) recorded at 3:15 p.m., with commencement of CPB. A single two-stage venous cannula was used for CPB. With rotation of the heart, venous return to the oxygenator decreased and JVP approached MAP values. *SVC,* superior vena cava. (Modified from Murkin JM. Intraoperative management. In: Estaphanous FG, Barash PG, Reves JG, eds. *Cardiac anesthesia: principles and clinical practice.* Philadelphia: J.B. Lippincott Company, 1994:326, with permission.)

IV. Pathophysiology of neuronal ischemia.
  A. Lactic acidosis. Glucose is essentially the sole substrate for energy production by the brain, being metabolized to produce 36 moles of adenosine triphosphate (ATP) per mole glucose. Oxygen is essential for oxidative phosphorylation and in the presence of ischemia, anaerobic glucose metabolism yields only 2 moles of ATP and results in lactate production with accumulation of hydrogen ion (H^+). Anaerobic glycolysis is the primary cause of acidosis during ischemia, and the severity of lactic acidosis is directly related to preischemia glucose concentrations. Hyperglycemia is associated with worsening of neurologic injury after cerebral ischemia, and tight blood sugar levels should be maintained during CPB [9].
  B. Ion gradients. Neuronal function and structural integrity are dependent on ionic gradients, such that up to 75% of ATP produced by resting neurons is utilized by sodium-potassium ATPase and for extrusion of calcium by calcium-dependent ATPase. With ischemia, decreased ATP production and evolving lactic acidosis impair transmembrane ionic pumps and consequently diminish cellular electrochemical gradients leading to cell depolarization. Extraneuronal leakage of K^+ depolarizes adjacent neurons, thereby decreasing synaptic transmission and, along with calcium, promoting vasospasm in adjacent vasculature.
  C. Calcium. With ischemia, ATP depletion causes loss of ionic gradients, resulting in cell membrane depolarization and influx of calcium ion (Ca^{2+}) through voltage-sensitive channels. Intracellular accumulation of Ca^{2+} is likely the final common pathway leading to neuronal death through enhanced protein and lipid catabolism.

Influx of Ca^{2+} can be minimized by calcium antagonists. Nimodipine has shown clinical benefit in decreasing vasospasm after subarachnoid hemorrhage, but it increases bleeding and mortality in cardiac surgical patients.

    D. Free fatty acids. Some of the earliest cell membrane changes with ischemia involve production of free fatty acids (FFAs) from membrane phospholipids. Intracellular Ca^{2+} activates calcium-dependent phospholipases C and A2, transforming membrane phospholipids into FFAs, which themselves are neurotoxic. FFAs are powerful uncouplers of oxidative phosphorylation and can undergo further oxidation from arachidonic acid, with resultant free radical formation. During cerebral ischemia, FFA production is decreased by administration of calcium antagonists, and 21-aminosteroids *(lazaroids)* are potent inhibitors of lipid peroxidation.

    E. Excitotoxicity. Glutamate and aspartate are excitatory amino acid (EAA) neurotransmitters, with three distinct postsynaptic receptor subtypes: *N*-methyl-D-aspartate (NMDA); kainate (KA); and quisqualate/α-methyl propionic acid (AMPA), responsible for mediating Ca^+ and Na^+/K^+ passage. Ischemia produces enhanced presynaptic EAA release and decreased reuptake, which causes activation of postsynaptic NMDA and AMPA receptors and produces massive efflux of K^+ and influx of Na^+ and Ca^+ and resultant osmolysis and calcium-related damage. EAAs also are increasingly implicated in free radical formation.

    F. Reperfusion injury. With reperfusion, mitochondrial cyclooxygenase and lipooxygenase pathways, in conjunction with oxidation of FFAs, are primarily responsible for heightened free radical (e.g., superoxide anion) formation and produce oxidative cellular destruction. Experimentally, lazaroids ameliorate neuronal ischemic damage when administered for ischemic stress, but results of clinical trials have not yet been positive.

V. Intraoperative cerebral monitoring

    A. Brain temperature. Accurate monitoring of brain temperature is essential because temperature profoundly influences cerebral metabolic rate and thus tolerance for ischemia. Mild hypothermia (<35°C) is disproportionately effective in decreasing ischemia-related injury due to inhibition of EAA release (see previous sections). During CPB, thermal gradients exist between various tissues; thus, brain temperature must be measured independently of other sites. Because of the small risk of trauma associated with placement of a tympanic thermistor, nasopharyngeal temperature (NPT) is the preferred site for clinical monitoring of brain temperature. Thermistor insertion should be through the nares to the level of the midpoint of the zygoma, a depth of 7 to 10 cm in an adult. Insertion of the thermistor before heparinization, using lubrication and exerting gentle pressure parallel to the floor of the nose, will prevent epistaxis and trauma to mucosa and turbinates. Esophageal temperature is a poor substitute for NPT because it variously reflects aortic inflow temperature, temperature of surrounding tissue, and the influence of residual ice or cooled fluid within the pericardial sac. For DHCA and high-risk patients, a thermistor/oximetric catheter can be placed retrograde into the jugular bulb, thus providing the most sensitive clinical measure of global brain temperature and oxygenation.

    B. Electroencephalogram. EEG represents the amplified, summated, spontaneous electrical activity of the superficial cerebral cortex. Each electrode reflects microcurrent (10 to 200 μV) generated by electrical gradients across layers of neurons aligned at right angles to the monitored cortical surface in a 2- to 3-cm radius. Electrode placement should be based on the standard 10- to 20-electrode system and modified according to the number of channels being monitored (Fig. 23.6). EEG activity commonly is divided into four bands according to frequency: δ less than 4 Hz; θ4 to 8 Hz; α 9 to 12 Hz; and β greater than 13 Hz. In general, slower frequencies indicate a deeper level of anesthesia. Use of the bispectral index (BIS) measures the degree of synchronization of component EEG waveforms, with lower BIS numbers associated with greater EEG synchronization and thus deeper levels of hypnosis.

    Several factors can confound interpretation of intraoperative EEG (Table 23.3). Recordings are potentially made in the presence of various anesthetic agents, during profound changes in body temperature, and in the electrically hostile environment

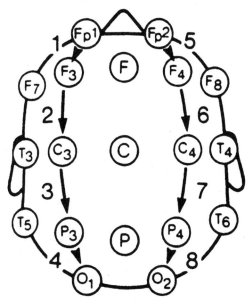

FIG. 23.6 Standard bipolar parasagittal montage based on the international 10–20 system. F_{P1} and F_{P2} refers to frontal pole; F_3, F_4, F_7, and F_8 refer to frontal; C_3 and C_4 refer to central; P_3 and P_4 refer to parietal; O_1 and O_2 refer to occipital; and T_3, T_4, T_5, and T_6 refer to temporal positions. (From Murkin JM, et al. Absence of seizures during induction of anesthesia with high-dose fentanyl. *Anesth Analg* 1984;63:489–494, with permission.)

found in an operating room. Although subtle EEG changes may be difficult to interpret, development of asymmetric EEG activity should be considered to represent hemispheric compromise (Table 23.4).

    1. Processed EEG. After initial electronic filtering, analog EEG voltages are rapidly digitized (150/s) and analyzed over "epochs" (generally 2 to 4 seconds in duration) using analyses based on either frequency-domain or time-domain processing.

        a. Compressed spectral assay (CSA), density-modulated display of power spectrum analysis (DSA). For frequency-domain processing, many EEG applications use power spectral analysis. In this application, each EEG epoch is converted into a series of sine wave components using

Table 23.3 Electroencephalogram confounds

Anesthetic agents (e.g., propofol, isoflurane, thiopental, etomidate) producing EEG burst
    suppression (Fig. 23.10)
High-dose enflurane (EEG pattern indistinguishable from electrocortical seizure activity)
High-dose narcotics or cerebral ischemia (similar EEG δ wave activity)
Biopotentials [e.g., cardiac depolarization (electrocardiogram), skeletal muscle (shivering),
    eye movement myopotentials, blood flow through aortic cannula]
60-Hz activity from electrical equipment (e.g., cardiopulmonary bypass pump motor,
    electrocautery)

EEG, electroencephalogram.

Table 23.4 Causes of electroencephalographic asymmetry

Unilateral carotid perfusion from aortic miscannulation
Cerebral venous hypertension from kinking of atrial cannulas
Cerebral hypoperfusion from low pump flow or systemic arterial hypotension
  unmasking unilateral unilateral cerebrovascular disease
Cerebral ischemia from embolus
Unmasking of previous cerebrovascular accident
Artifact from proximity of arterial inflow cannula to certain electroencephalographic
  electrodes

Fourier transformation that treats the digitized EEG as a sum of sine waves of variable frequency and power. The amplitude (power) of each of the sine wave components is indicated as a function of its frequency, and in the CSA each EEG epoch is shown over time in a three-dimensional representation (frequency vs power vs time) with the most current epoch in the foreground. The vertical displacement, representing both power and time, hinders recognition of low-amplitude activity followed by high-amplitude activity in the same frequency band (Fig. 23.7). DSA is a representation in which each epoch is displayed using gray-scale intensity or dot size proportional to the power of the individual frequency band plotted. Consequently, it can be difficult to recognize small changes in frequency using this display (Fig. 23.7).

   b. **Spectral edge frequency (aperiodic analysis).** Aperiodic analysis is time-domain–based processing and does not use Fourier transformation. Instead it is based on assessing voltage versus time of the raw EEG. For each component EEG wave in an epoch, the frequency is determined as the reciprocal of the time interval measured between zero axis voltage crossings, the zero-crossing frequency (ZXF), while the amplitude is the square root of the sum of squares of the voltages of the wavelets. Fast- and slow-wave components are analyzed separately, then combined for display (Fig. 23.7). This model of analysis also is used to calculate the burst-suppression ratio, which can be an indicator of anesthetic depth and cerebral metabolism depression. Epileptiform activity and artifact have been reported to be most readily identified by time-domain processing. EEG frequency carrying the median power (median frequency power) correlates with plasma levels of several narcotics. The spectral edge frequency (frequency below which 95% of summated EEG power is contained) correlates with clinical assessment of anesthetic depth achieved with barbiturates or volatiles anesthetics.

   c. **Bispectral index.** Most frequency-domain processing (CSA, DSA) treats as independent those component waveforms resulting from Fourier transformation. Bispectral analysis measures potential interactions between the waves to determine the presence of interactive components (harmonics) indicative of phase coupling (biocoherence), information that is not present in power spectral analysis. It has been recognized that EEG slowing and synchrony often occur in relation to increasing depth of anesthesia. The BIS measurement is the first device specifically for the measurement of the hypnotic effects of drugs approved by the U.S. Food and Drug Administration. There is increasing evidence that *BIS number correlates inversely with depth of anesthesia and degree of biocoherence.*

2. **Evoked potentials.** Metabolic and hemodynamic homeostasis determines the state of cerebral functional integrity. The latter can be inferred from EEG changes in response to repeated stimulation of intact afferent pathways. Separated from raw EEG and averaged, these evoked potentials (EPs) are described in terms of latency (time between the stimulus and respective EEG change) and amplitude (cortical microcurrent 1 to 5 μV). Reduction in CBF

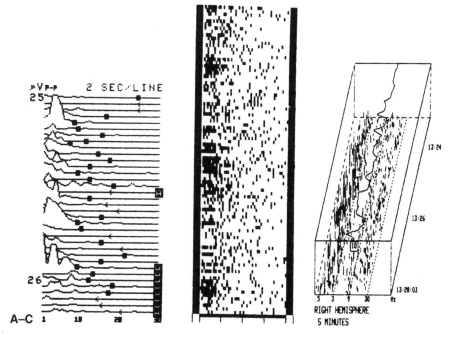

FIG. 23.7 Electroencephalographic (EEG) information from the same patient depicted in three different formats. Only one lead is presented for each format. In actual practice, multiple leads (2 to 4) usually are displayed. **A:** Compressed spectral array (CSA). Peaks on a line are used to represent amplitude of cerebral electrical activity across a frequency axis. Information is updated at a preselected interval by adding new lines that progress down the recording. Large peaks may obscure previous data. A *square* is used to mark the spectral edge (frequency below which a preselected percentage of electrical activity occurs). The symbol *A* indicates recording artifact. **B:** Density modulation spectral array (DSA). A color gradient or gray scale is used to depict amplitude on a frequency axis so that data are not obscured. Precision is lost in amplitude interpretation. **C:** Aperiodic analysis. Spikes are recorded on a frequency axis to depict amplitude data. These spikes appear in a parallelogram so that new data can be added without obscuring previous data. A line on the top of the parallelogram plots the activity edge, which is the frequency below which a preselected percentage of the cerebral electrical activity occurs. (From Wickey GS, Hickey RR. Brain protection during cardiac surgery. In: Hensley FA, Martin DE, eds. *The practice of cardiac anesthesia.* Boston: 1990: 716, with permission.)

below 18 mL/(100 g · min) causes progressive decrease of the latter, which disappears at CBF below 15 mL/(100 g · min). In clinical practice, only the response of sensory neurons of gray matter can be tested in this way. More commonly, EPs serve to monitor the function of sensory tracts. Certain anesthetic agents complicate the recognition of specific effects of changing metabolic environment on EPs (e.g., isoflurane increases latency and decreases amplitude of somatosensory EPs) and have opposite effects on different EPs (visual somatosensory) (Table 23.5).

    C. Transcranial Doppler. Insonation of blood moving within a vessel produces a characteristic shift in signal frequency (Doppler shift) that is proportional to the flow velocity. Use of low-frequency sound waves (2 to 4 MHz) from depth-gated,

Table 23.5 Evoked potential applications

Visual EPs can monitor the integrity of the optic nerve and chiasm during procedures in the anterior fossa, and auditory EPs can be used during posterior fossa operations to assess auditory nerve integrity
Somatosensory EPs are used to monitor for spinal cord ischemia during thoracic aortic surgery or spinal reconstruction
Auditory EPs are being investigated for assessing depth of anesthesia

EP, evoked potential.

direction-sensitive probes allows transmission through thin areas of skull (e.g., *temporal window located above zygomatic arch between ear and orbit*). This transmission enables continuous assessment of blood flow velocity within major intracerebral arteries (e.g., proximal middle cerebral artery) (Table 23.6). Cerebral perfusion characteristics also can be assessed using TCD insonation for demonstration of laminar versus pulsatile flow or for detection of emboli. Because dissimilar acoustic echoes reflect inhomogeneities in the insonated substrate, microaggregate or microgaseous emboli can be detected within the bloodstream. Because TCD essentially functions as a microphone, artifactual noise transients can register as emboli. However, certain characteristics that distinguish embolic signals from noise artifact are discernible when interpreting the output of the TCD monitor (Table 23.7). Much greater acoustic resonance of gas emboli relative to formed elements creates limits of TCD detection for formed elements greater than 100 µm. Additionally, the amplitude of signal is proportional to the size of the embolus, whereas for bubble emboli, limits of resolution are 50µm and the amplitude of the reflected signal is unrelated to size of bubble. *Distinction between small bubble or large formed element emboli currently is not readily achieved with TCD.* Algorithms developed by using both maximal amplitudes of individual signals as well as the sum of the amplitudes of a particular signal's component spectral lines can help differentiate particulate from gaseous emboli with high sensitivity and specificity experimentally and may be useful clinically.

D. Jugular oximetry. The characteristic attenuation of 650 to 1,100 nm infrared light by a few specific light-absorbing chromophores (primarily oxyhemoglobin, deoxyhemoglobin, and oxidized cytochrome c oxydase) imparts wavelength (color) shift on the incident light. This spectral shift is proportionate to the degree of oxygenation enabling quantification of tissue oxygenation using optical spectroscopic devices. Placement of a fiberoptic oximetric catheter into the jugular bulb provides continuous monitoring of the hemoglobin saturation of effluent cerebral venous blood and reflects global cerebral O_2 supply and demand balance. *Jugular oximetry may provide an appropriate endpoint for termination of cooling before DHCA* (see above). Once jugular saturation has increased maximally and stabilized, $CMRo_2$ is at its lowest. Such monitoring has identified an association between rewarming after hypothermic CPB and significant cerebral venous blood desaturation. This indicates mismatching between cerebral O_2 supply and metabolic rate, and increasing either hemoglobin concentration or depth of anesthesia (greater metabolic suppression) may be appropriate.

E. Noninvasive optical spectroscopy. Similar principles of light absorbance are used during noninvasive cerebral optical spectroscopy using a scalp-attached probe. For this application, narrow wave band, near-infrared incident light is emitted

Table 23.6 Transcranial Doppler assessment of cerebral blood flow

Constant transcranial Doppler probe angle (fixed probe holder)
Constant vessel diameter (proximal middle cerebral artery)
Insonation via temporal window (accessible in 80% of adults)

Table 23.7 Transcranial Doppler characteristics of emboli versus noise

	Emboli	Noise
Duration(s)	<0.1	0.5
Directionality	Unidirectional	Bidirectional
Frequency range (db)	3–60	1–20
Sound	Chirpy	Noisy
Time delay (ms; bigate, 10-mm distance)	11	0.08

through one fiberoptic cable attached to the scalp, and the resulting scattered light is reflected back through two or more sensor cables. Spacing of the sensor cables is such that the reflected light is propagated primarily through either skull and extra-cerebral tissue (Fig. 23.8), and total cortical O_2 saturation (ScO$_2$; venous, capillary, and arteriolar) is represented by the intensity difference between the superficial and deep sensors. Because cerebral hypoxia affects reduction and oxidation equilibrium of neuronal mitochondrial enzyme cytochrome aa$_3$, which in turn affects near-infrared light absorption, continuous monitoring of cortical oxygenation is possible. Preliminary clinical studies in cardiac surgical patients indicate a correspondence between low ScO$_2$ and poor outcomes. Prospective studies are awaited.

F. **Cerebral perfusion pressure.** CPP represents the difference between driving pressure, or MAP, and downstream pressure, or intracranial pressure. During CPB direct measure of intracranial pressure is not available, thus CVP often is used as a surrogate. In the presence of impaired drainage from the SVC, which is possible during dislocation of the heart (particularly with use of a single two-stage cannula), cerebral venous hypertension may occur. Because atrial drainage is unimpaired, CVP measured from the atrium will be low; hence, this condition may be unrecognized. If sustained, cerebral venous hypertension can lead to cerebral edema and

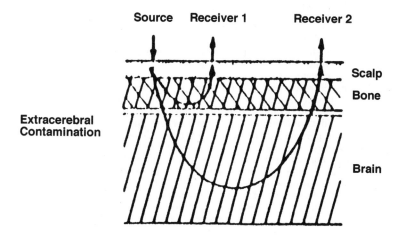

FIG. 23.8 Schematic representation of tissue layers through which light must propagate to reach the brain. Light propagating from source to receiver 1 has a mean tissue path length such that it predominantly samples superficial tissue (scalp and skull), whereas light propagating to receiver 2 has a deeper mean path length into brain. The signal from receiver 1 is used to correct the signal from receiver 2 for superficial tissue contamination. (From McCormick PW, et al. Noninvasive optical spectroscopy for monitoring cerebral oxygen delivery and hemodynamics. *Crit Care Med* 1991;19:89–97, with permission.)

substantially decreased CPP, despite apparently adequate MAP (Fig. 23.5). **During CPB, cerebral venous pressure should be monitored by a catheter placed proximally (usually pulmonary artery catheter introducer sheath) in the SVC and by visual inspection of the face.**

VI. Prevention of central nervous system injury

A. Embolic load

1. **Aortic instrumentation**

   a. Although still the standard of care, palpation of the aorta has not proven sensitive to detect aortic atherosclerosis. Direct EAS scan of ascending aorta is the most sensitive technique for assessment of atherosclerotic burden. Alternatively, initial TEE screening of descending aorta, followed by EAS if TEE detects descending aortic atherosclerosis, represents an acceptable screening strategy. With extensive aortic atherosclerosis, distal aortic arch or axillary artery cannulation should be considered.

   b. Minimize the number of aortic clampings. Use of all arterial grafts (e.g., mammary, gastroepiploic) or sutureless proximal anastomotic devices eliminates the need for aortic side clamping for proximal anastomoses. In cases of severe atherosclerosis, aortic exclusion techniques are recommended.

2. **Perfusion equipment and techniques**

   a. Precirculation of CPB circuit for a minimum of 30 minutes with a 5-μm filter before usage removes plasticizers and other manufacturing microdebris.

   b. Incorporation of a micropore (20- to 40-μm) filter into the cardiotomy return line keeps tissue and other particulate debris from the surgical field out of the CPB circuit.

   c. Retransfusion of unwashed cardiotomy suction blood is associated with increased cerebral lipid microemboli [7].

   d. Use of a 40-μm filter on the arterial inflow line decreases delivery of emboli into the arterial circulation.

   e. To minimize gas bubble formation due to decreased solubility with rewarming, the temperature gradient between the arterial inflow blood and the patient must be less than 10°C, particularly with use of a bubble oxygenator.

   f. During rewarming, arterial blood inflow temperature must not exceed 37°C.

3. **De-airing techniques**

   a. Before ventricular ejection, needle aspiration of the LV and LA, combined with manual agitation of the heart, to dislodge air entrapped in trabeculae. This process should be combined with concomitant manual ventilation of the lungs to mobilize residual air within the pulmonary veins.

   b. Use of TEE to detect residual intracavitary air and to direct needle aspirations.

   c. Tilting the patient's head down. This procedure achieves a dependent position of the great vessels of the head and minimizes entry of gas bubbles.

   d. Transient bilateral carotid compression during defibrillation and initial filling and commencement of heart ejection.

B. Cerebral perfusion.
During moderate hypothermia, hypotension is well tolerated because cerebral autoregulation is preserved down to CPP 20 mm Hg with α-stat blood gas management. As assessed by NPT, the brain rewarms rapidly; therefore, hypotension (MAP less than 50 mm Hg) should be avoided after commencement of rewarming. Inadvertent compromise of CPP should be avoided by monitoring proximal SVC pressure to detect cerebral venous hypertension. Diabetics and patients with previous CVA have impaired cerebral autoregulation and CBF is directly dependent on MAP. Such patients may benefit from close CNS monitoring (see previous discussion) and maintenance of higher perfusion pressures.

C. Euglycemia.
There is considerable evidence from experimental models and from patients with CVA that hyperglycemia increases the magnitude and extent of neurologic injury during ischemia [9]. Although there are limited clinical outcome data in cardiac patients, blood glucose level should be maintained within the normal range in patients during cardiac surgery because they are at increased risk for ischemic injury. Hyperglycemia should be avoided as a basic approach. *Glucose-free infusions and a glucose-free prime should be used for CPB circuit,* because in-

sulin resistance develops during CPB (partially as a result of increased endogenous catecholamines), producing glucose intolerance and increasing the tendency for refractory hyperglycemia.

D. **Mild hypothermia.** There is increasing evidence showing that the release of EAA and excitotoxicity are pivotal in the genesis of ischemic neurologic injury (see preceding discussion). Because EAA release is critically temperature dependent and is significantly inhibited below 35°C, brain temperature (degrees NPT; see previous sections) should be monitored continuously during rewarming, *hyperthermia (NPT greater than 37°C) must be avoided,* and brain temperature should be maintained less than 37°C until after separating from CPB and decannulation [10].

VII. Pharmacologic cerebral protection. Over the last decade there has been a profound increase in our understanding of the mechanisms involved in ischemic neuronal injury. Many new classes of drugs have been developed, and the most promising are undergoing clinical development. Currently, none represent standards of practice, but these or related compounds may become part of the therapeutic armamentarium in the near future [11].

  A. **Metabolic suppression**
  1. **Rationale and limitations.** Metabolic activity is temperature dependent, and hypothermia produces an exponential decrease in cerebral metabolic rate. Unlike pharmacologic metabolic suppressants, hypothermia decreases metabolic activity related both to functional activity (e.g., EEG activity) and basal activity (e.g., ion pumps). Hypothermia prolongs the tolerance for global ischemia (Fig. 23.9) and is undertaken particularly for circulatory arrest (see following discussion). During cardiac surgery, however, greatest risk for cerebral emboli occurs during normothermia with cannulation and decannulation; hence, pharmacologic metabolic suppressants have been investigated. One clinical study reported that administration of high-dose thiopental resulted in

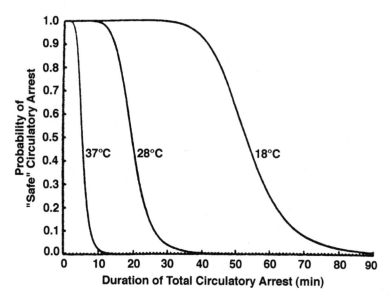

FIG. 23.9 Nomogram of probability of "safe" total circulatory arrest according to duration of total arrest time as nasopharyngeal temperatures of 37°C, 28°C, and 18°C, defined as the duration of total arrest after which no structural or functional damage has occurred. (From Kirklin JK, Kirklin JW, Pacifico AD. Deep hypothermia and total circulatory arrest. In: Arciniegas E, ed. *Pediatric cardiac surgery.* Chicago: Year Book, 1985:79–85, with permission.)

significantly fewer persisting neurologic deficits in patients undergoing open chamber cardiac surgery at mild hypothermia (32°C), but using a similar protocol in closed chamber cardiac surgery at moderate hypothermia (28°C) produced no demonstrable difference in CNS outcome. It had been believed that any benefit resulting from such therapy was derived from the profound suppression of cerebral metabolic rate associated with suppression of synaptic activity (EEG burst suppression), and that this practice resulted in increased tolerance for ischemia. As described previously, this would likely result only in an ischemic tolerance prolongation of a very few minutes. Decreases in CBF secondary to cerebral metabolic suppression (EEG burst suppression) using propofol also have been unsuccessful in ameliorating brain injury.

2. **Agents.** Various anesthetics have the ability to produce EEG burst suppression (Fig. 23.10) and result in profound decreases in cerebral metabolic rate to approximately 50% of awake $CMRo_2$, averaging 1.5 mL/(100 g · min).

    a. **Thiopental.** A dosage of 5 to 8 mg/kg results in 5 minutes of EEG suppression at normothermia. Proportional decreases in both CBF and $CMRo_2$ are produced. An infusion at 0.5 to 1.0 mg/(kg · min) is required for prolonged EEG suppression; results in prolonged recovery and extubation times; and may increase the need for inotropic support because of myocardial depression.

    b. **Propofol.** Transient EEG burst suppression is obtained at dosages of 2 to 3 mg/kg and results in proportional decreases in CBF and $CMRo_2$.

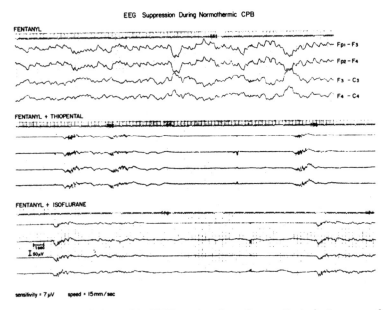

FIG. 23.10 Electroencephalographic (*EEG*) tracings from three patients during normothermic cardiopulmonary bypass (*CPB*). The *top tracing* demonstrates characteristic low voltage activity occurring during high-dose fentanyl anesthesia. The *middle tracing* shows the burst-suppression pattern resulting from thiopental administration. The *lower pattern* demonstrates burst suppression occurring during isoflurane administration. (From Woodcock TE, et al. Pharmacologic EEG suppression during cardiopulmonary bypass: cerebral hemodynamic and metabolic effects of thiopental or isoflurane during hypothermia and normothermia. *Anesthesiology* 1987;67:218–224, with permission.)

Infusion at 0.1 to 0.3 mg/(kg · min) produces sustained EEG suppression and is rapidly metabolized; therefore, it does not prolong recovery and extubation times. Hypotension from systemic vasodilation may require administration of phenylephrine or other such vasoconstrictor.

    c. Isoflurane. At inspired concentrations of 2% to 3% (1.5 to 2 MAC), burst suppression is produced. Unlike the intravenous agents, EEG suppression with isoflurane is not accomplished by any decrease in CBF, although $CMRo_2$ is significantly reduced. Rapid elimination is characteristic of volatile anesthetics.

B. Calcium channel blockers. Massive calcium influx is likely the final common pathway of ischemic neuronal injury (see preceding comments). In clinical trials, calcium channel antagonists (nimodipine) have demonstrated efficacy in decreasing vasospasm after subarachnoid hemorrhage; however, nimodipine also has been associated with increased bleeding and higher mortality in cardiac surgical patients.

C. Glutamate antagonists. Because excitotoxicity is recognized as central to ischemic neuronal injury (see previous discussion), EAA receptor antagonists are being actively investigated. Remacemide, a competitive glutamate antagonist, has been shown superior to placebo in improving neuropsychologic outcome after CABG [3]. A development has been the experimental use of antibodies to the NMDA receptor [5].

D. Lazaroids and other 21-aminosteroid compounds. Free radical scavengers (including allopurinol and methylprednisolone) have not consistently demonstrated benefit in experimental ischemic brain injury. Lazaroids (21-aminosteroids) are inhibitors of lipid membrane peroxidation and they act as free radical scavengers. The most extensively studied of these agents is tirilazad. Promising results in experimental stroke have failed to translate into improved outcome in clinical trials [5].

E. Aprotinin. A bovine serine protease inhibitor, aprotinin has been shown to significantly reduce intraoperative bleeding and transfusion requirements in a variety of settings, including cardiac surgery with CPB. High-dose aprotinin increasingly appears to be associated with a decreased incidence of perioperative stroke, possibly resulting from its antiinflammatory properties.

VIII. Deep hypothermic circulatory arrest

  A. Clinical indications. DHCA sometimes is used for major surgical procedures because it provides a motionless, cannula-free, bloodless field. By allowing unobstructed surgical access, DHCA facilitates repair of complex congenital anomalies in neonates and infants. In adults, DHCA allows temporary interruption of cerebral perfusion, primarily for aortic arch reconstruction or for resection of giant cerebral aneurysms.

  B. Technique

    1. Core and external cooling. In most North American centers, active external cooling (e.g., ice baths) has been eliminated. Core cooling using CPB allows efficient and controlled onset of hypothermia, and cooling persists until core temperature (bladder, rectal) is stable at 15° to 20°C. Cooling must be continued until stable brain temperature (e.g., NPT, jugular thermistry) has been achieved.

    2. Decannulation. Before circulatory arrest, administration of long-acting muscle relaxants (e.g., pancuronium 0.1 mg/kg) is essential to ensure profound paralysis in order to minimize systemic O_2 consumption. With cessation of perfusion, venous cannulas are unclamped, allowing passive exsanguinations into the CPB circuit and decreasing distention of the heart and bleeding into the surgical site. For pediatric surgery, venous cannulas usually are removed to facilitate surgical exposure. Often passive circulation of blood within the CPB circuit is continued *ex vivo* to avoid stasis and setting of blood with platelet clumping.

  C. Brain protection

    1. Temperature. Hypothermia is the primary component of brain protection during circulatory arrest. *Over a range of 20°C (37° to –17°C), the temperature coefficient (Q_{10}) of the brain averages 3.65;* thus, cerebral tolerance for ischemia is greatly enhanced (Fig. 23.9). Minimizing rewarming of the brain is essential; therefore, external heat sources (e.g., overhead lights, ambient room temperature) should be minimized. Application of external ice packs to the head have been shown experimentally to delay brain rewarming and increase ischemic tolerance. Thiopental and/or steroids are administered before circulatory arrest in some centers, although any beneficial effect is unproved.

2. **Anterograde and retrograde perfusion.** Because of cerebral autoregulation with preferential shunting of blood to the brain, even low perfusion rates (e.g., 10 to 25 mL · kg · min) during deep hypothermia have been shown experimentally to significantly improve cerebral ischemic tolerance in comparison to total circulatory arrest. For aortic arch procedures in which arterial inflow is restricted, selective cerebral perfusion via brachiocephalic or carotid cannulation has been used successfully [12]. Increasing interest is developing in retrograde cerebral perfusion through SVC cannula, although prospective clinical outcome studies are not yet available. Retrograde cerebral perfusion does not provide sufficient substrate supply to maintain brain metabolic demand but may help prevent rewarming and help further cool the brain [12].

A prospective randomized study has shown that continuous low-flow perfusion (0.7l/min · m²) at 18°C for pediatric patients younger than 3 months old undergoing arterial switch operations results in significantly lower incidences of clinical seizures and brain creatinine kinase isoenzyme release than does hypothermic circulatory arrest.

3. **pH Management.** Experimental studies have demonstrated more homogeneous brain cooling with pH-stat. A prospective study of the influence of pH management on developmental outcome after DHCA concluded that pH-stat is associated with better cerebral protection and clinical outcomes than α-stat when used in infants.

D. **Summary**
1. **Administer muscle relaxants prior to DHCA.**
2. **Cool until stable core (NPT) is achieved.**
3. **Eliminate glucose from solutions and pump prime.**
4. **Minimize ambient room temperature.**
5. **Place external ice packs around head.**
6. **Continuously monitor NPT and EEG during DHCA.**
7. **Use intermittent or low-flow perfusion when possible.**
8. **Minimize duration of DHCA.**

IX. **Cardiac surgery in patients with cerebrovascular disease.**
A. **Incidence.** Coronary atherosclerosis increases the likelihood of coexisting carotid arteriopathy. The incidence of hemodynamically significant carotid stenosis among patients requiring CABG is reported as high as 15% and increases with advancing age. Carotid bruits are a poor predictor of carotid stenosis or the risks of perioperative stroke. Among CABG candidates, noninvasive (ultrasonography) and invasive (contrast arteriography) investigations usually are reserved for patients who have had symptoms of cerebrovascular insufficiency (e.g., transient ischemic attacks or stroke) during the previous 3 to 6 months [3].
B. **Morbidity.** Neurologic injury associated with cardiovascular surgery using CPB is primarily due to emboli. Risk of stroke is greatly increased by an atherosclerotic aorta. Whereas carotid stenosis increases risk of stroke after cardiac surgery, it is not clear that concomitant endarterectomy is prophylactic because the mechanism of stroke is likely rather related to a greater incidence of aortic atherosclerosis than hemodynamic cerebral ischemia. Potential for global cerebral hypoperfusion is reduced by collateral flow via the circle of Willis, preservation of adequate CPP, and MAP within the patient's autoregulatory range (e.g., preexisting hypertension). CPB-related hemodilution improves blood flow through stenotic lesions of the cerebral vasculature.
C. **Combined carotid and cardiac procedures**
1. **Rationale.** Indications for carotid endarterectomy (CEA) and CABG should be considered independently. There is no compelling evidence that, in the absence of significant symptomatology, CEA decreases perioperative stroke risk.

If a patient is a candidate for both procedures, then a combined (one-stage) operation appears to offer better overall outcome than a two-stage approach performed in either order (two anesthetics), given the experience of centers with extensive experience with the combined approach.

2. **Monitoring.** TCD insonation of a major cerebral artery (e.g., proximal MCA) can help assess relative volume of cerebral flow during changes in MAP. EEG can aid in recognition of profound cerebral hypoperfusion.

3. **Morbidity.** A combined CEA and CABG procedure offers a 5-year 80% survival rate (93% for CABG alone). Marginal improvement is achieved in some centers that use DHCA for the combined procedure.

References

1. Llinas R, Barbut D, Caplan LR. Neurologic complications of cardiac surgery. *Prog Cardiovasc Dis* 2000;43:101–112.
2. Nussmeier NA. Adverse neurologic events: risks of intracardiac versus extracardiac surgery. *J Cardiothorac Vasc Anesth* 1996;10:31–37.
3. **Arrowsmith JE, Grocott H, Reves JG, et al. Central nervous system complications of cardiac surgery. *Br J Anaesth* 2000;84:378–393.**
4. **Murkin JM, Martzke JS, Buchan AM, et al. A randomized study of the influence of perfusion technique and pH management strategy in 316 patients undergoing coronary artery bypass surgery: (part 2) neurological and cognitive outcomes. *J Thorac Cardiovasc Surg* 1995;110:349–362.**
5. Gelb AW, Cowie DA. Perioperative stroke prevention. *IARS Review Course Lectures,* February 2001.
6. Gill R, Murkin JM. Neuropsychologic dysfunction after cardiac surgery: what is the problem? *J Cardiothorac Vasc Anesth* 1996;10:91–98.
7. Brooker RF, Brown WR, Moody DM, et al. Cardiotomy suction: a major source of brain lipid emboli during cardiopulmonary bypass. *Ann Thorac Surg* 1998;65:1651–1655.
8. Murkin JM, Baird DL, Martzke JS, et al. Cognitive dysfunction after ventricular fibrillation during implantable cardioverter/defibrillator procedures is related to duration of the reperfusion interval. *Anesth Analg* 1997;84:1186–1192.
9. **Murkin JM. Intraoperative tight glucose control improves outcome in cardiovascular surgery: pro. *J Cardiothorac Vasc Anesth* 2000;14:475–478.**
10. Newman MF, Croughwell ND, Blumenthal JA, et al. Cardiopulmonary bypass and the central nervous system: potential for cerebral protection. *J Clin Anesth* 1996;8:53S–60S.
11. **Murkin JM. Attenuation of neurologic injury during cardiac surgery. *Ann Thorac Surg* 2001;72:S1838–S1844.**
12. **Griepp RB, Juvonen T, Griepp EB, et al. Is retrograde cerebral perfusion an effective means of neural support during deep hypothermic circulatory arrest? *Ann Thorac Surg* 1997;64:913–916.**

IV. THORACIC ANESTHESIA AND PAIN MANAGEMENT

24. ANESTHETIC MANAGEMENT FOR THORACIC ANEURYSMS AND DISSECTIONS

Thomas M. Skeehan and John R. Cooper, Jr.

In the management of thoracic aortic surgery, the anesthesiologist may face a marked variability in the problems associated with etiology, type, and anatomic location of the surgical procedure. This chapter gives a concise overview of the pathophysiology of thoracic aortic surgery, an understanding of its surgical approaches and results, and a rational approach to the management of the patient undergoing thoracic aortic surgery.

I. **Classification and natural history**
   A. **Dissections.** An **aortic dissection** occurs when blood penetrates the aortic intima and forms an expanding hematoma within the vessel wall, usually separating the intima and media to create a so-called false lumen or dissecting hematoma. The vessel lumen is not dilated and often is compressed by the advancing hematoma. In contrast, an **aortic aneurysm** involves dilation of all three layers of the vessel wall and has a highly different pathophysiology and implications for management. The term **dissecting aneurysm,** although commonly used, is often a misnomer.
      1. **Incidence and pathophysiology**
         a. **Incidence.** Aortic dissections have been estimated to cause one of every 10,000 hospital admissions. In large autopsy series, aortic dissection has been found in one of every 600 cases, and it was believed that dissections may have caused or contributed significantly to the mortality in up to 1% of these autopsy cases.
         b. **Predisposing conditions.** The medical conditions predisposing to aortic dissection are listed in Table 24.1 in their order of importance. Interestingly, **atherosclerosis** by itself may not contribute to the risk of subsequent dissection.
         c. **Inciting event.** The onset of aortic dissections has been associated with increased physical activity or emotional stress. Dissections also have been associated with blunt trauma to the chest; however, the temporal relationship of blunt trauma and subsequent dissections has not been well established. Dissections can occur without any physical activity. They also may occur during cannulation for cardiopulmonary bypass (CPB).
         d. **Mechanism of aortic tear.** An intimal tear is the initial event in aortic dissection. The intimal tear of aortic dissections usually occurs in the presence of a weakened aortic wall, predominantly involving the middle and outer layers of the media. In this area of weakening, the aortic wall is more susceptible to shear forces produced by pulsatile blood flow in the aorta. The most frequent locations of intimal tears are the areas experiencing the greatest mechanical shear forces, as listed in Table 24.2. The ascending and isthmic (just distal to the left subclavian artery) segments of the aorta are relatively fixed and thus subject the aortic wall to the greatest amount of mechanical shear stress. This explains the high incidence of intimal tears in these areas.

            In large autopsy series, however, up to 4% of dissections had no identifiable intimal disruption. In these cases, rupture of the **vasa vasorum,** the vessels that supply blood to the aortic wall, has been implicated as an alternative cause of dissections. The thin-walled vasa vasorum are located in the outer third of the aortic wall, and their rupture would cause the formation of a medial hematoma and propagation of a dissection in the presence of an already diseased vessel, without formation of an intimal tear.

Table 24.1 Conditions predisposing to aortic dissections

History of hypertension	Present in ≈90% of patients
Advanced age	>60 years
Sex	Male preponderance age <60 years
Arachnodactyly (Marfan syndrome)	Also other connective tissue diseases
Congenital heart disease	Coarctation of aorta, bicuspid aortic valve
Pregnancy	Uncommon
Other causes	Toxins and diet

Table 24.2 Sites of primary intimal tears in acute dissections of the aorta (398 autopsy cases)

Site	Percent incidence
Ascending	61
Descending	24
Isthmus	16
Other	8
Arch	9
Abdominal	3
Other	1

Modified from Hirst AE Jr, Johns VJ Jr, Kime W Jr. Dissecting aneurysm of the aorta: a review of 505 cases. *Medicine* 1958; 37:243.

e. **Propagation.** Propagation of an aortic dissection can occur within seconds. The factors that contribute to propagation are the hemodynamic forces inherent in pulsatile flow: pulse pressure and ejection velocity of blood.

f. **Exit points.** Exit points of dissections are found in a relatively small percentage of cases. Exit point tears usually occur distal to the intimal tear and represent points at which blood from the false lumen reenters the true lumen. The presence or absence of an exit point does not appear to have an impact on the clinical course.

g. **Involvement of arterial branches.** The origins of the major branches of the aorta, including the coronary arteries, may be involved in aortic dissections. Their involvement ranges from the occlusion of their lumens by mechanical compression by the false lumen or propagation of the dissecting hematoma into the arterial branch. The incidence of involvement of arterial branches gathered from a large autopsy series is listed in Table 24.3.

2. **DeBakey classification of dissections** (Fig. 24.1). This classification comprises three different types, depending on where the intimal tear is located and which section of the aorta is involved.

a. **Type I.** The intimal tear is located in the ascending portion, but the dissection involves all portions (ascending, arch, and descending) of the thoracic aorta.

b. **Type II.** The intimal tear is in the ascending aorta, but the dissection involves the ascending aorta only, stopping before the takeoff of the innominate artery.

Table 24.3 Involvement of major arterial branches in aortic dissections

Artery	Percent incidence
Iliac	25.2
Common carotid	14.5
Innominate	12.9
Renal (either)	12.0
Left subclavian	10.9
Mesenteric	8.2
Coronary (either)	7.5
Intercostal	4.0
Celiac	3.2
Lumbar	1.6

Modified from Hirst AE Jr, Johns VJ Jr, Kime W Jr. Dissecting aneurysm of the aorta: a review of 505 cases. *Medicine* 1958; 37:243.

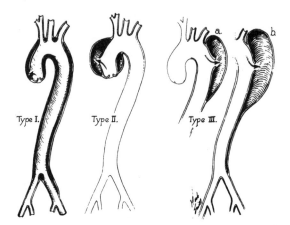

FIG. 24.1 DeBakey classification of aortic dissections by location: type I, with intimal tear in the ascending portion and dissection extending to descending aorta; type II, ascending intimal tear and dissection limited to ascending aorta; type III, intimal tear distal to left subclavian, but dissection extending for a variable distance, either to the diaphragm (*a*) or to the iliac artery (*b*). (From DeBakey ME, Henly WS, et al. Surgical management of dissecting aneurysms of the aorta. *J Thorac Cardiovasc Surg* 1965;49:131, with permission.)

    c. Type III. The intimal tear is located in the descending segment, and the dissection almost always involves the descending portion of the thoracic aorta only, starting just distal to the origin of the left subclavian artery. By definition, type III dissections can propagate proximally into the arch, but this is rare.

  3. Stanford (Daily) classification of dissections (Fig. 24.2). This classification is simpler than the DeBakey classification and has more clinical relevance.

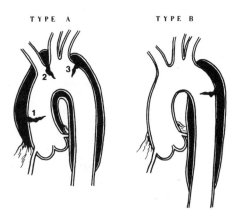

FIG. 24.2 Stanford (Daily) classification of aortic dissections. Type A describes a dissection involving the ascending aorta regardless of site of intimal tear (*1*, ascending; *2*, arch; *3*, descending). In type B, both the intimal tear and the extension are distal to the left subclavian. (From Miller DC, Stinson EB, et al. Aortic dissections. *J Thorac Cardiovasc Surg* 1979;78:367, with permission.)

      a. Type A. Type A dissections are those that have any involvement of the ascending aorta, regardless of where the intimal tear is located and regardless of how far the dissection propagates. Clinically, type A dissections run a more virulent course.

      b. Type B. Type B dissections are those that involve the aorta distal to the origin of the left subclavian artery.

    4. Natural history

      a. Mortality—untreated. The survival rate of untreated patients with aortic dissections is dismal, with a 2-day mortality of up to 50% in some series and a 6-month mortality approaching 90%. The usual cause of death is rupture of the false lumen and fatal hemorrhage. Other causes of death include progressive cardiac failure (aortic valve involvement), myocardial infarction, stroke, irreversible coma, and bowel gangrene (mesenteric artery occlusion).

      b. Surgical mortality. The overall surgical mortality is approximately 30%, but surgical therapy is often the only viable option for most of these patients.

B. Aneurysms

    1. Incidence. Thoracic aortic aneurysms account for 1% to 4% of aneurysms seen at autopsy. Currently, approximately 60% involve the ascending aorta and 30% are localized to the descending aorta. Aneurysms involving the aortic arch exclusively make up less than 10% of the total.

    2. Classification by location and etiology. In general, the etiology and pathophysiology of aortic aneurysms are site dependent. The most common causes by region are medionecrosis in the ascending aorta and atherosclerosis in the arch and descending aorta. Other etiologies are listed in Table 24.4.

    3. Classification by shape

      a. Fusiform. Fusiform aneurysmal dilation involves the entire circumference of the aortic wall.

      b. Saccular. Saccular aneurysms involve only one portion of the aortic wall. **Aortic arch aneurysms** are commonly of this type.

    4. Natural history. The usual history of aortic aneurysms is that of progressive dilation and, in more than 50% of cases, rupture. The untreated 5-year survival

Table 24.4 Etiology of aneurysms based on location in the aorta

Ascending	
Medionecrosis	Accumulation of mucoid material between elastic elements in the outer third of aortic wall, eventually involving the entire media
Syphilis	Major cause before 1950, distinguished by invasion of the aortic wall by *Treponema pallidum*
Congenital	Secondary to inborn errors in metabolism (Marfan syndrome, Ehlers-Danlos syndrome) leading to generalized defect of connective tissue
Poststenotic dilation	Secondary to long-standing aortic stenosis
Atherosclerosis	Not a major cause in ascending pathology
Arch	
Isolated	Atherosclerosis
Associated with ascending disease	Same etiologies as for disease in ascending aorta
Descending	
Atherosclerosis	Begins as intimal disease; major cause of thoracoabdominal and abdominal aneurysms
Congenital	See under Ascending, above
Trauma	Causal relationship difficult to prove; history of blunt trauma may be distant
Infection	Syphilis, *Salmonella,* tuberculosis

Etiologies are listed in order of frequency.

is approximately 13%, depending on the size of the aneurysm at diagnosis. Other complications include mycotic infection, atheroembolism to peripheral vessels, and dissection. This last complication is rare, probably occurring in fewer than 10% of cases. Some predictors of poor prognosis are large size (greater than 10-cm maximum transverse diameter), presence of symptoms, and associated cardiovascular disease, especially coronary artery disease, myocardial infarction, or cerebral vascular accident.

C. Thoracic aortic rupture (tear)

1. **Etiology.** The overwhelming majority of thoracic ruptures are secondary to trauma and almost always involve a **deceleration injury** in a motor vehicle accident. Sudden deceleration places large mechanical stresses on the aortic wall at points where the aorta is relatively immobile. Rupture of the aorta in many cases leads to immediate exsanguination and death. However, in approximately 10% to 15% of cases, the integrity of the lumen is maintained by the adventitial covering of the aorta, and these patients are able to reach emergency care. Surgical treatment of these survivors is often successful.

2. **Location.** The location of most ruptures of the thoracic aorta is the area just distal to the origin of the left subclavian artery (isthmus), due to the relative fixation of the aorta at this point by the ligamentum arteriosum (Fig. 24.3). The aorta also is fixed in the ascending portion just distal to the aortic valve, and this is the second most common site of rupture.

II. Diagnosis

A. Clinical signs and symptoms (Table 24.5)

1. **Dissections.** The clinical presentation of aortic dissection usually is characterized by a dramatic onset and a fulminant course. Differences and clinical presentation of Stanford types A and B are listed in Table 24.5.

2. **Aneurysms.** Aneurysms of the ascending, arch, or descending thoracic aorta often are asymptomatic until late in their course. In many circumstances, the presence of an aneurysm is not diagnosed until medical evaluation is conducted for an unrelated problem or for a problem related to a complication of the aneurysm.

3. **Traumatic rupture.** Ruptures most commonly occur just distal to the left subclavian artery. In this setting, signs and symptoms are similar to those

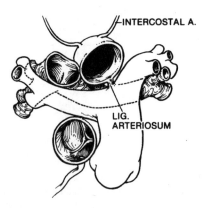

FIG. 24.3 The heart and great vessels are relatively mobile in the pericardium, whereas the descending aorta is relatively fixed by its anatomic relations. The attachment of the ligamentum arteriosum enhances this immobility and increases the risk of aortic tear due to deceleration injury. (From Cooley DA, ed. *Surgical treatment of aortic aneurysms.* Philadelphia: WB Saunders, 1986:186, with permission.)

seen with aneurysms of the descending thoracic aorta if the patient survives the initial event.
B. **Laboratory diagnosis**
1. **Electrocardiogram.** A common finding for many patients with aortic disease is that of **left ventricular hypertrophy,** a condition correlating with a history of accompanying hypertension. The electrocardiogram (ECG) may show a pattern associated with ischemia or pericarditis caused by coronary artery occlusion or hemopericardium, respectively, in the setting of ascending aortic dissection.
2. **Chest x-ray film.** A **widened mediastinum** is a classic x-ray finding in the presence of thoracic aortic pathology. Widening of the aortic knob is often seen, with **disparate ascending-to-descending diameter.** A double shadow has been described in the setting of aortic dissection, in which the false lumen actually is visualized.
3. **Serum chemistries.** There are no specific laboratory findings with asymptomatic aneurysm. Dissection or rupture will produce a fall in hemoglobin. Dissections may cause elevation of cardiac enzymes (coronary artery occlusion), elevation of blood urea nitrogen and creatine (renal artery occlusion), and acidosis (low cardiac output or bowel ischemia).
4. **Computed tomographic scans and magnetic resonance imaging.** Computed tomography is a useful tool for diagnosing aneurysm size and has replaced angiography in some instances. Magnetic resonance imaging has been found to be extremely sensitive and specific in terms of identifying the entry tear, false lumen, aortic regurgitation, and pericardial effusion associated with aortic dissections [1].
5. **Angiography.** This technique remains the "gold standard" for determining the severity and extent of aneurysm and dissection. It can be used to determine the site of an intimal tear in the setting of dissecting hematoma, to assess aortic valve function, and to identify the distal and proximal spread of the lesion. In the case of ascending aortic pathology that will require CPB, the coronary anatomy can be delineated. Patients with disease of the thoracic aorta usually have concurrent coronary disease. Bypassing significant lesions would help to improve ventricular function for weaning from CPB. Aortography can diagnose the involvement of major vessels but rarely can identify the critical intercostal vessels that provide blood supply to the spinal cord (see Section **IV.G**).
6. **Transesophageal echocardiography.** Transesophageal echocardiography (TEE) has a role in diagnosing and screening patients who are suspected of having an aortic dissection. It can be diagnostic if adequate images are obtained. Pulsed Doppler and color Doppler imaging will aid in diagnosing the presence, extent, and type of dissection in most cases. TEE has been found to be highly sensitive and specific in the diagnosis of aortic dissection. Identification of a mobile intimal flap provides a prompt bedside diagnosis that can be lifesaving. In addition, (a) entry and reentry tears can be defined; (b) aortic regurgitation can be identified and quantified; (c) assessment of left ventricular (LV) function can be made; (d) presence of pericardial effusion or cardiac tamponade can be identified; and (e) follow-up studies of the false lumen can be made after therapeutic intervention.
7. **Recommendation for diagnostic strategies.** Nienaber et al. [2] and colleagues proposed a noninvasive imaging strategy for the diagnosis of thoracic aortic dissection. Magnetic resonance imaging, because of its high degree of sensitivity (98.3%) and specificity (97.8%), was recommended as the preferred diagnostic method in hemodynamically stable patients. For patients deemed unstable for this rather lengthy procedure (40 to 45 minutes), TEE, which has an average duration of about 15 minutes and sensitivity and specificity of 97.7% and 76.9%, respectively, is recommended for the unstable patient. Aortography, because of its inability to provide more critical information than the noninvasive methods and its higher incidence of complications, should remain as a diagnostic tool to be used only in select cases.

Table 24.5 Presenting clinical signs and symptoms by location and type of aortic pathology

	Aneurysm	Dissection	Aortic tear
General presentation	Chronic symptoms, but leaking or ruptured aneurysm can lead to fulminant course (see aortic tear for symptoms and signs)	Dramatic onset and fulminant course. Symptoms depend on location (type A or type B). Patient presents in shock, anxious, diaphoretic	History of deceleration injury; usually fulminant course (good chance of survival if patient gets to treatment center). Patient can present in hypovolemic shock.
Symptoms and signs			
Ascending and arch			
Location of pain	Anterior chest pain secondary to compression of (1) Coronary arteries (2) Sensory mediastinal nerves	**Type A dissection**[a] Anterior chest pain secondary to (1) Extension of dissection (ripping or tearing sensation) (2) Angina, from dissection of coronaries	Chest pain secondary to compression of structures by enlarging adventitia (the only structure maintaining aortic integrity)
Cardiovascular	CHF symptoms secondary to aortic annular enlargement (1) Widened pulse pressure (2) Diastolic murmur Facial and upper trunk venous congestion secondary to superior vena cava compression Blood pressure usually elevated chronically	CHF symptoms: (1) Murmur of aortic valve insufficiency (2) Narrowing of true lumen (increased afterload) systolic ejection murmur Blood pressure (1) Hypotension secondary to rupture into the retroperitoneum, intraabdominal, intrathoracic, or pericardial spaces (2) Hypertension secondary to pain, anxiety Asymmetry of pulses, or pulseless extremity	Blood pressure (1) Hypotension from hypovolemia (2) Hypertension from pain
Respiratory	Hoarseness secondary to compression of recurrent laryngeal nerve Dyspnea or stridor due to tracheal compression Hemoptysis due to erosion into trachea Rales secondary to CHF	Hoarseness secondary to compression of recurrent laryngeal nerve Dyspnea and stridor due to tracheal compression Hemoptysis due to erosion into trachea (chronic) Rales secondary to CHF	Lung contusion if chest trauma is significant

continued

Gastrointestinal	Not usually affected	See under Descending,[a] below	Not usually affected
Renal	Not usually affected	See under Descending,[a] below	Decreased function secondary to hypotension Symptoms related to hypoperfusion
Neurologic	Possible due to emboli to carotid artery from aortic valve or aneurysmal segment (see Dissection, at right)	Hemiparesis or hemiplegia secondary to involvement of single carotid artery Reversible or progressive coma	
Descending Location of pain	Chronic back pain may occur	**Type B dissection** Located in back, midscapular region	Located in midscapular region
Cardiovascular	Blood pressure usually normal or elevated (chronic hypertension)	Blood pressure (1) Elevated secondary to pain (common) (2) Hypotension if rupture of dissection has occurred	Blood pressure (1) Elevated secondary to pain (especially with other injuries from trauma) (2) Hypotension if hypovolemic Sequelae of lung contusion or rib fracture
Respiratory	Dyspnea from left main stem bronchial obstruction Hemoptysis due to erosion into left bronchus Hemorrhagic pleural effusion	Dyspnea due to left main stem bronchial obstruction Hemorrhagic pleural effusion	Usually normal
Gastrointestinal	Usually normal	Mimics an acute abdomen (1) Pain, rigid abdomen, nausea and vomiting (2) Gastrointestinal bleeding Bowel ischemia secondary to compression or dissection of mesenteric or celiac artery	
Renal	Renal insufficiency or renovascular hypertension if occlusive aortic disease develops	Ischemia due to involvement of renal arteries in dissection: (1) Infarction and renal failure (2) Renal insufficiency	Renal hypofunction from hypoperfusion or hypovolemia
Neurologic	Usually not affected	Paraparesis or paraplegia possible secondary to occlusion of critical spinal cord blood flow	Paraplegia possible

[a] Type A dissections may involve the entire aorta; therefore, symptoms of both ascending and descending pathology may be present. CHF, congestive heart failure.

C. Indications for surgical correction
1. Ascending aorta
  a. Dissections. Currently, any acute type A dissection should be corrected surgically, given the virulent course and high mortality if left untreated.

  b. Aneurysms. Surgical indications for resection include the following:
  (1) Presence of persistent pain despite a small aneurysm
  (2) Involvement of the aortic valve producing aortic insufficiency
  (3) Presence of angina due either to LV strain from aortic valve involvement or coronary artery involvement by the aneurysm
  (4) Rapidly expanding aneurysm or an aneurysm greater than 10 cm in diameter, because the chance of rupture increases with increasing size

2. Aortic arch
  a. Dissections. Acute dissection limited to the aortic arch is an indication for surgery (rare).

  b. Aneurysms. Because even elective surgical treatment for these types of aneurysms is more difficult and is associated with a higher morbidity and mortality, management tends to be more conservative. Surgical indications include the following:
  (1) Persistence of symptoms
  (2) Aneurysm greater than 10 cm in transverse diameter
  (3) Progressive expansion of an aneurysm

3. Descending aorta
  a. Dissection. Some controversy remains concerning the best treatment for an acute type B dissection. Due to similar mortality statistics for medical or surgical intervention, type B dissections often are treated medically in the acute phase, especially if the patient's concurrent disease would make surgical mortality prohibitively high. However, in patients with a type B dissection, the following complications should be treated surgically as they occur:
  (1) Failure to control hypertension medically
  (2) Continued pain (indicating progression of the dissection)
  (3) Enlargement on chest x-ray film, computed tomographic scan, or angiogram
  (4) Development of a neurologic deficit
  (5) Evidence of renal or gastrointestinal ischemia
  (6) Development of aortic insufficiency
      It should also be noted, as shown in Table 24.6, that 10-year survival for patients with medically managed type B dissections is similar to surgical survival for type A and B dissections together. Both of these managements compare favorably with the 10-year survival of patients with untreated aortic dissections.

  b. Aneurysm. Surgical indications include the following:
  (1) Chronic aneurysm of the descending thoracic aorta that causes persistent pain or other symptoms
  (2) Aneurysm greater than 10 cm in diameter
  (3) Expanding aneurysm
  (4) Leaking aneurysm (more fulminant symptoms)

Table 24.6 Surgical versus medical therapy for aortic dissections

	Hospital mortality (%)	
	Surgical	Medical
Type A	32	72
Type B	32	27
10-yr survival	20–25 (A and B)	33 (B only)

Modified from Miller DC, Stinson EB, Oyer PE, et al. Operative treatment of aortic dissection. *J Thorac Cardiovasc Surg* 1979;78:365.

III. Preoperative management of patients requiring surgery of the thoracic aorta.
Emergency preoperative management of **aortic dissections** is discussed below. However, emergency preoperative management for a **leaking thoracic aneurysm** and a **contained thoracic rupture** would be similar.

    A. Prioritizing: making the diagnosis versus controlling blood pressure. In the setting of a suspected dissecting hematoma, aortic tear, or leaking aneurysm, the first priority must always be to control the blood pressure (BP). **Making the diagnosis with chest x-ray film or angiogram should occur only when proper monitoring, intravenous (IV) access, and therapy have been established.** During the diagnostic procedure, the patient should be monitored closely, with a physician present as the clinical situation dictates. The anesthesiologist should become involved as early as possible to lend expertise in monitoring and in airway and hemodynamic management, should clinical deterioration occur before the patient reaches the operating room. Rapid diagnosis using TEE may save critical minutes in initiating definitive surgical treatment in this setting.

    B. BP control. The ideal drug to control BP would be a rapid acting, IV administered drug that has an ultra-short half-life and few if any side effects. Not only systolic and diastolic pressures but also the ejection velocity must be reduced because both of these factors have been shown to be important in the propagation of dissecting hematomas.

        1. Monitoring. It is imperative that these patients have the following: an ECG for detection of ischemia and dysrhythmias; two large-bore IV catheters; an arterial catheter in the proper location (to be discussed); and, if time permits, a central venous catheter or pulmonary artery (PA) catheter to follow filling pressures and to allow drug infusion.

        2. Agents

            a. Vasodilators

                (1) Nitroprusside has emerged as the agent of choice for controlling the BP, because it is effective and easily regulated because of its short duration of action. It is given as an IV infusion, and central administration is optimal. The usual starting dose is 0.5 to 1 μg/kg/min, titrated to effect. Doses of 8 to 10 μg/kg/min have been associated with toxicity (see Chapter 2).

                (2) Nitoglycerin causes direct vasodilation, but it is less potent than nitroprusside. It can be useful in the setting of myocardial ischemia with ascending aortic pathology. Dosages usually range from 1 to 4 μg/kg/min.

                (3) Fenoldopam is a newer rapid-acting vasodilator that is a D_1-like dopamine receptor agonist. It has little affinity for the D_2-like, α_1, or β adrenoreceptors. Fenoldopam causes vasodilation in many vascular beds, but it increases renal blood flow to a significant degree. Therefore, it may have some renal sparing effects while treating acute hypertension. Dosing starts at 0.05 to 0.1 μg/kg/min and can be incrementally increased to a maximum of 0.8 μg/kg/min.

            b. Decreasing ejection velocity. Decreasing ejection velocity becomes an important therapeutic consideration, especially if nitroprusside is used as the agent to lower BP. Nitroprusside will increase ejection velocity by increasing dP/dt and heart rate. For this reason, β-adrenergic blockade should be used with nitroprusside not only to decrease tachycardia but also to decrease contractility (see Chapter 2).

                (1) Propranolol can be administered as an IV bolus of 1 mg, and doses of up to 4 to 8 mg may be required until the effect is seen.

                (2) Labetalol, a combined α- and β-blocker, may offer a single alternative to the nitroprusside–propranolol combination. It should be given initially as a 20-mg loading bolus, and several minutes should be allowed for its effect to be seen. If no effect is seen, the dose should be doubled and several minutes allowed again for onset of effect. This process should be repeated up to a maximum dose of 40 to 80 mg every 10 minutes until a total dose of 300 mg is reached or until BP is controlled. Continuous infusion starting at 1 mg/min may be used, or a small bolus dose can be repeated every 10 to 30 minutes to maintain BP control.

   (3) **Esmolol** is a short-acting β-blocking agent with a very short half-life that may be useful in this setting. It is administered as a bolus loading dose of 500 µg/kg over 1 minute and then continued as an infusion starting at 50 µg/kg/min, titrated to effect, to a maximum of 300 µg/kg/min. This drug is particularly advantageous in a patient with obstructive lung disease because it is β_1-selective and its action can be terminated quickly if respiratory symptoms ensue.

   3. **Desired endpoints.** BP should be lowered to approximately 105 to 115 mm Hg systolic, and heart rate should be kept at 60 to 80 beats/min. If a PA catheter is in place, the cardiac index may be lowered to the 2 to 2.5 L/(min·m²) range because a hyperdynamic myocardium may promote the progression of a dissecting hematoma.

C. **Transfusion.** A total of 8 to 10 units of blood should be typed and cross-matched before surgery. Use of blood scavenging devices has decreased the amount of banked blood used, but the logistics of processing scavenged blood, plus the clinical situation, may require that homologous transfusion still be used.

D. **Assessment of other organ systems**

   1. **Neurologic.** The patient should be monitored closely to detect signs of any change in neurologic status, because deterioration in function is an indication for immediate surgical intervention.

   2. **Kidneys.** Renal function should be followed closely with insertion of a urinary catheter. If aortic dissection has been diagnosed, the development of anuria or oliguria in the setting of euvolemia is an indication for immediate surgical intervention.

   3. **Gastrointestinal.** Serial abdominal examinations should be performed. In addition, blood gas analysis should be done routinely to assess changes in acid–base status, because ischemic bowel can produce significant acidosis.

E. **Use of pain medications.** Patients with aortic dissections may be anxious and in severe pain. Pain relief should be given not only to lessen suffering but also to aid in control of BP. It is important to avoid obtundation; otherwise, important changes in patient status will be missed. Worsening of back or abdominal pain may indicate expansion of the lesion or further dissection and is regarded by many surgeons as an emergent situation. In addition, propagation of a dissection into a head vessel may lead to a change in mental status that may be undetected if the patient is oversedated.

IV. **Surgical and anesthetic considerations**

A. **Goal of surgical therapy (for dissections, aneurysms, aortic rupture).** The first major goal of treating acute aortic disruption must be to control hemorrhage. Once control is achieved, the objectives of management of both acute and chronic lesions are similar: to repair the diseased aorta and to restore relationships of major arterial branches.

   Elective repair of a thoracic aneurysm most often is accomplished by replacing the diseased segment of aorta with a synthetic graft and then implanting major arterial branches into the graft. With a dissection, in contrast, the major goal is to resect the segment of aorta containing the intimal tear. When this segment is removed, it is possible to obliterate the false lumen and interpose graft material. It may not be possible or necessary to replace *all* of the dissected portion of the aorta because, if the origin of dissection is controlled, reexpansion of the true lumen may compress and obliterate the false lumen. With contained aortic tears, the objective is to resect the area of the tear and either reanastomose the natural aorta to itself in an end-to-end fashion or use graft material for the anastomosis if there is insufficient natural aorta remaining.

B. **Overview of intraoperative anesthetic management (for dissections, aneurysms, aortic rupture)**

   1. **Key principles**

      a. **Managing BP.** BP control must be maintained during the transition from the preoperative to the intraoperative period. Such control is important in light of the surgical and anesthetic manipulations that will profoundly affect BP.

   b. **Monitoring of organ ischemia.** The organs that must be monitored continuously for adequacy of perfusion are the central nervous system, heart, kidney, and lungs. The liver and gut cannot be monitored continuously, but their metabolic functions can be checked periodically.

   c. **Treating coexisting disease.** Patients with aortic pathology often have associated cardiovascular and systemic diseases, as outlined in Table 24.7.

   d. **Controlling bleeding.** Achieving hemostasis after CPB or with graft material in place poses special challenges, especially when the native tissue is damaged or diseased. Coagulation abnormalities and their treatment are discussed in Chapter 18.

2. **Induction and anesthetic agents.** Because many of these patients come to surgery emergently, most are considered to have a full stomach and require rapid securing of the airway. On the other hand, these patients also require a smooth induction, because wide swings in hemodynamics may worsen the clinical situation. Usually a compromise is made using a controlled induction with cricoid pressure and manual ventilation. This "modified" rapid sequence induction allows some airway protection and expeditious titration of anesthetic drugs to control BP, the main goal being to secure the airway as quickly as possible with a minimum of hemodynamic perturbation. Use of nonparticulate antacids, H_2-blockers, and metoclopramide should be considered before induction of anesthesia. Anesthetic considerations and agents are described more fully in Section **IV.D.** Despite all precautions, marked changes in hemodynamics are common and should be expected [3].

3. **Importance of site of lesion** (Table 24.8). Although the principles of anesthetic induction and choice of anesthetic agents are similar for all aortic lesions, practical intraoperative management depends almost entirely on the site of the lesion.

C. **Ascending aortic surgery**
   1. **Surgical approach.** The approach used for ascending aortic surgery is a midline sternotomy.
   2. **Cardiopulmonary bypass.** Because of the proximal involvement of the aorta and because the surgery often includes repair or replacement of the aortic valve, CPB is required.
      a. If the aneurysm ends in the proximal or midportion of the ascending aorta, the arterial cannula for CPB can be placed in the upper ascending aorta or arch.
      b. The usual site of cannulation is the femoral artery. This is required if the entire ascending aorta is involved because an **aortic cannula cannot be placed distal to the pathology without jeopardizing perfusion to the great vessels.**

Table 24.7 Incidence of coexisting diseases in patients with aortic pathology presenting for surgery

Coronary artery disease	66%
Hypertension	42%
Chronic obstructive pulmonary disease	23%
Peripheral vascular disease	22%
Cerebrovascular disease	14%
Diabetes mellitus	8%
Other aneurysms	4%
Chronic renal disease	3%

Modified from Romagnoli A, Cooper JR Jr. Anesthesia for aortic operations. *Cleve Clin Q* 1981;48:148.

Table 24.8 Anesthetic and surgical management for thoracic aortic surgery

	Surgical site		
	Ascending	Arch	Descending
Surgical approach	Median sternotomy	Median sternotomy	Left thoracotomy
Perfusion	CPB—aortic cannula distal to lesion, or in femoral artery	CPB—femoral artery cannula	Simple cross-clamp Heparinized Gott shunt ECC with cannulas proximal and distal to lesion
Involvement of			
Aortic valve	Sometimes	No	No
Coronary arteries	Sometimes	No	No
Pericardium	Sometimes	No	No
Invasive monitoring	Left radial or femoral arterial catheter PA catheter[b]	Arterial catheter—either arm, or femoral[a] PA catheter[b]	Proximal arterial (right radial or brachial) Distal arterial (femoral)[b] PA catheter[b]
Special techniques	Renal preservation EEG	Deep hypothermic circulatory arrest Cerebral protection (DHCA, DHCA with RCP, or anterograde cerebral perfusion) Renal preservation EEG	Motor evoked potentials[b] One-lung ventilation Renal preservation CSF drainage[b]
Common complications	Bleeding Cardiac dysfunction	Bleeding Hypotension from cerebral protective doses of thiopental Neurologic deficits	Bleeding Paralysis Renal failure Cardiac dysfunction

[a] Depends on whether the left subclavian or innominate arteries are involved in the pathologic process. If there is uncertainty preoperatively, use a femoral artery catheter.
[b] Optional, depending on physician's preferences.
CPB, cardiopulmonary bypass; CSF, cerebrospinal fluid; DHCA, deep hypothermic circulatory arrest; ECC, extracorporeal circulation; EEG, electroencephalogram; PA, pulmonary artery; RCP, retrograde cerebral perfusion.

      c. Venous cannulation usually can be performed through the right atrium; however, femoral venous cannulation may be necessary if the aneurysm is especially large.

3. **Aortic valve involvement.** Frequently, either aortic valvuloplasty or aortic valve replacement is necessary with ascending aortic dissections or aneurysms. Which procedure is used depends on the degree of involvement of the sinuses of Valsalva and the aortic annulus.

4. **Coronary artery involvement.** With an acute dissecting hematoma, the coronary arteries may be involved. Coronary occlusion usually takes the form of compression of the coronary lumen by the expanding false lumen and will require bypass grafting. Displacement of the coronary arteries from their normal position with enlargement of the aortic annulus will require reimplantation of their orifices into the graft wall or a vein bypass.

5. **Surgical techniques.** An example of the usual cross-clamp placement used in surgery of the ascending aorta is shown in Figure 24.4. Note that placement of the distal clamp is more distal than would be the case for simple cross-clamping for coronary surgery and at times might even include a part of the innominate artery. If aortic insufficiency is present, a large portion of the cardioplegic solution infused into the aortic root will flow through the incompetent aortic valve instead of the coronaries, causing distention of the LV and loss of the myocardial preservative effects of cardioplegia. For these reasons, an immediate aortotomy must be performed and the coronary vessels infused individually with cold cardioplegia. Many centers use retrograde coronary perfusion for cardioplegia administration as an alternative technique to obviate this problem.

    If the aortic valve and annulus both are normal, the diseased section of aorta is replaced with graft material. If the annulus is normal and the valve is incompetent, the valve may be resuspended or replaced. If both valve incompetence and annular dilation are present, either a composite graft (i.e., a tube graft

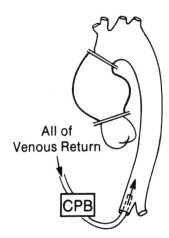

FIG. 24.4 Circulatory support and clamp placement for surgery of the ascending aorta. Femoral arterial cannula usually is required, and distal clamp must be beyond the extent of pathology. Proximal clamp would be needed to provide cold cardioplegia to the aortic root, but placement of this clamp is not possible if the proximal aorta is involved. CPB, cardiopulmonary bypass. (From Benumof JL. Intraoperative considerations for special thoracic surgery cases. In: Benumof JL, ed. *Anesthesia for thoracic surgery.* Philadelphia: WB Saunders, 1987:384, with permission.)

with an integral artificial valve) or an aortic valve replacement with a graft sewn to the native annulus can be used. The coronary arteries must be reimplanted into the wall of the composite graft and may not require reimplantation when separate aortic valve replacement and grafts are used, depending on whether enough of the native sinus of Valsalva remains (Fig. 24.5). The posterior wall of the old aneurysm can be wrapped around the graft material and sewn in place to maximize hemostasis.

In patients with ascending dissections, the aortic root is opened and the site of the intimal tear is located. A section of the aorta that includes the intimal tear is excised, and the edges of the true and false lumens are sewn together. A section of graft is used to replace the excised portion of the aorta.

6. **Complications.** Complications are those that occur with any procedure involving CPB and an open ventricle and include the following:

a. Air emboli

b. Atheromatous or clot emboli

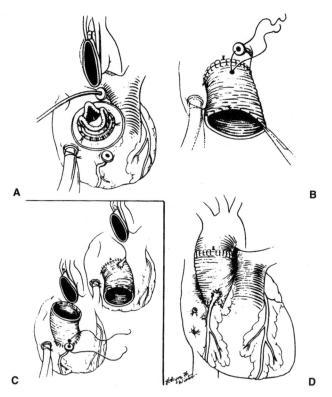

FIG. 24.5 Surgical repair of ascending aortic aneurysm or dissection. **A:** Aortic valve has been replaced and the aorta is transected at native annulus, leaving "buttons" of aortic wall around coronary ostia. **B:** Graft material anastomosed to the annulus, with left coronary reimplantation. **C:** Completion of left and beginning of right coronary reimplantation. **D:** Completion of distal graft anastomosis. (From Miller DC, Stinson EB, Oyer PE, et al. Concomitant resection of ascending aortic aneurysm and replacement of the aortic valve— operative results and long-term results with "conventional" techniques in ninety patients. *J Thorac Cardiovasc Surg* 1980;79:394, with permission.)

    c. LV dysfunction secondary to ischemia

    d. Myocardial infarction or myocardial ischemia secondary to technical problems with reimplantation of the coronaries

    e. Renal or respiratory failure

    f. Clotting abnormalities

    g. Surgical hemostasis; bleeding from suture lines can be especially difficult to control.

D. Anesthetic considerations for ascending aortic surgery

  1. Monitoring

    a. Arterial catheter placement. Because the right subclavian artery may be involved in either the disease process or the surgical repair, a left radial or femoral arterial catheter is inserted for monitoring BP.

    b. ECG. Five-lead, calibrated ECG should be used to monitor both leads II and V_5.

    c. PA catheter. Because of the advanced age of many of these patients and the presence of severe systemic disease, a PA catheter can be a useful aid in management preoperatively and postoperatively, but it is not mandatory.

    d. Two-dimensional echocardiography. In addition to its preoperative diagnostic importance, TEE is a useful adjunct in the intraoperative management of these patients. The diagnosis of hypovolemia, hypocontractility, myocardial ischemia, intracardiac air, and valvular dysfunction can be made with TEE. Caution should be exercised when placing this probe in the presence of a large ascending aortic aneurysm.

    e. Neurologic monitors

      (1) Electroencephalogram. For evaluating brain function, either raw or processed electroencephalographic data may be helpful for judging the adequacy of cerebral perfusion during CPB. Newer monitors such as the bispectral index may help to assess the depth of anesthesia during these procedures.

      (2) Temperature. When correctly placed, a nasopharyngeal temperature probe gives the anesthesiologist an approximation of brain temperature. Rectal temperature also should be monitored.

    f. Renal monitors. As with all cases involving bypass, urine output should be monitored.

  2. Induction and anesthetic agents. See Table 24.9.

  3. Cooling and rewarming. Hypothermic CPB is used in most cases of ascending aneurysms. Deep hypothermic circulatory arrest (DHCA) is needed if the proximal arch is involved. If femoral cannulation is used and the femoral artery is small, a smaller cannula may be needed. This probably will delay cooling and rewarming, because lower blood flows are used to avoid excessive arterial line pressures. Extra time for cooling and rewarming must be allowed in this setting.

E. Aortic arch surgery

  1. Surgical approach. The aortic arch is approached through a median sternotomy.

  2. Cardiopulmonary bypass. CPB is required, and femoral cannulation must be used in almost all cases.

  3. Technique. Typical placement of clamps for this procedure is shown in Figure 24.6. Note that the surgical technique dictates that the cerebral vessels be clamped to resect the aneurysmal or dissected section of aortic arch.

    The attachments of the arch vessels usually are excised *en bloc* so that all three vessels are located on one "button" of tissue, as shown in Figure 24.7. This facilitates rapid reimplantation of vessels and reestablishment of blood flow. Once the distal anastomosis is completed, the surgeon sutures the button of arch vessels to the graft material. The clamp can be replaced more proximally, the arch portion of the graft de-aired, the distal aortic clamp removed, and flow reestablished to the cerebral vessels from the femoral CPB aortic cannula. Thus, the time of brain ischemia is minimized. The proximal anastomosis then is completed.

Table 24.9 Anesthetic considerations and choice of anesthetic agent for surgery of the aorta

Patient variables	Opioids[a]	Volatile agent[b]	Other intravenous agents
Full stomach	Rapid acting (especially sufentanil, alfentanil)	Prolonged induction	Rapid acting if tolerated
Hemodynamic instability	Minimal myocardial depression Potent analgesics useful for treating intraoperative hypertension	Dose-dependent myocardial depression Indicated if hypertensive with adequate cardiac output	T,P: Myocardial depression M, E: Minimal myocardial depression K: Worsens hypertension
Ventricular function (VF)	Indicated with poor VF	Use only in patients with good VF	M, E, and K maintain VF Avoid T,P if VF is poor
Neurologic function	Decrease $CMRo_2$	Decrease $CMRo_2$, especially isoflurane; unclear *in vivo* protective effects	T,P decrease $CMRo_2$, probably protective, used with hypothermic arrest or open ventricle
Myocardial ischemia (coronary involvement)	Oxygen balance: Increases supply/demand ratio and therefore will have adverse effects in presence of hypertension	Decrease supply/demand ratio but will have negative effect in presence of hypotension	T,P: Adversely affects supply secondary to hypotension K: Increases oxygen demand, decreases supply (secondary to tachycardia)

[a] Refers to fentanyl, sufentanil, and alfentanil.
[b] Halothane, sevoflurane, desflurane, and isoflurane.
$CMRo_2$, cerebral metabolic rate of oxygen consumption; E, etomidate; K, ketamine; M, midazolam; P, propofol; T, thiopental.

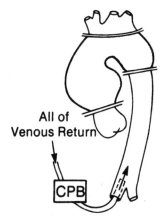

FIG. 24.6 Representation of cannula and clamp placement for surgery of the aortic arch. Femoral bypass is used. Proximal clamp is placed to arrest the heart. Distal clamp isolates the arch so that the distal anastomosis can be performed. Middle clamp on major branches isolates the head vessels so that *en bloc* attachment to graft is possible. CPB, cardiopulmonary bypass. (From Benumof JL. Intraoperative considerations for special thoracic surgery cases. In: Benumof JL, ed. *Anesthesia for thoracic surgery*. Philadelphia: WB Saunders, 1987:384, with permission.)

4. **Cerebral protection.** Resection of aortic arch aneurysms involves interruption or alteration of cerebral blood flow. Various surgical techniques have been used to prevent cerebral ischemia. All involve cooling the brain to reduce metabolic rate and the buildup of toxic metabolites.
   a. DHCA has been adopted by many surgeons as a technically advantageous way to repair aortic arch pathology, because blood flow is stopped and exposure maximized. DHCA requires core cooling to 15° to 22°C, depending on the exact technique used. Turning off the pump and partially draining the patient's blood volume into the pump provide a bloodless field with hypothermic brain protection for up to 45 minutes. This has improved results but is associated with longer bypass runs.
   b. Because of the time limits inherent with DHCA, some groups began using DHCA in conjunction with retrograde cerebral perfusion (RCP) through the superior vena cava as a method of brain protection. This technique has gained acceptance in many centers because it prolongs the "safe time" allowed for what can be a complicated reconstruction of the aortic arch and its vessels. Advantages of RCP include uniform cooling, efficient de-airing of the cerebral vessels (thus reducing the risk of embolism), and provision of oxygen and energy substrates. Outcome studies have identified the following risk factors for mortality and morbidity in RCP during DHCA: time on CPB, urgency of surgery, and patient age [4].
   c. Another technique that has been used with success is continuous anterograde cold blood cerebral perfusion. With this technique, the brain is selectively perfused via the brachiocephalic arteries with cold blood (6° to 12°C) while the patient is maintained at moderate core temperature. As shown in Figure 24.8, the cerebral perfusate is derived from the oxygenator and distributed via a separate roller pump, much the same as anterograde blood cardioplegia. This technique has largely supplanted the older technique of individual cannulation and perfusion of the carotid vessels because of technical considerations. Anterograde perfusion takes advantage of autoregulation of cerebral blood flow, which is thought to remain intact even

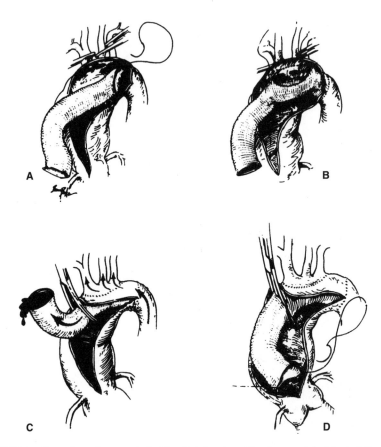

FIG. 24.7 Aortic arch replacement. **A:** The distal suture line is completed first, followed by (**B**) reattachment of the arch vessels. **C:** Flow is reestablished to these vessels by moving the clamp more proximally. **D:** The proximal suture line is completed. (From Crawford ES, Saleh SA. Transverse aortic arch aneurysm—improved results of treatment employing new modifications of aortic reconstruction and hypokalemic cerebral circulatory arrest. *Ann Surg* 1981;194:186, with permission.)

at low temperature. With intact autoregulation, physiologic protection against ischemia of hyperperfusion will be active. One of the chief advantages of this technique is that DHCA is required only for completion of the distal anastomosis. Because of these advantages, some groups believe that continuous anterograde perfusion is the safest method of brain protection during aortic arch surgery [5].

    5. Complications. Complications from this operation are similar to those with any procedure using CPB. Irreversible cerebral ischemia is a distinct possibility with this type of surgery. Hemostatic difficulties may be increased secondary to the multiple suture lines and long bypass time.

  F. Anesthetic considerations for aortic arch surgery
    1. Monitoring
      a. Arterial BP. An intraarterial catheter can be placed in either the right or left radial artery for prebypass management if the innominate or left

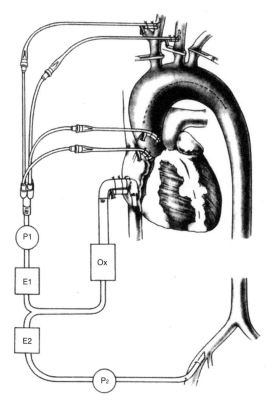

FIG. 24.8 Perfusion circuit for anterograde cerebral perfusion for aortic arch surgery. Venous blood from the right atrium drains to the oxygenator (*Ox*), and cooled to 28°C by heat exchange (*E2*) before passing via the main roller pump (*P2*) to a femoral artery. A second circuit derived from the oxygenator with a separate heat-exchanger (*E1*) and roller pump (*P1*) provides blood at 6° to 12°C to the brachiocephalic and coronary arteries. (From Bachet J, Guilmet D, Goudot B, et al. Antegrade cerebral perfusion with cold blood: a 13 year experience. *Ann Thorac Surg* 1999;67:1875, with permission.)

subclavian arteries, respectively, are not involved. If both are involved, the femoral artery should be catheterized.
   b. Neurologic monitors
      (1) Electroencephalography can be useful not only for ensuring that adequate cooling has been achieved but also for titration of the thiopental dose for brain protection.
      (2) Nasal temperature will verify adequate brain cooling.
   c. Transesophageal echocardiography. TEE provides useful information similar to that for ascending aortic surgery (see Section **IV.D.1**), but care should be taken when placing the probe.
2. Choice of anesthetic agents. See Table 24.9.
3. Management of hypothermic circulatory arrest. The technique involves core cooling to 15° to 20°C, packing the head in ice, using other cerebral protective agents, avoiding glucose-containing solutions, and using proper monitoring. More details are provided in Chapter 23.

4. **Complications.** Complications related to anesthesia for this procedure are uncommon. One is myocardial depression secondary to the use of thiopental for cerebral protection, and inotropic agents may be needed to wean the patient from CPB.

G. **Descending thoracic aortic surgery**

1. **Surgical approach.** Exposure of the descending aorta is accomplished through a left thoracotomy incision, usually between the fourth and fifth ribs. A double intercostal incision may be necessary for complete exposure (Fig. 24.9). The patient is placed in a full right lateral decubitus position with the hips slightly rolled to the left to allow access to the femoral vessels. When positioning the patient, it is important to provide protection to pressure points, including use of axillary roll, pillows between the knees, and pads for the head and elbows. It is important to maintain the occiput in line with the thoracic spine to prevent traction on the brachial plexus.

2. **Surgical techniques.** Whether an aneurysm, dissection, or rupture is being treated, the surgical technique involves placing cross-clamps above and below the lesion, opening the aorta, and replacing the diseased segment with a graft.

   a. **Simple cross-clamping.** Many groups report success with cross-clamping the aorta above and below the lesion without adjuncts to maintain distal perfusion. This technique has the advantage of simplifying the operation and reducing the amount of heparin needed (Fig. 24.10).

   Clamping the descending aorta produces marked hemodynamic changes: profound **hypertension** in the proximal aorta and **hypotension** below the distal clamp. The increase in afterload that occurs when the majority of the cardiac output goes only to the great vessels causes acute elevations in LV filling pressures and a progressive fall in cardiac output. The presumption is that LV failure will result if this afterload is maintained for

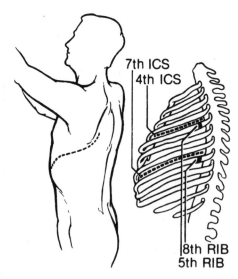

FIG. 24.9 Surgical approach to an extensive aneurysm or dissection involving the descending thoracic aorta. A single musculocutaneous incision and a double intercostal incision are used. The standard proximal and distal intercostal incisions are made through the fourth and seventh intercostal spaces (*ICS*), respectively. A traumatic aortic rupture at the isthmus usually can be reached through a single intercostal incision. (From Cooley DA, ed. *Surgical treatment of aortic aneurysms.* Philadelphia: WB Saunders, 1986:63, with permission.)

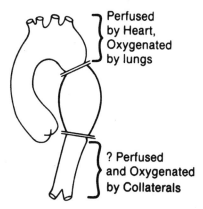

Perfused
by Heart,
Oxygenated
by lungs

? Perfused
and Oxygenated
by Collaterals

FIG. 24.10 Illustration of simple cross-clamp placement for repair of descending aortic aneurysm or dissection. Distal clamp placement dictates that flow to the spinal cord and major organs proceeds through collateral vessels. (From Benumof JL. Intraoperative considerations for special thoracic surgery cases. In: Benumof JL, ed. *Anesthesia for thoracic surgery.* Philadelphia: WB Saunders, 1987:384, with permission.)

any significant length of time. The acute increase in pressure proximal to the clamp can precipitate a catastrophic cerebral event (e.g., rupture of a cerebral aneurysm).

Mean arterial pressure distal to the cross-clamp decreases to less than 10% to 20% of control. This decrease is paralleled by a decrease in renal blood flow and spinal cord blood flow. The presence of a chronic obstruction to flow and the resultant well-developed collateral flow (i.e., coarctation) will lessen the hemodynamic changes that usually are seen. Examples of BPs above and below a cross-clamp from a series of patients with different aortic pathologies are listed in Table 24.10.

The use of an "open" technique of simple aortic cross-clamping has been advocated. With this technique, no distal cross-clamp is used, thereby

Table 24.10 Proximal versus distal blood pressure in simple aortic clamp

	Proximal systolic to diastolic (mm Hg)	Distal mean (mm Hg)
Coarctation	160/85	23
	145/80	54
	150/85	18
	155/80	36
Average	152/82	33
Thoracic aneurysm	260/160	12
	240/135	8
	245/150	24
	235/140	4
	240/155	10
	255/160	6
Average	245/150	10

Modified from Romagnoli A, Cooper JR Jr. Anesthesia for aortic operation. *Cleve Clin Q* 1983;48:150.

allowing direct inspection of the distal aorta for thrombus or debris. More importantly, graft material can be anastomosed in an oblique fashion that incorporates the maximal number of intercostal arteries.

b. **Shunts.** A method that provides decompression of the proximal aorta and perfusion of the distal segment involves placement of a heparin-bonded (Gott) extracorporeal shunt from the LV, aortic arch, or left subclavian artery to the femoral artery (Fig. 24.11). Systemic heparinization is not required. The advantage with this technique is that distal perfusion can be maintained while decompression of the proximal aorta is achieved. The major problems with this technique are technical difficulties with placement and kinking with inadequate distal flows. Two sizes of these shunts are available: 7 mm (5-mm inner diameter) and 9 mm (6-mm inner diameter). The limitations on flow imposed by these relatively small diameters interfere with the actual proximal ventricular decompression and augmentation of distal perfusion pressure that can be achieved.

c. **Extracorporeal circulation.** Historically the first method used for distal perfusion and proximal decompression, extracorporeal circulation (ECC) is being used more often after a period of being out of favor at many centers. There are several ways to perform ECC; all involve removal of blood, passage of blood to an extracorporeal pump, and reinfusion of blood into the femoral artery to perfuse the aorta below the distal cross-clamp (Fig. 24.12). Blood can be returned to the pump from the femoral vein, which is technically the easiest site to use. However, this site requires placement of an oxygenator in the circuit. Alternatively, the left atrium or LV apex may be cannulated for blood return to the pump. The pump may be a standard double roller (positive displacement) or a centrifugal (kinetic) type.

Each of these variations has disadvantages. Use of an oxygenator requires complete systemic heparinization, which is associated with increased incidence of hemorrhage, especially into the left lung. Left atrial or ventricular cannulation without an oxygenator may allow use of less heparin but carries an increased risk of air embolism. Table 24.11 summarizes the

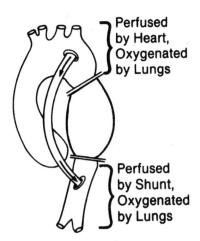

Perfused
by Heart,
Oxygenated
by Lungs

Perfused
by Shunt,
Oxygenated
by Lungs

FIG. 24.11 Placement of a heparin-coated vascular shunt from proximal to distal aorta during repair of descending aneurysm or dissection. (From Benumof JL. Intraoperative considerations for special thoracic surgery cases. In: Benumof JL, ed. *Anesthesia for thoracic surgery.* Philadelphia: WB Saunders, 1987:384, with permission.)

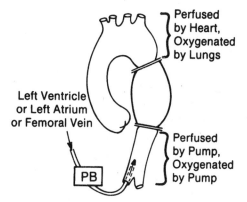

Left Ventricle
or Left Atrium
or Femoral Vein

Perfused
by Heart,
Oxygenated
by Lungs

Perfused
by Pump,
Oxygenated
by Pump

PB

FIG. 24.12 Partial bypass *(PB)* [or extracorporeal circulation (ECC)] method for maintaining distal perfusion pressure and preventing proximal hypertension. Oxygenated blood can be taken directly from the left ventricle or atrium (or aortic arch) and pumped either by roller head or centrifugal pump into the femoral artery. Alternatively, unoxygenated blood can be taken from the femoral vein, passed through a separate oxygenator, and pumped into the femoral artery. Use of an oxygenator dictates the use of a full heparinizing dose. (From Benumof JL. Intraoperative considerations for special thoracic surgery cases. In: Benumof JL, ed. *Anesthesia for thoracic surgery.* Philadelphia: WB Saunders, 1987:384, with permission.)

possible cannulation sites and major differences between heparinized shunts and ECC for distal perfusion.

3. **Complications of repair**

   a. **Cardiac.** Cardiac disorders (myocardial infarction, dysrhythmia, or low-output syndrome) are a significant (20% to 40%) cause of death in patients with all types of descending aortic repair.

   b. **Hemorrhage.** This is a common cause of death (20% to 30%) in all types of repair of the descending aorta.

   c. **Renal failure.** The incidence of renal failure ranges from 4% to 9% among survivors, with a much higher incidence among nonsurvivors. The etiology is presumed to be a decrease in renal blood flow during aortic cross-clamping. However, renal failure may occur in the presence of apparently adequate perfusion (heparinized shunt or ECC). Preexisting impairment of renal blood flow from a dissection involving the renal arteries increases the incidence of renal failure.

   d. **Paraplegia.** Most case reviews report the incidence of paraplegia as being in the range from 6% to 10%. [6] This is probably the most devastating morbid event because it is irreversible. The cause is either interruption or prolonged hypoperfusion (more than 30 minutes) of the blood supply to the anterior spinal artery. The anterior spinal artery is formed from the vertebral arteries rostrally. As it descends, it also receives blood from radicular arteries, which arise from the intercostal arteries (Fig. 24.13). In a majority of patients, one of these radicular arteries, the great radicular artery (of Adamkiewicz), contributes a major portion of the supply to the midportion of the anterior spinal artery. Unfortunately, this vessel is almost impossible to identify angiographically or by inspection at operation. It may arise anywhere from T_5 to below L_1. These anatomic considerations place blood flow in this artery at higher risk intraoperatively and postoperatively. Interruption of flow in this vessel may lead to paraplegia, depending on the contribution available from other collaterals. An anterior

Table 24.11 Options for increasing distal perfusion in descending aortic surgery

| Blood removed from | Blood infused into | Heparinized shunt | Perfusion apparatus | | Extracorporeal bypass | |
			Roller	Centrifugal	Oxygenator	Heparin (ACT)[a]
LV, AoA, LSA	FA, DAo	Yes	No	No	No	None (nl)
FV	FA, DAo	No	Either		Yes	Full (>480)
LA, AoA, LSA, LV	FA, DAo	No	No	Yes	No	Minimum (nl–250)[b]

[a] Refers to the activated clotting time (in seconds); if used, optimum ACT is controversial.
[b] Some groups will not use heparin when using a centrifugal pump.

AoA, aortic arch; DAo, descending aorta; FA, femoral artery; FV, femoral vein; LA, left atrium; nl, normal; LSA, left subclavian artery; LV, left ventricle.

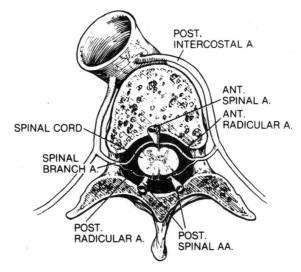

FIG. 24.13 Anatomic drawing of the contribution of the radicular arteries to spinal cord blood flow. If the posterior intercostal artery is involved in a dissection or is sacrificed to facilitate repair of aortic pathology, critical blood supply may be lost, causing spinal cord ischemia. (From Cooley DA, ed. *Surgical treatment of aortic aneurysms.* Philadelphia: WB Saunders, 1986:92, with permission.)

spinal syndrome can result, in which motor function is lost (anterior horns) but some sensation remains intact (posterior columns).

    e. Miscellaneous. Many other complications may arise. Some are a function of the type of pathology. For example, death from multiple organ trauma is a major factor in patients who survive traumatic rupture. Respiratory failure alone and as a component of multiple organ failure is more common with thoracic aortic disease than with abdominal aortic disease. Cerebrovascular accidents are seen in a small number of patients, as is left vocal cord paralysis due to recurrent laryngeal nerve damage.

H. Anesthetic considerations in descending aortic surgery

    1. General considerations. Anesthesia for descending aortic surgery can be one of the most demanding cases because of the profound changes in numerous organ systems. This topic is summarized in several good reviews [7,8].

    2. Monitoring

        a. Arterial BP. A right radial or brachial arterial catheter is needed to monitor pressures above the cross-clamp because the left subclavian artery may be compromised by the cross-clamp. To assess perfusion distal to the lower aortic clamp, many anesthesia and surgical teams prefer to monitor pressure below the clamp also, which requires placement of a femoral arterial catheter. Should a partial bypass technique be used, the left femoral artery is cannulated for distal perfusion and the right femoral artery is used for BP monitoring.

        b. Ventricular function. Some operative teams prefer to monitor LV function during proximal cross-clamping and therefore insert a PA catheter to follow filling pressures and cardiac output.

        c. Other monitors. Additional monitors used are similar to those used for other thoracic procedures: ECG (standard lead V_5 cannot be used because of the surgical approach), pulse oximetry, core temperature, and urine output. TEE would be useful to assess ventricular function and filling volumes during these cases, but anatomic interference by the probe in the surgical field may preclude its use.

3. **One-lung anesthesia.** Double-lumen endobronchial tubes are recommended not only to improve surgical exposure but also to provide an element of patient safety. By collapsing the left lung, trauma to that lung is decreased. If manipulation during surgery causes hemorrhage into the airway, the contralateral (right) lung is protected from blood spillage. A left-sided tube is technically easier to place and is used often, but it may be impossible to insert in some patients because of aneurysmal distortion of the trachea or left main stem bronchus. Patients with aortic rupture may have a distorted left main stem bronchus. Right-sided tubes may be used, but proper alignment with the right upper lobe bronchus should be checked with a fiberoptic bronchoscope. Alternatively, tubes with an endobronchial blocker should be considered in cases where adequate placement of a double-lumen tube cannot be achieved. For a detailed description of double-lumen or endobronchial blocker tube placement and single-lung ventilation, see Chapter 25.

4. **Conduct of anesthesia before and during cross-clamping.** Before the aorta is cross-clamped, mannitol (0.5 g/kg) should be infused to provide some renal protection during clamping. Even though a shunting procedure will be used, changes in the distribution of renal blood flow make mannitol administration prudent. In addition, sodium nitroprusside should be mixed and ready for infusion.

After the clamp is applied, it is important to closely monitor acid–base status with serial arterial blood gas measurements. It is common for metabolic acidosis to develop due to hypoperfusion of critical organ beds, and this should be treated aggressively if the patient is normothermic. If simple cross-clamping without adjuncts is used, proximal hypertension should be controlled, again with the realization that distal organ flow may be diminished. In treating proximal hypertension, regional blood flow studies have shown that nitroprusside infusion may decrease renal and spinal cord blood flow in a dose-related fashion. Ideally, cross-clamp time (regardless of technique) should be less than 30 minutes, because the incidence of complications, especially paraplegia, begins to increase above this limit.

If a heparinized shunt has been placed and proximal **hyper**tension cannot be treated without producing subsequent distal **hypo**tension (less than 60 mm Hg), the surgeon should be made aware that there may be a technical problem with shunt placement. If partial bypass (ECC) is used, the pump speed or venous return can be adjusted so that control of proximal hypertension can be maintained by adequate unloading while the lower body is simultaneously perfused. Usually little or no pharmacologic intervention is necessary in this case because the pump speed and manipulation of venous return provide rapid control of proximal and distal pressures. Table 24.12 lists the treatment options for several clinical scenarios during ECC.

Before removal of the cross-clamp, a vasopressor should be available. The anesthesiologist must be constantly aware of the stage of operation so that major events such as clamping and declamping may be anticipated.

5. **Declamping shock.** When **simple cross-clamping** of the aorta is used, subsequent unclamping can lead to serious and even life-threatening consequences, usually severe hypotension or myocardial depression. There are several theoretical causes of this declamping syndrome, including washout of acid metabolites, vasodilator substances, sequestration of blood in the lower extremities, and reactive hyperemia. The usual cause, however, is relative or absolute hypovolemia. To attenuate the effects of clamp removal, in the 10 to 15 minutes before unclamping of the thoracic aorta, the volume status of the patient should be optimized. This includes elevating filling pressures by infusing blood products, colloid, or crystalloids. Some advocate prophylactic bicarbonate administration just before clamp removal to minimize the myocardial depression caused by the acidosis that occurs following removal. It is advisable for the surgeon to release the cross-clamp slowly over a period of 1 to 2 minutes to allow enough time for compensatory changes to occur.

Table 24.12 Management of extracorporeal circulation for surgery of the descending aorta

Proximal arterial pressure	Distal arterial pressure	Pulmonary wedge pressure	Treatment
↑	↓	↓	Volume; increase pump flow
↑	↓	↑	Increase pump flow
↑	↑	↓	Volume; vasodilator
↑	↑	↑	Vasodilator; diuretic; maintain pump flow, hold volume in pump reservoir (if in use)
↓	↓	↓	Volume; look for partial occlusion of arterial outflow cannula (if reservoir in use)
↓	↓	↑	Increase pump flow; inotrope
↓	↑	↑	Decrease pump flow; inotrope; diuretic
↓	↑	↓	Decrease pump flow; may need volume

Vasopressors may be needed to compensate for hypotension but must be used with care because even transient hypertension may result in significant bleeding. With a volume-loaded patient and slow clamp release, any significant hypotension usually is short lived and well tolerated. If hypotension is severe, the easiest maneuver is reapplication of the clamp to allow further volume infusion.

If shunts or ECC is used, declamping hypotension usually is attenuated because the vascular bed below the clamp is less "empty." ECC also provides a means of rapid volume infusion if a reservoir is used.

6. **Fluid therapy and transfusion.** Even patients undergoing elective repair of a descending aneurysm may be relatively hypovolemic, and fluid therapy should have the following aims: correct this fluid deficit, provide maintenance fluids, compensate for evaporative and "third space" losses, decrease red cell loss by mild hemodilution, and replace blood loss as needed.

Despite proximal and distal control of the aorta, blood loss can be considerable in these cases due to back-bleeding from the intercostal arteries. These collateral vessels often are ligated on opening the aorta. Use of cell-scavenging devices has become common and has reduced the need for banked blood, but because massive losses may occur, banked blood may still be needed. As long as liver perfusion is adequate, even with a large blood loss, citrate toxicity usually is not a problem because of rapid "first pass" metabolism in the liver. Repair of a thoracic aneurysm with simple clamping, however, presents a unique situation—the liver is not perfused. In this circumstance, transfusion of large amounts of banked blood may rapidly produce citrate toxicity, resulting in myocardial depression that requires calcium chloride infusion.

7. **Spinal cord protection.** Several methods have been espoused to provide protection of the spinal cord during cross-clamping in addition to ECC, shunts, and expeditious surgery [9].

   a. **Maintaining perfusion pressure.** Some groups prefer to maintain perfusion pressure of the distal aorta in the range from 40 to 60 mm Hg to increase blood flow to the middle and lower spinal cord. This practice should be regarded as controversial because at present there are few data on outcome supporting this position. **No method used to maintain blood flow to the distal aorta (i.e., shunt or partial bypass) guarantees that spinal cord blood flow, and therefore function, will be maintained.** Proximal and distal clamp placement to isolate the diseased aortic segment may include critical intercostal vessels that provide flow to the cord and whose loss is not compensated by distal perfusion. In addition, distal perfusion may be hindered by the presence of atherosclerotic disease in the abdominal aorta, a condition that may prevent significant flow to the kidneys and spinal cord. Last, these crucial vessels may be disrupted in gaining surgical exposure. One should never assume that the cord and kidneys are absolutely "protected" because a shunt or partial bypass has been used. The largest studies have shown no difference in the incidence of paraplegia regardless of the surgical adjunct used.

   b. Somatosensory-evoked potentials. Somatosensory-evoked potentials (SEPs) have been promoted as a means of assessing functional status of the spinal cord during periods of possible ischemia [10]. Briefly, SEPs monitor spinal cord function by stimulating a peripheral nerve and monitoring the response in the brainstem and cerebral cortex. Normal SEPs seem to ensure the integrity of the posterior (sensory) columns. However, SEPs have several shortcomings. First, during aortic surgery, it is the *anterior* (motor) horns that are more at risk. Perhaps for this reason, there have been reports of patients who had normal SEPs during cross-clamping and who subsequently were found to have paraplegia. Second, it must be remembered that many anesthetics, including all of the halogenated drugs, nitrous oxide, and several IV drugs (e.g., thiopental and propofol) will alter the amplitude and latency of the evoked potential. In addition, if simple cross-clamping is used, ischemia of the peripheral nerves will interfere with SEP interpretation.

   Other than being used as an intraoperative tool to help identify intercostal arteries that should be reimplanted to preserve spinal cord perfusion, SEP monitoring has not been shown to decrease the incidence of paraplegia.

   c. Motor-evoked potentials. Because of the noted deficiencies in SEP monitoring, the use of motor evoked potentials has been advocated as a superior monitor of spinal cord ischemia [11]. Motor evoked potentials can accurately monitor the integrity of the anterior horn of the spinal cord and currently are used during procedures of the spinal column. However, because access to the central nerve roots for direct stimulation is not possible in thoracic surgery, transcranial stimulation over the motor cortex has been used. In addition to being cumbersome, this method has been reported to trigger seizures in susceptible patients. However, some groups have experienced success in the application of this method.

   d. Hypothermia. Allowing the core temperature to be reduced to approximately 33° to 34°C will lower the metabolic rate of the spinal cord tissue and may provide some protection from reduced or interrupted blood flow. Adequate temperature reduction usually can be accomplished with topical cooling agents (cooling blankets, bags of crushed ice). Iced saline gastric lavage also may be used. Administration of even 1 or 2 units of cool banked blood (only if indicated) will lower the core temperature. Precise control of temperature is difficult. At temperatures below 32°C, the myocardium may become more irritable and prone to ventricular arrhythmias. These facts, plus the lack of improved outcome data, have resulted in sparse use of this technique.

   e. Spinal drains. Experimental data show that spinal cord damage may be mediated through the increase in cerebrospinal fluid (CSF) pressure that accompanies the reduction in spinal cord blood flow during cross-clamping. CSF pressure may be increased to as high as the mean distal **arterial** pressure. Because spinal cord blood flow is proportional to the mean arterial pressure minus the higher of the CSF or venous pressure, perfusion in this circumstance may be reduced to zero. A spinal drain would allow not only for measurement of the intraspinal pressure but also for therapeutic reduction of CSF pressure by its removal and an increase in spinal cord blood flow. As a note of caution, removal of CSF in the presence of an elevated intraspinal pressure may provide a gradient for herniation of cerebral structures. In addition, placement of a spinal drain followed by systemic heparinization may lead to the formation of an epidural hematoma as a rare complication. The use of spinal drains has increased because of the associated low morbidity and possible significant benefits [12]. To date, no controlled study has demonstrated a reduction in morbidity associated with the use of spinal drains.

    f. Other. Additional "protective" measures, such as IV steroids, pharmacologic suppression of spinal cord function through IV or intrathecal drug administration, local hypothermia, and free radical scavengers, are not widely used or are considered experimental.

  8. Prevention of renal failure. The etiologic cause of renal failure is thought to be ischemia from interruption of blood flow by clamping, although embolism remains another possibility. Use of CPB or a shunt may be protective, but superior outcome data are lacking, and renal failure still occurs despite these surgical adjuncts. Adequate volume loading should be used and probably is most important in renal protection. Mannitol may help, and because its use is innocuous in most patients it is recommended.

V. Future trends. Just as the past 40 years of treatment of aortic diseases have been highlighted by innovation and the refinement of surgical and anesthetic techniques, so also will the future. The most promising surgical developments have been made in the area of intraluminal stenting of aneurysmal segments of the thoracoabdominal aorta [13]. Anesthetic developments will focus on refinements in the pharmacology and physiology of organ preservation. Advances in both areas should continue to improve survival in patients with what once was considered to be a lethal disease [14,15].

References

1. Hartnell GG. Imaging of aortic aneurysms and dissection: CT and MRI. *J Thorac Imaging* 2001;16:35–46.
2. Nienaber CA, Von Kodolitsch Y, Nicolas V. The diagnosis of thoracic aortic dissection by noninvasive imaging procedures. *N Engl J Med* 1993;328:1–9.
3. Cooper JR Jr, Skeehan TM, Cooley DA. Resection of a thoracic aneurysm in a 57-year-old male [case conference]. *J Cardiothorac Vasc Anesth* 1991;5:390–398.
4. Ueda Y, Okita Y, Aomi S, et al. Retrograde cerebral perfusion for aortic arch surgery: analysis of risk factors. *Ann Thorac Surg* 1999;67:1879–1882.
5. Bachet J, Guilmet D, Goudot B, et al. Anterograde cerebral perfusion with cold blood: a 13-year experience. *Ann Thorac Surg* 1999;67:1874–1878.
6. **Shenaq SA, Svensson LG. Paraplegia following aortic surgery. *J Cardiothorac Vasc Anesth* 1993;7:81–94.**
7. **O'Connor CJ, Rothenberg DM. Anesthetic considerations for descending thoracic aortic surgery: part I. *J Cardiothorac Vasc Anesth* 1995;9:581–588.**
8. **O'Connor CJ, Rothenberg DM. Anesthetic considerations for descending thoracic aortic surgery: part II. *J Cardiothorac Vasc Anesth* 1995;9:734–737.**
9. Robertazzi RR, Cunningham JN Jr. Intraoperative adjuncts of spinal cord protection. *Semin Thorac Cardiovasc Surg* 1998;10:29–34.
10. **Robertazzi RR, Cunningham JN Jr. Monitoring of somatosensory evoked potentials: a primer on the intraoperative detection of spinal cord ischemia during reconstructive surgery. *Semin Thorac Cardiovasc Surg* 1998;10:11–17.**
11. DeHaan P, Kalkman CJ, Jacobs MJ. Spinal cord monitoring with myogenic motor evoked potentials: early detection of spinal cord ischemia as an integral part of spinal cord protective strategies during thoracoabdominal aneurysm surgery. *Semin Thorac Cardiovasc Surg* 1998;10:19–24.
12. Ling E, Arellano R. Systematic overview of the evidence supporting the use of cerebrospinal fluid drainage in thoracoabdominal aneurysm surgery for prevention of paraplegia. *Anesthesiology* 2000;93:1115–1122.
13. Mitchell RS. Endovascular solutions for diseases of the thoracic aorta. *Cardiol Clin* 1999; 17:815–825.
14. **Oliver WC Jr, Nuttall G, Murray MJ. Thoracic aortic disease. In: Kaplan JA, ed. *Cardiac anesthesia*, 4th ed. Philadelphia: WB Saunders, 1999;821–860.**
15. Gewertz BL, Schwartz LB, eds. *Surgery of the aorta and its branches.* Philadelphia: WB Saunders, 2000.

25. ANESTHETIC MANAGEMENT FOR SURGERY OF THE LUNGS AND MEDIASTINUM

Peter Slinger and Erin A. Sullivan

I. Preoperative assessment

A. Overview. Advances in anesthetic management, surgical techniques, and perioperative care have expanded the envelope of patients now considered to be operable. The principles described apply to all types of pulmonary resections and other chest surgery. In patients with malignancy, the risk/benefit ratio of canceling or delaying surgery pending other investigation/therapy is always complicated by the risk of further spread of cancer during any interval before resection.

A patient with a "resectable" lung cancer has a disease that is still local or locoregional in scope and can be encompassed in a plausible surgical procedure. An "operable" patient is one who can tolerate the proposed resection with acceptable risk.

1. Risk assessment. It is the anesthesiologist's responsibility to use the preoperative assessment to identify patients at elevated risk and then to use that risk assessment to stratify perioperative management and focus resources on the high-risk patients to improve their outcome. This is the primary function of the preanesthetic assessment.

2. Initial and final assessments. Commonly, the patient is initially assessed in a clinic and often not by the member of the anesthesia staff who will administer the anesthesia. The actual contact with the responsible anesthesiologist may be only 10 to 15 minutes before induction. It is necessary to organize and standardize the approach to preoperative evaluation for these patients into two temporally disjoint phases: the initial (clinic) assessment and the final (day-of-admission) assessment.

3. "Lung-sparing" surgery. Postoperative preservation of respiratory function has been shown to be proportional to the amount of functioning lung parenchyma preserved. To assess patients with limited pulmonary function, the anesthesiologist must understand these surgical options in addition to conventional lobectomy and pneumonectomy.

Prethoracotomy assessment naturally involves all of the factors of a complete anesthetic assessment: past history, allergies, medications, and upper airway. The major cause of perioperative morbidity and mortality in the thoracic surgical population is respiratory complications. Atelectasis, pneumonia, and respiratory failure occur in 15% to 20% of patients. Cardiac complications, such as arrhythmia and ischemia, occur in 10% to 15% of the thoracic population.

B. Risk stratification

1. Assessment of respiratory function. The best assessment of respiratory function comes from a history of the patient's quality of life. An asymptomatic American Society of Anesthesiologists (ASA) class I or II patient with full exercise capacity does not need screening cardiorespiratory testing. Assess respiratory function in three related but independent areas: respiratory mechanics, gas exchange, and cardiopulmonary interaction. These three factors give the "three-legged stool" of prethoracotomy respiratory assessment (Fig. 25.1).

a. Lung mechanics. The most valid single test for postthoracotomy respiratory complications is the predicted postoperative forced expiratory volume in 1 second (ppoFEV$_1$%) [1], which is calculated as:

$$\text{ppoFEV}_1\% = \text{preoperative FEV 1}\% \times \frac{1 - \%\ \textbf{functional lung tissue removed}}{100}$$

Consider the right upper and middle lobes combined as approximately equivalent to each of the other three lobes and the right lung 10% larger than the left lung.

Low risk   = >40% ppoFEV$_1$
Moderate risk = 30% to 40% ppoFEV$_1$
High risk   = <30% ppoFEV$_1$

b. Pulmonary parenchymal function. Traditionally arterial blood gas (ABG) data such as P$_a$O$_2$ less than 60 mm Hg or P$_a$CO$_2$ greater than 45 mm Hg have been used as cutoff values for pulmonary resection. Cancer resections

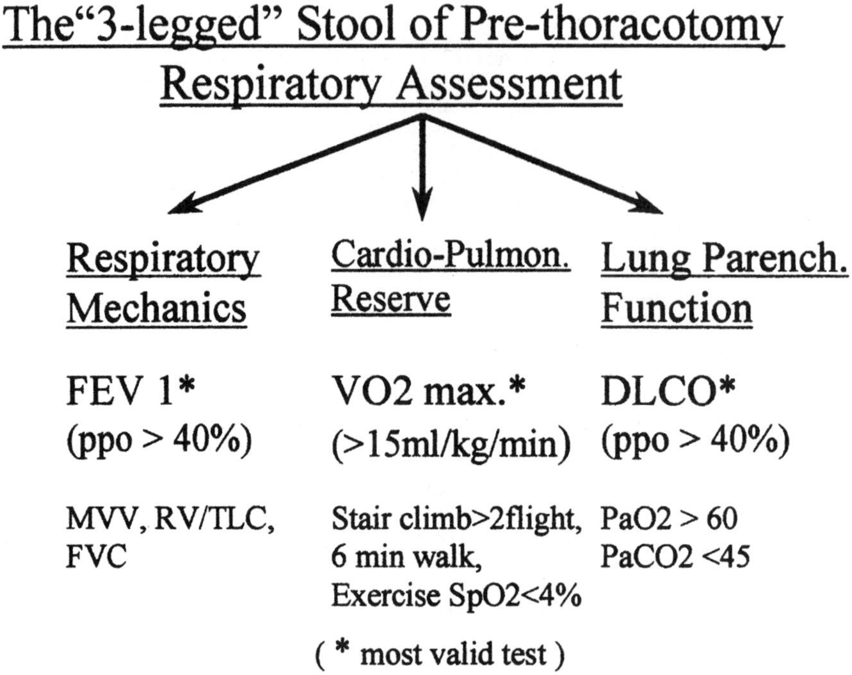

The "3-legged" Stool of Pre-thoracotomy Respiratory Assessment

Respiratory Mechanics	Cardio-Pulmon. Reserve	Lung Parench. Function
FEV 1* (ppo > 40%)	VO2 max.* (>15ml/kg/min)	DLCO* (ppo > 40%)
MVV, RV/TLC, FVC	Stair climb>2flight, 6 min walk, Exercise SpO2<4%	PaO2 > 60 PaCO2 <45

(* most valid test)

FIG. 25.1 "Three-legged" stool of prethoracotomy respiratory assessment.

now have been successfully done or even combined with volume reduction in patients who do not meet these criteria, although they remain useful as warning indicators of increased risk. The most useful test of the gas exchange capacity of the lung is the diffusing capacity for carbon monoxide (DLCO). DLCO correlates with the total functioning surface area of alveolar–capillary interface. A ppoDLCO less than 40% correlates with both increased respiratory and cardiac complications [2].

c. **Cardiopulmonary interaction.** The traditional, and still extremely useful, test in ambulatory patients is stair climbing. The ability to climb three flights or more is closely associated with decreased mortality. Less than two flights is very high risk. Formal laboratory exercise testing is currently the "gold standard" for assessment of cardiopulmonary function. The maximal oxygen consumption Vo$_2$max is the most valid exercise predictor of postthoracotomy outcome.

Low risk   = Vo$_2$max > 20 mL/kg/min
Moderate risk = Vo$_2$max 15 to 20 mL/kg/min
High risk   = Vo$_2$max < 15 mL/kg/min

The 6-minute walk test and exercise oximetry also correlate with Vo$_2$max.

d. **Ventilation–perfusion scintigraphy** is particularly useful in pneumonectomy patients and should be considered for any patient who has ppoFEV$_1$ less than 40%. Assessments of ppoFEV$_1$, DLCO, and Vo$_2$max can be upgraded if the lung region to be resected is nonfunctioning.

e. **Split-lung function studies.** These tests have not shown sufficient predictive validity for universal adoption in potential lung resection patients.

     f. **Flow–volume loops.** Flow–volume loops can help identify the presence of a variable intrathoracic airway obstruction by evidence of an exacerbation of an abnormal plateau of the expiratory limb with a change in the patient's position from sitting to supine. This can occur due to compression of a main conducting airway by a tumor mass. Such a problem may warrant induction airway management with awake intubation or maintenance of spontaneous ventilation. In an adult patient capable of giving a complete history who does not describe supine exacerbation of cough or dyspnea, flow–volume loops are not required as a routine preoperative test.

     g. **Combination of tests** (Fig. 25.2). If a patient has ppoFEV$_1$ greater than 40%, it should be possible for the patient to be extubated in the operating room at the conclusion of surgery, assuming the patient is alert, warm, and comfortable ("AWaC"). If ppoFEV$_1$ is greater than 30% and exercise tolerance and lung parenchymal function exceed the increased risk thresholds, then extubation in the operating room should be possible depending on the status of associated diseases. Patients with ppoFEV$_1$ 20% to 30% and favorable predicted cardiorespiratory and parenchymal function can be considered for early extubation if thoracic epidural analgesia is used [3].

2. Intercurrent medical conditions

    a. **Age.** For patients older than 80 years, the rate of respiratory complications (40%) is double that expected in a younger population, and the rate of cardiac complications (40%), particularly arrhythmias, is nearly triple. The mortality from pneumonectomy (22% in patients older than 70 years), particularly right pneumonectomy, is excessive.

    b. **Cardiac disease**

       (1) **Ischemia.** Pulmonary resection is generally regarded as an intermediate risk procedure for perioperative ischemia. Beyond the standard history, physical examination, and electrocardiogram, routine screening testing for cardiac disease does not appear to be cost effective for all prethoracotomy patients. Noninvasive testing is indicated in patients with major (unstable ischemia, recent infarction, severe valvular disease, significant arrhythmia) or intermediate (stable angina, remote infarction, previous congestive failure, or diabetes) clinical predictors of myocardial risk and in the elderly. Timing of lung resection surgery

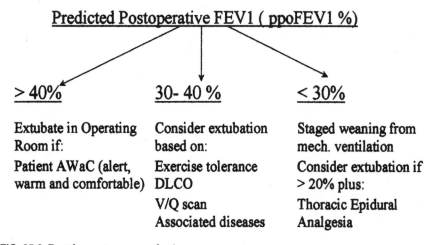

FIG. 25.2 Postthoracotomy anesthetic management.

after a myocardial infarction is always a difficult decision. Limiting the delay to 4 to 6 weeks in a medically stable and fully investigated and optimized patient seems acceptable.

   (2) **Arrhythmia.** Atrial fibrillation is a common complication (10% to 15%) of pulmonary resection surgery. Factors correlating with an increased incidence of arrhythmia are the amount of lung tissue resected, age, intraoperative blood loss, and intrapericardial dissection. Prophylactic digoxin does not prevent these arrhythmias, but diltiazem may.

   c. **Renal dysfunction.** Renal dysfunction after pulmonary resection surgery is associated with a high incidence of mortality [4]. The factors that are highly associated with an elevated risk of renal impairment are listed in Table 25.1.

   d. **Chronic obstructive pulmonary disease.** Assessment of the severity of chronic obstructive pulmonary disease (COPD) is based on FEV_1 % predicted, as follows—stage I: greater than 50%; stage II: 35% to 50%; and stage III: less than 35%. The following factors in COPD need to be considered.

   Respiratory drive. Many stage II or III COPD patients have an elevated P_aCO_2 at rest. It is not possible to differentiate "CO_2 retainers" from nonretainers on the basis of history, physical examination, or spirometry. These patients need an ABG preoperatively. Supplemental oxygen causes the P_aCO_2 to increase in CO_2 retainers by a combination of decreased respiratory drive and increased dead space.

   Nocturnal hypoxemia. COPD patients desaturate more frequently and severely than normal patients during sleep. This is due to the rapid/shallow breathing pattern that occurs during rapid eye movement sleep.

   Right ventricular (RV) dysfunction. Cor pulmonale occurs in 40% of adult COPD patients with FEV_1 less than 1 L and in 70% with FEV_1 less than 0.6 L. COPD patients who have resting P_aO_2 less than 55 mm Hg should receive supplemental home oxygen and those who desaturate to less than 44 mm Hg with exercise. The goal of supplemental oxygen is to maintain P_aO_2 60 to 65 mm Hg. Pneumonectomy candidates with ppoFEV_1 less than 40% should have transthoracic echocardiography to assess right heart function. Elevation of right heart pressures places these patients in a very high-risk group.

3. **Preoperative therapy of COPD.** The four treatable complications of COPD that must be actively sought and therapy begun at the initial prethoracotomy assessment are atelectasis, bronchospasm, chest infection, and pulmonary edema (Table 25.2). Patients with COPD have fewer postoperative pulmonary complications when a perioperative program of chest physiotherapy is initiated preoperatively. Pulmonary complications are decreased in thoracic surgical patients who are not smoking versus those who continue to smoke up until the time of surgery.

4. **Lung cancer considerations.** At the time of initial assessment, cancer patients should be assessed for the "4 M's" associated with malignancy: **M**ass effects, **M**etabolic abnormalities, **M**etastases, and **M**edications. Prior use of medications that can exacerbate oxygen-induced pulmonary toxicity, such as bleomycin, should be considered (Table 25.3).

Table 25.1 Factors associated with an increased risk of postthoracotomy renal impairment

1. Previous history of renal impairment
2. Diuretic therapy
3. Pneumonectomy
4. Postoperative infection
5. Blood loss requiring transfusion

Table 25.2 Step-by-step pharmacologic therapy for chronic obstructive pulmonary disease

1. For mild, variable symptoms:
   - Selective β_2-agonist MDI aerosol, 1–2 puffs every 2–6 h as needed, not to exceed 8–12 puffs per 24 h
2. For mild-to-moderate continuing symptoms:
   - Ipratropium MDI aerosol, 2–6 puffs every 6–8 h; not to be used more frequently
   plus
   - Selective β-agonist MDI aerosol, 1–4 puffs as required four times daily for rapid relief, when needed, or as regular supplement
3. If response to step 2 is unsatisfactory or there is a mild-to-moderate increase in symptoms:
   - Add sustained release theophylline 200–400 mg twice daily or 400–800 mg at bedtime for nocturnal bronchospasm
   and/or
   - Consider use of sustained release albuterol, 4–8 mg twice daily, or at night only
   and/or
   - Consider use of mucokinetic agent
4. If control of symptoms is suboptimal:
   - Consider course of oral steroids (e.g., prednisone), up to 40 mg/d for 10–14 d
   If improvement occurs, wean to low daily or alternate-day dose
   - If steroid appears to help, consider possible use of aerosol MDI, particularly if patient has evidence of bronchial hyperactivity
5. For severe exacerbation:
   - Increase β_2-agonist dosage, e.g., MDI with spacer 6–8 puffs every 30 min to 2 h or inhalant solution, unit dose every 30 min to 2 h or subcutaneous administration of epinephrine or terbutaline, 0.1–0.5 mL
   and/or
   - Increase ipratropium dosage, e.g., MDI with spacer 6–8 puffs every 3–4 h or inhalant solution of ipratropium 0.5 mg every 4–8 h
   and
   - Provide theophylline dosage intravenously with calculated amount to bring serum level to 10–12 µg/mL
   and
   - Provide methylprednisolone dosage intravenously giving 50–100 mg immediately, then every 6–8 h; taper as soon as possible
   and add:
   - An antibiotic, if indicated
   - A mucokinetic agent if sputum is very viscous

MDI, metered dose inhaler.

5. **Postoperative analgesia.** The risks and benefits of the various forms of post-thoracotomy analgesia should be explained to the patient at the time of initial preanesthetic assessment. Potential contraindications to specific methods of analgesia should be determined, such as coagulation problems, sepsis, and neurologic disorders. If the patient is to receive prophylactic anticoagulants and it is elected to use epidural analgesia, appropriate timing of anticoagulant

Table 25.3 Anesthetic considerations in lung cancer patients (the "4 M's")

1. **Mass effects:** Obstructive pneumonia, superior vena cava syndrome, tracheobronchial distortion, Pancoast syndrome, recurrent laryngeal nerve or phrenic nerve paresis
2. **Metabolic effects:** Lambert-Eaton syndrome, hypercalcemia, hyponatremia, Cushing syndrome
3. **Metastases:** Particularly to brain, bone, liver, and adrenal
4. **Medications:** Chemotherapy agents, pulmonary toxicity (bleomycin, mitomycin), cardiac toxicity (doxorubicin), renal toxicity (cis-platinum).

administration and neuraxial catheter placement need to be arranged. American Society of Regional Anethesia guidelines suggest an interval of 2 to 4 hours before or 1 hour after catheter placement for prophylactic heparin administration. Low-molecular-weight heparin precautions are less clear, but an interval of 12 to 24 hours before and 24 hours after catheter placement is recommended.

6. **Premedication.** Avoid inadvertent withdrawal of drugs that are being taken for concurrent medical conditions (bronchodilators, antihypertensives, β-blockers). For esophageal reflux surgery, oral antacid and H_2-blockers are routinely ordered preoperatively. Mild sedation, such as an intravenous (IV) short-acting benzodiazepine, often is given immediately before placement of invasive monitoring lines and catheters. In patients with copious secretions, an antisialagogue (e.g., glycopyrrolate 0.2 mg) is useful to facilitate fiberoptic bronchoscopy (FOB) for positioning of a double-lumen tube (DLT) or bronchial blocker (BB).

7. **Final preoperative assessment.** The final preoperative anesthetic assessment is made immediately before the patient is brought to the operating room. Review the data from the initial prethoracotomy assessment (Table 25.4) and the results of tests ordered at that time. Two other concerns for thoracic anesthesia need to be assessed: (i) the potential for difficult lung isolation and (ii) the risk of desaturation during one-lung ventilation (OLV).

   a. **Assessment of difficult endobronchial intubation.** The most useful predictor of difficult endobronchial intubation is the chest x-ray film. Clinically important tracheal or bronchial distortions or compression from tumors or previous surgery usually can be detected on plain chest films. Distal airway problems not detectable on the plain x-ray film may be visualized on chest computed tomographic (CT) scans. These abnormalities often will not be mentioned in a written or verbal report from the radiologist or surgeon. The anesthesiologist must examine the chest image before placing a DLT or BB.

   b. **Prediction of desaturation during OLV.** It is possible to determine patients who are most at risk for desaturation during OLV for thoracic surgery [5]. The factors that correlate with desaturation during OLV are listed in Table 25.5. The most useful prophylactic measure is the use of continuous positive airway pressure (CPAP) 2 to 5 cm H_2O of oxygen to the nonventilated lung.

   The most important predictor of P_aO_2 during OLV is the P_aO_2 during two-lung ventilation in the lateral position before OLV. The proportion of perfusion or ventilation to the nonoperated lung on preoperative ventilation–perfusion (V/Q) scans also correlates with the P_aO_2 during OLV. The side of the thoracotomy has an effect on P_aO_2 during OLV. With the left lung being 10% smaller than the right lung, there is less shunt when the left lung is collapsed. The degree of obstructive lung disease correlates in an

Table 25.4 Summary of preanesthetic assessment

Initial preanesthetic assessment for pulmonary resection
1. All patients: exercise tolerance, ppoFEV$_1$%,? postoperative analgesia, D/C smoking
2. Patients with ppoFEV$_1$ <40%: DLCO, V/Q scan, Vo$_2$ max
3. Cancer patients: the "4 M's": mass effects, metabolic effects, metastases, medications
4. Chronic obstructive pulmonary disease patients: Arterial blood gas, physiotherapy, bronchodilators
5. Increased renal risk: Serum creatinine, blood urea nitrogen

Final preanesthetic assessment for pulmonary resection
1. Review initial assessment and test results
2. Assess difficulty of lung isolation: Chest x-ray film, computed tomographic scan
3. Assess risk of hypoxemia during one-lung ventilation

D/C, discontinue DLCO, diffusing capacity for carbon monoxide; ppoFEV$_1$, predicted postoperative forced expiratory volume in 1 second; V/Q, ventilation/perfusion.

Table 25.5 Factors that correlate with an increased risk of desaturation during one-lung ventilation

---

1. High percentage of ventilation (V) or perfusion (Q) to the operative lung on preoperative V/Q scan
2. Poor P_aO_2 during two-lung ventilation, particularly in the lateral position intraoperatively
3. Right-sided surgery
4. Good preoperative spirometry (FEV_1 or FVC)

FEV_1, forced expiratory volume in 1 second;
FVC, forced vital capacity.

inverse fashion with P_aO_2 during OLV. Patients with more severe airflow limitation on preoperative spirometry tend to have a better P_aO_2 during OLV. This is related to the development of auto positive end-expiratory pressure (PEEP) during OLV in the obstructed patients.

Stratifying the perioperative risks allows the anesthesiologist to develop a systematic focused approach to these patients at the time of initial contact and immediately before induction, which can be used to guide anesthetic management (Fig. 25.2) [2].

II. Intraoperative management

A. Lung separation.
There are three basic options for lung separation: single-lumen endobronchial tubes (EBTs), DLTs, and BBs (Fig. 25.3). The second half of the twentieth century has seen refinements of the DLT from that of Carlens to a tube specifically designed for intraoperative use (Robertshaw) with larger, D-shaped lumens and without a carinal hook. Current disposable polyvinyl chloride DLTs have incorporated high-volume/low-pressure tracheal and bronchial cuffs. These recent DLT refinements have two major drawbacks: (i) the tubes require FOB for positioning; and (ii) a satisfactory right-sided DLT has not yet been designed that can deal with the short (average 2 cm) and variable length of the right main stem bronchus. Recently, there has been a revival of interest in BBs due to several factors: design advances such as the Univent tube and Arndt catheter [6]; greater familiarity of anesthesiologists with fiberoptic placement of BBs; and cost.

1. Indications for lung separation.
Absolute indications for lung isolation include purulent secretions, massive pulmonary hemorrhage, and bronchopleural fistula, blebs, and bullae (blood, pus, and air). More commonly, lung separation is provided intraoperatively to facilitate surgical exposure.

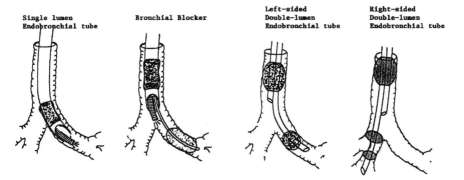

Single lumen
Endobronchial tube

Bronchial Blocker

Left-sided
Double-lumen
Endobronchial tube

Right-sided
Double-lumen
Endobronchial tube

FIG. 25.3 Methods of lung isolation.

2. **Techniques of lung separation.** The optimal methods for lung isolation are listed in Table 25.6. Because it is impossible to describe one technique as best in all indications for OLV, the various indications are considered separately.

   a. **Elective pulmonary resection, right-sided.** The first choice is a left DLT. The widest margin of safety in positioning is with left DLTs. With blind positioning, the incidence of malposition can exceed 20% but is correctable in virtually all cases by fiberoptic adjustment. There is continuous access to the nonventilated lung for suctioning, fiberoptic monitoring of position, and CPAP. There are two possible alternatives. (i) Single-lumen EBT: A standard 7.5-mm diameter, 32-cm long endotracheal tube (ETT) can be advanced over an FOB into the left main stem bronchus. (ii) Univent tube or BB: The BB can be placed external to or intraluminally with an ETT.

   b. **Elective pulmonary resection, left-sided.**

     (1) **Not pneumonectomy.** There is no obvious best choice between a BB and a left DLT. Use of a left DLT for a left thoracotomy can be associated with obstruction of the tracheal lumen by the lateral tracheal wall and subsequent problems with gas exchange in the ventilated lung. A right DLT is an alternate choice.

     (2) **Left pneumonectomy.** When a pneumonectomy is foreseen, a right DLT is the best choice. A right DLT will permit the surgeon to palpate the left hilum during OLV without interference from a tube or blocker in the left main stem bronchus. The disposable right DLTs currently available in North America vary greatly in design, depending on the manufacturer (Mallinckrodt, Rusch, Kendall). The Mallinckrodt design currently is the most reliable. All three designs include a ventilating side slot in the distal bronchial lumen for right upper lobe ventilation. If left lung isolation is impossible despite extremely high pressures in the right DLT bronchial cuff, a Fogarty catheter can be passed into the left main bronchus as a BB. As an alternative, there is no clear preference between a left DLT or BB. These all require repositioning before clamping the left main stem bronchus.

Table 25.6 Selection of airway device for lung isolation

Surgery	Primary choice[a]	Secondary options (in order of preference)
Pulmonary resection, right sided	Left DLT	EBT, BB
Pulmonary resection, left sided, not pneumonectomy	Left DLT	BB, right DLT
Pulmonary resection, left sided pneumonectomy/ left main bronchial surgery	Right DLT	BB, left DLT,
Thoracoscopy	Left DLT	Right DLT, BB, EBT
Pulmonary hemorrhage	DLT/BB/EBT	
Bronchopleural fistula/abscess	Left DLT	Right DLT, BB, EBT
Esophageal, thoracic aortic, transthoracic vertebral surgery	Left DLT/BB	Right DLT, EBT
Lung transplantation, bilateral/right single	Left DLT	EBT, BB
Lung transplantation, left single	Right DLT	BB, left DLT
Abnormal upper airway, left thoracotomy	BB	Right DLT/left DLT, EBT
Abnormal upper airway, right thoracotomy	EBT	BB, left DLT/right DLT

[a] Options separated by a slash (/) are equivalent choices.

BB, bronchial blocker ipsilateral to side of surgery; EBT, single-lumen tube placed endobronchial contralateral to surgery; Left DLT, left-sided double-lumen tube; Right DLT, right-sided double-lumen tube.

   c. **Thoracoscopy.** Lung biopsies, wedge resection, bleb/bullae resections, and some lobectomies can be done using video-assisted thoracoscopic surgery (VATS). During open thoracotomy, the lung can be compressed by the surgeon to facilitate collapse before inflation of a BB. A left DLT is preferred for thoracoscopy of either hemithorax because it gives more rapid deflation of the nonventilated lung.

   d. **Pulmonary hemorrhage.** Instances of life-threatening pulmonary hemorrhage can occur due to a wide variety of causes, such as aspergillosis, tuberculosis, and pulmonary artery (PA) catheter trauma. The primary risk for these patients is asphyxiation, and first-line treatment is lung isolation and suctioning the lower airways. Lung isolation can be with a DLT, BB, or single-lumen EBT, depending on availability and the clinical circumstances. Tracheobronchial hemorrhage from blunt chest trauma usually resolves with suctioning; only rarely is lung isolation necessary. PA catheter-induced hemorrhage during weaning from cardiopulmonary bypass (CPB) should be dealt with by resumption of full bypass, bronchoscopy, and lung isolation. Weaning then may proceed without pulmonary resection in some cases.

   e. **Bronchopleural fistula.** The anesthesiologist is faced with the triple problem of avoiding tension pneumothorax, ensuring adequate ventilation, and protecting the healthy lung from the fluid collection in the involved hemithorax. Management depends on the site of the fistula and the urgency of the clinical situation. For a peripheral bronchopleural fistula in a stable patient, a BB may be acceptable. For a large central fistula and in urgent situations, the most rapid and reliable method of securing one-lung isolation and ventilation is a DLT. In life-threatening situations, a DLT can be placed in awake patients with direct FOB guidance.

   f. **Purulent secretions** (lung abscess, hydatid cysts). Lobar or segmental blockade is ideal. Loss of lung isolation in these cases is not merely a surgical inconvenience but may be life threatening. Univent tubes can be used for lobar blockade. A secure technique in these cases is the combined use of a BB and a DLT.

   g. **Nonpulmonary thoracic surgery.** Thoracic aortic and esophageal surgeries require OLV. Because there is no risk of ventilated-lung contamination, a left DLT and a BB are equivalent choices.

   h. **Bronchial surgery.** An intrabronchial tumor, bronchial trauma, or bronchial sleeve resection during a lobectomy requires that the surgeon have intraluminal access to the ipsilateral main stem bronchus. Either a single-lumen EBT or a DLT in the ventilated lung is preferred.

   i. Unilateral lung lavage, independent lung ventilation, and lung transplantation are all best accomplished with a left DLT.

3. **Upper airway abnormalities.** It occasionally is necessary to provide OLV in patients who have abnormal upper airways due to previous surgery or trauma or in patients who are known for unanticipated difficult intubations. There are four basic options for these patients: (i) fiberoptic-guided intubation with a DLT; (ii) secure the airway with an ETT and then use a "tube exchanger" to place a DLT; (iii) use a BB; and (iv) use an uncut single-lumen tube as an EBT.

   The optimal choice will depend on the patient and the operation. At all times it is best to maintain spontaneous ventilation and to do nothing blindly in the presence of blood or pus. Awake FOB intubation with a DLT requires thorough topical anesthesia of the airway. Rigid fiberoptic laryngoscopes, such as the Bullard and Wu scopes, or a lighted stylet can be used with some DLTs. It is important when using a tube exchanger to have a second person perform a direct laryngoscopy to expose as much of the glottis as possible during the tube change. Direct laryngoscopy decreases the angles between the oropharynx and trachea and reduces the chance of trauma to the airway from the DLT.

   BBs are often the best choice for some of these patients [7]. If the ET tube is too narrow to easily accommodate both a bronchoscope and a BB, the BB can be introduced through the glottis independently external to the ET tube with fiberoptic guidance. Bilateral BBs can be used for bilateral resections or the same blocker can be manipulated from side to side. Bilateral single-lumen EBTs or BBs can be used for lung isolation in patients with tracheal fistulas, trauma, or other abnormalities in the region of the carina. Smaller DLTs (32, 28, and 26 Fr) are available, but they will not permit passage of an FOB of the diameter commonly available to monitor positioning (3.5 to 4.0 mm). An ETT designed for microlaryngoscopy [5 to 6 mm inner diameter (ID) and greater than 30 cm long] can be used as an EBT, with FOB positioning. If the patient's trachea can accept a 7.0-mm ETT, a Fogarty catheter (8 Fr venous thrombectomy catheter with a 10-mL balloon) can be passed through the ETT via an FOB adapter for use as a BB.

4. **Chest trauma.** It is common in both open and closed chest trauma to have some hemoptysis from alveolar hemorrhage. The majority of these cases can be managed without lung isolation after bronchoscopy and suction. The majority of the deaths in these patients are due to their other injuries and not from airway hemorrhage or air embolus. Lung isolation may be helpful in some of these cases, but if resources and time are limited the priority must be the resuscitation of the patient.

5. **Avoiding iatrogenic airway injury.** Iatrogenic injury has been estimated to occur in 0.5 to 2 per 1,000 cases with DLTs.
   a. **View the chest x-ray film or CT scan,** which can help predict the majority of difficult endobronchial intubations.
   b. **Use an appropriate size tube.** Too small a tube will make lung isolation difficult. Too large a tube is more likely to cause trauma. Useful guidelines for DLT sizes in adults are as follows:

   Females height < 1.6 m (63 inch): 35 Fr
   Females > 1.6 m: 37 Fr
   Males < 1.7 m (67 inch): 39 Fr (possibly 37 Fr if < 1.6 m)
   Males > 1.7 m: 41 Fr

   c. **Depth of insertion of DLT.** Tracheobronchial dimensions correlate with height. The average depth at insertion, from the teeth, for a left DLT is 29 cm in an adult and varies ± 1 cm for each 10 cm of patient height above/below 170 cm.
   d. **Avoid nitrous oxide.** Nitrous oxide 70% can increase the bronchial cuff volume from 5 to 16 mL intraoperatively.
   e. **Inflate the bronchial cuff/blocker only to the minimal volume required for lung isolation and for the minimal time.** This volume usually is less than 3 mL. Inflating the bronchial cuff does not stabilize the DLT position when the patient is turned to the lateral position.
      (1) Endobronchial intubation must be done gently and with fiberoptic guidance if resistance is met [8]. A significant number of case reports are from cases of esophageal surgery, where the elastic supporting tissue may be weakened and predisposed to rupture from DLT placement.

6. **Other complications of lung separation**
   a. **Malpositioning.** Initial malpositioning of DLTs with blind placement can occur in greater than 30% of cases. Verification and adjustment with FOB immediately before initiating OLV is mandatory because these tubes will migrate during patient positioning. Malpositioning after the start of OLV due to dislodgment is more of a problem with BBs than DLTs.
   b. **Airway resistance.** The resistance from a 37 Fr DLT exceeds that of a no. 9 Univent by less than 10% over the range of airflows seen with spontaneous ventilation. These flow resistances both are less than that of an 8.0-mm ID ETT but exceed that of a 9.0-mm ETT. For short periods of postoperative ventilation and weaning, airflow resistance is not a problem with a DLT.

7. The **ABC's** of lung separation will always apply:
   a. Know the tracheobronchial **A**natomy
   b. Use the fiberoptic **B**ronchoscope [9]
   c. Look at the **C**hest x-ray film and **C**T scan in advance.

B. Positioning. The majority of thoracic procedures are performed with the patient in the lateral position, but, depending on the surgical technique, a semisupine or semiprone lateral position may be used. It is awkward to induce anesthesia in the lateral position; thus, monitors will be placed and anesthesia usually will be induced in the supine position and the anesthetized patient then will be repositioned for surgery. It is possible to induce anesthesia in the lateral position. This may rarely be indicated with unilateral lung diseases, such as bronchiectasis or hemoptysis, until lung isolation can be achieved. However, even these patients will have to be repositioned and the diseased lung turned to the nondependent side. Due to the loss of venous vascular tone in the anesthetized patient, it is not uncommon to see hypotension when the patient is turned to or from the lateral position.

All lines and monitors will have to be secured during position change and their function reassessed after repositioning. The anesthesiologist should take responsibility for the head, neck, and airway during position change and must be in charge of the operating team to direct repositioning. It is useful to make an initial "head-to-toe" survey of the patient after induction and intubation, checking oxygenation, ventilation, hemodynamics, lines, monitors, and potential nerve injuries. This survey must be repeated after repositioning. It is nearly impossible to avoid some movement of a DLT or BB during repositioning. The patient's head, neck, and EBT should be turned *en bloc* with the patient's thoracolumbar spine. The margin of error in positioning EBTs or blockers often is so narrow that even small movements can have significant clinical implications. EBT/blocker position and adequacy of ventilation must be rechecked by auscultation and FOB after patient repositioning.

1. **Neurovascular complications.** The brachial plexus is the site of the majority of intraoperative nerve injuries related to the lateral position. The brachial plexus is fixed at two points: proximally by the transverse process of the cervical vertebrae and distally by the axillary fascia. This two-point fixation plus the extreme mobility of neighboring skeletal and muscular structures make the brachial plexus extremely liable to injury (Table 25.7). The patient should be positioned with padding under the dependent thorax to keep the weight of the upper body off the dependent arm brachial plexus. This padding will exacerbate the pressure on the brachial plexus if it migrates superiorly into the axilla.

The brachial plexus of the nondependent arm is at risk for traction injuries if it is suspended from an arm support or "ether screen." Vascular compression of the nondependent arm in this situation is possible, and it is useful to monitor pulse oximetry in the nondependent hand. The arm should not be abducted beyond 90 degrees and should not be extended posteriorly beyond the neutral position nor flexed anteriorly greater than 90 degrees. Anterior flexion of the arm at the shoulder (circumduction) across the chest or lateral flexion of the neck toward the opposite side can cause a traction injury of the suprascapular nerve, which causes a deep, poorly circumscribed pain of posterior and lateral aspects of the shoulder. Lateral flexion of the cervical spine

Table 25.7 Factors contributing to brachial plexus injury in the lateral position

---

A. Dependent arm (compression injuries)
   1. Arm directly under thorax
   2. Pressure on clavicle into retroclavicular space
   3. Cervical rib
   4. Cephalad migration of thorax padding into the axilla[a]
B. Nondependent arm (stretch injuries)
   1. Lateral flexion of cervical spine
   2. Excessive abduction of arm (>90%)
   3. Semiprone or semisupine repositioning after arm fixed to a rigid support

---

[a] Unfortunately, this padding under the thorax sometimes is referred to an "axillary roll." This padding absolutely should **not** be placed in the axilla.

because of improper positioning of the patient's head can cause a "whiplash" syndrome and is difficult to appreciate from the head of the operating table. It is useful to survey the patient from the side of the table immediately after the patient is turned to ensure that the entire vertebral column is aligned properly.

The dependent leg should be slightly flexed with padding under the knee to protect the peroneal nerve lateral to the proximal head of the fibula. The nondependent leg is placed in a neutral extended position and padding placed between it and the dependent leg. The dependent leg must be observed for vascular compression. Excessively tight strapping at the hip level can compress the sciatic nerve of the nondependent leg. A "head-to-toe" protocol to monitor for possible neurovascular injuries related to the lateral decubitus position is given in Table 25.8.

2. **Physiologic changes in the lateral position**
    a. **Ventilation.** Significant changes in ventilation develop between the lungs when the patient is placed in the lateral position. The compliance curves of the two lungs are different because of their difference in sizes. The lateral position, anesthesia, paralysis, and opening the thorax all combine to magnify these differences between the lungs.

    In a spontaneously breathing patient, the ventilation of the dependent lung will increase approximately 10% when the patient is turned to the lateral position. Once the patient is anesthetized and paralyzed, the ventilation of the dependent lung will decrease 15%. The compliance of the entire respiratory system will increase once the nondependent hemithorax is open.

    Applying PEEP to both lungs in the lateral position, PEEP preferentially goes to the most compliant lung regions and hyperinflates the nondependent lung without causing any improvement in gas exchange. In the lateral position, atelectasis will develop in a mean of 5% of lung volume, all in the dependent lung.

    b. **Perfusion.** Turning the patient to the lateral position decreases the blood flow of the nondependent lung due to gravity by approximately 10% of the total pulmonary blood flow.

    The matching of ventilation and perfusion usually will decrease in the lateral position compared to the supine position. Pulmonary arteriovenous shunt usually increases from approximately 5% in the supine position to 10% to 15% in the lateral position.

C. **Intraoperative monitoring**
    1. **General to all pulmonary resections.** The majority of these are major operative procedures of moderate duration (2 to 4 hours) and performed in the lateral position with the hemithorax open. Consideration for monitoring and maintenance of body temperature and fluid volume should be given to all of these cases. All cases should have standard ASA monitoring. Additional monitoring is guided by a knowledge of which complications are likely to occur (Table 25.9).

Table 25.8 Avoiding neurovascular injuries specific to the lateral position

---

Routine "head-to-toe" survey
1. Dependent eye
2. Dependent ear pinna
3. Cervical spine alignment
4. Dependent arm: (i) brachial plexus, (ii) circulation
5. Nondependent arm[a]: (i) brachial plexus, (ii) circulation
6. Nondependent leg sciatic nerve
7. Dependent leg: (i) peroneal nerve, (ii) circulation

---

[a] Neurovascular injuries of the nondependent arm are more likely to occur if the arm is suspended or held in an independently positioned armrest.

Table 25.9 Intraoperative complications that occur with increased frequency during thoracotomy

Complication	Etiology
1. Hypoxemia	Intrapulmonary shunt during one-lung ventilation
2. Sudden severe hypotension	Surgical compression of the heart or great vessels
3. Sudden changes in ventilating pressure or volume	Movement of endobronchial tube/blocker, air leak
4. Arrhythmias	Direct mechanical irritation of the heart
5. Bronchospasm	Direct airway stimulation, increased frequency of reactive airways disease
6. Massive hemorrhage	Surgical blood loss from great vessels or inflamed pleura
7. Hypothermia	Heat loss from the open hemithorax

2. **Specific to certain types of resection.** There are complications that are more prone to occur with certain resections, such as hemorrhage from an extrapleural pneumonectomy, contralateral lung soiling with resection of a cyst or bronchiectasis, air leak hypoventilation, or tension pneumothorax with a bronchopleural fistula.

3. **Oxygenation.** Significant arterial oxygen desaturation (less than 90%) during OLV occurs in approximately 10% of the surgical population despite a high FIO_2 of 1.0. Pulse oximetry (S_pO_2) has not negated the need for direct measurement of arterial P_aO_2 via intermittent blood gases in the majority of thoracotomy patients. P_aO_2 offers a more useful estimate of the margin of safety above desaturation than S_pO_2. The rapidity of the fall in P_aO_2 after the onset of OLV is an indicator of the risk of subsequent desaturation. Measure P_aO_2 by ABG before OLV and 20 minutes after the start of OLV. There are significant differences among manufacturers in the accuracy of S_pO_2. Although the trends are reliable, in order to use a specific cutoff S_pO_2 value as a guideline for treatment of hypoxemia, the accuracy of the oximeter should be verified intraoperatively with ABG measurement. Also, during hypoxemia, S_pO_2 sensor malpositioning can cause significant underestimation of saturation.

4. **Capnometry.** End-tidal CO_2 ($P_{et}CO_2$) is a less reliable indicator of the P_aCO_2 during OLV than during two-lung ventilation and the $P_{a-et}CO_2$ gradient increases during OLV. As the patient is turned to the lateral position, the $P_{et}CO_2$ of the nondependent lung falls relative to the dependent lung because of increased perfusion of the dependent lung and increased dead space of the nondependent lung. At the onset of OLV, the $P_{et}CO_2$ of the dependent lung usually falls transiently as all the minute ventilation is transferred to this lung. The $P_{et}CO_2$ then rises as the fractional perfusion is increased to this dependent lung by collapse and pulmonary vasoconstriction of the nonventilated lung. If there is no correction of minute ventilation, the net result will be increased baseline P_aCO_2 and $P_{et}CO_2$ with an increased gradient. Severe (greater than 5 mm Hg) or prolonged falls in $P_{et}CO_2$ indicate a maldistribution of perfusion between ventilated and nonventilated lungs and may be an early warning of a patient who will desaturate during OLV.

5. **Invasive hemodynamic monitoring**

   a. **Arterial line.** There is a significant incidence of transient severe hypotension from surgical compression of the heart or great vessels during intrathoracic procedures. For this reason, plus the utility of intermittent ABG sampling, it is useful to have beat-to-beat assessment of systemic blood pressure during the majority of thoracic surgery cases. Exceptions are limited procedures such as thorascopic resections in younger/healthier patients.

For most thoracotomies, placement of a radial artery catheter can be in either the dependent or nondependent arm.

   b. **Central venous pressures.** Central venous pressure (CVP) readings obtained intraoperatively with the chest open are not completely reliable. The CVP is a useful monitor postoperatively, particularly for cases where fluid management is critical (e.g., pneumonectomies). It is our practice to routinely place CVP lines in pneumonectomy patients but not for lesser resections unless there is significant other concurrent illness. Our choice is to use a high anterior approach to the right internal jugular vein to minimize the risk of pneumothorax for CVP access unless there is a contraindication. Internal jugular CVP data are not reliable in patients with superior vena cava obstruction.

   c. **PA catheters.** Intraoperative PA pressure may be a less accurate indicator of true left heart preload in the lateral position with the chest open than in other clinical situations. It often is not known initially if the catheter tip lies in the dependent or nondependent lung. Thermodilution cardiac output data may be unreliable if there are significant transient unilateral differences in perfusion between the lungs, as can occur during positive-pressure OLV. Complications from the use of PA catheters, including arrhythmias, hemorrhage, and pulmonary infarction, are well documented. If a PA catheter is in the nonventilated lung, it frequently becomes wedged as the lung collapses. The risk/benefit ratio for the routine use of PA catheters for pulmonary resection surgery favors their use only in certain specific cases, such as patients with major coexisting disease (cardiac, renal) and/or patients undergoing particularly extensive procedures (e.g., extrapleural pneumonectomy).

 6. Fiberoptic bronchoscopy. Significant malpositions of left-sided or right-sided DLTs that can lead to desaturation during OLV often are not detected by auscultation or other traditional methods of confirming placement. Positioning of DLTs or BBs should be confirmed after placing the patient in the surgical position because a large number of the tubes/blockers migrate during repositioning of the patient [9].

 7. Continuous spirometry. Side-stream spirometry monitors inspiratory and expiratory pressure, volume, and flow interactions during anesthesia. The adequacy of lung isolation can be monitored by breath-to-breath comparison of inspiratory and expiratory tidal volumes. This also gives a sense of the magnitude of air leaks from the ventilated lung. Changes in the position of a DLT can be detected by changes in the pressure–volume loops.

D. Anesthetic technique. Any anesthetic technique that provides safe and stable general anesthesia for major surgery can and has been used for lung resection. Many centers use combined thoracic epidural and general anesthesia for thoracic surgery.

 1. IV fluids. Because of hydrostatic effects, excessive administration of IV fluids can cause increased shunt and lead to pulmonary edema of the dependent lung. Because the dependent lung is the lung that must carry on gas exchange during OLV, it is best to be as judicious as possible with fluid administration. IV fluids are administered to replace volume deficits and for maintenance only during lung resection anesthesia. No volume is given for theoretical third space losses during thoracotomy. There is no good evidence that such third space losses occur during lung resection as they do during abdominal or other types of major surgery (Table 25.10).

 2. Nitrous oxide. Nitrous oxide/oxygen mixtures are more prone to cause atelectasis in poorly ventilated lung regions than oxygen by itself. The optimal method to prevent dependent lung atelectasis is the use of air/oxygen mixtures during both two-lung ventilation and OLV, titrating the FIO_2 to avoid hypoxemia. Nitrous oxide also tends to increase PA pressures in patients who have pulmonary hypertension.

 3. Temperature. Maintenance of body temperature can be a problem during thoracic surgery because of heat loss from the open hemithorax. This is par-

Table 25.10 Fluid management for pulmonary resection surgery

1. Total positive fluid balance in the first 24 hours perioperatively should not exceed 20 mL/kg.
2. For an average adult patient, crystalloid administration should be limited to <3 L in the first 24 hours.
3. No fluid administration for "third space" fluid losses during pulmonary resection.
4. Crystalloids should be used in preference to colloids.
5. Urine output >0.5 mL/kg/h is unnecessary.
6. If increased tissue perfusion is needed postoperatively, it is preferable to use invasive monitoring and inotropes rather than to cause fluid overload.

ticularly a problem at the extremes of the age spectrum. Most of the body's physiologic functions, including hypoxic pulmonary vasoconstriction (HPV), are inhibited during hypothermia. Increasing the ambient room temperature and using a lower-limb forced-air patient warmer are the best methods to prevent inadvertent intraoperative hypothermia.

4. **Prevention of bronchospasm.** Due to the high incidence of coexisting reactive airways disease in the thoracic surgical population it is generally advisable to use an anesthetic technique that decreases bronchial irritability. This is particularly important because the added airway manipulation caused by placement of a DLT or BB is a potent trigger for bronchoconstriction. Avoid manipulation of the airway in a lightly anesthetized patient, use bronchodilating anesthetics and avoid drugs which release histamine.

   For IV induction of anesthesia, either Propofol or Ketamine diminish bronchospasm. For maintenance of anesthesia, propofol and/or any of the volatile anesthetics will diminish bronchial reactivity. Sevoflurane may be the most potent bronchodilator of the volatile anesthetics.

5. **Coronary Artery Disease.** Since the lung resection population are largely elderly and smokers there is a high coincidence of coronary artery disease. This consideration will be a major factor in the choice of the anesthetic technique for most thoracic patients. The anesthetic technique should optimize the myocardial oxygen supply/demand ratio by maintaining arterial oxygenation and diastolic blood pressure while avoiding unnecessary increases in cardiac output and heart rate. Thoracic epidural anesthesia (TEA)/analgesia may aid in this.

E. **Management of one-lung ventilation**

1. **Hypoxemia.** There is an incidence of <10% of hypoxemia (arterial saturation <90%) during OLV for thoracic surgery. Hypoxemia is more likely to occur when OLV is in the supine position.

2. **Hypoxic pulmonary vasoconstriction.** HPV is thought to decrease the blood flow to the nonventilated lung by 50%. The stimulus for HPV is primarily the alveolar oxygen tension (P_aO_2), which stimulates precapillary vasoconstriction redistributing pulmonary blood flow away from hypoxemic lung regions via a pathway involving nitric oxide (NO) and/or cyclooxygenase synthesis inhibition. All of the volatile anesthetics inhibit HPV. This inhibition is dose dependent. Isoflurane, sevoflurane, and desflurane cause less inhibition than other volatiles [7]. No clinical benefit has been shown for total IV anesthesia beyond that seen with isoflurane 1 MAC (minimum alveolar concentration) or less. HPV is decreased by all vasodilators such as nitroglycerin and nitroprusside. In general, vasodilators can be expected to cause a deterioration in P_aO_2 during OLV.

3. **Cardiac output.** The net effects of an increase in cardiac output during OLV tend to favor an increase in P_aO_2. Elevation of cardiac output beyond physiologic needs tend to oppose HPV and may cause P_aO_2 to fall.

4. **Ventilation during one-lung anesthesia.** Many anesthesiologists use the same tidal volume during OLV as during two-lung ventilation. This strategy is adequate for the majority of cases. It is possible to improve gas exchange for selected individual patients by altering the ventilatory variables that are under

Table 25.11 Ventilation parameters for one-lung ventilation

Parameter	Suggested	Exceptions
1. Tidal volume	10 mL/kg	Maintain: Peak airway pressure <35 cm H_2O Plateau airway pressure <25 cm H_2O
2. Positive end-expiratory pressure (PEEP)	0 cm H_2O	Patients with good spirometry and large a-A O_2 gradient during two-lung ventilation in the lateral position (5 cm H_2O PEEP)
3. Respiratory rate	12/min	Maintain normal P_aCO_2. $P_{a\text{-}et}CO_2$ gradient usually will increase 1–3 mm Hg during one lung ventilation
4. Mode	Volume control	Patients with moderate/severe chronic obstructive pulmonary disease: pressure control ventilation to deliver tidal volume 10 mL/kg (ventilation pressure approximately 20–25 cm H_2O)

the control of the anesthesiologist: tidal volume, rate, inspiratory/expiratory ratio, P_aCO_2, peak and plateau airway pressures, and PEEP (Table 25.11).

a. **Respiratory acid–base status.** The overall efficacy of HPV is optimal with normal pH and P_aCO_2

b. **Positive end-expiratory pressure.** Most patients do not increase P_aO_2 with added PEEP during OLV. The minority of patients with either normal or supranormal (restrictive lung disease) lung elastic recoil will benefit from low levels (5 cm H_2O) of PEEP during OLV. Auto PEEP is most prone to occur in patients with decreased lung elastic recoil, such as the elderly or those with emphysema. Auto PEEP is difficult to detect using currently available anesthetic ventilators. Many patients show surprising high levels of auto PEEP, often greater than 10 cm H_2O, during OLV. Applied PEEP combines with auto PEEP in an unpredictable fashion.

c. **Tidal volume.** 10 mL/kg tidal volume for both two-lung ventilation and OLV is a reasonable starting point. The tidal volume should be adjusted during OLV to keep the airway peak pressure less than 35 cm H_2O and the plateau airway pressure less than 25 cm H_2O.

d. **Volume control versus pressure control.** Pressure-control OLV is useful in patients with severe obstructive disease and to limit airway pressure in patients with blebs, bullae, or fresh resections in the lung.

e. **FIO_2.** The FIO_2 should be increased at the start of OLV to 80% to 100% and then can be decreased as tolerated over the next 30 minutes.

5. **Treatment of hypoxemia during OLV (Table 25.12)**

a. **Increase FIO_2.** The first-line therapy is to increase the FIO_2, which is an option in essentially all patients except those who received bleomycin or similar therapy that potentiates pulmonary oxygen toxicity.

Table 25.12 Treatment options for hypoxemia during one-lung ventilation

1. Increase FIO_2
2. Continuous positive airway pressure to the nonventilated lung
3. Positive end-expiratory pressure to the ventilated lung
4. Manipulation of tidal volume
5. Pharmacologic
6. Alternative ventilation methods

b. **Continuous positive airway pressure.** CPAP with oxygen to the non-ventilated lung is the most useful ventilatory manipulation. CPAP must be applied to a fully inflated or reinflated lung for optimal effect. When CPAP is applied to a fully inflated lung, as little as 2 to 3 cm H_2O can be used. All that is required is a CPAP valve and an oxygen source. Ideally the circuit should permit variation of the CPAP level and should include a reservoir bag to allow easy reinflation of the nonventilated lung and a manometer to measure the actual CPAP supplied. Such circuits are commercially available or can be readily constructed. When the bronchus of the operative lung is obstructed or open to atmosphere, CPAP will not improve oxygenation. During thoracoscopic surgery, CPAP can significantly interfere with surgery.

c. **Positive end-expiratory pressure.** PEEP to the ventilated dependent lung may help in some patients.

d. **Pharmacologic manipulations.** Increasing cardiac output will result in a small but clinically useful increase in both P_vO_2 and P_aO_2 if cardiac output has decreased. Eliminating potent vasodilators, such as nitroglycerin and halothane, will improve oxygenation during OLV. Selective pulmonary vasodilators such as NO have not yet proven to be reliable.

e. **Alternative ventilation methods.** Several alternative methods of OLV, all of which involve partial ventilation of the nonventilated lung, have been described and improve oxygenation during OLV (Table 25.13). These techniques are useful in patients who are particularly at risk for desaturation, such as those with previous pulmonary resections of the contralateral lung.

(1) Selective lobar collapse of only the operative lobe in the open hemithorax by placement of a blocker in the appropriate lobar bronchus of the ipsilateral operative lung.

(2) Differential lung ventilation by only partially occluding the lumen of the DLT to the operative lung.

(3) Intermittent reinflation of the nonventilated lung by regular reexpansion of the operative lung via an attached CPAP circuit.

(4) Two-lung high-frequency positive-pressure ventilation (HFPPV).

(5) Conventional OLV of the nonoperative lung and high-frequency jet ventilation of the operative lung.

f. **Mechanical restriction of pulmonary blood flow.** It is possible for the surgeon to directly compress or clamp the blood flow to the nonventilated lung. This can be done temporarily in emergency desaturation situations or definitively in cases of pneumonectomy. Another technique is inflation of a PA catheter balloon in the main PA of the operative lung.

6. **Prevention of hypoxemia.** The treatments outlined as therapy for hypoxemia can be used prophylactically to prevent hypoxemia in patients who are at high risk for desaturation during OLV. Desaturation during bilateral lung procedures is particularly a problem during the second period of OLV. It is advisable to operate first on the lung that has better gas exchange. For the majority of patients this means operating on the right side first.

III. **Specific procedures**

A. **Thoracotomy**

1. **Operations**

a. **Lobectomy.** Lobectomy is the most common pulmonary resection for lung cancer. Early functional loss exceeds the amount of lung tissue resected,

Table 25.13 Alternative ventilation methods for problematic one-lung anesthesia

A. Selective lobar collapse
B. Differential lung ventilation
C. Intermittent reinflation
D. Two-lung high-frequency positive-pressure ventilation
E. One-lung high-frequency jet ventilation

but function recovers over a period of 6 weeks so that the final net loss of respiratory function is equivalent to the amount of functioning lung tissue excised. The recovery of pulmonary function after thoracotomy is unique because it shows a plateau with no early recovery during the first 72 hours postoperatively. This period coincides with the occurrence of the majority of postthoracotomy respiratory complications (atelectasis, pneumonia), which are the major causes of mortality after pulmonary resection. These complications are particularly associated with lobectomy and its variations, probably due to the transient dysfunction that occurs in the remaining lobe(s). The right middle lobe is particularly at risk for these complications after a right upper lobectomy and can develop torsion about its bronchovascular pedicle or lobar bronchial kinking as it expands into the apex of the right hemithorax.

   b. **Sleeve lobectomy.** A sleeve lobectomy is the excision of a lobe plus the adjacent segment of main stem bronchus with bronchoplastic repair of the bronchus by end-to-end anastomosis to preserve the distal functioning pulmonary parenchyma. It is done to preserve functioning lung tissue when the tumor encroaches to less than 2 cm from the lobar bronchial orifices, precluding simple lobectomy. This procedure usually is done for right upper lobe tumors but can be used for other lobes. The anesthetic implications of this procedure are that no airway catheter (single-lumen or DLT) or BB can be placed in the ipsilateral main stem bronchus. Mucus clearance across the bronchial anastomosis may be impaired after sleeve resection, and local tumor recurrence is a problem.

   c. **Bilobectomy.** In the right lung, a bilobectomy may be used to conserve either a functioning upper or lower lobe when the tumor extends across the lobar fissure or for malignancies involving the bronchus intermedius (the portion of the right main stem bronchus distal to the right upper lobe orifice). The complication rate is slightly higher than for a simple lobectomy but is less than for a pneumonectomy. The incidence of cardiac dysrhythmias increases postoperatively versus lobectomy, whereas the incidence of respiratory complications remains the same. The residual lobe cannot completely fill the hemithorax, and all patients will have a degree of pneumothorax that can be expected to resolve gradually.

   d. **Pneumonectomy.** Complete removal of the lung is required when a lobectomy or its modifications is not adequate to remove the local disease and/or ipsilateral lymph node metastases. Atelectasis and pneumonia occur after pneumonectomy as they do after lobectomy but may be less of a problem because of the absence of residual parenchymal dysfunction on the operative side. The mortality rate after pneumonectomy exceeds that for lobectomy because of complications that are more likely with pneumonectomy.

      (1) **Postpneumonectomy pulmonary edema.** The syndrome presents clinically with dyspnea and an increased alveolar–arterial oxygen gradient on the second or third postoperative day [10]. Radiologic changes precede clinical symptoms by approximately 24 hours. The factors that are known about this syndrome are listed in Table 25.14. This syndrome has such a high case of fatality rate (greater than 50%) that it represents a large portion of mortality after lung resection.

Table 25.14 Postpneumonectomy pulmonary edema

Incidence 2%–4% of pneumonectomies
Case fatality >50%
Incidence right > left pneumonectomy (3–4:1)
Clinical onset 2–3 days postoperatively
Not associated with increased pulmonary artery pressures
Possible exacerbation by fluid overload

Excessive perioperative administration of IV crystalloids or colloids can exacerbate this syndrome. There is no evidence that judicious amounts of fluids cause this problem. The residual nonoperated lung has an increased pulmonary capillary permeability after pneumonectomy that is not seen in the nonoperated lung after lobectomy. The cause of this increased permeability may be related to surgical lymphatic damage, capillary stress injury from increased flow, or increased airway pressure and hyperinflation of the ventilated lung during OLV.

The majority of lobectomies have the potential to become a pneumonectomy, so caution is needed with fluids in most thoracic cases.

(2) **Atrial fibrillation.** Up to 50% of postpneumonectomy patients will develop supraventricular arrhythmias in the first week postoperatively and the majority of these are atrial fibrillation. The perioperative mortality is 17% in patients who develop arrhythmias versus 2% in those without this complication. The etiology of these arrhythmias seems to depend on two factors: RV strain and increased sympathetic nervous activity. Similar arrhythmias occur after lesser pulmonary resections with a lower incidence. Prophylactic digoxin is not effective in preventing these arrhythmias. Diltiazem 10 mg IV every 8 hours is of some benefit [11].

(3) **Mechanical effects.** A variety of potentially lethal intrathoracic mechanical derangements of cardiorespiratory function can occur after pneumonectomy. The most important of these is cardiac herniation through an incompletely closed pericardium. This is particularly a risk after right pneumonectomy and presents with acute severe hypotension in the immediate postoperative period. The only useful therapy is immediate reoperation to return the heart into the pericardium. A subacute form of cardiac herniation can occur after a left pneumonectomy and presents with a picture of myocardial ischemia as the apex of the heart herniates through the pericardial defect and compresses the coronary blood flow. Less acute presentations of cardiovascular or respiratory symptoms may develop related to shifts of the mediastinum that can compress the great vessels or airways after pneumonectomy.

e. **Sleeve pneumonectomy.** Tumors involving the most proximal portions of the main stem bronchus and the carina may require a sleeve pneumonectomy. These are performed most commonly for right-sided tumors and usually can be performed without CPB via a right thoracotomy. A long single-lumen EBT can be advanced into the left main stem bronchus during the period of anastomosis, or the lung can be ventilated via a separate sterile ETT and circuit that is passed into the operating field and used for temporary intubation of the open distal bronchus. HFPPV also has been used for this procedure.

Because the carina is surgically more accessible from the right side, left sleeve pneumonectomies are commonly performed as a two-stage operation, first a left thoracotomy and pneumonectomy, and then a right thoracotomy for the carinal excision. The complication rate and mortality are higher and the 5-year survival significantly lower than for other pulmonary resections.

f. **Lesser resections (segmentectomy, wedge).** These procedures are commonly performed in the elderly or in patients with limited cardiopulmonary reserves to preserve functioning pulmonary parenchyma. These lesser resections are associated with a lower 5-year survival rate compared to lobectomy due to locoregional recurrence of cancer.

The decrease of pulmonary function (FEV_1) for lesser resections is in proportion to the amount of lung tissue removed. Lesser resections are acceptable therapy for nonmalignant lung lesions.

g. **Extended resections.** Portions of the chest wall, diaphragm, pericardium, left atrium, venae cavae, brachial plexus, or vertebral body may be excised with adjacent lung tumor. Resection of any of these structures has important anesthetic implications for choice and placement of intraoperative monitors and lines and for postoperative management.

h. Subsequent pulmonary resections. Lung resection surgery after previous lung resection is not infrequent. These operations can be performed for either benign or malignant disease. Ten percent of lung cancer patients can be expected to develop a second primary tumor. Prediction of postoperative lung function for these patients is accurate based on the assessment of preoperative function (lung mechanics, gas exchange, and cardiopulmonary reserve) and estimation of the amount of functional lung tissue removed at surgery (Fig. 25.1). Lobectomy after pneumonectomy can be performed safely if the patient meets minimal standards for predicted postoperative pulmonary function. Intraoperative collapse of the ipsilateral lung is not possible, but surgery can be facilitated by selective lobar or segment bronchial blockade or the use of HFPPV.

Completion pneumonectomy after a previous ipsilateral resection for cancer has a greater than 40% 5-year survival rate. Intraoperative hemorrhage is the specific anesthetic concern with this procedure, and more than 50% of patients experience blood loss of greater than 1,000 mL. Hemorrhage is particularly a problem in completion pneumonectomy for nonmalignant lung disease (lung abscess, bronchiectasis, tuberculosis). Inflammatory lung disease tends to destroy the tissue planes around the hilum and makes the surgical dissection more difficult, with an attendant increase in perioperative mortality.

i. Incomplete resections. In general, a lung cancer patient's prognosis is not improved from an incomplete resection. There are several exceptions. Incompletely resected tumors with direct mediastinal invasion or tumors of the superior sulcus may benefit if the resection is combined with adjuvant brachytherapy or external irradiation. Also, if the residual tumor is limited to microscopic involvement of the cut mucosal margin of the bronchus, 5-year survival is increased beyond that seen without surgery. Incomplete resections may be indicated for palliation in cases of airway obstruction or hemoptysis if these are not amenable to endoscopic or radiologic procedures.

j. Adjuvant and neoadjuvant therapy. The benefits of postoperative prophylactic chemotherapy or radiotherapy are unclear for lung cancer patients who have undergone complete resections. Thoracic irradiation usually is given to patients with resected N_2 node involvement disease. Chemotherapy may be of some benefit after resection of advanced adenocarcinoma. Neoadjuvant cisplatin-based regimens for marginally resectable stage IIIa or IIIb disease currently are under investigation. Preoperative radiotherapy does not appear to offer any survival benefits and makes the surgery technically more difficult.

2. Surgical approaches. Any given pulmonary resection can be accomplished by a variety of different surgical approaches. The approach used in an individual case depends on the interaction of several factors, which include the site and pathology of the lesion(s) and the training and experience of the surgical team. Each approach has specific anesthetic implications. Common thoracic surgical approaches and their generally accepted advantages and disadvantages are listed in Table 25.15.

a. Posterolateral thoracotomy. This is the most common incision in thoracic surgery. The patient is placed in the lateral decubitus position. Chest access is usually via the fifth or sixth intercostal space. The left seventh or eighth space may be used for access to the esophageal hiatus. The serratus anterior, latissimus dorsi, and trapezius muscles all will be partially divided during incision, with subsequent postoperative pain and disability. Chest access may be obtained directly through an intercostal space or by excision of a rib. Exposure to all ipsilateral intrathoracic structures is excellent.

Table 25.15 Surgical approaches for pulmonary resections

Incision	Pro	Con
Posterolateral thoracotomy	Excellent exposure to entire operative hemithorax	Postoperative pain; ± respiration dysfunction (short and long term)
Lateral muscle-sparing thoracotomy	Decreased postoperative pain	Increased incidence of wound seromas
Anterolateral thoracotomy	Better access for laparotomy, resuscitation, or contralateral thoracotomy, especially in trauma	Limited access to posterior thorax
Axillary thoracotomy	Decreased pain; adequate access for first rib resection, sympathectomy, apical blebs, or bullae.	Limited exposure
Sternotomy	Decreased pain; bilateral access	Decreased exposure of left lower lobe and posterior thoracic structures
Transsternal bilateral thoracotomy ("clamshell")	Good exposure for bilateral lung transplantation	Postoperative pain and chest wall dysfunction
Video-assisted thoracoscopic surgery	Less postoperative pain and respiratory dysfunction	Increased local recurrence of lung cancer

b. **Muscle-sparing lateral thoracotomy.** The lateral muscle-sparing thoracotomy has been advocated to reduce the pain and disability associated with a standard posterolateral thoracotomy. The skin incision is basically the same, but an extensive subcutaneous dissection is required to mobilize the latissimus and serratus muscles. A randomized controlled study has shown significantly decreased pain and opioid use and improved shoulder girdle strength up to 1 week postoperatively in the muscle-sparing group. However, wound seromas were significantly more frequent in the muscle-sparing group. There were no differences between groups after 1 month and no difference in perioperative morbidity.

c. **Anterolateral thoracotomy.** This is a particularly useful incision in trauma because it allows complete access to the patient for ongoing resuscitation and does not require repositioning for laparotomy or exploration of the contralateral chest. Exposure to the posterior hemithorax is limited in comparison to a posterolateral incision. Because this approach requires incision of only the pectoralis muscles, pain and shoulder disability may be less than with a standard thoracotomy.

d. **Axillary thoracotomy.** The transaxillary approach provides limited access, only to the apical areas of the hemithorax. The ipsilateral arm must be draped free or suspended and access to this arm will be limited intraoperatively. Thus, it is preferable for vascular access and monitoring to use the contralateral arm. Postoperative pain and disability are less than with a standard thoracotomy. This is an adequate incision for first rib resection, resection of apical bullae/blebs, or thoracic sympathectomy.

e. **Median sternotomy.** This incision, which is the standard for cardiac surgery, has potential benefits for certain thoracic procedures. Bilateral excisions for metastases and bullae are best performed via this incision. It has been demonstrated that postoperative spirometry is superior and pain is less after median sternotomy than thoracotomy. Most pulmonary resections can be performed via a median sternotomy, which obviates the need for a separate incision in cases of combined cardiac and thoracic surgery (see section **III.J**). Certain procedures are more difficult via a median sternotomy, including procedures performed for superior sulcus tumors, tumors with posterior chest wall extension and left lower lobe tumors. OLV is more of a necessity for surgical exposure than for lateral thoracotomies because of the limited surgical access.

   f. **Transsternal bilateral thoracotomy (the "clamshell" incision).** This is the common incision for bilateral lung transplantation. Because of increased pain and postoperative chest wall dysfunction, it is not commonly used for other intrathoracic procedures. It has been used for resection of bilateral metastases, pericardiectomy, resection of a posterior ventricular aneurysm, and cardiac surgery in a patient with a tracheotomy.

B. **Video-assisted thoracoscopic surgery.** Essentially any surgical procedure that is performed via thoracotomy has been attempted by VATS. VATS has been advocated for pulmonary resection of lung cancer in patients with limited respiratory reserves because of decreased postoperative pain and loss of early postoperative spirometric respiratory function that is only approximately half of that seen when the same operation is performed by thoracotomy. However, an increased rate of local recurrence of lung tumors excised by VATS has led to the consensus that this is not an optimal first choice as a surgical approach for lung cancer. VATS is the procedure of choice in many centers for resection of nonmalignant pulmonary lesions (blebs, bullae, granulomas). VATS also is used for sympathectomy for palmar hyperhidrosis and for the intrathoracic portion of esophagogastrectomy. Bilateral VATS can be performed in the supine position for apical lesions, but for most operations bilateral VATS requires change from one lateral position to the other intraoperatively.

   Many procedures are attempted by VATS initially with conversion to thoracotomy if the surgery proves impractical. OLV with complete collapse of the operative lung is more of a priority than for thoracotomy, and application of CPAP to the nonventilated lung is more detrimental to surgery than in open thoracotomy. To aid collapse of the lung, particularly in patients with COPD and poor lung elastic recoil, it is best to ventilate with oxygen instead of air/oxygen mixtures during the period of two-lung ventilation before lung collapse. Postoperative management is essentially the same as for thoracotomy, and most patients initially will have chest drains. The amount of postoperative pain after VATS varies greatly depending on the surgical procedure performed. Simple wedge excisions will have only the pain of several small intercostal incisions and the chest drain(s), and this can usually be easily managed with oral medications. Pleural abrasions or instillation of pleural sclerosing agents, which often are done for recurrent pneumothoraces or effusions, are extremely painful and may require full postoperative analgesic management, up to and including thoracic epidural analgesia, in patients with limited pulmonary function.

C. **Bronchopleural fistula.** A persistent communication between the airway and the interpleural space can develop after medical conditions, such as rupture of a bleb or bulla, infection, or malignancy. Bronchopleural fistula can develop as a postoperative complication after lung surgery. The large majority of persistent lung air leaks will heal with drainage and conservative management.

   Surgical intervention is indicated when conservative therapy is unable to permit adequate gas exchange (this is more likely to occur in the immediate postoperative period, particularly after pneumonectomy) or when conventional chest tube drainage and suction are unable to reexpand the ipsilateral lung, or for a second ipsilateral or first contralateral pneumothorax.

   There are three specific **anesthetic goals** in all patients with a bronchopleural fistula:

   1. Healthy lung regions must be protected from soiling by extrapleural fluid from the affected hemithorax.
   2. The ventilation technique must avoid development of a tension pneumothorax in the affected hemithorax.

3. The anesthetic technique must ensure adequate alveolar gas exchange in the presence of a low-resistance air leak.

To achieve these goals there are two **management principles** that should be used in essentially all cases:

1. A functioning chest drain should be placed before the induction of anesthesia and connected to an underwater seal without suction.
2. A method of lung separation should be placed so that the fistula can be isolated as necessary intraoperatively.

After placement of a chest drain there are three **options for induction** of anesthesia [12]:

1. A single-lumen or double-lumen EBT or blocker can be placed in an awake patient with topical anesthesia and its position checked fiberoptically before induction. This often is not the best choice in a patient with severely compromised gas exchange because maintaining adequate oxygenation in an already hypoxemic patient can be a problem during awake intubation.
2. Induction of anesthesia maintaining spontaneous ventilation until lung isolation is secured. A spontaneous-ventilation induction may not be desirable if there is a risk of aspiration and in patients with compromised hemodynamics.
3. IV induction of general anesthesia and muscle relaxation after meticulous preoxygenation and manual ventilation using small tidal volumes and low airway pressures until the lung isolation is confirmed. The efficiency of this technique can be improved by using a bronchoscope to guide DLT placement during intubation.

The air leak through a bronchopleural fistula is dependent on the pressure gradient between the mean airway pressure at the site of the fistula and the interpleural space. High-frequency ventilation, with and without lung or lobar blockade, has been used in certain cases. High-frequency techniques may permit relatively lower proximal mean airway pressures than conventional mechanical ventilation and may be more useful in large central air leaks.

D. **Bullae and blebs.** Whenever positive-pressure ventilation is applied to the airway of a patient with a bulla or bleb, there is the risk of lesion rupture and development of a tension pneumothorax that will require drainage and may progress to a bronchopleural fistula. The anesthetic considerations are similar to those for a patient with a bronchopleural fistula, except that it is best not to place a chest drain prophylactically because the chest tube may enter the bulla and create a fistula and there is not the risk of soiling healthy lung regions from extrapleural fluid that exists with fistulas. For induction of anesthesia it usually is optimal to maintain spontaneous ventilation until the lung or lobe with the bulla or bleb is isolated. When there is a risk of aspiration or it is believed that the patient's gas exchange or hemodynamics may not permit spontaneous ventilation for induction, the anesthesiologist will need to use small tidal volumes and low airway pressures during positive-pressure ventilation until the airway is isolated. Nitrous oxide will diffuse into a bleb or bulla, causing it to enlarge, and must be avoided.

E. **Abscesses, bronchiectasis, cysts, and empyema.** As with bronchopleural fistulas, there is the risk of soiling healthy lung regions by uncontrolled spillage from these lesions. Lung isolation is a primary requirement for anesthesia and the anesthetic principles and management are similar to those described for fistulas. When an intrathoracic space-occupying lesion is removed, there is the potential for reexpansion pulmonary edema to develop after reinflation of the ipsilateral lung. A slow and gradual reinflation may decrease the severity of this complication.

F. **Mediastinoscopy.** Cervical mediastinoscopy is a diagnostic sampling of the mediastinal nodes to assess if a pulmonary resection will improve outcome. Basically it is an attempt to differentiate between stage I or II and stage III lung cancer because the benefits of surgery vary tremendously between these stages. Mediastinoscopy can avoid some but not all unnecessary exploratory thoracotomies. Mediastinoscopy often is omitted from the cancer staging if the CT scan of the mediastinum is negative (mediastinal nodes less than 1 cm in the short axis). Because there are a significant number of false-positive results on cancer staging with CT scan, all patients with positive mediastinal nodes on CT should have a mediastinoscopy.

Mediastinoscopy can be done at a separate anesthetic before pulmonary resection, often as an outpatient, or immediately after induction as part of the same procedure before the pulmonary resection. Apart from the specific anesthetic considerations of mediastinoscopy itself, the anesthetic implication of starting the case with these diagnostic procedures is that the resection may be aborted based on the initial mediastinoscopy findings. Consider avoiding the use of long-acting nondepolarizing muscle relaxants until the biopsy results indicate that the resection will proceed. The likelihood of not proceeding to thoracotomy must enter into each individual assessment of risk/benefit when considering placing an epidural catheter before induction.

Mediastinoscopy most commonly is done via a cervical approach with an incision in the suprasternal notch. Any structure in the upper chest can be injured during the procedure, including great vessels, pleura (pneumothorax), nerves (recurrent laryngeal), and airways.

Hemorrhage is the most frequent major complication, particularly due to inadvertent PA biopsy, and this must always be considered with respect to vascular access, monitoring, and the availability of means for resuscitation. Fortunately, significant hemorrhage during mediastinoscopy usually can be tamponaded temporarily by the surgeon when resuscitation is required. In only a minority of mediastinoscopy hemorrhages is it necessary to proceed to thoracotomy for surgical control of bleeding.

A frequent complication of cervical mediastinoscopy is transient compression of the brachiocephalic artery by the mediastinoscope. The surgeon usually is unaware that this is occurring, and it is part of the anesthetic considerations to always continuously monitor the circulation in the right arm (pulse oximetry or arterial line or palpation) so that the surgeon can be notified and avoid the risk of cerebral ischemia in patients who may not have good collateral cerebral circulation.

Because of the different pattern of lymphatic drainage of the left upper lobe, patients with left upper lobe tumors often will have an anterior left parasternal mediastinoscopy or median sternotomy instead of or in addition to a cervical mediastinoscopy. The serious complications associated with cervical mediastinoscopy are not as frequent with parasternal mediastinoscopy.

G. **Anterior mediastinal mass.** Patients with anterior mediastinal masses present unique problems to the anesthesiologist. A large number of such patients require anesthesia for biopsy of these masses by mediastinoscopy or VATS, or they may require definitive resection via sternotomy or thoracotomy. Tumors of the anterior mediastinum include thymoma, teratoma, lymphoma, cystic hygroma, bronchogenic cyst, and thyroid tumors. Anterior mediastinal masses may cause obstruction of major airways, main pulmonary arteries, atria, and superior vena cava. Any one of these complications can be life threatening. During induction of general anesthesia in patients with an anterior mediastinal mass, airway obstruction is the most common and feared complication.

It is important to note that the point of tracheal compression usually occurs distal to the ETT. A history of supine dyspnea or cough should alert the clinician to the possibility of airway obstruction upon induction of anesthesia. Life-threatening complications may occur in the absence of symptoms. The other major complication is cardiovascular collapse secondary to compression of the heart or major vessels. Symptoms of supine syncope suggest vascular compression. Deaths upon induction of general anesthesia in patients with an anterior mediastinal mass is always a risk. Anesthetic deaths have mainly been reported in children. The deaths may be the result of the more compressible cartilaginous structure of the airway in children or because of the difficulty in obtaining a history of positional symptoms in children.

The most important diagnostic test in the patient with an anterior mediastinal mass is the CT scan of the trachea and chest. Children with tracheobronchial compression greater than 50% on CT cannot be safely anesthetized [13]. Flow–volume loops, specifically the appearance of a variable intrathoracic obstruction pattern

Table 25.16 Grading scale for symptoms in patients with an anterior mediastinal mass

A. Asymptomatic
B. Mild: Can lie supine with some cough/pressure sensation
C. Moderate: Can lie supine for short periods but not indefinitely
D. Severe: Cannot tolerate supine position

when supine, are useful, particularly in the patient unable to give an adequate history. Echocardiography is indicated for patients with vascular compressive symptoms.

1. **Management.** General anesthesia will exacerbate extrinsic intrathoracic airway compression in at least three ways. First, reduced lung volume occurs during general anesthesia; second, bronchial smooth muscle relaxes during general anesthesia allowing greater compressibility of large airways; and third, paralysis eliminates the caudal movement of the diaphragm seen during spontaneous ventilation. This eliminates the normal transpleural pressure gradient that dilates the airways during inspiration and minimizes the effects of extrinsic intrathoracic airway compression.

Management of these patients is guided by their symptoms (Tables 25.16–25.18) and the CT scan. All of these patients requiring general anesthesia need a step-by-step induction of anesthesia with continuous monitoring of gas exchange and hemodynamics. This **"NPIC" (Noli Pontes Ignii Consumere; i.e., don't burn your bridges)** anesthetic induction can be an inhalation induction with a volatile agent such as sevoflurane or IV titration of propofol with or without ketamine, which maintains spontaneous ventilation until either the airway is definitively secured or the procedure is completed [14]. Awake intubation of the trachea before induction is a possibility in some adult patients if the CT scan shows an area of noncompressed distal trachea to which the ETT can be advanced before induction. If muscle relaxants are required, ventilation should first be gradually taken over manually to assure that positive-pressure ventilation is possible and only then can a short-acting muscle relaxant be administered. Development of airway or vascular compression requires that the patient be awakened as rapidly as possible and then other options for the surgery to be explored. Intraoperative life-threatening airway compression usually has responded to one of two therapies: either **repositioning** of the patient (which should be determined before induction if there is one side or

Table 25.17 Stratification of patients regarding safety for NPIC general anesthesia

A. **Safe**	(I)	Asymptomatic adults
	(II)	Asymptomatic children with normal supine and upright flow–volume loops
	(III)	CT min. tracheal/bronchial diameter >50% of normal
B. **Unsafe**	(I)	Severely symptomatic adults
	(II)	Children with abnormal supine/upright flow–volume loops
	(III)	Children with CT tracheal/bronchial diameter <50% of normal
C. **Uncertain**	(I)	Mild/moderate symptomatic adult
	(II)	Asymptomatic adult with CT tracheal/bronchial diameter <50% of normal
	(III)	Asymptomatic adult with abnormal supine/upright flow–volume loops
	(IV)	Symptomatic child with CT tracheal/bronchial diameter >50% of normal
	(V)	Adult or child unable to give history

CT, computed tomography.

Table 25.18 Management for all "uncertain" patients for NPIC general anesthesia

1. Secure airway beyond stenosis awake if feasible
2. Rigid bronchoscope and surgeon available at induction
3. Laryngeal mask airway available
4. Determine optimal positioning of patient
5. Monitor for airway compromise postoperatively

position that causes less compression) or **rigid bronchoscopy** and ventilation distal to the obstruction (this means that an experienced bronchoscopist and equipment must always be immediately available in the operating room with these cases).

Femorofemoral CPB before induction of anesthesia is a possibility for some patients who are considered "unsafe" for NPIC general anesthesia. The concept of CPB "standby" during attempted induction of anesthesia is fraught with danger because there is not enough time after a sudden airway collapse to establish CPB before hypoxic cerebral injury occurs. Other options for "unsafe" patients include local anesthetic biopsy of the mediastinal mass or biopsy of another node (e.g., supraclavicular), preoperative radiotherapy with a non-radiated "window" for subsequent biopsy, preoperative chemotherapy or short-course steroids, and CT-guided biopsy of mass or drainage of a cyst.

H. **Tracheal and bronchial stenting.** Regional narrowing of the trachea or bronchi can be treated temporarily or definitively by placement of tracheal or bronchial stents [15]. The only previous options for these lesions were dilation, laser excision, or surgical excision. Airway stenting is an option for palliation of patients with mediastinal masses pending other therapy. There are two major varieties of stent: metallic and Silastic (Dumon). Both are commonly placed during rigid bronchoscopy, although there is an option to place the self-expanding metallic stents with flexible FOB. The metallic stents are more stable and more resistant to dislocation in the airway but are more difficult (often impossible) to remove once placed.

Anesthetic management for tracheal stenting is similar to management of patients with mediastinal masses. General anesthesia with muscle relaxation is optimal, but in patients with severe symptoms of airway obstruction, induction of anesthesia should follow a step-by-step NPIC protocol as discussed above.

I. **Tracheal resection.** Anatomically, the trachea has a necessary structural rigidity and a segmental blood supply that complicate its resection and repair. Many different prosthetic designs and materials have been evaluated as tracheal substitutes. Because of unresolved problems with anatomic disruption, poor healing, and infection, end-to-end anastomosis of the trachea remains the ideal method of repair.

Endotracheal intubation and resulting strictures were the primary cause of the need for tracheal resection, but using less irritating ETT materials and limiting the duration of prolonged endotracheal intubation have decreased this complication. Benign and malignant tumors (e.g., adenocarcinomas and cylindromas) constitute the remaining indications for tracheal resection.

For a controlled and methodical operation on the trachea, full control of the airway must be maintained at all times. Cooperation between the surgeon and anesthesiologist is of utmost importance. Both should visualize the lesion preoperatively (CT and bronchoscopy). With preoperative planning and discussions, they can avoid unnecessary hasty procedures that might compromise the end result or worse. Benign lesions can be dilated preoperatively to allow the passage of a small ETT through the lesion. Operatively, the area below the lesion is addressed first. If the degree of obstruction increases, a sterile ETT can be placed directly. The patient should be spontaneously ventilating at the end of the case to allow for extubation. Some surgeons will temporarily place a Montgomery "T" tube distal to the anastomosis with the side arm of the "T" brought out anteriorly through the neck incision to ensure gas exchange in case of proximal tracheoglottic obstruction or edema. Some surgeons will leave a temporary "chin retention" suture for several days postoperatively. This heavy suture between the chin and the sternum restricts head extension and limits traction on the fresh tracheal anastomosis. CPB greatly complicates the conduct of the operation and has largely been unnecessary.

J. Combined pulmonary resection and cardiac surgery. Potentially, most cardiac operations (aortocoronary bypass, valve repair/replacement, congenital defects) can be combined with thoracic procedures for either malignant or benign disease (pneumonectomy, lobectomy, wedge resection). There is no agreement about the surgical management of patients found to have both cardiac and thoracic surgical lesions.

The one-stage combined procedure avoids a second anesthetic and incision and may reduce hospital stay. The two-stage procedure may be associated with less blood loss than with pulmonary resection in heparinized patients and may allow better operative exposure and staging of mediastinal nodes for malignant lung lesions. Preferred management at this institution is a one-stage combined procedure because of the documented comparable long-term survival with a low incidence of short-term morbidity and mortality.

Patients with combined surgical lesions present in one of three patterns:

1. An asymptomatic lung lesion is discovered during evaluation for cardiac surgery.
2. A patient being investigated for lung pathology is found to have significant cardiac disease.
3. A previously undetected lung lesion is discovered intraoperatively after sternotomy.

In the first or second scenario, adequate pulmonary assessment can be arranged preoperatively to guide perioperative anesthetic management. When a lesion is discovered intraoperatively, anesthetic management will be more *ad hoc*. Many of these "surprise" lesions are benign (granulomas) and require only simple wedge resection without intraoperative lung isolation or loss of postoperative pulmonary function.

Due to the difficulty assessing subcarinal nodes for staging via a sternotomy, all known lung cancer patients should have a mediastinoscopy as the first step of a combined procedure. For cardiac valvular surgery, because of the risk of contamination of the operative field from an open bronchus, it is recommended to complete the cardiac procedure, wean from CPB, and close the pericardium before the pulmonary resection. Lung isolation and OLV are necessary for lung resection in these cases. A double-lumen EBT placed at induction is the preferred airway management.

For aortocoronary bypass, lung isolation and OLV may not be necessary. It is optimal to perform the pulmonary resection at the end of CPB after the aortic cross-clamp is removed. For cases where difficult weaning from CPB is anticipated (poor ventricular function, prolonged CPB, redo), the preferred management is to wean from CPB and stabilize the patient, then perform the pulmonary resection. Lung isolation will aid in these cases. Because problems weaning from CPB are not always predictable, a BB may be useful in these cases. Because of the increased incidence of phrenic nerve injury and diaphragmatic paralysis associated with topical cooling (slush) of the heart during CPB, topical cooling is not advised during combined cardiac and thoracic procedures.

K. Combined cancer and emphysema surgery. The combination of lung volume reduction surgery (LVRS) or bullectomy in addition to lung cancer surgery has been reported in emphysematous patients who previously would not have met minimal criteria for pulmonary resection because of their concurrent lung disease. Although the numbers of patients reported are small, the expected improvements in postoperative pulmonary function have been seen and the outcomes are encouraging. This offers an extension of the standard indications for surgery in a small, well-selected number of patients.

IV. Lung transplantation. End-stage pulmonary disease (ESPD) is one of the five leading causes of mortality and morbidity in adults in the United States. ESPD results from destruction of the pulmonary parenchyma and vasculature. Lung transplantation is the definitive treatment for these patients. Depending on the patient's pathophysiology, there are several surgical options: single-lung transplantation (SLT), bilateral sequential lung transplantation (BSLT), *en bloc* double-lung transplantation (DbLT), heart-lung transplantation (HLT), and living-related lobar transplantation (LRT). Due to a severe shortage of suitable donor lungs, other therapeutic options were developed that may offer alternatives to those patients who otherwise might succumb to their disease while awaiting lung transplantation. Several improvements in the management of a highly selected group of patients with emphysema via LVRS, patients with cystic fibrosis (CF) via newer antibiotic agents, and patients with pulmonary hypertension via long-term prostacyclin therapy have been reported as viable options.

A. **Epidemiology**
  1. **Total candidates.** There are in excess of one million potential lung transplant recipients among those suffering from ESPD.
  2. **Survival of candidates.** Because the number of lung transplant recipients far exceeds the number of suitable lung donors, up to one third of recipients die while awaiting transplantation. Statistics from April 2001 indicate that there are 3,748 lung recipients and 215 heart-lung recipients awaiting transplantation (United Network Organ Sharing Critical Data, *http://www.unos.org*).
  3. **Total procedures.** The number of reported lung transplants performed from 1994 through 1999 has quadrupled, peaking in 1997. Although the number of centers performing lung transplants has remained stable or increased, continued growth in the number of procedures has reached a plateau despite the rising use of older donors.
      According to the most recent data supplied by the International Society of Heart and Lung Transplant (ISHLT) Registry, a total of 7,204 SLT, 5,420 BSLT, and 2,861 HLT have been performed to date [16].

B. **Pathophysiology of end-stage pulmonary disease**
  1. **Parenchymal ESPD** is classified as obstructive, restrictive, or infectious.
      a. **Obstructive diseases** are characterized by elevation of airway resistance, diminished expiratory flow rates, severe V/Q mismatching, and pronounced air trapping. The most common cause is smoking-induced emphysema; however, other causes include asthma and several comparatively rare congenital disorders. Among these, α_1-antitrypsin deficiency is associated with severe bullous emphysema that manifests in the fourth or fifth decade of life.
      b. **Restrictive diseases** are characterized by interstitial fibrosis that results in a loss of lung elasticity and compliance. Most fibrotic processes are idiopathic in nature but they also may be caused by an immune mechanism or inhalation injury. Interstitial lung diseases may affect the pulmonary vasculature as well; therefore, pulmonary hypertension frequently is present. Functionally, diseases in this category are associated with diminished lung volumes and diffusion capacities, albeit with preserved airflow rates. Respiratory muscle strength usually is adequate because of the increased work of breathing experienced by this patient population.
      c. The common **infectious etiologic factors** are associated with CF and bronchiectasis.
          (1) CF produces mucous plugging of peripheral airways leading to the development of pneumonia, chronic bronchitis, and bronchiectasis. The incidence of CF is 0.2% of live births in the United States.
          (2) Smoking, α_1-antitrypsin deficiency and environmental exposures may lead to the development of bronchiectasis.
  2. **Etiologic factors of end-stage pulmonary vascular diseases** are (a) diffuse arteriovenous malformations, (b) congenital heart disease with Eisenmenger syndrome, or (c) primary pulmonary hypertension (PPH). PPH is rare and most frequently idiopathic. It is characterized by marked elevation of pulmonary vascular resistance secondary to hyperplasia of the muscular pulmonary arteries combined with fibrosis and obliteration of the smallest arterioles.

C. **Recipient selection criteria: indications and contraindications**
  1. **Recipient selection criteria and indications** for lung transplantation are listed in Table 25.19 [17]. Referral and listing of potential candidates are based on the progression of the patient's disease; however, each patient must be considered on an individual basis and be subject to standardized selection criteria.

Table 25.19 Indications and contraindications for lung transplantation

Indications
  Untreatable end-stage pulmonary, parenchymal, and/or vascular disease
  Absence of other major medical illnesses
  Substantial limitation of daily activities
    Projected life expectancy <2 years
    NYHA class III or IV functional level
    Rehabilitation potential
    Satisfactory psychosocial profile and emotional support system
    Acceptable nutritional status
    Disease-specific mortality exceeding transplant specific mortality over 1–2 years
Relative contraindications
  Tobacco use within the past 6 months
  Physiologic age (years)
    >65 for single lung transplantation
    >60 for bilateral lung transplantation
    >55 for heart-lung transplantation
  Psychosocial instability
  Weight <70% or 130% predicted
  Prednisone use >20 mg/d or 40 mg every other day
  Mechanical ventilation
  Major dysfunction of other organs
  Coronary disease or left ventricular dysfunction
  Significant peripheral vascular disease
  Symptomatic osteoporosis
  Severe chest wall deformity
  Sputum with pan-resistant bacteria, fungus, or atypical mycobacterium
  Active hepatitis B or C infection
Absolute contraindications
  Dysfunction of other organs (e.g., renal)
  Current smoking, alcohol or drug abuse
  Bone marrow failure
  Hepatic cirrhosis
  Active malignancy
  HIV infection

HIV, human immunodeficiency virus; NYHA, New York Heart Association.
From DeMeo DL, Ginns LC. Clinical status of lung transplantation: overview. *Transplantation* 2001;72:1717, with permission.

The average waiting period for lung transplantation after the initial referral for evaluation is 1 to 2 years after completion of the screening process.

2. **Relative and absolute contraindications** to lung transplantation are listed in Table 25.19. Although candidates for organ transplantation frequently have abnormal physical or laboratory findings, such information must be distinguished from concurrent primary organ failure or a systemic disease that otherwise might disqualify candidacy. The relative contraindications to lung transplant have changed as improvements in the medical management of potential recipients have evolved. For example, coronary artery disease and corticosteroid usage, once absolute contraindications, are now not prohibitive, particularly if left ventricular function is preserved and corticosteroid doses are moderate [18]. Another highly controversial and debated issue is the transplantation of patients with multiple or pan-resistant bacteria, in particular, patients with CF who concurrently have been diagnosed with *Burkholderia cepacia*. Although the international guidelines do not regard the presence of *B. cepacia* as an absolute contraindication to lung transplantation, there are multiple transplant centers that limit organ allocation and treatment to these

patients. It has been reported in the literature that triple antimicrobial therapy can be bacteriocidal toward multiresistant *B. cepacia* [19]. The decision to ultimately transplant CF patients with this microbe rests with each transplant center because the previous data indicate a much higher incidence of preoperative and postoperative morbidity and mortality in this population.

D. Medical evaluation of lung transplant candidates. All candidates are systematically evaluated by history, physical examination, and the laboratory studies discussed in Section **I.B.** Additionally, evaluation includes chest radiographs; ABG values; spirometric and respiratory flow studies; ventilation and perfusion scanning; and right heart catheterization. Based on studies of the natural history of ESPD, specific laboratory criteria for referral to most lung transplantation programs have been developed and depend on the specific underlying disease (e.g., cardiac index less than 2 L/min/m² in patients with PPH and FEV_1 less than 30% predicted in patients with COPD or CF). Most centers provide documentation of the evaluation results on a summary sheet that is readily available to the anesthesiology team on short notice.

E. Choice of lung transplant procedure is based upon (a) the consequences of leaving a native lung *in situ;* (b) the procedure most likely to yield the best functional outcome for a given pathophysiologic process; and (c) the relative incidence of perioperative complications associated with a particular procedure.

  1. Single-lung transplantation

    a. SLT is commonly selected for transplant recipients with nonseptic lung pathophysiology. SLT is a frequent option for patients with end-stage emphysema; however, in patients with severe bullous emphysema, SLT may exacerbate native lung hyperinflation and result in severe acute and or chronic allograft compromise secondary to compression atelectasis. Preoperative measurement of the recipient static lung compliance has been suggested as a screening technique to determine whether SLT alone, SLT plus LVRS, or BSLT is most beneficial.

    b. SLT offers several advantages over the less frequently used *en bloc* DbLT: (a) allograft availability is optimized to the lung transplant recipient population; (b) SLT is feasible in many patients without the use of CPB, so complications arising from coagulopathic states are less frequent; and (c) bronchial anastomoses used in SLT show a decreased rate of dehiscence compared to tracheal anastomosis used for *en bloc* DbLT.

    c. SLT can be used to treat PPH and postoperative survival is similar when compared to DbLT and BSLT [16]. Because of the hemodynamic instability of these patients, CPB often is used during SLT, DbLT, or BSLT. In this setting, SLT frequently results in severe reperfusion injury to the allograft secondary to its increased pulmonary compliance. There are some data suggesting that early intervention with extracorporeal membrane oxygenation and NO administration intraoperatively and postoperatively may attenuate the effects of reperfusion injury.

    d. SLT involves pneumonectomy and implantation of the lung allograft. The choice of the native lung to be extracted is determined preoperatively. The lung with the poorest pulmonary function as delineated by V/Q scanning is generally chosen for replacement by the allograft. If the native lungs are equally impaired and pleural scarring is absent, the left lung is chosen for relative technical simplicity.

      (1) The native left pulmonary veins are more accessible than those on the right.

      (2) The left hemithorax can more easily accommodate an oversized donor lung.

      (3) The recipient's left main stem bronchus is longer.

  2. Double-lung transplantation

    a. BSLT is the procedure of choice for septic lung disease and other pathophysiologic conditions where BSLT is the preferred technique (e.g., CF). In contrast to *en* bloc DbLT, the BSLT procedure offers several advantages:

(a) it permits two lungs to be implanted without CPB; (b) it decreases the incidence of bronchial anastomotic complications; and (c) it is less technically difficult.

    b. In some instances, BSLT may lead to better functional outcomes in the treatment of end-stage pulmonary hypertension.

3. Heart-lung transplantation

    a. The indications for HLT are diminishing as experience with isolated lung transplantation evolves. The latter operation will suffice in most cases when it is performed before irreversible heart failure occurs or in concert with intracardiac repair of simple congenital defects. The total number of centers performing HLT has decreased from 62 in 1993 to 30 in 1998 [16].

    b. HLT is **indicated** for patients with ESPD complicated by irreversible heart failure or end-stage congenital heart disease with secondary pulmonary vascular involvement (Eisenmenger syndrome). Specific pathologic diagnoses in recipients include PPH, emphysema, multiple pulmonary emboli, CF, and fibrotic and granulomatous diseases of the lung.

4. Living-related donor lobar transplantation

    a. As of December 2000, 139 living-donor lobar transplants have been performed in the United States. Although outcomes in adult recipients are similar to cadaveric transplants, results in the pediatric recipient population are reported to be superior to those who receive cadaveric allografts [20]. Improved function and a decrease in the incidence of bronchiolitis obliterans have been noted.

    b. Although lobar donation is considered to be a relatively safe procedure, one group noted a 61% postoperative complication rate in the living donors. Complications included pleural effusions, bronchial stump fistulas, phrenic nerve injury, and bronchial strictures.

F. Selection criteria for donor lungs

    1. Suitable lung allografts are characterized by P_aO_2 **greater than 300 mm Hg during mechanical ventilation with** FIO_2 **of 1.0 and PEEP of 5 cm** H_2O.

    2. Unilateral pneumonia or trauma does not preclude use of the contralateral lung. In general, the donor **ideally should be younger than 60 years with a smoking history of no more than 20 to 30 pack-years.** Smoking criteria for donor lungs have been liberalized in some incidences, particularly if there is strong evidence indicating that a recipient's death is imminent should there be a prolonged waiting period. Outcomes have been similar when the more liberal smoking criteria have been used for donor lung selection [21].

    3. In an attempt to provide a larger pool of suitable lung donors, the lungs from **non–beating heart donors** have been transplanted and reported to produce a successful recipient outcome [22].

    4. As experience in the field of genetic therapy continues to grow, **cytokine profiling** has come to represent a significant method to identify organs suitable for donation and transplantation. Fisher et al. [23] reported that elevated levels of interleukin-8 in donor lungs were associated with early graft failure and decreased recipient survival. These data suggest that cytokine profiles could be an early indicator of recipient outcome.

    5. Harvesting procedure. Because both the heart and lungs often are harvested from the same donor for different recipients, a method has been developed to perform cardiectomy and reduce the risk of lung injury. During cardiectomy, a residual atrial cuff is left attached to the donor lungs. The trachea is stapled and divided at its midpoint, and the lungs are removed *en bloc*. Subsequently, the pulmonary vasculature is flushed and immersed in a hypothermic preservative (most commonly Euro-Collins or University of Wisconsin solution).

    6. Lung allograft preservation

        a. There are several relevant issues surrounding donor lung preservation; however, all focus on methods to provide ready sources of energy and cryoprotection and to prevent vasospasm, cellular swelling, and accumulation of toxic metabolites. For example, free radical scavengers such as superoxide dismutase and catalase can be added to prevent oxygen-derived free radicals from damaging key intracellular constituents after reperfusion; and prostaglandin E_1 (PGE_1) can be added to promote even cooling and distribution of preservative solutions.

   b. Standard preservation techniques allow a reported **maximum allograft ischemic time of 6 to 8 hours.**

7. **Clinical immunology of organ matching.** ABO matching is essential before transplantation because the donor-specific major blood group isoagglutinins have been implicated as a cause of allograft hyperacute rejection. Once procured, the practical matter of a 6- to 8-hour donor lung ischemic time limit severely restricts prospective matching of histocompatibility antigens, percentage of reactive antibody screens, and the geography of organ donation. One study suggests that the total ischemic time alone is not predictive of a poor outcome after transplantation. Rather, the additive effects of increased donor age (older than 55 years) plus increased ischemic allograft time (more than 6 to 7 hours) are a more reliable indicator of poor posttransplantation survival [24].

G. Preanesthetic considerations

1. Because of a chronic shortage of suitable lungs available for transplantation, many patients experience long waiting periods ranging from several months to several years. **Interval changes** may occur since completion of the initial medical evaluation (see Section **IV.D**). Specifically, reduction in exercise tolerance; new drug regimens or requirements for oxygen and steroids; appearance of purulent sputum; signs or symptoms indicative of right heart failure (e.g., hepatomegaly, peripheral edema); or presence of fever are among the most common occurrences that should be explored in the immediate preoperative period.

2. Lung transplants are always performed as emergency procedures because of the relatively short, safe ischemic time for allografts. As is customary for any emergent surgical procedure, the time of **last oral intake** should be ascertained before induction of general anesthesia.

3. Patients undergoing lung transplantation may exhibit signs and symptoms of anxiety. They usually have not received the benefit of anxiolytic **premedication** before their arrival in the operating room. One should be vigilant when administering anxiolytic agents to these patients so that their impaired respiratory drive is not further compromised.

4. Insertion of a **thoracic epidural catheter** for both intraoperative and postoperative analgesia may be performed before induction of general anesthesia. The catheter should be inserted at a spinal level that provides appropriate anesthesia and analgesia in concordance with the surgical incision site (e.g., T-4 to T-5 or T-5 to T-6). Placement of a thoracic epidural catheter when anticoagulation is anticipated for CPB remains controversial.

5. Chronically cyanotic patients frequently are severely polycythemic (hematocrit greater than 60%) and may manifest clotting abnormalities. In these instances, phlebotomy and hemodilution may be beneficial in minimizing the occurrence of end-organ infarction.

6. **Size matching** between donor and recipient is facilitated by comparing the vertical and transverse radiologic chest dimensions of the donor and recipient. Organs also are matched on the basis of ABO compatibility, because the value of histocompatibility matching still is unknown and requires time in excess of the tolerable ischemic time for the lung allograft.

7. Some **transfusion practices** are specific for transplantation. For example, cytomegalovirus (CMV) seronegative blood products must be available for seronegative recipients if CMV sepsis is to be avoided. When transplantation of CMV negative donors and recipients occurs, leukocyte-poor filters are used to reduce exposure to CMV during transfusion of blood and blood products. Likewise, if human leukocyte antigen alloimmunization is to be avoided, leukocyte-poor blood is necessary for transplant candidates, particularly if they require transfusion before organ transplantation.

8. Close **coordination and effective communication** between the transplant team and the organ harvesting team is vital so that excess allograft ischemic time is avoided.
9. Arrangements should be made for intraoperative availability of a multimodality ventilator for patients with the most severe forms of lung disease. Useful **ventilator settings** include the ability to deliver minute volumes greater than 15 L/min (especially helpful if airway leaks are present); adjustable inflation pressure "popoffs" (to allow high inflation pressures to be delivered to non-compliant lungs); adjustable respiratory cycle waveforms; and availability of high levels of PEEP (e.g., 15 to 20 cm H_2O during reperfusion pulmonary edema).
10. NO and inhaled nebulized prostacyclin have been shown to be effective therapies for treatment of pulmonary hypertension and early reperfusion injury in some patients.

H. **Induction and maintenance of anesthesia**
1. **Preoperative laboratory studies.** These studies are useful to predict difficulties during the induction of general anesthesia. For example, air trapping and diminished expiratory flow rates may exacerbate hypercapnia and lead to hemodynamic instability during mask ventilation and after endotracheal intubation. Elevated PA pressures may indicate the likelihood that CPB may be necessary.
2. **Intraoperative monitoring**
   a. Both **systemic and PA pressure monitoring** are essential during lung transplant procedures. Dyspnea, arrhythmias, RV dilation, and pulmonary hypertension may complicate PA catheter insertion before induction of general anesthesia. Oximetric PA catheters are useful in this setting to evaluate tissue oxygen delivery in patients who are subject to sudden cardiac instability. Some suggest that RV ejection fraction catheters may be useful for the diagnosis of right heart failure. Radial arterial cannulation with or without femoral artery cannulation is appropriate for monitoring of systemic arterial blood pressure. Femoral arterial catheters may interfere with groin cannulation for CPB.
   b. **Pulse oximetry** is useful for continuous monitoring of S_pO_2 during stressful intervals, such as the onset of OLV or cross-clamping of the PA.
   c. **Transesophageal echocardiography** (TEE) is perhaps the most useful monitor available. TEE allows for (a) direct visualization of RV and left ventricular wall motion and function as well as assessment of intracardiac valvular function; (b) assessment of PA and pulmonary vein anastomoses and blood flow; (c) assessment of the elimination of intracardiac air that occurs during pulmonary venous anastomosis; and (d) calculation of PA pressure as measured by color Doppler flow velocity.
3. **IV access.** Large-caliber IV catheters inserted peripherally and centrally (e.g., 14-gauge peripheral IV; 8.5 to 9.0 Fr central venous introducer), supplemented by a rapid infusion device, are essential for lung transplant operations where massive transfusion requirements are anticipated (e.g., HLT for congenital heart disease with Eisenmenger syndrome; BSLT for CF with pleural scarring). When the clamshell incision is used for BSLT, placement of IV catheters in the antecubital fossae should be avoided.
4. **Positioning.** Full lateral decubitus position typically is used during SLT, even when CPB is anticipated (e.g., SLT for PPH). One groin usually is prepped into the field to allow for the option of femoral cannula insertion for CPB. General considerations for the thoracotomy position are reviewed in Section **II.B.** The supine position is used for BSLT, facilitating either median sternotomy or the clamshell incision.
5. **"Pump standby."** This safeguard is prudent for patients with pulmonary hypertension or borderline ABG values, even when SLT is planned.
6. **Selection of anesthetic agents**
   a. Agents that promote hemodynamic homeostasis are preferred for induction of general anesthesia. One example is etomidate and a nondepolarizing neuromuscular blocking agent such as rocuronium, which may be used

during a rapid sequence induction technique. Modest amounts of fentanyl (5 to 10 µg/kg) administered IV may be used if indicated to control cardiovascular responses to endotracheal intubation.

   b. For **maintenance** using conventional anesthetic agents, moderate-to-high doses of opioids (e.g., fentanyl 20 to 75 µg/kg) supplemented with low doses of a potent inhaled agent (e.g., isoflurane, 0.2% to 0.6%) and a long-acting neuromuscular blocking agent are recommended. **Thoracic epidural** anesthesia, in addition to providing excellent postoperative analgesia, may be used to enhance general anesthesia intraoperatively. Continuous infusions of a local anesthetic, such as 0.25% to 0.5% bupivacaine, provide ideal surgical anesthesia and analgesia and allow for reduced doses of both IV opioids and inhaled agents.

   c. **Nitrous oxide** generally is avoided for the following reasons: (a) 100% oxygen almost always is required to maintain an acceptable arterial saturation during OLV; (b) bullae may expand and compress the residual normal lung parenchyma, thus exacerbating V/Q mismatching; and (c) occult pneumothoraces may occur.

7. Securing the airway. Lung isolation is required for optimal surgical exposure. Both double-lumen EBTs and BBs are useful for this purpose. A general discussion of these choices is given in Section **II.A.**

   a. Advantages of double-lumen EBTs in the setting of lung transplantation include the following:

      (1) Facilitation of lung isolation
      (2) Ability to suction the nonventilated lung
      (3) Ability to apply CPAP to the nonventilated lung
      (4) Provision for postoperative independent lung ventilation

   b. Left-sided EBTs (Robertshaw) are recommended for both right and left SLT as well as for BSLT. There is a higher incidence of right upper lobe obstruction when right-sided double-lumen EBTs are used because the right upper lobe orifice is relatively close to the right main stem bronchus.

   c. **Selecting the correct size of EBT** was discussed in Section **II.A.5.B.** In general, the largest sized EBT that can be placed without causing airway trauma is preferred to facilitate therapeutic flexible bronchoscopy both intraoperatively and postoperatively.

   d. Many lung transplant recipients have limited pulmonary reserve, and desaturation during intubation may occur rapidly. Therefore, **initial EBT positioning** can be accomplished quickly and accurately with the aid of a flexible FOB. A complete discussion of bronchoscopic placement is given in Section **II.A.**

8. Management of ventilation

   a. **Lateral decubitus positioning** may be associated with significant alterations in oxygenation and ventilation, depending on the underlying pulmonary pathophysiology. Positional improvement or deterioration in blood gas values sometimes is predictable on the basis of the patient's preoperative V/Q scan.

   b. General strategies for supporting oxygenation during OLV (i.e., during SLT and BSLT) are discussed in Section **II.E.5.**

   c. Alteration of the inspired to expired ratios during mechanical ventilation may be useful during SLT of patients with emphysema. Increasing the expiratory time during each respiratory cycle allows for adequate exhalation, thus reducing the possibility of overinflation of the native lung and subsequent compromise of the allograft.

   d. Similarly, **independent or differential ventilation** often is used during SLT for emphysema recipients, particularly those with gross V/Q mismatching.

   e. After allograft implantation, **the lowest possible F_{IO_2}** to maintain adequate oxygenation is used in concert with **5 to 10 cm H_2O PEEP.** In patients with emphysema, independent lung ventilation allows PEEP to be selectively delivered to the allograft and avoid air trapping and overinflation of the native lung.

    f. Frequent **suctioning and lavage** via **flexible FOB** is helpful to maintain airway patency during BSLT for CF or whenever airway bleeding and secretions are sufficient to cause obstruction and impair gas exchange.

I. Surgical procedures and anesthesia-related interventions

    1. Surgical dissection is complicated by extensive pleural adhesions, vascular anomalies, vascular collaterals, or previous cardiac or thoracic surgery.

    2. OLV almost always is used during SLT to facilitate dissection. The relevant physiology was reviewed in Section **II.A** and **II.E.** With the onset of OLV, acute deterioration in gas exchange and hemodynamics must be anticipated. Strategies for improving oxygenation under these circumstances include the following:

        a. PEEP applied to the dependent (ventilated) lung provided that bullous disease or emphysema is absent

        b. CPAP or high-frequency jet ventilation in the nondependent (nonventilated) lung

        c. Ligation of the branch PA of the operative lung

    3. Clamping the branch PA when PA pressures are low usually is well tolerated and improves V/Q matching and ABG values. If elevated PA pressures exacerbate right heart failure, vasodilators and inotropes may improve systemic hemodynamics; however, gas exchange may be further impaired, depending on the agents that are selected (e.g., nitroprusside may worsen V/Q mismatching). Should the patient's condition deteriorate despite pharmacologic intervention, implementation of CPB should be considered.

    4. Immediately before single-lung implantation, the donor hilar structures are trimmed to match the size of the recipient bronchus, branch PA, and atrial cuff containing the pulmonary venous orifices. While the allograft is kept scrupulously cold, the atrial PA, and bronchial anastomoses are completed in sequence.

    5. The **ischemic interval** ends with the removal of vascular clamps, but until ventilation is restored, systemic arterial saturation remains unchanged. Immediately before vascular unclamping, **methylprednisolone** (500 to 1,000 mg) is administered IV to minimize the potential for hyperacute allograft rejection.

    6. Reinflation of the allograft follows, sometimes with the aid of a flexible FOB to clear airway secretions. This procedure allows for direct viewing of the airway anastomosis to ensure patency.

    7. After SLT for emphysema, independent lung ventilation can be instituted if indicated using the anesthesia ventilator for the native lung (increased expiratory time, low tidal volume, no PEEP) and an intensive care unit-quality ventilator for the allograft (increased respiratory rates, low tidal volumes, 5 to 10 cm H_2O PEEP).

    8. Reperfusion injury, characterized by increasing alveolar–arterial gradients, deteriorating compliance, and gross pulmonary edema, may follow allograft reperfusion within minutes to hours. The most effective treatments are PEEP and strict limitation of volume infusion, both crystalloid and colloid. Rarely, reperfusion injury may be accompanied by pulmonary hypertension. Treatment consists of continuous IV infusion of PGE_1 (0.05 to 0.2 µg/kg/min). Inhaled NO (40 to 80 ppm) also can be used for this purpose. If evidence of right heart failure occurs, continuous IV infusion of norepinephrine (0.05 to 0.2 µg/kg/min), milrinone (0.375 to 0.5 µg/kg/min), or a combination of the two may prove efficacious.

    9. After the patient is returned to the supine position, the EBT can be exchanged for a standard single-lumen ETT or retained for independent lung ventilation in the intensive care unit.

    10. BSLT is used to treat the same spectrum of patients as those treated by the *en bloc* DbLT procedure. BSLT is the preferred technique in many centers. BSLT often can be accomplished without the use of CPB. Its major disadvantage is that serial implantation prolongs the ischemic time for the second allograft lung.

J. Postoperative management and complications

1. The immediate priorities are acute, intensive **respiratory and cardiovascular support.**

   a. Early **respiratory insufficiency** usually is due to reperfusion injury, which is characterized by large alveolar–arterial O_2 gradients, poor pulmonary compliance, and parenchymal infiltrates despite low cardiac filling pressures. Mechanical ventilation with PEEP is essential, but inflation pressures are kept to a minimum in consideration of the new airway anastomoses.

   b. FIO_2 is maintained at the lowest levels compatible with an acceptable arterial oxygen saturation.

   c. Fifteen percent of lung transplant recipients may develop severe lung injury secondary to reperfusion injury and lymphatic disruption during the surgical procedure. This pattern of lung injury can be treated with extracorporeal membrane oxygenation, NO, or selective lung ventilation if indicated.

   d. Acute allograft dysfunction can occur and is associated with a mortality rate of up to 60%.

   e. **Cardiovascular deterioration** may be secondary to hemorrhage, PA or pulmonary venous anastomotic obstruction, tension pneumothorax, or pneumopericardium. TEE may be a useful diagnostic tool in the setting of vascular obstructive lesions. Hemorrhage most frequently occurs after HLT or *en bloc* DbLT, particularly in patients with pleural disease and Eisenmenger syndrome. Tension pneumothorax occurs more frequently in patients with concomitant end-stage emphysema.

2. **Immunosuppression drug regimens** have been developed to control the recipient's immune response and prevent allograft rejection [25]. Most centers use a triple-drug regimen that includes steroids, cyclosporine, and azathioprine. Although these regimens may adequately control acute rejection, chronic rejection still accounts for a majority of long-term morbidity and mortality.

   a. **Cyclosporine** is a small peptide derived from a soil fungus. Its major actions are to inhibit macrophage and T-cell production of interleukins and to block activation of helper T cells.

   b. **Azathioprine blocks** *de novo* purine biosynthesis, which is important to both DNA and RNA production, thus inhibiting both T- and B-cell proliferation.

   c. **Prednisone** is an antiinflammatory drug that suppresses helper T-cell proliferation and interleukin production by T cells.

   d. **FK506 (tacrolimus)** is a macrolide antibiotic with immunosuppressant properties that blocks interleukin production and proliferation of T lymphocytes. It is used as a substitute for cyclosporine in the setting of acute allograft rejection. FK506, in comparison to cyclosporine, has been associated with a lower rate of rejection, similar infection rates, and increased incidence of new-onset diabetes mellitus. It is effective in slowing progression of bronchiolitis obliterans. Some suggest using FK506 as a primary immunosuppressive agent for these reasons.

   e. **Antibodies** include antithymocyte globulin, a polyclonal immunoglobulin G antibody that rapidly reduces circulating T lymphocytes and promotes formation of suppressor T cells. OKT3 is a murine monoclonal antibody directed against the CD3 surface antigen on mature T lymphocytes that blocks the recognition of MHC antigens on foreign cells and the subsequent immune response.

3. The rate of **postoperative infectious complications** is higher in lung transplant patients compared with other solid organ transplant recipients. Therefore, one must be able to differentiate **infection versus allograft rejection.**

   a. Several factors increase the susceptibility of transplanted lungs to infection: (a) exposure to the external environment; (b) pulmonary lymphatic disruption; (c) impairment of mucociliary function; (d) prolonged mechanical ventilation predisposing the patient to nosocomial infection and airway colonization; and (e) presence of airway foreign bodies (e.g., sutures).

   b. Proper diagnosis is crucial to successful outcome and usually is performed via a transbronchial biopsy using flexible FOB. Occasionally, open lung biopsy is necessary.
   c. During the initial 2 postoperative months, nosocomial Gram-negative bacteria are the most frequent **causes of pneumonia.** Thereafter, CMV pneumonitis becomes more common and is associated with progression to a state of chronic allograft rejection.
4. The **vagus, phrenic, and recurrent laryngeal nerves** are jeopardized during lung transplantation. Their injury complicates weaning from mechanical ventilation.
5. **Tracheal anastomotic leaks** often lead to fatal mediastinitis. In contrast, **bronchial fistulas** lead to the development of strictures that are treated by placing silicone stents and repeated airway dilation procedures. Airway complications have decreased as experience with successful lung transplants has increased. Although telescoping of the donor bronchus into the recipient has decreased the incidence of anastomotic dehiscence, the occurrence of anastomotic stenosis remains and varies with the surgical technique used at each center.
K. **Outcome**
   1. **Survival.** Recent reports from the ISHLT Registry indicate that the current 30-day mortality after SLT and DbLT is between 10% and 15% [16]. Specialized lung transplant centers (e.g., Washington University) report even lower mortality (87.1% 1-year survival after SLT and 86.9% after BSLT) [26].
      a. Independent predictors of an adverse outcome at 1 year after transplantation are (a) pretransplant ventilator requirement, (b) retransplant, (c) pretransplant diagnosis other than emphysema, and (d) recipient age.
      b. Post lung transplant morbidity factors include (a) hypertension, (b) renal dysfunction, (c) hyperlipidemia, (d) diabetes mellitus, (e) bronchiolitis obliterans, and (f) development of malignancy (predominantly skin and lymphatics).
      c. Donor age and total allograft ischemic time appear to be significant risk factors for development of bronchiolitis obliterans.
   2. **Exercise tolerance has** been shown to improve after lung transplantation, as has the quality-of-life factors for survivors.
L. **Special considerations for pediatric lung transplantation**
   1. **Epidemiology**
      a. Since 1994, there have been 381 isolated lung transplant procedures reported in children younger than 17 years.
      b. Congenital heart disease, CF, and vascular ESPDs account for almost all diagnoses in pediatric lung recipients. DbLT/BSLT is the most frequent procedure (in contrast to adults in whom SLT is most common).
   2. **Outcome.** One-year survival currently is in excess of 80% when the BSLT procedure is used [16].
   3. **Pathophysiology.** In children with severe developmental anomalies of the lung (e.g., congenital diaphragmatic hernia with pulmonary hypoplasia, and cystadenomatous malformations), isolated lung transplantation may offer the only chance for survival. Rarely, HLT may be indicated during childhood for PPH, CF, or Eisenmenger syndrome.
   4. **Donor lungs.** Size considerations place additional limitations on organ matching for pediatric recipients and thereby exacerbate shortages. The scarcity of suitable donor organs has propagated living-related lung lobe donation; however, the success of this approach is somewhat uncertain. In addition, donor and recipient morbidity and mortality inherent for this operation have sparked considerable controversy.
   5. **Intubation.** In smaller children, using DLTs is not feasible; instead, **selective endobronchial intubation** with a conventional cuffed single-lumen tube is the most frequent choice.
M. **Anesthesia for the post lung transplant patient.** In addition to certain specific considerations, several general principles apply to all patients who have undergone successful lung transplantation, including the toxicity of immunosuppressants,

potential for infectious and malignant complications, and interactions between immunosuppressants and other pharmacologic agents (including anesthetics).

1. **Cardiac denervation** may result after *en bloc* DbLT because extensive retrocardiac dissection often is necessary.
2. Airway anastomoses may be associated with chronic strictures and **inadequate clearance of secretions.**
3. **Toxic systemic effects of immunosuppressants**
   a. **Cyclosporine** is a potent nephrotoxin. Blood urea nitrogen and creatinine levels increase and most patients develop systemic hypertension. Cyclosporine can produce hepatocellular injury, hyperuricemia, gingival hypertrophy, hirsutism, and tremors or seizures (at high serum levels).
   b. **Azathioprine** suppresses all formed elements in the bone marrow. Anemia, thrombocytopenia, and occasionally aplastic anemia may result. Azathioprine is associated with hepatocellular and pancreatic impairment, alopecia, and gastrointestinal distress. There may be an increased requirement in the dosage of nondepolarizing neuromuscular blocking agents in this patient population.
   c. **Prednisone** produces adrenal suppression, glucose intolerance, peptic ulceration, aseptic osteonecrosis, and integument fragility. Controversy surrounds the need to administer intraoperative "stress doses" of glucocorticoids to patients with chronic adrenal suppression.
   d. **FK506 (tacrolimus)** exhibits a spectrum of toxicities including nephrotoxicity similar to cyclosporine.
   e. **Antithymocyte globulin and OKT3** use may be accompanied by fever and other mild systemic symptoms, and rarely by pulmonary edema or aseptic meningitis.
4. **Infections**
   a. Early posttransplantation bacterial infections typically are related to **pneumonia** (*Streptococcus pneumoniae;* Gram-negative bacilli), **wound infection** (*Staphylococcus aureus*), and use of **urinary catheters** (*Escherichia coli*). Because of the particular susceptibility of pneumonia, early extubation of the trachea after general anesthesia is highly recommended.
   b. CMV is the most frequent viral pathogen in lung transplant recipients and results either from primary infection (after contaminated allograft implantation or blood transfusion in seronegative recipients) or secondary to reactivated infection in a seropositive patient.
   c. After the first few months of immunosuppression, vulnerability to **opportunistic pathogens** increases (CMV, *Pneumocystis carinii,* herpes zoster). If diagnosis is rapid and treatment decisive, survival prevails. Prophylactic antibiotic regimens are available and have been successful in reducing the prevalence of some of these infections (e.g., trimethoprim-sulfamethoxazole for *P. carinii*).
5. **Posttransplant lymphoproliferative disorders** are more likely to develop in immunosuppressed patients. Posttransplant lymphoproliferative disorder is the third leading cause of death outside the perioperative period, with an incidence ranging from 1.8% to 20%. Other neoplasms have been associated with immunosuppression, including (a) non-Hodgkin lymphoma; (b) squamous cell carcinoma of the skin and lip; (c) Kaposi sarcoma; and (d) carcinoma of the vulva, perineum, kidney, and hepatobiliary tree.
6. **Drug interactions**
   a. Both cyclosporine and prednisone are metabolized by the cytochrome P450 enzyme system in hepatocytes. Drugs that inhibit those enzymes (e.g., calcium channel blockers) may increase their serum concentrations and promote toxic side effects.
   b. Other drugs (e.g., barbiturates and phenytoin) may induce the P450 enzymes and decrease cyclosporine levels below therapeutic range.

N. **The future of lung transplantation.** Lung transplantation has been a viable therapeutic option for many patients with ESPD. Obstacles with regard to graft availability, allograft function, and prolongation of patient survival remain to be overcome. New therapies, such as LVRS and nebulized prostacyclin for patients with end-stage pulmonary hypertension, may eliminate the need for transplantation altogether [27]. Living-related pulmonary lobar transplantation and gene therapy for transplant-related injuries show much promise. Refinements of current methods for organ harvest and preservation, along with the development of improved techniques to evaluate donor organs, are important obstacles yet to be overcome. Ultimately, further technologic advances may lead to the success of xenotransplantation and the development of pulmonary organogenesis, providing a solution to the ongoing shortage of suitable organs available for transplantation

V. Lung volume reduction surgery. Approximately 15 million persons in the United States are afflicted with COPD, and two million of these patients have emphysema. Airflow obstruction associated with chronic bronchitis or emphysema occurs due to a loss of the elastic recoil properties of the lung and chest wall. As the disease progresses, patients become increasingly debilitated. Patients exhibit symptoms of severe dyspnea, require supplemental oxygen, and display poor exercise tolerance. LVRS offers a select group of patients the possibility of improved exercise tolerance, reduction in dyspnea, improved quality of life, and extended life span. It has been suggested that LVRS may provide these patients with a benefit that otherwise cannot be achieved by any means other than lung transplantation.

    A. History of lung volume reduction surgery

        1. In 1957, Otto Brantigan, M.D., described a surgical technique for patients with end-stage emphysema that was designed to alleviate symptoms of severe dyspnea and exercise intolerance. It was Brantigan's intent to remove functionally useless areas of the lung in order to restore pulmonary elastic recoil, thus increasing the outward traction on small airways and subsequently improve airflow. Brantigan believed that this technique could restore diaphragmatic and thoracic contours that would improve respiratory excursion. Additionally, he reasoned that by excising the nonfunctional lung tissue, the compressive effects exerted on normal lung tissue could be relieved and result in improved V/Q matching. Unfortunately, the operative mortality was significant and no objective measures of benefit could be documented. Thus, early LVRS was abandoned as a viable therapy for patients with end-stage emphysema until 1993.

        2. In 1996, Joel Cooper, M.D., authored an editorial advocating the technique of LVRS as a "logical, physiologically sound procedure of demonstrable benefit for a selected group of patients with no alternative therapy [28]." He further stated that the successful application of LVRS was "made possible through an improved understanding of pulmonary physiology, improved anesthetic and surgical techniques, and lessons learned from experience with lung transplantation." Although Dr. Cooper touted the benefits of LVRS for certain patients, he did not minimize the surgical risk and suggested that this was not a procedure to be performed in all health care centers across the country. He made the following proposal:

        1) health care providers should restrict the application of this (LVRS) procedure to a limited number of centers of excellence; 2) such centers should be required to document and report specified information regarding morbidity, mortality and objective measures of outcome; and 3) these data should be periodically reviewed and evaluated by a scientific panel before approval to continue performing the procedure is approved.

        Additionally, he advocated that the patients who would otherwise qualify for lung transplantation should be simultaneously evaluated for LVRS so that they would receive the procedure proving to be most appropriate. Although Dr. Cooper did not necessarily advocate a long-term prospective randomized trial to validate the benefit of LVRS, his proposals led to the design and implementation of the National Emphysema Treatment Trial (NETT).

    B. The NETT commenced in October 1997. It is a prospective, randomized, multicenter trial sponsored by the National Heart, Lung, and Blood Institute in conjunction with Health Care Financing Administration [now known as Center for Medicare and Medicaid Services (CMS)] that has a duration of 4.5 years and includes a total of

4,700 patients. Patients who are considered for entry into the study must have Medicare insurance unless their private insurer is willing to cover the costs.

1. The **primary objective** of the NETT is to determine if the addition of LVRS to medical therapy improves patient survival and increases exercise capacity.

2. **Secondary objectives** include defining the profile of patients likely to benefit from LVRS and determining if LVRS improves quality of life, reduces debilitating symptoms, and improves overall pulmonary function.

3. Patients are randomized to either medical therapy alone or medical therapy plus surgery. Surgical patients are further randomized to intervention via either **median sternotomy** or **bilateral thoracoscopy**.

4. A successful procedure is defined as a **60% to 70% increase in FEV₁ by 3 months postoperatively that is sustained for at least 1 year; decreased total lung capacity and residual volume; improved exercise tolerance; and significant reduction in supplemental oxygen requirement**.

C. **Results**. At the time of this writing, the final results of the NETT were not known; however, there are several reports based on early LVRS that were published before the start of the NETT as well as a preliminary outcomes report by the NETT Research Group.

1. Gaissert et al. [29] compared the outcome of patients who received either LVRS or a lung transplant. In their series, they found that although the patients who received either a single or bilateral lung transplant exhibited superior pulmonary function, LVRS achieved satisfactory improvement of disabling symptoms early after operation and avoided the immunosuppression and transplant-specific complications. They also found that LVRS was a suitable procedure for selected patients who also were eligible for lung transplantation and that LVRS provided an earlier option of treatment for those awaiting lung transplant. Finally, they concluded that LVRS might be the only alternative for some patients with debilitating emphysema who would not otherwise qualify as a transplant candidate.

2. Cooper et al. [30] reported another series of 150 consecutive bilateral lung volume reduction procedures in 1996. Patients between the ages of 36 and 77 years with severe emphysema were selected to undergo LVRS based on the following criteria: (a) severe dyspnea; (b) an increased total lung capacity (142% of predicted value) and decreased FEV₁ (25% of predicted value); and (c) a pattern of emphysema that included regions of severe destruction, hyperinflation, and poor perfusion. Ninety-three percent of these patients were oxygen dependent. The results of this series of patients significantly impacted the future of LVRS. The 90-day mortality was 4%; hospital stay decreased with the increased experience of the health care team; prolonged air leak was the major complication; and patients displayed a significant reduction in dyspnea and improvement in their overall quality of life compared to the preoperative state. At 6 months there was an increase in FEV₁, decreased residual volume, an average increase in P₍ₐ₎O₂ of 8 mm Hg, and 70% of all patients no longer required supplemental oxygen. This same series of patients was reevaluated 1 and 2 years after LVRS, and the group maintained benefit from their surgery at both periods.

3. Brenner et al. [31] described the result of the largest study reported to date. This series of 256 patients who had bilateral LVRS for emphysema focused on the survival data. Patients had a 1-year survival of 85% ± 2.3% and a 2-year survival of 81% ± 2.7%. They also found that the survivors tended to be younger than 70 years and had higher baseline FEV₁ (greater than 0.5 L) and P₍ₐ₎O₂ (greater than 54 mm Hg). Patients with the greatest short-term improvement in FEV₁ postoperatively (greater than 0.56 L) had overall significantly better long-term survival.

4. In 2001, the NETT Research Group [32] released a preliminary outcomes report on a group of 1,033 patients. They reported that caution is warranted when using LVRS in emphysema patients with a low FEV₁ (at least 20% of predicted value) and either homogenous emphysema or a very low carbon monoxide diffusing capacity (at least 20% of predicted value). Furthermore, they concluded

that this group of patients was unlikely to benefit from LVRS and they were at high risk for postoperative death.

D. Anesthetic management for lung volume reduction surgery. Anesthesiologists and their expertise are essential to the continued successful outcomes for patients undergoing LVRS. Our expertise in cardiopulmonary physiology, pharmacology, and pain management allows us to minimize complications in the postoperative period.

    1. Preoperative assessment. All patients scheduled for LVRS within the confines of the NETT receive the following preoperative physiologic studies: (a) standard pulmonary function studies; (b) plethysmographic measurement of lung volumes; (c) standardized 6-minute walk test; (d) ABG values; (e) quantitative nuclear lung perfusion scans; and (f) radionuclide cardiac ventriculogram and/or dobutamine stress echocardiogram.

    2. Preoperative pulmonary rehabilitation program. After the initial preoperative evaluation, all patients are enrolled into a pulmonary rehabilitation program for a minimum of 6 weeks before surgical intervention.

    3. Monitors. In addition to the standard monitors, large-bore IV access and an arterial line are recommended. The use of central venous catheters and PA catheters should be considered on an individual patient basis.

    4. The judicious use of **TEA,** both intraoperatively and postoperatively, affords advantages as follows: (a) preserved ability to cough and clear secretions, thus decreasing atelectasis and possibly reducing pulmonary infection; (b) decreased airway resistance; (c) improved phrenic nerve function; (d) stabilization of coronary endothelial function; (e) improved myocardial perfusion; (f) earlier return of bowel function; (g) preservation of immunocompetence; and (h) decreased cost of perioperative care through reduction of perioperative complications. Best results are obtained with catheters placed at the T-4 to T-5 or T-5 to T-6 spinal level.

        a. Intraoperative TEA. TEA can be used as an adjunct to general anesthesia. Local anesthetics, such as 2% lidocaine, 0.25% bupivacaine, or 0.5% bupivacaine, provide optimal surgical conditions. The local anesthetics can be delivered via intermittent bolus or as continuous infusion.

            (1) Because persistent air leaks may be a problem in the postoperative period and may be exacerbated by positive-pressure ventilation, it is optimal to extubate the patients either at the conclusion of surgery or as soon as possible thereafter.

            (2) Caution must be exercised if opioids are added to the infusate because they have the potential to severely depress the patient's respiratory efforts.

        b. Postoperative TEA. TEA provides superior postoperative analgesia for both median sternotomy and bilateral thoracoscopic surgical procedures. A reduced concentration of local anesthetic plus a small dose of opioids delivered by continuous infusion is suggested (e.g., 0.125% bupivacaine plus 0.01 mg/mL hydromorphone).

    5. A left-sided double-lumen EBT should be used to secure the patient's airway.

    6. General anesthesia. Induction of general anesthesia can be conducted with agents that promote hemodynamic homeostasis. An example is etomidate 0.2 mg/kg plus an easily reversible nondepolarizing neuromuscular blocking agent such as rocuronium. Maintenance anesthesia may consist of low doses of a volatile agent (e.g., 0.2% to 0.4% isoflurane) and oxygen in addition to TEA. The anesthetic plan for each patient should be individualized appropriately.

    7. Postoperative management. Problems that should be anticipated in the postoperative period include (a) oversedation, (b) accumulation of airway secretions, (c) pneumothorax, (d) bronchospasm, (e) pulmonary embolism, (f) pneumonia, and (g) persistent air leaks. Reintubation and mechanical ventilation are associated with high morbidity and mortality. Several measures can be taken to minimize these adverse side effects:

        a. Judicious pulmonary toilet

        b. Bronchodilators

        c. Effective analgesia with TEA

E. Conclusions. In summary, we need to consider the following points. What is the future for LVRS? Should patients who can potentially benefit from LVRS be excluded because of an inability to pay? Can anesthesiologists make a difference in the outcome of patients undergoing LVRS? It is the opinion of the authors that LVRS is a viable and valuable therapy that shows clear benefit for a highly select group of patients with end-stage emphysema. Many of these patients have no other therapeutic options available to them, and some who would qualify for lung transplantation may die in the interim period. Because LVRS has been demonstrated to be of benefit to some patients, insurers should no longer consider this form of therapy as experimental or investigational. The final results of the NETT may support this position. If LVRS is to continue to prove beneficial to patients with end-stage emphysema, it is essential that anesthesiologists continue to be intimately involved in the perioperative care. Our expertise does make a difference!

References

 1. Kearney DJ, Lee TH, Reilly JJ, et al. Assessment of operative risk in patients undergoing lung resection. *Chest* 1994;105:753.
 2. Slinger PD, Johnston MR. Preoperative assessment for pulmonary resection. *J Cardiothorac Vasc Anesth* 2000;14:202–211.
 3. **Cerfolio RJ, Allen MS, Trastak VF, et al. Lung resection in patients with compromised pulmonary function. *Ann Thorac Surg* 1996;62:348.**
 4. Golledge J, Goldstraw P. Renal impairment after thoracotomy: incidence, risk factors and significance. *Ann Thorac Surg* 1994;58:524.
 5. Slinger P, Suissa S, Triolet W. Predicting arterial oxygenation during one-lung ventilation. *Can J Anaesth* 1992;39:1030–1035.
 6. Arndt GA, DeLessio ST, Kranner PW. One-lung ventilation when intubation is difficult—presentation of a new endobronchial blocker. *Acta Anaesthesiol Scand* 1999;43:356.
 7. Slinger P, Scott WAC. Arterial oxygenation during one-lung ventilation: a comparison of enflurane and isoflurane. *Anesthesiology* 1995;82:940.
 8. Hogue CW Jr. Effectiveness of low levels of non-ventilated lung continuous positive airway pressure in improving oxygenation during one-lung ventilation. *Anesth Analg* 1994; 79:364.
 9. **Slinger P. Fiberoptic bronchoscopic positioning of double lumen tubes. *J Cardiothorac Anesth* 1989;3:486–496.** For photographs see "Double-Lumen Tubes" in the Review Articles section at the web site *www.thoracicanesthesia.com.*
10. Slinger P. Post-pneumonectomy pulmonary edema: is anesthesia to blame? *Curr Opin Anesthesiol* 1999;12:49–54.
11. Amar D, Roistacher N, Burt ME, et al. Effects of diltiazem versus digoxin on dysrhythmias and cardiac function after pneumonectomy. *Ann Thorac Surg* 1997;63:1374.
12. Riley RH, Wood BM. Induction of anesthesia in a patient with a bronchopleural fistula. *Anaesth Intens Care* 1994;22:625.
13. **Shamberger RC, Hozman RS, Griscom NT, et al. Prospective evaluation by computed tomography and pulmonary function tests of children with mediastinal masses. *Surgery* 1995;118:468.**
14. Frawley G, Low J, Brown TCK. Anaesthesia for an anterior mediastinal mass with ketamine and midazolam infusion. *Anaesth Intens Care* 1995;23:610–612.
15. Licker M, Schweizer A, Nicolet G, et al. Anesthesia of a patient with an obstructing tracheal mass: a new way to manage the airway. *Acta Anaesthesiol Scand* 1997;41:84–86.
16. **Hosenpud JD, Bennett LE, Keck BM, et al. The Registry of the International Society for Heart and Lung Transplantation: eighteenth official report—2001. *J Heart Lung Transplant* 2001;20:805–815.**
17. **Demeo DL, Ginns LC. Clinical status of lung transplantation: overview. *Transplantation* 2001;72:1713–1724.**
18. Snell GI, Richardson M, Griffiths AP, et al. Coronary artery disease in potential lung transplant recipients greater than 50 years old: the role of coronary intervention. *Chest* 1999;116:874.
19. Aris RM, Gilligan PH, Neuringer IP, et al. The effects of pan-resistant bacteria in cystic fibrosis patients on lung transplant outcome. *Am J Respir Crit Care Med* 1997;155:1699.
20. Starnes VA, Woo MS, MacLaughlin EF, et al. Comparison of outcomes between living donor and cadaveric lung transplantation in children. *Ann Thorac Surg* 1999;68:2279.

21. **Bhorade SM, Vigneswaran W, McCabe MA, et al. Liberalization of donor criteria may expand the donor pool without adverse consequence in lung transplantation.** *J Heart Lung Transplant* **2000;19:1199.**
22. Shennib H, Kuang JQ, Giaid A. Successful retrieval and function of lungs from non-heart-beating donors. *Ann Thorac Surg* 2001;71:458.
23. Fisher AJ, Donnelly SC, Hirani N, et al. Elevated levels of interleukin-8 in donor lungs is associated with early graft failure after lung transplantation. *Am J Respir Crit Care Med* 2001;163:259.
24. **Novik RJ, Bennett LE, Meyer DM, et al. Influence of graft ischemic time and donor age on survival after lung transplantation.** *J Heart Lung Transplant* **1999; 18:425.**
25. **Hausen B, Morris RE. Review of immunosuppression for lung transplantation: novel drugs, new uses for conventional immunosuppressants, and alternative strategies.** *Clin Chest Med* **1997;18:353.**
26. **Meyers BF, Lynch J, Trulock E, et al. Lung transplantation: a decade of experience.** *Ann Surg* **1999;230:362–371.**
27. **Meyers BF, Yusen RD, Guthrie TJ, et al. Outcome of bilateral lung volume reduction in patients with emphysema potentially eligible for lung transplantation.** *J Thorac Cardiovasc Surg* **2001;122:10–17.**
28. Cooper JD, Lefrak SS. Is volume reduction surgery appropriate in the treatment of emphysema? Yes. *Am J Respir Crit Care Med* 1996;153:1201–1204.
29. Gaissert HA, Trulock EP, Cooper JD, et al. Comparison of early functional results after volume reduction or lung transplantation for chronic obstructive pulmonary disease. *J Thorac Cardiovasc Surg* 1996;111:296–307.
30. Cooper JD, Patterson GA, Sundaresan RS, et al. Results of 150 consecutive bilateral lung volume reduction procedures in patients with severe emphysema. *J Thorac Cardiovasc Surg* 1996;112:1319–1330.
31. Brenner, Matthew MD, et al. Survival following bilateral staple lung volume reduction surgery for emphysema. *Chest* 1999;115:390–396.
32. National Emphysema Treatment Trial Research Group. Patients at high risk of death after lung-volume-reduction surgery. *N Engl J Med* 2001;345:1075–1082.

26. PAIN MANAGEMENT FOR CARDIOTHORACIC PROCEDURES

Mark Stafford-Smith and Thomas M. McLoughlin, Jr.

I. Introduction
A. Incidence and severity of pain after cardiothoracic procedures
It is generally accepted that surgeries requiring sternotomy and particularly thoracotomy incisions are some of the most debilitating of all surgeries for postoperative patients, both from a pain and a respiratory function viewpoint. In addition to incisional skin pain, other sources of discomfort are important after cardiothoracic surgery. Additional rib and sternal fractures and costovertebral joint pain from vigorous spreading of the ribs all may contribute to postoperative pain. Chronic pain due to intercostal nerve injury develops in approximately 50% of postthoracotomy patients; in 5% the pain becomes severe and disabling. Despite much early speculation that minimally invasive thoracic and cardiac procedures involving smaller incisions would reduce the incidence and severity of postoperative pain compared to traditional cardiac surgery, clinical experience has not borne out this assumption in most cases. No single thoracotomy technique has been shown to reduce the incidence of chronic postthoracotomy pain, and patients should be warned of this potential complication.

B. Transmission pathways for nociception
An understanding of the anatomy and physiology of pain pathways underpins the logical use of analgesic strategies for cardiothoracic surgery. Multimodal approaches take advantage of numerous therapeutic targets in the signaling chain to optimize pain control while minimizing side effects.

In the thoracic region, pain signals are relayed through myelinated Aδ and unmyelinated C fibers in peripheral intercostal nerves. The ventral, posterior, and visceral branches of each intercostal nerve innervate the anterior chest wall, posterior chest wall, and visceral aspects of the chest, respectively. These branches join together just before entering the paravertebral space and then pass through the intervertebral foramina into the spinal canal. Sensory intercostal nerve fibers form a dorsal root that fuses with the spinal cord dorsal horn to enter the central nervous system (CNS). Somatic pain is mediated predominantly through myelinated Aδ fibers in the ventral and posterior branches. Sympathetic (visceral) pain is mediated by unmyelinated C fibers in all three branches. Sympathetic afferent pain signals are directed from intercostal nerve branches through the sympathetic trunk (a paravertebral structure found just beneath the parietal pleura in the thorax), and then pass back into peripheral nerves to enter the CNS from T-1 to L-2. In addition, the vagus nerve provides parasympathetic visceral innervation of the thorax. This cranial nerve enters the CNS through the medulla oblongata and, therefore, is not affected by epidural or spinal methods of pain control.

The spinal cord and spinal canal are considerably different in length, and consequently spinal cord segments do not always sit opposite their respective vertebrae. Thus, knowledge of spinal anatomy is essential if regional analgesia techniques are to be successful. This is particularly true with the use of lipid-soluble epidural opioids, because the targeted dorsal horn often is significantly cephalad relative to the associated intervertebral foramen and nerve.

Most spinal pain signals are transmitted to the brain after crossing from the dorsal horn to contralateral spinal cord structures (e.g., spinothalamic tract). Distribution of nociceptive messages occurs to numerous locations in the brain, resulting in cognitive, affective, and autonomic responses to the noxious stimulus.

Endogenous modification of pain signals starts at the site of tissue trauma, including hyperalgesia related to inflammation, and other CNS-mediated phenomena such as "windup." The substantia gelatinosa of the dorsal horn is an important location for pain signal modulation, including effects that are mediated through opioid, adrenergic, and N-methyl-D-aspartate (NMDA) receptor systems.

C. Analgesia considerations: the procedure, patient, and process
The degree and location of surgical trauma, particularly in relation to the site of skin incisions and route of bony access to the chest, are particularly important in anticipating analgesic requirements after cardiothoracic surgery. Notably, minimally invasive procedures that reduce surgical trauma but relocate it to more pain-sensitive regions (e.g., minithoracotomy vs sternotomy) may not translate into reduced postoperative pain. Analgesic strategies must be individualized, particularly

for high-risk patients in whom outcome benefits may be the greatest. Application of "fast track" principles to cardiothoracic surgery has become common and requires a rational approach to postoperative analgesia. This includes not only appropriate postoperative analgesia delivery but also preoperative education regarding pain reporting, analgesia procedures, and devices, and expectations for postoperative transition to oral analgesics and home administration.

D. Adverse consequences of pain

In addition to the unpleasant cognitive aspects of pain, nociceptive signals have several other effects that can be harmful and delay patient recovery. These include activation of CNS neuroendocrine reflexes that constitute the surgical stress response, a catabolic state involving the release of numerous humoral substances (e.g., cortisol, vasopressin, renin, angiotensin) that is characterized by increased circulating catecholamines, decreased vagal tone, and increased oxygen consumption. Spinal reflex responses to pain include localized muscle spasm and activation of the sympathetic nervous system.

The pathophysiologic consequences of local and systemic responses to pain include respiratory complications related to diaphragmatic dysfunction, myocardial ischemia, ileus, urinary retention and oliguria, thromboembolism, and immune impairment [1].

E. Outcome benefits of good analgesia for cardiothoracic procedures

A primary benefit of effective pain control is patient satisfaction. Studies have documented additional advantages of optimizing analgesia. Outcome benefits that involve perioperative complications appear to be highly related to the analgesia technique used, particularly in relation to the effectiveness in blocking the surgical stress response and nociceptive spinal reflexes. In this regard, neuraxial and regional analgesia appear to be the most effective. The outcome benefits of regional analgesia are nicely summarized in a review by Lui et al. [2]. In general, the benefits reflect the avoidance of the adverse consequences of pain outlined in Section **I.D.** In addition, effective analgesia, established before surgery, appears in some settings to provide a preemptive advantage and may protect against the development of chronic pain syndromes.

F. Economic and acute pain service issues, and Joint Commission on Accreditation of Healthcare Organizations pain management standards

In 2001, the Joint Commission on Accreditation of Healthcare Organizations (JCAHO) integrated pain evaluation and management into its standards for accreditation of health care organizations. This reflects the general increasing awareness of the importance of pain for patients, both in the unpleasantness of the experience and the adverse influence on outcome. Six standards assert a patient's right to have appropriate in-hospital education, assessment and treatment of pain, and, as necessary, postdischarge provisions for pain management. The goal of these standards is to make pain the fifth vital sign; they can be reviewed at the JCAHO web site (*www.jcaho.org*).

Whereas many institutions already have acute pain services that are well established, the consequence of the JCAHO standards on perioperative service planners and funding agencies has been to further emphasize the importance of dedicating resources and financial support to the pain relief specialist.

II. Pain management pharmacology

A. Opioid analgesics

1. Mechanisms

Opioid analgesics are a broad group of compounds that includes naturally occurring extracts of opium (e.g., morphine, codeine); synthetic surrogates (e.g., fentanyl, hydromorphone); and endogenous peptides (e.g., endorphins, enkephalins). They are linked through their interaction with opioid receptors; however, individual drugs may function as agonists, antagonists, or partial agonists at different receptor populations. Opioid receptors are widely distributed, but they are concentrated within the substantia gelatinosa of the dorsal horn of the spinal cord, as well as regions of the brain including the rostral ventral medulla, locus ceruleus, and midbrain periaqueductal gray area. Stimulation of opioid receptors inhibits adenyl cyclase, closes voltage-dependent calcium channels, and opens calcium-dependent inwardly rectifying potassium channels, resulting in inhibitory effects characterized by neuronal hyperpolarization and decreased excitability [3]. Opioid receptor subtypes have been sequenced and cloned, and they belong to the growing list of G-protein–coupled receptors. The effects of agonist binding at different opioid receptor subtypes are summarized in Table 26.1.

  2. **Perioperative use**

Opioids are commonly administered throughout the perioperative period for cardiothoracic procedures. Preoperatively, they can be given orally, intramuscularly (IM), or intravenously (IV) in order to provide anxiolysis and analgesia for transport and placement of intravascular catheters. Intraoperatively, they are given IV as either the primary anesthetic agent or, more commonly, as an adjunct to a mixed anesthetic technique that includes potent inhaled anesthetics, benzodiazepines, and other agents. Finally, they can be injected directly into the thecal sac or included as a component of epidural infusions, to provide intraoperative and postoperative analgesia. An individual opioid for epidural administration is best chosen with knowledge of the position of the epidural catheter relative to the dermatomes involved in the pain and the relative lipophilicity of the drug [4]. Highly lipophilic drugs, such as fentanyl, are best used with catheters placed near the involved dermatomes. Hydrophilic drugs, such as morphine, are best used with remote catheters. Drugs with intermediate lipophilicity, such as hydromorphone, can be used for more balanced spread.

  3. **Side effects and cautions**

  a. Respiratory depression (increased risk with higher dosing, coadministration of other sedatives, opioid-naïve patients, advanced age, central neuraxial administration of hydrophilic opioid agents).

  b. Pruritus

  c. Nausea

  d. Urinary retention, especially common in males receiving spinal opioids

  e. Inhibition of intestinal peristalsis/constipation

  f. CNS excitation/hypertonia, much more notable with rapid IV administration of lipophilic agents

  g. Miosis

  h. Biliary spasm

  i. All of the above effects can be reversed with administration of opioid antagonist drugs (e.g., naloxone)

B. **Nonsteroidal antiinflammatory drugs**

  1. **Mechanisms**

Nonsteroidal antiinflammatory drugs (NSAIDs) act principally through both central and peripheral inhibition of cyclooxygenase, resulting in decreased synthesis of prostaglandins. Prostaglandins are short-lived molecules that are formed throughout the body in response to specific stimuli. They are involved in the physiology of numerous systems, including renal blood flow, bronchial smooth muscle, hemostasis, the gastric mucosa, and the inflammatory response. Specifically, prostaglandin E_2 is the eicosanoid produced in greatest

Table 26.1 Opioid receptors

Type	Mediated effects
μ_1	Analgesia
μ_2	Respiratory depression, euphoria, physical dependence, pruritis, nausea and vomiting
κ	Spinal analgesia, sedation, miosis, diuresis
σ	Dysphoria, hypertonia
δ	Spinal analgesia, Mu-receptor modulation

quantity at sites of trauma and inflammation. It is an important mediator of pain. The full therapeutic effects of NSAIDs are complex and likely involve mechanisms that are independent of prostaglandin effects. For example, prostaglandin synthesis is effectively inhibited with low doses of most NSAIDs; however, much higher doses are required to produce antiinflammatory effects.

2. Perioperative use

NSAIDs are useful for postoperative analgesia. There are preparations for oral, rectal, IM, and IV administration. They are most commonly administered in cardiothoracic surgical patients as a complement to neuraxial techniques. Their principal advantage is the absence of respiratory depression and other opioid side effects.

3. Side effects and cautions
   a. Decreased renal blood flow/parenchymal ischemia
   b. Gastrointestinal mucosal irritation
   c. Impaired primary hemostasis

C. COX-2 inhibitors

1. Mechanisms

The effects of cyclooxygenase are mediated by two distinct isoenzymes, termed COX-1 and COX-2. COX-1 is the constitutive form, responsible for production of prostaglandins involved in homeostatic processes of the kidney, gut, endothelium, and platelets. COX-2 is predominantly an inducible isoform, responsible for production of prostaglandins during inflammation. A few constitutive roles of COX-2 are being investigated, including mediation of renal sodium balance and control of glomerular filtration. Highly selective COX-2 inhibitors have been developed and are being used in clinical settings (e.g., celecoxib, rofecoxib). These drugs retain analgesic and antiinflammatory properties with less risk of adverse side effects attributable to the inhibition of COX-1 with nonselective NSAIDs.

2. Perioperative use

Current preparations of COX-2 inhibitors are at various stages of approval by the U.S. Food and Drug Administration (FDA) for treatment of acute pain. They are limited to oral administration, which precludes their use intraoperatively or immediately postoperatively. COX-2 inhibitors suitable for parenteral administration are being developed. If deemed safe and effective for treatment of acute pain in the perioperative setting, these agents are likely to become a popular choice for analgesia throughout the perioperative period.

3. Side effects and cautions
   a. Gastrointestinal complications are largely absent with COX-2 inhibitors, except with high doses and prolonged therapy.
   b. Platelets contain exclusively COX-1; thus, platelet impairment effects are absent with COX-2 inhibition.
   c. The risk of adverse renal effects may be reduced with COX-2 inhibitors versus traditional NSAIDs. However, reversible volume overload and renal failure have been reported with their use, and caution must be used for patients with congestive heart failure, liver disease, or preexisting renal insufficiency [5].

D. Local anesthetics

1. Mechanisms

Local anesthetics interrupt neural conduction, thus disrupting transmission of pain and other nerve impulses through blockade of neuronal voltage-gated sodium channels. This blockade does not change the resting potential of the nerve. However, altered sodium ion channel permeability slows depolarization such that, in the presence of a sufficient concentration of local anesthetic, threshold for propagation of an action potential cannot be reached.

2. Perioperative use

Local anesthetics are used throughout the perioperative period for topical, infiltration, peripheral nerve, or central neuraxial anesthesia. Their advantage lies in the capacity to provide profound analgesia without the undesired side effects seen with opioids or NSAIDs. Effective regional anesthesia is the best technique to most completely attenuate the neurohumoral stress response to pain. Thoracic epidural analgesia is particularly useful in treating pain, both somatic and visceral, for patients with occlusive coronary artery disease.

3. Side effects and cautions

a. Not surprisingly, side effects from sodium channel blockade due to local anesthetic toxicity resemble those observed with severe hyponatremia. Excessive blood concentrations, reached through absorption or inadvertent intravascular injection, predictably result in toxic effects on the CNS (seizures, coma) and the heart (negative inotropy, conduction disturbances, arrhythmias). Table 26.2 lists commonly accepted maximum local anesthetic dosing for infiltration anesthesia.

b. Caution must be exercised in the performance of any invasive regional anesthesia procedure in the setting of ongoing or proposed anticoagulation or thrombolysis.

c. Allergic reactions are not uncommon, particularly to the para-aminobenzoic acid metabolites of ester local anesthetics or to preservative materials in commercial local anesthetic preparations. True allergic reactions to preservative-free amide local anesthetics (e.g., lidocaine) are rare, and suspected cases often can be attributed in retrospect to inadvertent intravascular injection of epinephrine-containing solutions.

d. A concentration-dependent neurotoxic property of local anesthetics is now well described.

E. Analgesic adjuvants

1. α_2-Adrenergic agonists

Clonidine is the prototypical drug in this class, although dexmedetomidine also is approved for use. Both drugs produce analgesia through agonism at central α_2-receptors in the substantia gelatinosa of the spinal cord. They also may act at peripheral α_2-receptors located on sympathetic nerve terminals to decrease norepinephrine output in sympathetically mediated pain. The analgesic effect of these drugs is distinct and complementary to that of opioids when used in combination. Clonidine may be administered orally to provide sedation and analgesia as a premedication. Preservative-free clonidine may be included as a component of epidural infusions or intrathecal (IT) injections. Hypotension, sedation, and dry mouth are common side effects of these drugs.

2. Acetaminophen

Although not a potent analgesic, acetaminophen can be administered orally or via suppository to supplement other analgesic techniques in the early postoperative period. It is particularly useful in those patients in whom an NSAID would be contraindicated.

3. Ketamine

Ketamine has complex interactions with a variety of receptors, but it is thought to act primarily through blockade of the excitatory neurotransmitter,

Table 26.2 Maximum recommended dosing of local anesthetic agents for local infiltration

Drug	Maximum dose for 70-kg adult (mg)	
	Plain solution	Containing epinephrine (1:200,000)
Chloroprocaine	600–800	1,000
Lidocaine	300	500
Mepivacaine	300	500
Bupivacaine	175	225
Ropivacaine	200	250

Dose may be increased modestly for use in compartments where absorption will be delayed (e.g., brachial plexus) and decreased for use in more vascular regions (e.g., epidural space, intercostal).

glutamic acid, at the NMDA receptor in the CNS. It can be administered orally or parenterally to provide sedation, potent analgesia, and "dissociative anesthesia." The principal advantages of ketamine stem from its sympathomimetic properties and lack of ventilatory depression. Cautions include increased secretions and dysphoric reactions.

F. Nonpharmacologic

1. Cryoablation

A cryoprobe can be introduced into the intercostal space and used to produce transient (1 to 4 days) numbness in the distribution of the intercostal nerve. A cryoprobe circulates extremely cold gas, on the order of –80°C. When applied for two to three treatments of approximately 2 minutes each, it temporarily disrupts neural function. Cryoablation has been shown to reduce pain and the need for systemic analgesics after lateral thoracotomy for cardiac surgery [6].

2. Nursing Care

Empathic nursing care and nursing-guided relaxation techniques are important components to patient comfort throughout the perioperative period and should not be overlooked [6].

III. Pain management strategies

A. Oral

Gastrointestinal ileus is rarely a concern after routine cardiothoracic surgical procedures; therefore, transfer to oral administration of analgesics should be considered as soon as pain management goals are likely to be effectively achieved by this route. This is particularly important, because oral agents are currently the simplest, and cheapest, and most reliable way to continue effective analgesia after hospital discharge, and they should be used as the mainstay of any "fast track" analgesia protocol.

B. Subcutaneous/intramuscular

Subcutaneous (SC) and IM injections remain effective and inexpensive alternate routes to IV administration for delivery of potent systemic analgesia using opioid agents (e.g., morphine, hydromorphone, meperidine). SC or IM injection results in slower onset of analgesia compared to the IV route and, therefore, is more suitable for scheduled dosing (e.g., every 3 to 6 hours) rather than "as needed." A notable disadvantage of the IM route is injection-related discomfort, which can be largely avoided by slow injection through an indwelling SC butterfly needle.

C. Parenteral

In the absence of neuraxial analgesia, IV opioid analgesia is generally the primary tool to provide effective pain relief for the early postoperative patient. The advantages of this route include rapid onset and ease of titration to effect. In addition, for the awake patient, technology permitting patient-controlled IV delivery of opioids [i.e., patient-controlled analgesia (PCA)] has become widely available. PCA units combine options for baseline continuous opioid infusion with patient-administered bolus doses with lockout periods. Patient satisfaction using PCA analgesia rivals that with neuraxial analgesia.

Analgesic agents that have traditionally been available only for oral administration are becoming available for parenteral usage. IV ketorolac has gained widespread acceptance as an analgesic alternative for thoracic surgical patients that is devoid of respiratory depressant effects. Parenteral COX-2 inhibitor agents currently are in clinical trials and, if proven safe and effective, would appear to have potential advantages.

D. Interpleural

Interpleural analgesia requires placement of a catheter between the visceral and parietal pleura, for subsequent injection of local anesthetic agent. The effect obtained is thought to be a result of blockade of intercostal nerves in addition to local actions on the pleura. Disadvantages of this technique include requirement for relatively high doses of local anesthetic, poor effectiveness, and possible impairment of ipsilateral diaphragmatic function. For these reasons interpleural analgesia has been largely abandoned as a strategy for pain control in cardiothoracic surgery patients.

E. Intercostal

Sequential intercostal blocks (e.g., T-4 to T-10) can contribute to unilateral postoperative chest wall analgesia for cardiothoracic surgery. Intercostal nerve block

(ICB) requires depositing local anesthetic (e.g., 4 mL of 0.5% bupivacaine per nerve) at the inferior border of the associated rib near the proximal intercostal nerve. ICBs are generally performed through the skin before surgery or by the surgeon under direct vision within the chest. ICBs contribute to analgesia for up to 12 hours, but in general they do not include blockade of the posterior and visceral rami of the intercostal nerve; therefore, they often require additional NSAID or parenteral analgesia to be effective.

F. **Paravertebral**

Paravertebral blocks (PVBs) can provide unilateral chest wall analgesia for thoracic surgery. Sequential thoracic PVB injections (e.g., T-4 to T-10, 4 mL of 0.5% ropivacaine per space) are combined with "light" general anesthesia for thoracotomy procedures and last 18 to 24 hours postoperatively. Anticipated chest tube insertion sites usually dictate the lowest PVB level required. Although use of PVBs often significantly reduces intraoperative opioid requirements, NSAID analgesia and small doses of IV opioid generally are required after thoracotomy to achieve full comfort. "Emergence" from PVB analgesia on the day after surgery may result in rapidly increasing pain, often after discharge from intensive monitoring; therefore, it is essential that other analgesia alternatives be immediately available during this period. Potential advantages of PVBs compared to neuraxial techniques include avoidance of opioid side effects, risk of spinal hematoma, and hypotension related to bilateral sympathetic block. The paravertebral space, where peripheral nerves exit from the spinal canal, is limited superiorly and inferiorly by the heads of associated ribs, anteriorly by the parietal pleura, and posteriorly by the superior costotransverse ligament. Technical considerations for PVBs are well described elsewhere [7,8]. Similar advantages exist for ICBs and PVBs compared to neuraxial analgesia. Both of these procedures can be complicated by epidural spread of local anesthetic. However, when compared to PVBs, ICBs do not affect the posterior and visceral ramus of the intercostal nerve and recede more rapidly (6 to 12 hours) than PVBs.

G. **Intrathecal**

IT opioid analgesia is a suitable treatment for major pain after median sternotomy or thoracotomy incisions. The benefits and risks of a spinal procedure should always be carefully weighed before using this technique, particularly with regard to risk of spinal hematoma in patients with abnormal hemostasis. Small-caliber noncutting spinal needles (e.g., 27-gauge Whitacre needle) often are selected for lumbar spinal injection of preservative-free morphine. Age rather than weight predicts IT opioid dosing in adults; 0.7 to 1.0 mg IT morphine dosing is effective for cardiothoracic surgery in most adults, usually administered before anesthesia induction. Smaller doses (e.g., 0.3 to 0.5 mg) are required to reduce the likelihood of respiratory depression in elderly patients (older than 75 years). It is prudent to avoid the use of IT morphine in patients 85 years or older. Because rare patients will develop significant delayed respiratory depression, hourly monitoring of respiratory rate and consciousness for 18 to 24 hours is mandatory with this technique. Reduced doses of sedative and hypnotic agents during general anesthesia are required, to avoid excessive postoperative somnolence. Onset of thoracic analgesia is approximately 1 to 2 hours after injection, lasting up to 24 hours. Postoperative NSAID therapy complements IT morphine analgesia without sedative effects. Analgesia alternatives must be immediately available in anticipation of the resolution of IT morphine analgesia approximately 24 hours after injection, because significant pain may develop rapidly. IT administration of other drugs for cardiac and thoracic surgery, such as local anesthetic agents, or short-acting opioids (e.g., sufentanil) [9] has been reported, but the effects of these substances is mainly limited to the intraoperative period.

H. **Epidural**

1. **Epidural selection/technique**

Epidural anesthesia is ideal for thoracic surgery and is the most widely studied and used form of regional analgesia for this purpose. Although epidural catheter placement for use during and after cardiac surgery is reported to have benefits [10], this approach has not gained a similar level of acceptance.

Thoracic epidural catheter location (T-4 to T-10) is generally preferred over lumbar for thoracic surgery. Proponents cite the reduced local anesthetic dosing requirements, closer proximity to thoracic segment dorsal horns, and reduced likelihood of dislodgment postoperatively. Concern regarding the potential for increased spinal cord injury using a thoracic compared to lumbar approach to epidural catheter placement has not been borne out. Selection of the thoracic interspace should be dictated by surgical site. The epidural catheter should be placed 5 to 6 cm into the epidural space and securely taped.

Intraoperative use of an epidural catheter enhances the benefits of regional anesthesia for thoracotomy surgery by permitting a "light general" anesthetic technique with reduced residual respiratory depressant effects. Epidural local anesthetic block can be initiated before surgical incision using a "test dose" of epinephrine-containing local anesthetic to rule out intravascular or IT catheter placement. Administration of preincision epidural opioid may contribute to a preemptive analgesic effect, but it should not be administered unless at least 24 hours of postoperative observation can be assured. To minimize postoperative somnolence and the risk of respiratory depression, administration of potent IV sedatives and opioids should be reduced or avoided during surgery, and agents used to maintain general anesthesia should be easily reversible (e.g., volatile anesthetic agents). Monitoring inhaled volatile anesthetic concentrations or using a bispectral analysis monitor to assess level of consciousness may permit reduced exposure to sedative agents. A popular mixture for postoperative epidural analgesia is dilute local anesthetic (e.g., 0.125% bupivacaine) containing an opioid with intermediate solubility properties (e.g., 50 µg/mL hydromorphone); this is administered by continuous infusion at 3 to 5 mL/hour, ideally starting at least 15 minutes before the end of surgery. Because early titration of the epidural analgesic infusions often is required and pain is not effectively reported by the awakening patient, an initial analgesic dose of local anesthetic agent should be administered to the patient (e.g., 3 mL preservative-free 2% lidocaine) before emergence. IV ketorolac also can be administered at this time, when indicated. Titration of epidural analgesia to comfort should be completed in the postoperative recovery area, where transfer of care to the acute pain care team should occur.

IV. Pain management regimens for specific cardiothoracic procedures
A. Conventional coronary artery bypass and open chamber procedures

Over the past 2 decades, anesthetic design for cardiac surgery has commonly included large doses of potent opioids (e.g., fentanyl, sufentanil), thus assuring intraoperative hemodynamic stability and excellent analgesia but often requiring considerable periods of postoperative ventilation. Although this remains a useful approach for the management of selected high-risk patients, it has been recognized that most procedures are suitable for analgesia regimens compatible with more rapid recovery. Standard regimens for cardiac surgery currently include modest intraoperative opioid dosing, with postoperative bedside availability of parenteral opioids as required in the first 12 to 24 hours, either patient controlled or administered by a nurse. Transition to oral agents is encouraged as soon as food is tolerated.

The move away from traditional high-dose opioid anesthesia has increased interest in different approaches to analgesia after cardiac surgery. Routine NSAID therapy for uncomplicated patients is a safe and cost-effective way to complement opioid analgesia. Preoperative IT morphine has gained popularity in some centers. In experienced hands, imaginative combinations such as preoperative IT morphine and intraoperative IV remifentanil infusion provide reproducible excellent analgesia, with tracheal extubation often possible in the operating room [11].

B. Off-pump (sternotomy) cardiac procedures

One interpretation of "minimally invasive" cardiac surgery involves the avoidance of cardiopulmonary bypass (CPB). Theoretically, avoidance of the systemic inflammatory response associated with CPB may increase the perception of pain. Anecdotally, there is an impression that this is true. With the "fast track" approach to patient management that has accompanied off-pump cardiac surgery, analgesia regimens are challenged and inadequate pain control is more commonly a reason for delayed hospital discharge than in the past. Interest in analgesic approaches other than parenteral opioids has paralleled that for patients undergoing traditional cardiac surgery with CPB, as outlined above (see Section **IV.A**). Because reduced heparin administration and avoidance of CPB-related impairment of hemostasis occur with off-pump surgery, IT morphine, combined with NSAID or COX-2 inhibitor therapy, ultimately may gain a higher profile as a safe approach to analgesia in this patient group.

C. **Minimally invasive (minithoracotomy) cardiac procedures**

In contrast to off-pump procedures, a second interpretation of "minimally invasive" cardiac surgery involves port-access catheter-based CPB and very small incisions to achieve surgical goals. Although early hopes were that port-access procedures would be associated with less pain, this has not proven to be true, most likely because of the relocation of the smaller incisions to more pain sensitive areas (e.g., minithoracotomy). In addition to the alternate analgesic approaches outlined for patients undergoing traditional cardiac surgery with CPB (see Section **IV.A**), the possibility of using novel approaches to minithoracotomy analgesia including ICBs, PVBs and PVB continuous infusion now are being considered.

D. **Postthoracotomy (noncardiac)**

"Light" general anesthesia with regional blockade of the chest wall is a particularly suitable anesthetic approach for lung and other chest surgery. Using this technique, residual sedative/hypnotic effects can be minimized, early tracheal extubation reliably achieved, and the transition to postoperative pain management facilitated. Selection of regional blockade technique is best made after evaluation of both patient status and the demands of the surgery. American Society of Anesthesiologists class I to II patients anticipating postoperative hospital stays up to 48 hours may benefit from single-shot local anesthetic blocks (e.g., PVBs, ICBs); however, anxious patients in this group should not be overly pressured to undergo a regional procedure. In contrast, patients who are deconditioned or undergoing more extensive procedures are more likely to benefit from regional anesthesia, and placement of a thoracic epidural catheter unless contraindicated, should be strongly encouraged. Routine postoperative NSAID or COX-2 inhibitor therapy should be considered. These agents are devoid of sedation and are particularly effective analgesics in combination with regional analgesia. Local anesthetic/opioid mixtures are popular analgesic regimens for use as continuous epidural infusions (see Section **III.H**). However, in high-risk cases (e.g., lung volume reduction or lung transplant surgery) where avoidance of all respiratory depressants is desirable, analgesia can be achieved using a dilute local anesthetic agent alone. Tachyphylaxis is a common problem with this technique, requiring frequent rate readjustments. Removal of an epidural catheter is fraught with all the same risks of insertion. When transfer from epidural to oral analgesia is being considered, thromboprophylaxis protocols should be coordinated with epidural catheter removal to minimize the risk of epidural hematoma.

V. **Approach to specific complications and side effects of analgesic strategies**

A. **Complications of nonsteroidal antiinflammatory drugs**

1. **Renal toxicity**

   a. Normal patients exhibit a low rate of prostaglandin synthesis in renal vasculature, such that cyclooxygenase inhibition has little effect. However, vasodilatory prostaglandins may play an important role in preservation of renal perfusion in disease states.

   b. Nephrotoxicity secondary to vasoconstriction of both afferent and efferent renal arterioles, leading to reduced glomerular filtration rate, is commonly seen with NSAID administration in patients with dehydration, sepsis, congestive heart failure, or other causes of renal hypoperfusion.

   c. Avoiding NSAID-induced renal toxicity is best accomplished by limiting or avoiding their use in patients with decreased renal reserve and in those at risk for hypoperfusion.

   d. Risk appears to be low with perioperative ketorolac administration (1 : 1,000 to 1 : 10,000) [12].

      e. NSAID-induced nephrotoxicity usually is reversible with discontinuation of the drug.

  2. Gastrointestinal mucosal irritation

      a. Gastrointestinal mucosal irritation is the most common NSAID side effect. It can occur regardless of route of administration. It may result in erosion and severe gastrointestinal bleeding.

      b. Prostaglandins are involved in multiple aspects of gastric mucosal protection, including mucosal blood flow, epithelial cell growth, and surface mucus and bicarbonate production.

      c. Prophylaxis may involve administration of histamine (H_2) receptor antagonists, proton pump inhibitors (omeprazole), protective agents (sucralfate), or prostaglandin analogues (misoprostol). Each of these treatments appears to be effective in decreasing ulceration with NSAID treatment.

  3. Impaired primary hemostasis

      a. Cyclooxygenase inhibition leads to impaired platelet aggregation. It may increase intraoperative or postoperative bleeding.

      b. Duration of effect is highly variable depending on individual drug (reversible vs irreversible enzymatic inhibition).

      c. Only effective prophylaxis or treatment is to discontinue NSAIDs for a sufficient duration preoperatively (ibuprofen more than 3 days, aspirin more than 7 to 10 days).

B. Nausea and vomiting

Nausea and vomiting as a consequence of analgesia is most commonly associated with opioids. Opioids cause nausea primarily through activation of the chemoreceptor trigger zone of the brainstem in the floor of the fourth ventricle. A vestibular component also is postulated because it is clear that ambulation increases the incidence. Finally, the inhibitory effects of opioids on gastrointestinal motility may contribute. Nausea can accompany opioid therapy regardless of the route of administration. It occurs in roughly 25% to 35% of patients treated with spinal opioids and is more frequent with spinal use of hydrophilic drugs (e.g., morphine) secondary to enhanced rostral spread of these agents [13].

Treatment can include traditional antiemetic drugs such as prochlorperazine, chlorpromazine, promethazine, metoclopramide, or droperidol; however, most of these treatments can be complicated by excessive sedation and/or extrapyramidal side effects secondary to central dopamine receptor antagonism. In contrast, serotonin receptor agonists (e.g., ondansetron, dolasetron) are effective antiemetics with few side effects. Often, however, such symptomatic treatment is effective in reducing, but not eliminating, complaints of nausea. Scopolamine, administered via transdermal patch to deliver 0.5 mg/day, is an effective antiemetic in the setting of spinal opioids. Finally, IV naloxone in doses up to 5 µg/kg/hour is extremely effective in reversing complaints of nausea from spinal opioids, without apparent antagonism of analgesia.

C. Pruritus

Pruritus is a common side effect of opioids administered by any route, but it can be particularly problematic after central neuraxial administration. The mechanism is unclear and likely complex, but it is not secondary to preservatives within the opioid preparation or specifically to histamine release. Pruritus often improves as the duration of opioid treatment lengthens. Pruritus is most effectively treated with antihistamines, mixed agonist opioids such as nalbuphine, or naloxone infusion as outline above.

D. Respiratory depression

Hypoventilation is a potentially life-threatening complication of opioids. It can occur early after administration by any route, but it is particularly feared as a delayed presentation during spinal opioid administration. In either case, hypoventilation occurs secondary to elevated cerebrospinal fluid drug levels with depression of the medullary respiratory center, either from systemic absorption or rostral spread of spinally administered drug. Respiratory depression requiring naloxone administration is reported to occur in 0.2% to 1% of patients receiving epidural narcotics [14], but the incidence likely is higher in opioid-naïve patients being treated for acute pain. Other factors that may increase the risk include advanced age, poor overall medical condition, higher narcotic dosing (particularly of hydrophilic drugs), increased intrathoracic or intraabdominal pressure (as may occur during mechanical ventilation), and coincident administration of other CNS depressants. Patients who have received spinal narcotics in the prior 18 to 24 hours or in whom continuous infusions are being administered should have their ventilatory rate and level of alertness confirmed at least hourly. Caretakers should be aware that deteriorating levels of consciousness might portend severe respiratory depression, even if ventilatory rates appear preserved. Arterial blood gas analysis should be used early in the investigation of decreased alertness. Modest doses of naloxone (0.04 to 0.1 mg) usually are sufficient to temporarily reverse respiratory depression if it is discovered before it has become severe.

E. **Neuraxial procedures and anticoagulation**

Anticoagulation takes numerous forms during the perioperative period, especially in cardiothoracic procedures. Considerations for spinal and epidural blockade vary depending on the circumstances. This topic has prompted guidelines that have formed the current opinion on appropriate usage of neuraxial procedures in the setting of impaired hemostasis [15]. These guidelines are reviewed in the following.

1. **Heparin anticoagulation**

Spinal administration of opioids and placement of epidural catheters for perioperative use have been performed widely in circumstances where IV heparinization is to be delayed by at least 1 hour. This is accepted as safe practice providing this interim time is adhered to and the procedure is atraumatic. "Bloody tap" requires consideration of a delay of the proposed procedure.

2. **Heparin thromboprophylaxis**

Placement of a spinal needle and insertion or removal of an epidural catheter should precede SC heparin dosing (5,000 units every 8 to 12 hours) by at least 1 hour or be delayed for 4 to 6 hours after heparin administration.

3. **Low-molecular-weight heparin**

Since the introduction of low-molecular-weight heparin (LMWH, i.e., enoxaparin) into practice in the United States in 1993, neuraxial block in association with its administration has appeared to present a special risk to development of spinal hematoma. From May 1993 to February 1998, the U.S. FDA received reports of 43 such patients, 16 of whom suffered permanent paraplegia [16]. The plasma half-life of LMWH is two to four times that of standard heparin. Also, lack of a conventional clotting assay to assess the impact on factor Xa activity, recommended dosing that is not adjusted for weight, and twice daily dosing all may contribute to an increased risk of spinal bleeding after neuraxial block in patients receiving LMWH [17]. Consequently, the following precautions are recommended: (a) delay administration of LMWH for at least 12 hours after neuraxial block; (b) avoid neuraxial block in patients receiving LMWH in combination with other antiplatelet or anticoagulant medications; and (c) consider skipping a dose of LMWH before epidural catheter removal in patients receiving twice daily dosing, thus allowing 24 hours since the last dose and a true trough drug effect to develop [17].

4. **Nonsteroidal antiinflammatory drugs**

Although many clinicians advise caution in proceeding with neuraxial block in patients taking NSAIDs, there is no evidence of major increased risk of spinal hematoma with epidural or spinal anesthesia in patients taking aspirin or other NSAIDs.

5. **Warfarin**

Neuraxial block can be safely used in patients who have taken a single dose of oral anticoagulant and an epidural catheter can be removed safely up to 24 hours after an initial warfarin dose. Prothrombin time should be established before epidural catheter removal if more than 24 hours has elapsed or when repeat dosing has taken place.

6. **Fibrinolysis and antiplatelet agents**

Patients may present for urgent surgery after recently receiving activators of fibrinolysis or platelet glycoprotein IIb/IIIa receptor antagonists during treatment of acute myocardial infarction or in concert with interventional cardiology procedures. Experience with regional anesthesia in these settings is limited, and central neuraxial procedures should be avoided.

VI. Considerations in the establishment of fast tracking processes

Reliable postoperative analgesia is a key component in facilitating prompt tracheal extubation (within 6 hours) after cardiac surgery. Such "fast tracking" of low-risk cardiac surgery patients appears to be safe and has been adopted by many centers throughout the world as a process to decrease intensive care unit and hospital lengths of stay. Some patient benefits may accrue, such as improved cardiac function and reduced rates of respiratory infections and complications. IT morphine is used in many centers to provide analgesia and mild sedation in the early postoperative period. However, some studies have failed to demonstrate a beneficial effect of IT morphine, either in improving early analgesia or in facilitating early extubation [18]. NSAIDs complement opioid analgesia, regardless of how the opioid is administered. Indomethacin, administered rectally as 100-mg suppositories, is a common component of fast-tracking protocols for cardiac surgery. It reduces pain and early postoperative narcotic use. Some NSAIDs may antagonize opioid-induced respiratory depression [19]. Intraoperative and postoperative continuous infusions of remifentanil or alfentanil (with or without supplemental propofol infusion) are used in some centers to allow controlled analgesia and "scheduled extubation." Both a high-dose narcotic technique using the ultra–short-acting narcotic remifentanil [11] or an anesthetic incorporating high thoracic epidural conduction block [10] have been suggested as good methods that may improve outcome through inhibition of perioperative stress response while facilitating early extubation and fast tracking [20].

References

1. **Kehlet H. Manipulation of the metabolic response in clinical practice.** *World J Surg* 2000;24:690–695.
2. **Lui S, Carpenter RL, Neal JM. Epidural anesthesia and analgesia: their role in postoperative outcome.** *Anesthesiology* 1995;82:1474–1506.
3. **Bovill JG. Update on opioid and analgesic pharmacology.** *Anesth Analg* 2001; 92:S1–S5.
4. Perazella M, Eras J. Are selective COX-2 inhibitors nephrotoxic? *Am J Kidney Dis* 2000;35:937–940.
5. Bucerius J, Metz S, Walther T, et al. Pain is significantly reduced by cryoablation therapy in patients with lateral minithoracotomy. *Ann Thorac Surg* 2000;70:1100–1104.
6. Oates H. Non-pharmacologic pain control for the CABG patient. *Dimen Crit Care Nursing* 1993;12:296–304.
7. **Greengrass R, Steele S. Paravertebral blocks for breast surgery.** *Tech Region Anesth Pain Manage* 1998;2:8–12.
8. Richardson J, Lonnqvist PA. Thoracic paravertebral block. *Br J Anaesth* 1998;81:230–238.
9. Swenson JD, Hullander RM, Wingler K, et al. Early extubation after cardiac surgery using combined intrathecal sufentanil and morphine. *J Cardiothorac Vasc Anesth* 1994; 8:509–514.
10. **Scott N, Turfrey D, Ray D, et al. A prospective randomized study of the potential benefits of thoracic epidural anesthesia and analgesia in patients undergoing coronary artery bypass grafting.** *Anesth Analg* 2001;93:528–535.
11. Zarate E, Latham P, White PF, et al. Fast-track cardiac anesthesia: use of remifentanil combined with intrathecal morphine as an alternative to sufentanil during desflurane anesthesia. *Anesth Analg* 2000;91:283–287.
12. Myles P, Power I. Does ketorolac cause postoperative renal failure? *Br J Anaesth* 1998; 80:420–421.
13. **Carr D, Cousins M. Spinal route of analgesia. In: Cousins M, Bridenbaugh P, eds. *Neural blockade*, 3rd ed. Philadelphia: Lippincott-Raven Publishers 1998: 915–983.**
14. **Ready L. Regional analgesia with intraspinal opioids. In: Loeser J, ed. *Bonica's management of pain*. Philadelphia: Lippincott, Williams & Wilkins, 2001:1953–1966.**

15. **Horlocker T, Wedel D. Anticoagulation and neuraxial block: historical perspective, anesthetic implications, and risk management.** *Region Anesth Pain Med* **1998;23:129–134.**
16. Wysowski D, Talarico L, Bacsanyi J, et al. Spinal and epidural hematoma and low-molecular weight heparin. *N Engl J Med* 1998;338:1774–1775.
17. Horlocker T, Wedel D. Spinal and epidural blockade and perioperative low molecular weight heparin: smooth sailing on the Titanic. *Anesth Analg* 1998;86:1153–1156.
18. **Chaney M, Nickolov M, Blakeman B, et al. Intrathecal morphine for coronary artery bypass graft procedure and early extubation revisited.** *J Cardiothorac Vasc Anesth* **1999;13:574–578.**
19. Moren J, Francois T, Blanloeil Y, et al. The effects of a nonsteroidal antiinflammatory drug (ketoprofen) on morphine respiratory depression: a double-blind, randomized study in volunteers. *Anesth Analg* 1997;85:400–405.
20. **Royston D. Patient selection and anesthetic management for early extubation and hospital discharge: CABG.** *J Cardiothorac Vasc Anesth* **1998;12:11–19.**

SUBJECT INDEX.